color atlas
OF ORAL AND MAXILLOFACIAL DISEASES

Brad W. Neville, DDS
Distinguished University Professor
Director, Division of Oral and Maxillofacial Pathology
Department of Stomatology
James B. Edwards College of Dental Medicine
Medical University of South Carolina
Charleston, South Carolina

Douglas D. Damm, DDS
Emeritus Professor
Oral and Maxillofacial Pathology
College of Dentistry
University of Kentucky
Lexington, Kentucky

Carl M. Allen, DDS, MSD
Emeritus Professor
Division of Oral and Maxillofacial Pathology and Radiology
College of Dentistry
The Ohio State University
Columbus, Ohio;
Staff Oral and Maxillofacial Pathologist
Central Ohio Skin & Cancer, Inc.
Westerville, Ohio

Angela C. Chi, DMD
Professor
Division of Oral and Maxillofacial Pathology
Department of Stomatology
James B. Edwards College of Dental Medicine
Medical University of South Carolina
Charleston, South Carolina

ELSEVIER

ELSEVIER

1600 John F. Kennedy Blvd.
Ste 1600
Philadelphia, PA 19103-2899

COLOR ATLAS OF ORAL AND MAXILLOFACIAL DISEASES　　　　ISBN: 978-0-323-55225-7

Library of Congress Control Number: 2018952971

Content Strategist: Alexandra Mortimer
Content Development Specialist: Caroline Dorey-Stein
Publishing Services Manager: Catherine Jackson
Senior Project Manager: Kate Mannix
Design Direction: Amy Buxton

Printed in China

Last digit is the print number:　9　8　7　6　5　4　3　2　1

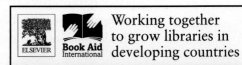

To our colleagues, many of whom have shared these cases with us.

Contents

Preface

By its very nature, the discipline of pathology encompasses not only the microscopic diagnosis of disease, but also the recognition and diagnosis of lesions on a clinical and radiographic basis. As oral and maxillofacial pathologists, we naturally spend a significant amount of our time in the laboratory examining tissue specimens for diagnosis. However, we also have the great opportunity and privilege to see many patients in a clinical setting for both the diagnosis and management of various oral diseases. As a matter of fact, it is this fascination with disease on a clinical basis that first stimulated our interest to enter the specialty of oral and maxillofacial pathology.

With this in mind, we are pleased to offer this collection of photographs and radiographic images of oral, head, and neck diseases. These illustrations represent a compilation of what we consider to be among the best clinical teaching material that we have accrued over the course of our careers. The book has been designed primarily with the dental professional in mind, but it also should be useful to other health care providers who treat oral diseases, such as otolaryngologists and dermatologists.

In keeping with an atlas format, we have decided to include more pictures rather than more words. The chapters are organized by broad disease categories, which match the sequence of how we initially lecture about these topics in the classroom. A wide variety of lesions has been included, but we have tried to emphasize more commonly occurring and important disorders. No photomicrographs are included in this book. Although we obviously recognize the importance of histopathology in the diagnosis of disease, we think that the purpose of this book is better served by limiting it to clinical photographs and radiographs.

Acknowledgments

We are deeply indebted to our friends and colleagues who have shared many of the images included in this atlas or who have referred patients for us to examine and photograph. We have attempted to be as thorough as possible in listing credit to these individuals in the figure legends. However, if anyone's name has been inadvertently omitted, please accept our apologies.

We would like to acknowledge some of the many teachers who have mentored us during our careers, particularly those individuals who stimulated and fostered our interest in clinical oral pathology. This list includes Drs. George Blozis, Jerry Bouquot, George Gallagher, Susan Müller, Charles Waldron, and Ronnie Weathers.

We also wish to thank Alexandra Mortimer, Jennifer Flynn-Briggs, Kate Mannix, Caroline Dorey-Stein, and Taylor Ball at Elsevier for their editorial expertise and patience as we worked on this project. Finally, our families deserve more personal thanks and praise for their love and support during the preparation of this book.

1

Developmental Defects of the Oral and Maxillofacial Region

Cleft Lip and Palate

Fig. 1.1

Cleft lip (CL) is a common congenital anomaly that is caused by defective fusion of the medial nasal and maxillary processes during embryologic development. Approximately 80% of cases are unilateral and 20% are bilateral. **Cleft palate** (CP), which results from failure of the lateral palatal shelves to fuse, often occurs in conjunction with CL, although it also may develop as an isolated defect. CL alone and CL with CP are etiologically related conditions that can be grouped together as CL ± CP (CL with or without CP). CP only (CPO) represents a separate entity from CL ± CP. Orofacial clefting is seen with greater frequency in a variety of specific genetic syndromes, although more often it occurs in a sporadic fashion due to a combination of environmental and genetic factors. Factors known to increase the risk for clefts include maternal smoking, alcohol consumption, and phenytoin usage.

The frequency of CL ± CP varies considerably among different racial/ethnic groups. Among whites, the frequency is estimated at 1 per every 700 to 1000 births. The prevalence in blacks is much lower, with a rate of 0.4 cases per 1000 births. In contrast, the rate in Asian populations is about 1.5 times that seen in whites. The highest rate occurs in Native Americans, with a frequency of 3.6 per 1000 births. CL ± CP is more common in males, whereas CPO is more common in females.

Orofacial clefting can result in a variety of problems related to appearance, feeding, speech, hearing, and socialization skills. Management involves a dedicated craniofacial team, which may include specialists in genetics, oral and maxillofacial surgery, orthodontics, otolaryngology, pediatric dentistry, pediatric medicine, plastic surgery, prosthodontics, psychology, and speech pathology. Treatment may require multiple surgeries, with repair of CL usually accomplished around 2 to 3 months after birth and surgical correction of CP undertaken between 6 and 12 months of life.

Bifid Uvula (Cleft Uvula)

Fig. 1.2

During the embryologic formation of the hard and soft palate, the lateral palatal shelves normally fuse in the midline. This fusion begins in the anterior region of the palate and progresses posteriorly to the uvula. If the fusion is not totally completed, then a **bifid uvula** may occur, which represents the most minimal manifestation of a cleft palate (CP). Sometimes a bifid uvula may be associated with a submucous palatal cleft in which the overlying mucosa is intact but there is a defect in the formation of the musculature of the soft palate. Submucous clefts also may be associated with a notched defect of the midline bone of the posterior hard palate. Bifid uvula is more common than complete CP, with an estimated overall prevalence of 1% to 2%. The frequency is much higher in Asian and Native American populations. In most instances, bifid uvula is an incidental finding that does not cause any problems. If an associated submucous CP is present, velopharyngeal insufficiency may be present, which can result in hypernasal speech. A bifid uvula can be associated with certain genetic conditions, such as van der Woude syndrome and Loeys-Dietz syndrome (hypertelorism, bifid uvula or CP, and aortic aneurysm with tortuosity).

Double Lip

Fig. 1.3

Double lip is an uncommon oral anomaly in which there is an excess fold of tissue along the mucosal surface of the lip. It either may be congenital or develop later in life. The upper lip is affected more frequently than the lower lip, although sometimes both lips are involved. The redundant tissue may be seen bilaterally in a symmetric fashion, or it may appear primarily on one side. When the lips are at rest, a double lip may not be noticeable; however, when the patient smiles, the excess tissue will become evident. Double lip occasionally may be a component of Ascher syndrome, which is characterized by the following triad: (1) double lip, (2) blepharochalasis (edema and sagging of the upper eyelid), and (3) nontoxic thyroid enlargement.

No treatment may be required for mild forms of double lip. However, more severe examples can be managed by surgical excision of the excess tissue for cosmetic purposes.

■ Figure **1.1**
Cleft Lip
Unilateral cleft of the left upper lip. (Courtesy Dr. Cathy Flaitz.)

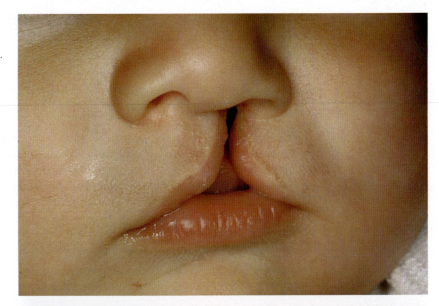

■ Figure **1.2**
Bifid Uvula
A midline cleft divides the uvula into two lobes.

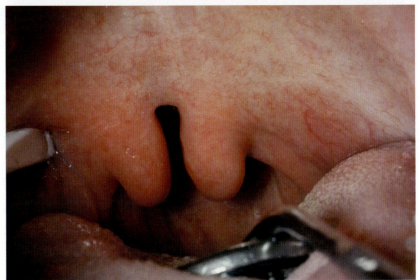

■ Figure **1.3**
Double Lip
An extra fold of tissue hangs down from the left upper lip.

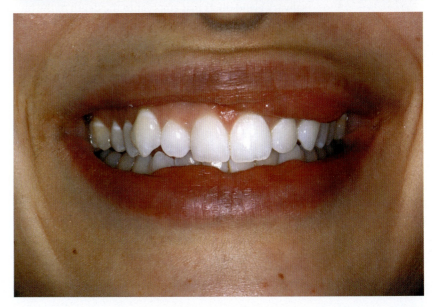

Commissural Lip Pits

Fig. **1.4**

Commissural lip pits are tiny mucosal invaginations at the corners of the mouth near the vermilion border. Such depressions have been noted in 12% to 20% of the adult population, whereas among children the reported prevalence is only about 0.2% to 0.7%. Although such pits often are considered to be congenital defects, their increased frequency in adult patients suggests that they usually do not appear until later in life. Commissural lip pits occur more often in males than in females.

Commissural lip pits are typically asymptomatic unilateral or bilateral lesions that are discovered as incidental findings. They appear as small punctate depressions extending to a depth of 1 to 4 mm on the lip vermilion at the commissures. Because ducts from minor salivary glands may empty into the depth of the pit, a small amount of mucoid secretion sometimes can be expressed. Commissural lip pits have been associated with a higher prevalence of preauricular pits, but they are not associated with orofacial clefting. Because of their asymptomatic nature, treatment rarely is required. However, if excessive salivary secretions occur or secondary infection develops in a deep pit, then surgical excision may be considered.

Paramedian Lip Pits and Van der Woude Syndrome

Figs. **1.5 and 1.6**

Paramedian lip pits are rare congenital invaginations that are seen on the vermilion border of the lower lip, lateral to the midline. Such lesions are usually bilateral, although in some instances a single pit may be found more centrally positioned or lateral to the midline. Paramedian lip pits are significant because they usually are associated with **van der Woude syndrome**, an autosomal dominant condition that also includes cleft lip (CL) and/or cleft palate (CP). Van der Woude syndrome is the most common form of syndromic orofacial clefting, occurring in 1 out of every 40,000 to 100,000 births. It is estimated that 2% of all CL and CP cases are part of van der Woude syndrome, which is caused by mutations of the gene that encodes interferon regulatory factor 6 (IRF6). Some people with paramedian lip pits and van der Woude syndrome may not demonstrate clefting or they may exhibit only a submucosal CP; however, such individuals can transmit the full syndrome to their offspring. Paramedian lip pits also can be a feature of two other syndromes that include orofacial clefting: popliteal pterygium syndrome and Kabuki syndrome.

Paramedian lip pits appear as blind sinuslike depressions that can extend to a depth of 1.5 cm. A humped swelling sometimes surrounds the central pore. Salivary secretions may be expressed because of minor salivary gland ducts that empty into the depth of the pit. If the pits are a cosmetic problem for the patient, then surgical excision can be performed.

■ Figure 1.4
Commissural Lip Pit

A punctate depression is present at the right labial commissure.

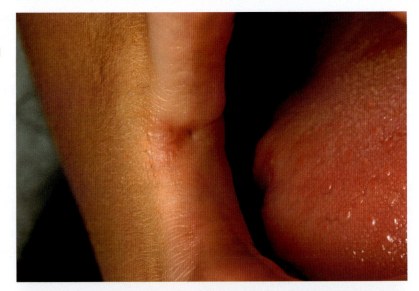

■ Figure 1.5
Paramedian Lip Pits in Van der Woude Syndrome

Bilateral pits are seen adjacent to the midline of the lower lip vermilion. (Courtesy Dr. Nadarajah Vigneswaran.)

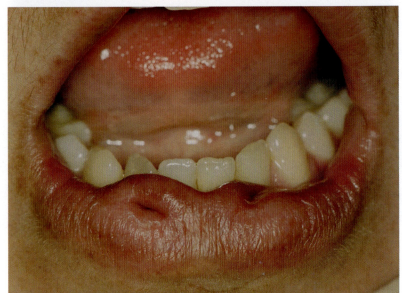

■ Figure 1.6
Cleft Palate in Van der Woude Syndrome

Same patient as depicted in Fig. 1.5 with a cleft of the soft palate. (Courtesy Dr. Nadarajah Vigneswaran.)

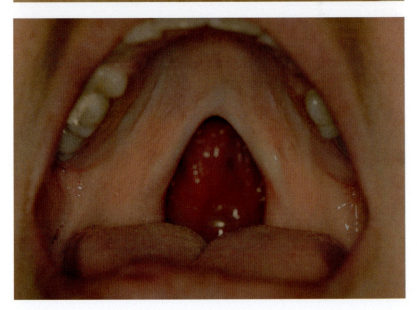

Figs. 1.7–1.9

Sebaceous glands are common adnexal structures on the skin, where they typically are associated with hair follicles. However, sebaceous glands also can be found on mucosal surfaces, where they are known as **Fordyce granules**. In the oral cavity, Fordyce granules are seen most frequently on the upper lip vermilion and buccal mucosa, although they also may appear on the retromolar pad and tonsillar pillars. The term *Fordyce granules* also is used to describe sebaceous glands found on the genitalia. Although oral Fordyce granules often are regarded as ectopic structures, they are found in over 80% of adults, suggesting that these glands represent a normal anatomic variation. Their prevalence is higher in adults than in children, probably because of hormonal influences. Clinically, they appear as tiny yellowish or chamois-colored papules ranging from 1 to 3 mm in diameter. Some patients may exhibit only isolated lesions, whereas others may have well over 100 such papules that focally may appear tightly packed and almost confluent. Because Fordyce granules are asymptomatic normal anatomic structures, no treatment is necessary. Occasionally such glands can become hyperplastic or form keratin-filled pseudocysts, which might prompt biopsy to confirm the diagnosis. Extremely rare examples of sebaceous tumors in the oral cavity, which may have arisen from Fordyce granules, have been described.

■ Figure 1.7
Fordyce Granules
Confluent yellow papules on the upper lip vermilion.

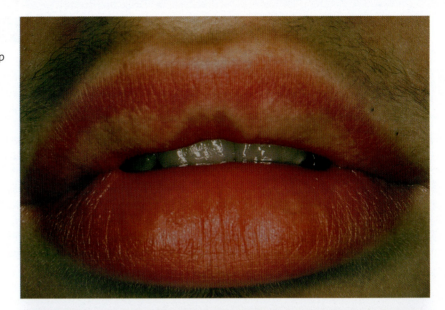

■ Figure 1.8
Fordyce Granules
Cluster of yellow papules on the left buccal mucosa.

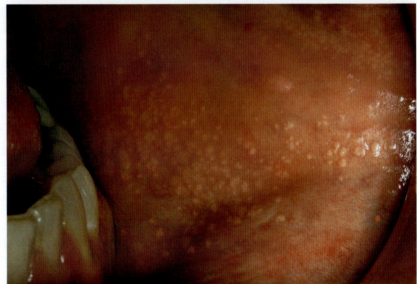

■ Figure 1.9
Fordyce Granules
Multiple prominent sebaceous glands on the right buccal mucosa. The parotid papilla is located near the center, and a varix can be seen toward the anterior buccal mucosa.

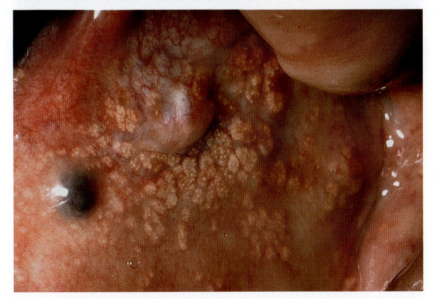

Leukoedema

Figs. **1.10 and 1.11**

Leukoedema is a bilateral, white, opalescent appearance of the buccal mucosa that may represent a normal variation in anatomy. The white appearance is created by an increase in thickness of the surface epithelium, which includes numerous cells with prominent intracellular edema. Leukoedema exhibits a predilection for blacks, among whom it has been described in 70% to 90% of adults and 50% of children. In whites, the condition often has a milder presentation and may be hardly noticeable. Leukoedema in blacks may appear more obvious because of the contrast between the edematous mucosa and background pigmentation. Although leukoedema is considered to be a developmental lesion, the white color can be more prominent in smokers and may become less severe after smoking cessation.

Leukoedema appears as a diffuse, milky, gray-white change in the color of the buccal mucosa, which should be bilateral and symmetric. Often, the mucosal surface appears somewhat folded, resulting in white streaks or wrinkles. The diagnosis can be confirmed easily by stretching and everting the cheek, which will result in disappearance of the opalescent white change. No treatment or biopsy is necessary.

Ankyloglossia

Fig. **1.12**

Ankyloglossia ("tongue-tie") refers to a short or tight attachment of the lingual frenum to the ventral tongue, which results in limited tongue mobility. Ankyloglossia has been reported in 2% to 16% of neonates, with a male predilection. However, because the tongue normally is short at birth and then grows longer at the tip, the prevalence is much lower in adults. The term *anterior ankyloglossia* is used for examples in which the attachment of the frenum extends toward the tip of the tongue. *Posterior ankyloglossia* is often more difficult to appreciate, being caused by short submucosal collagen fibers in the posterior midline floor of the mouth that prevent full tongue motion. Although tongue-tie has been thought to contribute to speech difficulties, most patients have only minor difficulties and can compensate for any limitation in tongue movement. It also has been theorized that ankyloglossia might contribute to gingival recession if the frenum attaches high on the lingual alveolar mucosa. With the increased prevalence of breast-feeding over the past several decades, lactation experts believe that tongue-tie can contribute to feeding difficulties, such as inability of the baby to attach to the nipple and nipple pain.

Because most cases of ankyloglossia do not result in significant clinical problems, treatment is often unnecessary. For infants with breast-feeding difficulty, frenotomy (clipping and freeing the frenum) may improve the ability to nurse. However, there is insufficient evidence to support prophylactic surgical correction of tongue-tie in an effort to improve speech development.

■ Figure **1.10**
Leukoedema
Milky white appearance affecting almost the entire buccal mucosa.

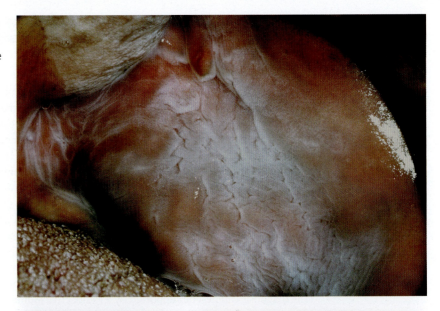

■ Figure **1.11**
Leukoedema
Same patient as seen in Fig. 1.10, showing disappearance of the white change when the cheek is stretched.

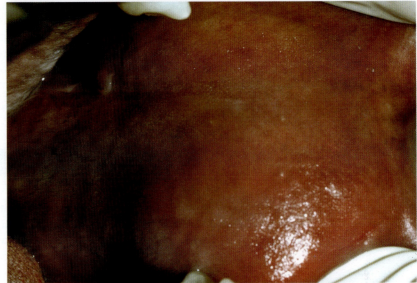

■ Figure **1.12**
Ankyloglossia
The lingual frenum attaches from the tip of the tongue to the lingual alveolar mucosa.

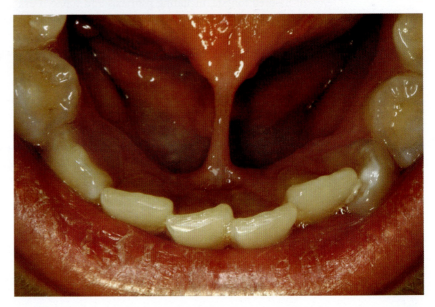

Figs. **1.13 and 1.14**

The thyroid gland originally develops at the base of the tongue in the foramen cecum area and then migrates to its normal pretracheal location during early embryologic life. However, if the embryonic gland does not undergo normal migration, then a **lingual thyroid** may develop at the midline of the dorsal tongue at the junction of the anterior two-thirds and posterior third. Other potential sites for ectopic thyroid tissue include the floor of the mouth and anterior neck. The prevalence of symptomatic or clinically evident lingual thyroid has been estimated at 1 in every 100,000 persons, with a female-to-male ratio of 5:1. However, autopsy studies have revealed incidental remnants of thyroid tissue on the posterior dorsal tongue in up to 10% of both men and women. Hypothyroidism will be present in 33% to 62% of patients with lingual thyroids, and some examples are discovered in newborns as part of screening for congenital hypothyroidism. Other cases may not be diagnosed until later in childhood or during adult life. In most instances, a lingual thyroid represents the only thyroid tissue that is present.

Many examples of lingual thyroid are asymptomatic and will be discovered incidentally upon routine oral examination or during evaluation for tonsillectomy or upper respiratory infections. Symptomatic patients may report the sensation of a mass or foreign body, hoarseness, cough, dysphagia, or snoring. The diagnosis can best be supported by a radioactive iodine scan. Other imaging tests may include magnetic resonance imaging (MRI), ultrasonography, or computed tomography (CT).

Asymptomatic lingual thyroids may not require treatment, although when associated hypothyroidism is present, thyroid hormone replacement is needed. Hormone replacement therapy sometimes results in shrinkage of a lingual thyroid. For symptomatic cases, radioactive iodine therapy or surgical resection may become necessary if hormone replacement therapy does not produce shrinkage. The risk of carcinoma development within a lingual thyroid is low, occurring in approximately 1% of cases.

Fig. **1.15**

Fissured tongue is a benign condition characterized by the presence of multiple grooves or fissures on the dorsal tongue. The cause is unknown, although genetic factors may play a role. Fissured tongue has a strong association with erythema migrans (geographic tongue), with many patients demonstrating both conditions simultaneously. It is possible that longstanding geographic tongue may contribute to the development of a fissured tongue. A variety of other factors also have been associated with a greater prevalence of fissured tongue, including psoriasis and tobacco usage. Fissured tongue also may be a component of Melkersson-Rosenthal syndrome (in association with orofacial granulomatosis and facial nerve paralysis). The reported prevalence of fissured tongue varies widely, probably related to the stringency of the criteria used to make the diagnosis. The frequency ranges from 2% to 5% of the overall population in some studies, whereas other studies indicate a prevalence in the range of 10% to 20%. Fissured tongue is uncommon in children, but it increases in frequency with age, reportedly reaching as high as 30% or more in older adults.

Patients with fissured tongue exhibit multiple grooves on the dorsal tongue, which may range from 2 to 6 mm in depth. Some patients may have a central midline fissure with smaller fissures branching off at 90-degree angles. Other patients may have numerous grooves crisscrossing the tongue, separating the surface into small islands. Sometimes one or more of these islands may develop into nodular fibroma-like growths. Fissured tongue is usually asymptomatic, although some patients may complain of mild burning or soreness. No treatment is necessary, although daily tongue brushing can help to remove any entrapped food or debris that might act as a source of irritation.

■ Figure **1.13**
Lingual Thyroid
Four-year-old girl with a mass of the posterior midline dorsal tongue.

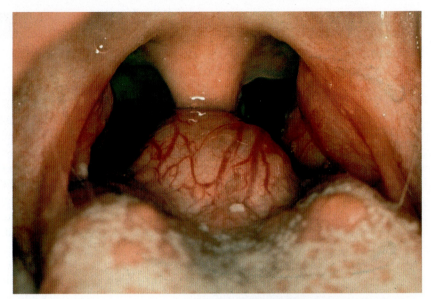

■ Figure **1.14**
Lingual Thyroid
Radioactive iodine scan of the patient seen in Fig. 1.13, showing strong uptake in the tongue mass *(center)* with minimal uptake in the lower neck.

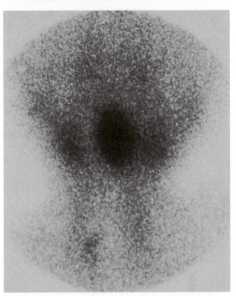

■ Figure **1.15**
Fissured Tongue
The tongue exhibits multiple cracks and grooves on the dorsal surface.

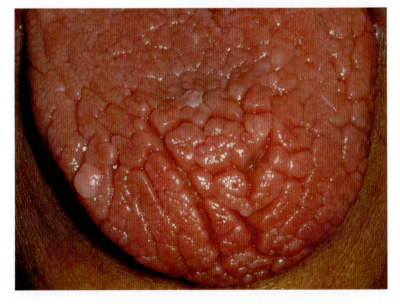

Figs. **1.16–1.19**

Hairy tongue is a common, benign condition of the dorsal tongue that is characterized by elongation and hyperkeratosis of the filiform papillae, mimicking the appearance of small hairs. Depending on the population studied, the prevalence ranges from 0.5% to 11.3%. Because the elongated papillae usually are pigmented secondary to smoking, coffee/tea consumption, or chromogenic bacteria, the condition often is referred to as *black hairy tongue*. However, many examples actually exhibit a brown or yellow color. The most common factor associated with the development of hairy tongue is smoking, although other causes include general debilitation, poor oral hygiene, xerostomia, and a history of radiation to the head and neck. Mild cases of hairy tongue will involve only the posterior midline region of the dorsal tongue. More severe examples can result in a generalized thick, matted appearance that involves most of the dorsal tongue surface. Hairy tongue is usually asymptomatic, although extreme elongation of the papillae has been known to cause gagging in some patients. Because of the accumulation of bacteria on the rough surface, halitosis is a possible sequela.

Some patients exhibit accumulation of bacteria and dead epithelial cells on the dorsal tongue surface without the development of hair-like elongation of the filiform papillae—a condition sometimes known as a *coated tongue*. Temporary "pseudo–black hairy tongue" can occur in patients who have used bismuth subsalicylate to treat upset stomach because the bismuth in such preparations can react with traces of sulfur in the saliva to produce bismuth sulfide.

Although hairy tongue is a benign condition, it is unsightly and can contribute to bad breath. Treatment includes elimination of causative factors (if possible) and improved oral hygiene. Periodic brushing/scraping of the tongue with a toothbrush or tongue scraper can promote desquamation of the excessive keratin layer and bacterial debris. Because hairy tongue is not caused by a yeast infection, clinicians should avoid unnecessary treatment with antifungal medications.

■ **Figure 1.16**
Hairy Tongue
The tongue exhibits multiple elongated filiform papillae with brown staining.

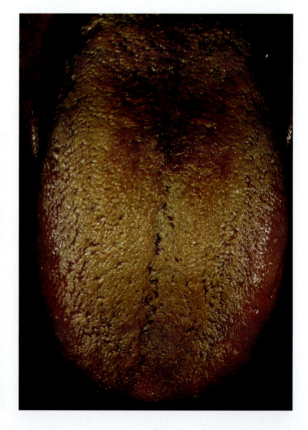

■ Figure **1.17**
Hairy Tongue
The filiform papillae show prominent elongation in the midline region of the posterior dorsal tongue. (Courtesy Dr. Scott Wietecha.)

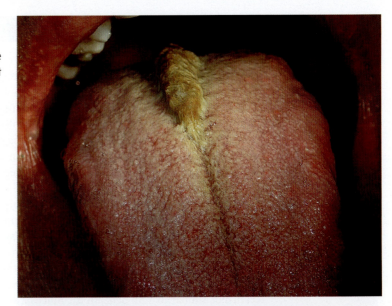

■ Figure **1.18**
Hairy Tongue
Same patient as seen in Fig. 1.17, showing resolution of the lesion after regular brushing of her tongue. (Courtesy Dr. Scott Wietecha.)

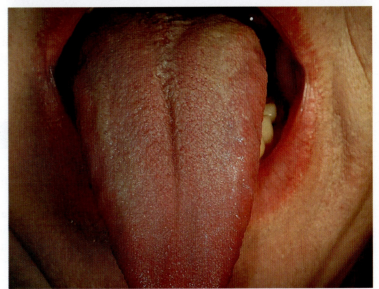

■ Figure **1.19**
Bismuth Staining
The dorsal tongue exhibits black staining, which developed after the patient used bismuth subsalicylate for an upset stomach.

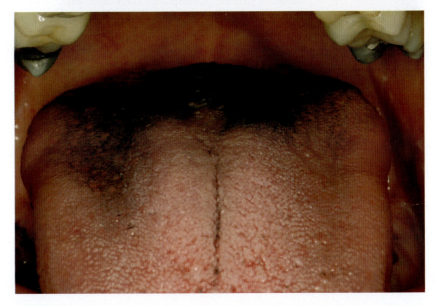

Varicosities (Varices)

Figs. **1.20 and 1.21**

A **varicosity**, or **varix**, is an abnormally dilated, tortuous vein. In the oral cavity, varicosities develop most frequently on the ventrolateral tongue, although such lesions can occur in other locations, especially the labial and buccal mucosa. They are rare in children but common in older adults, which suggests that age is an important factor in their development. Sublingual varicosities have been described in two-thirds of people over 60 years of age. Age-related weakening of blood vessel walls and loss of tone in the surrounding connective tissue may contribute to such vascular dilation. Also, oral varices have been reported to occur more often in patients with varicose veins of the legs and in those with a history of smoking, cardiovascular disease, and/or hypertension.

Clinically, oral varicosities appear as blue to purple blebs or soft nodules, which should blanch on compression. Blanching may be demonstrated clinically by pressing against the lesion with a glass slide, a technique known as *diascopy*. Sublingual varicosities usually are multiple and bilateral in distribution, although varices in other locations may occur as isolated lesions. Because the flow of blood will slow down within a dilated vessel, varicosities are prone to thrombosis. Such a lesion typically will not blanch under pressure because the thrombus cannot be pressed into the adjacent vasculature. A thrombosed varix will feel firmer, similar to a BB beneath the mucosal surface. However, unlike deep vein thromboses in the leg, a thrombosed oral varix poses minimal risk of embolism.

Oral varicosities are usually innocuous lesions that can be diagnosed clinically and, therefore, do not require treatment. However, surgical excision can be performed for thrombosed varices, for aesthetically displeasing varicosities on the lips, or in situations where the diagnosis must be confirmed.

Caliber-Persistent Artery

Fig. **1.22**

Larger arterial vessels normally are found within the deeper connective tissues. However, occasionally a large branch of an artery will extend close to the mucosal surface without a reduction in its diameter—a vascular anomaly known as a **caliber-persistent artery**. This lesion is seen most frequently in older adults, suggesting that it may represent an age-related phenomenon related to loss of tone within the surrounding connective tissues. Caliber-persistent arteries almost always occur on the lower or upper labial mucosa; some patients may develop lesions on both lips or bilaterally. The lesion appears as a curvilinear or papular elevation that can appear bluish in color. The artery may become less obvious when the lip is stretched. Pulsation may be noted within the vessel, although it may be difficult to feel this pulse through gloved fingers. The lesion is usually asymptomatic, although overlying mucosal ulceration has been reported in a few examples. Because of its benign nature, no treatment is necessary. However, sometimes a biopsy will be performed because the lesion is mistaken for a mucocele or hemangioma. In such instances, significant bleeding may be encountered.

■ Figure **1.20**
Varicosities

Multiple dilated purple veins found bilaterally on the ventrolateral tongue.

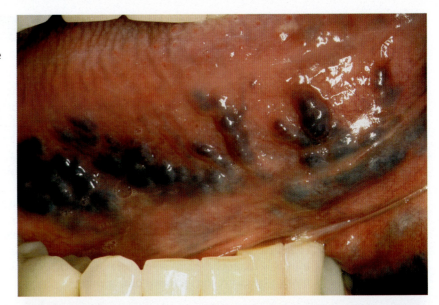

■ Figure **1.21**
Varicosities

Three separate varices can be seen on the skin and vermilion border of the upper lip.

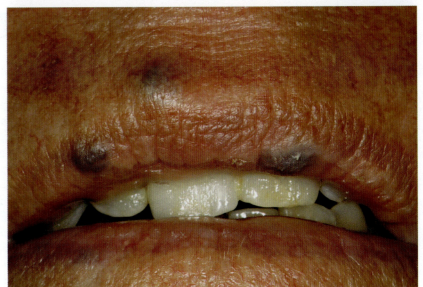

■ Figure **1.22**
Caliber-Persistent Artery

A slightly blue, arcuate vessel can be seen on the upper lip mucosa.

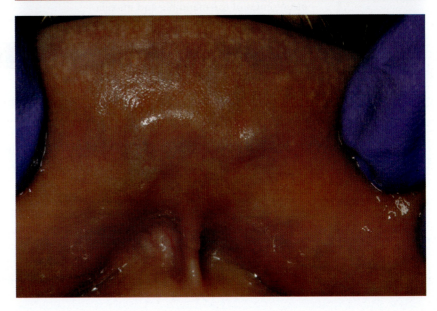

Coronoid Hyperplasia

Fig. **1.23**

Hyperplasia of the coronoid process of the mandible is an uncommon bony anomaly that limits the ability to open the mouth. As the jaw translates forward when the patient tries to open the mouth, the elongated coronoid process impinges on the body or arch of the zygomatic bone. **Coronoid hyperplasia** is diagnosed most frequently in teenagers, although some examples have been documented in newborns and older adults. The mean age at diagnosis is 23 to 25 years of age. Bilateral cases are four to five times more common than unilateral examples. Coronoid hyperplasia also is three to five times more common in males than in females, which suggests that there could be an endocrine influence. Heredity also may play a role because cases have been noted in siblings.

Bilateral coronoid hyperplasia presents with a progressively worsening ability to open the mouth, which typically develops over a period of several years. In unilateral examples, the mandible may deviate toward the affected side. Radiographic examination will reveal elongation of the coronoid process(es), which is often best demonstrated on CT imaging. Treatment consists of coronoidectomy or coronoidotomy, which usually is accomplished via an intraoral approach. Postoperative physiotherapy plays an important role in trying to preserve the increased oral opening.

Condylar Hyperplasia

Fig. **1.24**

Condylar hyperplasia is an uncommon bony malformation characterized by excessive growth of one or both of the mandibular condyles. The classification system developed by Wolford and associates describes four major categories: type 1—an accelerated and prolonged aberration of the "normal" condylar growth mechanism that can be either bilateral (type 1A) or unilateral (type 1B); type 2—unilateral enlargement caused by an osteochondroma; type 3—unilateral enlargement caused by other benign tumors of the condyle; and type 4—unilateral enlargement caused by malignant tumors of the condyle. Types 1 and 2 are the most common forms of condylar hyperplasia, with types 3 and 4 being much rarer. Approximately 60% of cases of type 1 condylar hyperplasia occur in females; this female predilection is even higher for type 2 cases (76%). The condition usually is discovered in teenagers and young adults.

Condylar hyperplasia classically presents as a progressively worsening asymmetry of the face, which may be associated with prognathism, crossbite, and open bite. In some cases, compensatory maxillary growth occurs with tilting of the occlusal plane. Radiographs will show elongation or enlargement of the affected condyle. In addition, some cases may exhibit some degree of expansion or asymmetry of the entire ramus. Treatment usually requires condylectomy, which may be combined with orthodontic therapy and osteotomies of the mandible and maxilla.

Bifid Condyle

Fig. **1.25**

A **bifid condyle** is an uncommon bony anomaly in which the head of the mandibular condyle is divided into two lobes by a central groove. The reported prevalence of bifid condyle varies from 0.02% to 4.5%, probably related to the criteria used and whether the study was performed on plain radiographs, cone beam CT, or dry mandibles. Regardless, the lesion usually is discovered as an asymptomatic, incidental radiographic finding. In some instances, the patient may report a popping or clicking noise in the temporomandibular joint.

Most bifid condyles have medial and lateral lobes that are divided by an anteroposterior groove. Less commonly, anterior and posterior heads are noted, which are separated by a transverse groove. Bifid condyles usually are unilateral, although occasionally both condyles may be affected. The etiology is uncertain, although various theories have been suggested. Some examples with anterior and posterior lobes may be due to trauma, such as a fracture during childhood. Because most bifid condyles are asymptomatic, no treatment is necessary. However, if the patient complains of joint problems, appropriate temporomandibular therapy may be considered.

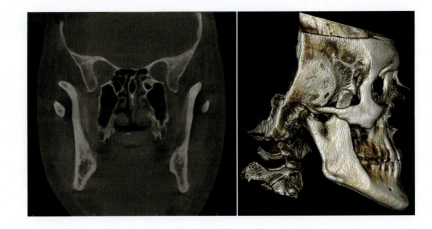

■ Figure **1.23**
Coronoid Hyperplasia
Coronal cone beam computed tomography and three-dimensional reconstruction showing elongation of the coronoid processes. (Courtesy Dr. Peter Green.)

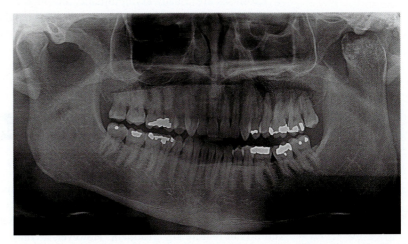

■ Figure **1.24**
Condylar Hyperplasia
The left mandibular condyle shows prominent enlargement.

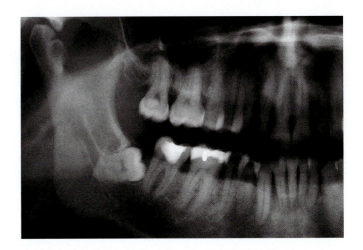

■ Figure **1.25**
Bifid Condyle
The right condylar head shows two lobes divided by a central groove.

An **exostosis** is a nodular protuberance of dense cortical bone. The most common and best-known exostoses of the jaws are the torus mandibularis and torus palatinus, which are discussed later in this chapter. However, exostoses can arise from the cortical surface in other areas of the jaws, especially along the buccal aspect of the alveolar processes or palatal to the maxillary molars. The specific cause of exostoses is uncertain, although they likely are related to both genetic factors and local stresses placed on the bone through occlusal function.

Buccal exostoses ("buttressing bone") appear as a bilateral row of smooth bony nodules along the facial alveolar process of the mandible and/or maxilla. The prevalence of buccal exostoses in different studies varies from 0.09% to nearly 19%, probably depending on the diagnostic criteria used and the population studied. Palatal exostoses occur along the lingual aspect of the maxillary molars. Such lesions are more common in males and may be unilateral or bilateral. The reported prevalence of palatal exostoses also varies widely, ranging from 8% to 69% in various studies. Many patients with buccal or palatal exostoses also have palatal and/or mandibular tori. If an exostosis is large enough, a relatively increased density of the bone might be noticed on radiographs.

Exostoses are usually asymptomatic, although trauma to the thin overlying mucosa sometimes can result in superficial ulceration. No treatment is required for most exostoses. However, surgical removal can be performed if repeated ulceration and pain occur or if the location of the lesion interferes with the fabrication of a dental prosthesis.

Reactive Subpontine Exostosis (Subpontic Osseous Hyperplasia)

Fig. **1.28**

The **reactive subpontine exostosis** is a rare type of osseous hyperplasia that develops beneath the pontic of a fixed bridge. In almost all instances, such lesions occur in association with a posterior mandibular bridge. It is theorized that occlusal stresses carried through the abutment teeth of the bridge may stimulate the formation of new cortical bone under the central pontic. Such exostoses usually are discovered incidentally and do not require any treatment. However, if continued growth of the exostosis places pressure against the pontic or if it interferes with oral hygiene, then surgical removal can be performed.

Figure **1.26**
Buccal Exostoses
Confluent bony nodules affect the maxillary and mandibular facial alveolar processes.

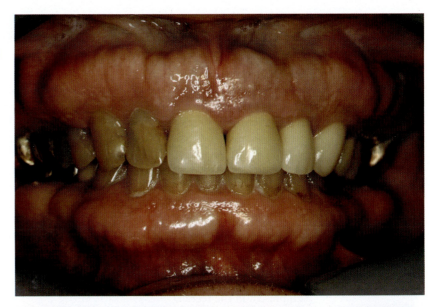

Figure **1.27**
Palatal Exostosis
A prominent nodular mass of dense bone is present lingual to the maxillary molars. The patient also has a midline torus palatinus.

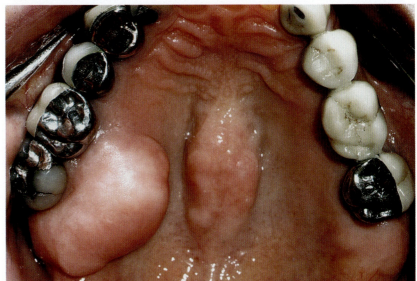

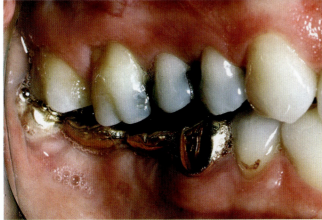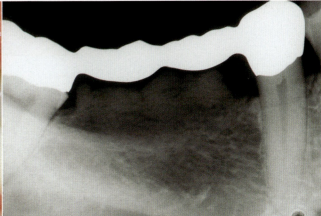

Figure **1.28**
Reactive Subpontine Exostosis
A nodular mass of bone has grown up beneath the pontics of this mandibular fixed bridge.

Figs. 1.29–1.32

The **torus mandibularis** is a common form of exostosis that develops along the lingual aspect of the mandible above the mylohyoid line. As with other jaw exostoses, the etiology is likely multifactorial, being related to genetic susceptibility and environmental factors (such as occlusal stresses). The reported prevalence of mandibular tori varies widely, which may be related to the population studied and the diagnostic criteria used. In various studies from around the world, the frequency has ranged from as low as 3% in Malaysia to as high as 58% in Japan.

Mandibular tori typically occur in the premolar region, but larger examples also can involve the canine and first molar areas. In most instances, they are bilateral and symmetric, although unilateral examples sometimes may be noted. Most lesions occur as single bony nodules; larger examples can appear as a row of variably sized lobules that may result in a radiopacity superimposed on the roots of the mandibular teeth. In rare instances, tori may grow so large that they actually meet in the midline ("kissing tori"). Mandibular tori usually are noted as incidental findings, although trauma may result in transient superficial ulceration or abrasion. Asymptomatic tori do not require any treatment, but surgical removal may be required to accommodate a mandibular prosthesis. On occasion, mandibular tori may recur if teeth are still present in the region.

■ **Figure 1.29**
Torus Mandibularis
Bilateral bony nodules are present on the lingual mandible in the premolar region.

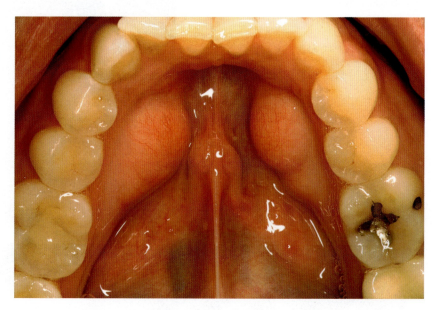

■ Figure **1.30**
Torus Mandibularis
Moderately large mandibular tori with a multilobulated appearance.

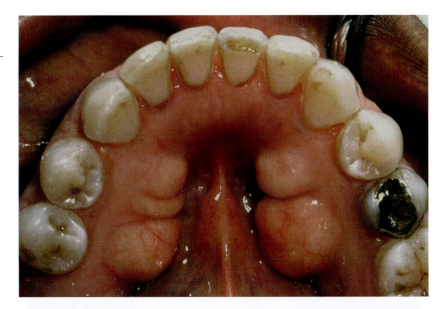

■ Figure **1.31**
Torus Mandibularis
Giant "kissing" mandibular tori.

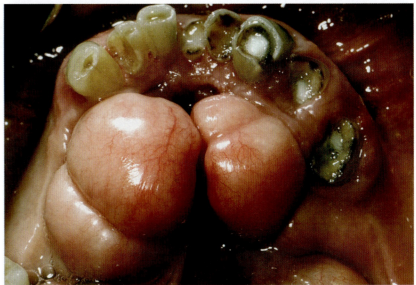

■ Figure **1.32**
Torus Mandibularis
Periapical radiograph showing a radiopaque shadow superimposed across the roots of the mandibular teeth.

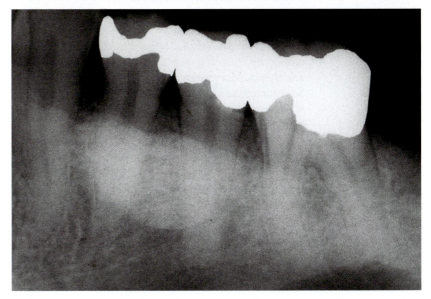

Fig. **1.33**

The **torus palatinus** is a common exostosis that develops in the midline region of the hard palate. The reported prevalence of palatal tori, like that of mandibular tori, varies considerably, ranging from as low as 4% to more than 60%. This variation may reflect genetic differences among populations, clinical criteria used to make the diagnosis, and whether the determination was made on live patients or dried skulls. There appears to be a higher prevalence in Asian and Inuit populations. Almost all studies show that the torus palatinus occurs more often in women (female-to-male ratio equals 2:1).

The torus palatinus has a spectrum of clinical appearances, ranging from slight midline elevation of the palatal bone to large, multilobular masses. Sometimes they have been categorized on the basis of morphology into *flat, spindle, nodular,* and *lobular* subtypes. Most palatal tori are asymptomatic, and some patients may be unaware of their presence. Larger tori are more susceptible to trauma from eating, which occasionally results in superficial abrasion or ulceration. Most palatal tori do not require any treatment. However, surgical removal may be required prior to fabrication of a maxillary denture or if repeated trauma is bothersome to the patient.

Eagle Syndrome (Stylohyoid Syndrome; Carotid Artery Syndrome; Stylocarotid Syndrome)

Figs. **1.34 and 1.35**

Eagle syndrome is an uncommon pain condition in which elongation of the styloid process or mineralization of the stylohyoid ligament results in a variety of clinical symptoms. The styloid process, a slender projection of bone arising from the inferior portion of the temporal bone, is connected to the hyoid bone in the neck by the stylohyoid ligament. The internal and external branches of the carotid artery are located on either side. Some degree of elongation of the styloid process or mineralization of the stylohyoid ligament is not unusual, although the reported prevalence varies widely, from 4% to greater than 40%. Regardless, only about 4% of individuals with radiographic evidence of such mineralization develop Eagle syndrome.

Eagle syndrome is characterized by unilateral pain in the anterior lateral neck, which may be precipitated by swallowing, turning the head, or yawning. This pain may radiate to the ear or temporomandibular joint. Other symptoms can include dysphagia and the sensation of a foreign body in the throat. In addition, compression of the adjacent carotid arteries can result in syncope, transient ischemic attacks, and even carotid artery dissection. Some authors distinguish between "classic" Eagle syndrome and stylohyoid syndrome. In classic Eagle syndrome, the symptoms develop after tonsillectomy, presumably due to development of scar tissue around the mineralized stylohyoid complex. **Stylohyoid syndrome (stylocarotid syndrome)** is not associated with a prior tonsillectomy but is thought to be due to direct impingement of the calcified stylohyoid complex upon the carotid arteries and adjacent sympathetic nerve fibers.

Treatment depends on the severity of the symptoms. Mild examples of Eagle syndrome may be managed conservatively using nonsteroidal antiinflammatory drugs and local injection of corticosteroids and anesthetics. More severe cases require partial surgical removal of the elongated styloid process, which can be accomplished by either a transoral tonsillar approach or an extraoral cervical approach. The prognosis after surgery is good.

■ Figure **1.33**
Torus Palatinus
Multilobulated bony growth of the hard palate.

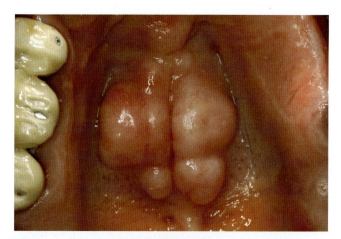

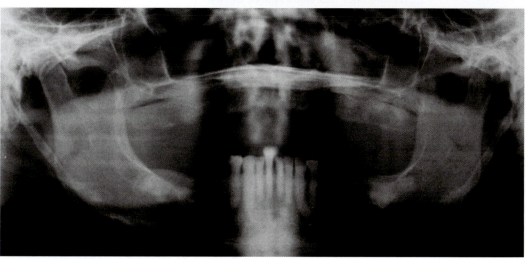

■ Figure **1.34**
Eagle Syndrome
Panoramic radiograph showing bilateral mineralization of the stylohyoid ligament.

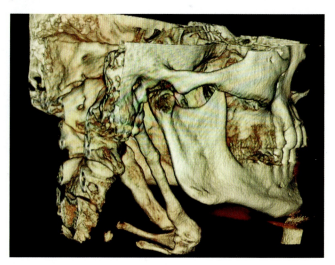

■ Figure **1.35**
Eagle Syndrome
Three-dimensional radiographic reconstruction showing complete ossification of the stylohyoid ligament, which attaches to the hyoid bone. (Courtesy Dr. Vicki Tatum.)

Stafne Defect (Lingual Mandibular Salivary Gland Depression; Latent Bone Cyst; Static Bone Cyst)

Figs. **1.36–1.39**

A **Stafne defect** is an uncommon radiographic anomaly of the mandible characterized by a cupped-out depression of the bony cortex adjacent to a major salivary gland. The lesion usually is related to the submandibular gland, although rare examples associated with the sublingual and parotid glands also have been described. Although Stafne defects generally are thought to be "developmental" in nature, they rarely are encountered in children, which indicates that these bony concavities gradually develop over time in adult patients. The posterior lingual submandibular type has been discovered on 0.08% to 0.48% of panoramic radiographs. There is a marked male predilection, with 80% to 90% of cases seen in men.

Stafne defects are asymptomatic lesions that typically are discovered as incidental findings on conventional dental radiographs. The classic posterior submandibular type appears as a well-circumscribed, corticated radiolucency near the angle of the mandible below the mandibular canal. On occasion, the lesion may involve the inferior border of the mandible, resulting in a palpable notch in this area. Anterior sublingual gland defects present as well-circumscribed radiolucencies located apical to the premolar or anterior teeth. Such a lesion may be mistaken for periapical pathosis. Exceedingly rare parotid examples may produce a radiolucency higher in the mandibular ramus. Computed tomography (CT), such as cone-beam CT, can be helpful to confirm that a suspected Stafne defect represents a cortical concavity rather than some other intrabony lesion.

Once discovered, a Stafne defect usually remains stable in size—hence the term *static bone cyst*. However, if discovered early enough in its formation, it is possible to see radiographic evidence of enlargement over time before the lesion becomes stable. No treatment is warranted for Stafne defects, and the prognosis is excellent.

■ Figure **1.36**
Stafne Defect
Circumscribed radiolucency located below the mandibular canal near the inferior border of the mandible. (Courtesy Dr. Caleb Poston.)

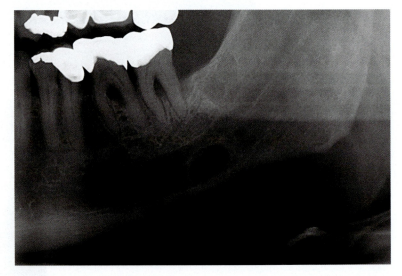

■ Figure **1.37**
Stafne Defect

Large radiolucency near the angle of the posterior mandible. (Courtesy Dr. Terry Day.)

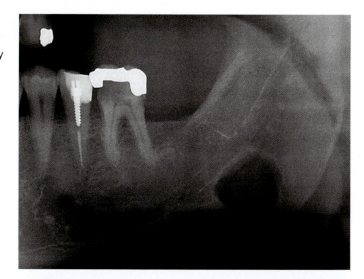

■ Figure **1.38**
Stafne Defect

Axial computed tomography image showing a cupped-out defect on the lingual surface of the mandible *(arrow)*. (Courtesy Dr. Kim Tambini.)

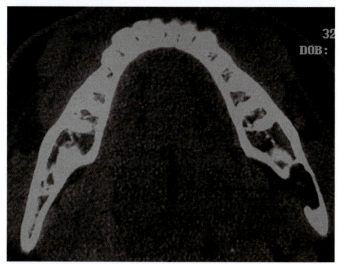

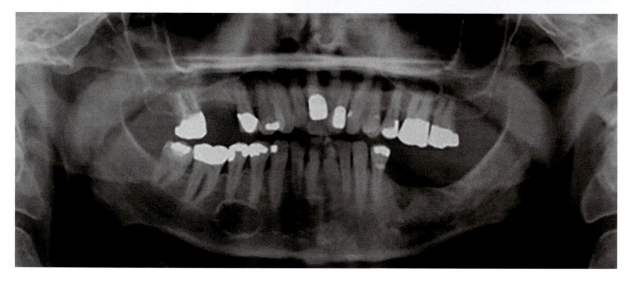

■ Figure **1.39**
Stafne Defect

Anterior Stafne defect associated with the sublingual gland. The lesion appears as a well-circumscribed corticated radiolucency apical to the right mandibular premolars.

Epstein Pearls

Fig. **1.40**

Epstein pearls are tiny, congenital, keratin-filled cysts found at the junction of the hard and soft palate near the midline. Such lesions are quite common, having been reported in 55% to 89% of newborns. The terminology associated with various congenital oral cysts is confusing. Theoretically, Epstein pearls develop from epithelium entrapped along the line of fusion of the lateral palatal shelves. The term *Bohn nodules* has been used to describe similar keratin-filled cysts scattered across the posterior hard/soft palate junction, presumably arising from epithelial remnants of the developing minor salivary glands. However, over the years these two terms have been used interchangeably, sometimes also in reference to gingival cysts of the newborn.

Epstein pearls appear as one to several white papules on the posterior midline region of the hard palate at the junction with the soft palate. No treatment is necessary because the lesions are asymptomatic and typically will disappear within a few weeks.

Nasopalatine Duct Cyst (Incisive Canal Cyst)

The most common nonodontogenic cyst of the oral cavity is the **nasopalatine duct cyst**, which is estimated to occur in 1% of the population. This developmental cyst arises from remnants of the nasopalatine ducts, which are paired embryonic passageways running through the incisive canal between the oral cavity and nasal cavity. Normally these ducts degenerate and disappear before birth, although epithelial remnants may remain in the incisive canal region and later give rise to a cyst. Nasopalatine duct cysts can develop at any age, but they are most commonly diagnosed in young to middle-aged adults. They occur twice as often in men as in women. Several examples have been reported to develop following placement of a dental implant in the area.

Small nasopalatine duct cysts may be discovered incidentally on dental radiographs, although larger lesions can produce symptoms such as swelling, pain, pressure, or drainage. Radiographically, the lesion appears as a well-circumscribed unilocular radiolucency that can range from less than 6 mm to more than 6 cm in diameter. Most examples are in the range of 1.0 to 2.5 cm. It is sometimes difficult to distinguish a small nasopalatine duct cyst from a large incisive canal. Generally a radiolucency smaller than 6 mm in diameter is considered to be a normal canal unless other signs or symptoms are present. Typically the radiolucency is found in the midline region of the maxilla superior to the apices of the central incisors, although some examples will extend laterally in an asymmetric fashion. In most cases, the radiolucency appears round to oval with a corticated rim. However, some examples may have the shape of an inverted pear or a heart because of resistance from the roots of the adjacent teeth or from superimposition of the nasal spine. Occasionally a nasopalatine duct cyst will occur solely in the soft tissue of the anterior palate ("**cyst of the incisive papilla**"). Such lesions may exhibit a bluish color due to the presence of fluid within the cyst lumen.

Nasopalatine duct cysts are treated by surgical enucleation, usually from a palatal approach. The lesion rarely recurs. Extremely rare examples of malignant transformation of the cystic lining have been reported.

■ Figure **1.40**
Epstein Pearls
Newborn infant with multiple white papules found in the midline region at the junction of the hard and soft palate.

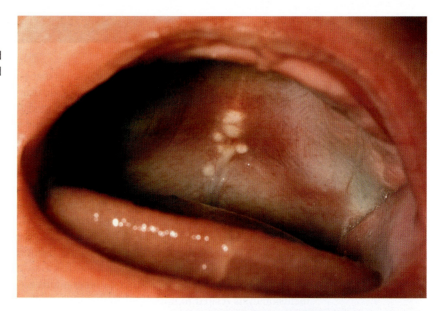

■ Figure **1.41**
Nasopalatine Duct Cyst
Well-circumscribed ovoid radiolucency of the anterior maxilla apical to the central incisors.

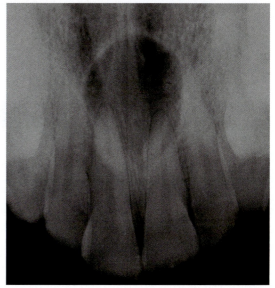

■ Figure **1.42**
Nasopalatine Duct Cyst ("Cyst of the Incisive Papilla")
Slight bluish soft tissue swelling located just behind the incisive papilla.

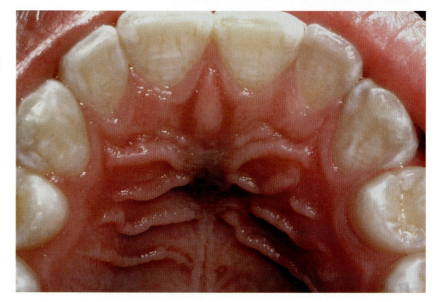

Epidermoid Cyst (Infundibular Cyst)

Figs. **1.43 and 1.44**

Keratin-filled cysts of the skin are common lesions that arise from hair follicles. The most common example is the **epidermoid cyst**, which is derived from the follicular infundibulum. Such lesions may develop secondary to inflammation of the hair follicle, and they are found most frequently in sites prone to acne, such as the head, neck, and back. Although follicular cysts of the skin often are referred to as *sebaceous cysts*, this term is a misnomer because neither the epidermoid cyst nor the pilar cyst (see next topic) arises from sebaceous glands. Another type of keratin-filled cyst of the skin is unrelated to hair follicles but instead arises secondary to traumatic implantation of the surface epithelium. Such lesions also can develop on oral mucosa and are designated as **epithelial** (or **epidermal**) **inclusion cysts**.

Epidermoid cysts on the skin occur more frequently in males than in females. They present as nodular subcutaneous growths that are often fluctuant to palpation. If the cyst becomes inflamed or infected, then the epidermal surface will appear red. Rupture of the cyst may release keratinaceous material, which typically will elicit a pronounced foreign-body response, resulting in pain and swelling. Epidermoid cysts rarely develop during childhood unless the patient has Gardner syndrome. Younger adults are more likely to develop these cysts on the face, whereas older adults are more likely to have them on the back. Epithelial inclusion cysts related to implanted epithelium usually appear as small, yellowish-white papules.

Epidermoid and epithelial inclusion cysts usually are treated by conservative surgical excision, and recurrence is uncommon. Extremely rare examples of malignant transformation of epidermoid cysts have been reported.

Pilar Cyst

Fig. **1.45**

In addition to the epidermoid cyst, the **pilar cyst** is the second type of follicular cyst that arises from the outer sheath of the hair follicle. Also known as a trichilemmal cyst or isthmus-catagen cyst, it comprises approximately 10% to 15% of skin cysts. Unlike the epidermoid cyst, the pilar cyst occurs most frequently on the scalp and exhibits a female predilection. A tendency to develop such cysts may run in families, and some patients will develop multiple lesions. Pilar cysts appear as movable nodules that typically shell out easily when surgically removed.

■ Figure **1.43**
Epidermoid Cyst
Yellow keratin-filled cyst located on the earlobe. (With appreciation to Dr. Kevin Riker.)

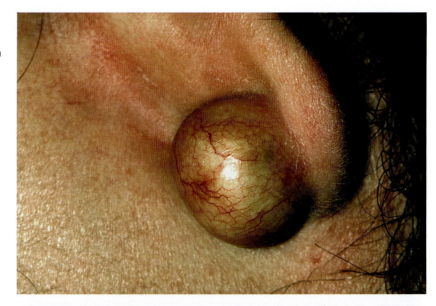

■ Figure **1.44**
Epithelial Inclusion Cyst
Yellowish-white papule on the lateral tongue secondary to traumatically implanted epithelium.

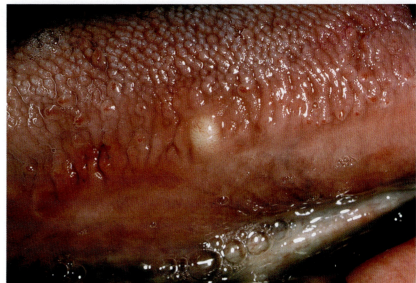

■ Figure **1.45**
Pilar Cyst
Nodular mass located at the edge of the scalp line.

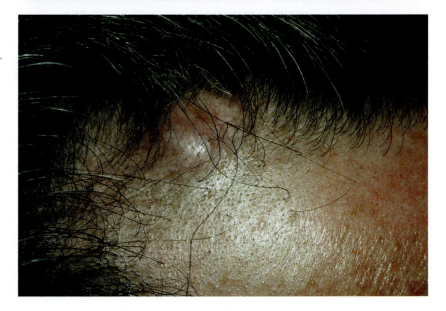

Dermoid Cyst

Fig. **1.46**

A **dermoid cyst** is a rare developmental malformation characterized primarily by a keratin-filled cavity lined by epithelium resembling epidermis. In addition, the surrounding cyst wall contains one or more dermal adnexal structures, such as hair follicles, sebaceous glands, or sweat glands. The lesion is generally considered to represent a simple cystic form in the *teratoma* spectrum, even though it does not contain tissue from all three germ layers.

Oral dermoid cysts develop most frequently in the midline floor-of-mouth region. They are seen most often in children and young adults, with 15% of reported cases being congenital. If the lesion occurs above the geniohyoid muscle, then it will present as an intraoral swelling that tends to elevate the tongue. Examples that develop below the geniohyoid muscle appear as submental masses. At presentation the lesion may vary from only a few millimeters to 12 cm in diameter. The mass often exhibits a soft, doughy, or rubbery consistency. CT scans or MRI scans may be helpful in determining the extent of the lesion. Treatment consists of surgical removal, which can be accomplished via an intraoral or extraoral approach, depending on the relationship of the cyst to the geniohyoid muscle. Recurrence is uncommon.

Thyroglossal Duct Cyst (Thyroglossal Tract Cyst)

Fig. **1.47**

During early embryonic life, the thyroid gland begins its development at the base of the tongue. It then descends to its normal anatomic location anterior to the trachea and below the thyroid cartilage. As it migrates downward, an epithelial tract or duct is formed, which maintains an attachment to the tongue at the foramen cecum. Although this duct typically involutes and disappears between 7 and 10 weeks of gestation, remnants of this epithelial tract may be found in as many as 7% of the population. These epithelial remnants are thought to be the source of a developmental cyst known as a **thyroglossal duct cyst** in the midline neck region.

Thyroglossal duct cysts occur most often in children and young adults. There is no sex predilection. The lesion presents as a painless fluctuant mass that may move vertically when the patient protrudes the tongue or swallows. The cyst can develop anywhere along the thyroglossal tract, but the most common location is in the region of the hyoid bone. Approximately 75% of cases will be infrahyoid in location, and 25% will be suprahyoid. Intralingual cysts are rare. Secondary infection or a draining sinus tract may develop in some cases. Treatment of thyroglossal duct cysts consists of surgical removal via a Sistrunk procedure, which includes removal of part of the hyoid bone. There is a low recurrence rate, estimated at around 3%, with this procedure. From 1% to 3% of thyroglossal duct cysts will show the development of carcinoma, usually papillary thyroid carcinoma.

Branchial Cleft Cyst (Cervical Lymphoepithelial Cyst)

Fig. **1.48**

The **branchial cleft cyst** is a developmental cyst thought to arise from remnants of the embryonic branchial arches. Because lymphoid tissue is found in the cyst wall, it also is known as a **cervical lymphoepithelial cyst**. About 70% to 95% of cases develop from the second branchial arch, with the remainder arising from the first, third, and fourth branchial arches. Second branchial cleft cysts typically are located anterior to the sternocleidomastoid muscle between the angle of the mandible and the clavicle. They are seen most frequently in young adults, although examples also can be found in children. The lesion presents as a painless compressible swelling that may wax and wane in size. Sometimes secondary inflammation and drainage to the skin surface will occur. Bilateral cysts are rare; however, these may be associated with an autosomal dominant condition known as branchio-oto-renal syndrome.

Branchial cleft cysts are treated by surgical excision, and recurrence is uncommon. Great care must be taken clinically and pathologically to distinguish this lesion from metastatic oropharyngeal carcinoma, which frequently produces cystic metastases to cervical lymph nodes.

■ Figure **1.46**
Dermoid Cyst
Large swelling in the floor of mouth, which is elevating the tongue. (Courtesy Dr. Michael Bobo.)

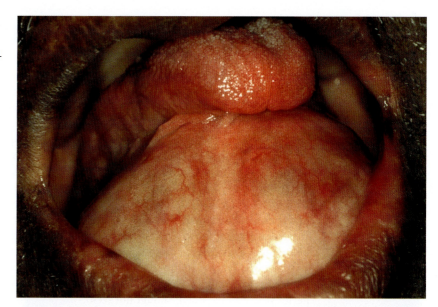

■ Figure **1.47**
Thyroglossal Duct Cyst
Nodular swelling in the midline of the neck.

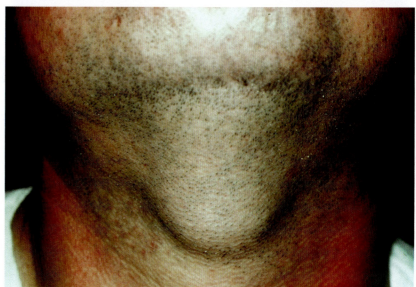

■ Figure **1.48**
Branchial Cleft Cyst
Axial computed tomography image showing a circumscribed, round, cystic mass in the lateral neck *(arrow)*. (Courtesy Dr. Seth Stalcup.)

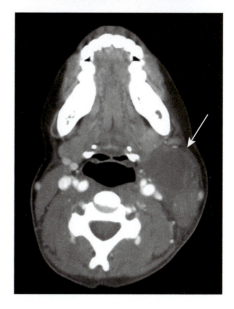

The **oral lymphoepithelial cyst** is an uncommon keratin-filled cyst that develops within tonsillar or accessory oral lymphoid tissue. Normal tonsillar tissue is situated immediately beneath the mucosal surface. The surface epithelium typically demonstrates invaginations into the underlying lymphoid tissue, known as *tonsillar crypts*. An epithelium-lined crypt may fill with keratinaceous debris and form a small keratin-filled cyst that becomes pinched off from the mucosal surface. However, it also has been theorized that some oral lymphoepithelial cysts could arise from excretory salivary gland ducts that either are entrapped within tonsillar tissue or induce an adjacent lymphoid reaction.

Oral lymphoepithelial cysts can occur at any age, but they are diagnosed most frequently in young adults. The lesion appears as a small, white or yellow, pearl-like nodule that is usually less than 1 cm in diameter. Oral lymphoepithelial cysts develop most often in the palatine tonsil or lingual tonsil, although some examples occur in the floor of the mouth in association with accessory lymphoid aggregates. The lesion often is discovered as an asymptomatic incidental finding.

Many oral lymphoepithelial cysts can be diagnosed on a clinical basis with reasonable certainty and may not require biopsy. However, if the diagnosis is uncertain, then conservative excisional biopsy can be performed, and the lesion should not recur.

Fig. **1.51**

Progressive hemifacial atrophy is a rare and poorly understood condition that results in atrophy of the tissues on one side of the face. Because the process shares many features with localized scleroderma, these may be related disorders. The disease usually has its onset during the first two decades of life, initially appearing as atrophy of skin and subcutaneous tissues in a localized area. The atrophic skin may have a shiny, hyperpigmented appearance. Some patients will develop a linear, scar-like depression near the middle of the forehead known as *linear scleroderma* "en coup de sabre" ("strike of the sword"). As the condition progresses, the face may show a caved-in appearance due to muscular atrophy, loss of fat, and hypoplasia of the underlying bone. Orbital involvement often results in enophthalmos. Other potential complications include alopecia, facial paresthesia, epilepsy, and trigeminal neuralgia. Intraorally, unilateral atrophy of the tongue can develop, and atrophy of the upper lip may result in exposure of the maxillary teeth. Teeth on the affected side may demonstrate an open bite, incomplete root formation, or root resorption.

Progressive hemifacial atrophy slowly progresses over a period of 2 to 20 years but then becomes stable. Active disease may be managed with methotrexate, which often is combined with systemic corticosteroids. Plastic surgery can be used to improve the cosmetic deformity, and orthodontic therapy is often necessary to treat any associated malocclusion.

■ Figure **1.49**
Oral Lymphoepithelial Cyst
Asymptomatic yellow papule on the left posterior lateral tongue.

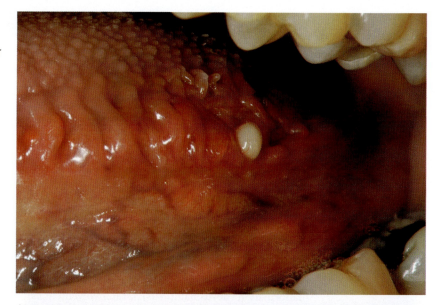

■ Figure **1.50**
Oral Lymphoepithelial Cyst
Small yellow nodule in the tonsillar fossa.

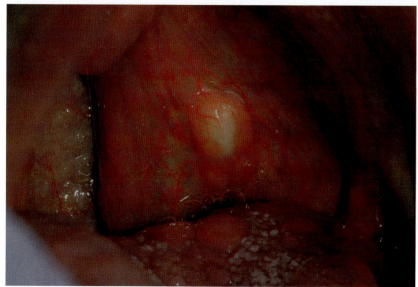

■ Figure **1.51**
Progressive Hemifacial Atrophy
Woman who developed atrophy of the skin and underlying bone of the left face during childhood.

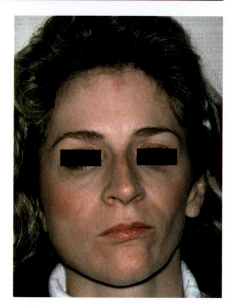

Figs. 1.52–1.55

Hemihyperplasia is a rare developmental condition that results in unilateral overgrowth of part of the body. Although it sometimes is referred to as *hemihypertrophy*, this process actually represents a hyperplasia (increase in the number of cells) rather than a hypertrophy (increase in the size of cells). The etiology of hemihyperplasia is uncertain, and most examples are sporadic. Various suggested causes include vascular abnormalities, neurologic disturbances, and endocrine dysfunctions. It should be noted that hemihyperplasia may be seen in a variety of syndromes, such as Beckwith-Wiedemann syndrome, neurofibromatosis type I, and Proteus syndrome.

Hemihyperplasia affects females twice as often as males, and it occurs more frequently on the right side of the body. Often the asymmetry is noted at birth, although some examples may not be noted until later in childhood. The condition can vary in severity from *simple hemihyperplasia*, which involves only a single limb, to *complex hemihyperplasia*, which may affect the entire body. When the enlargement occurs on one side of the face, it is termed *hemifacial hyperplasia*. The process often involves all tissues in the area, including the skin, subcutaneous tissues, and the underlying bone. The thickened skin sometimes demonstrates hyperpigmentation, hypertrichosis, telangiectatic blood vessels, or a port wine vascular malformation (nevus flammeus). Oral involvement can include unilateral macroglossia with enlargement of the tongue papillae on the affected side. Jaw expansion and asymmetry may be noted, including earlier development and enlargement of teeth in the region.

One of the most significant complications associated with hemihyperplasia is an increased risk for abdominal malignancies, such as Wilms tumor, hepatoblastoma, and adrenal cortical carcinoma. Such tumors have been reported in 5.9% of patients with isolated hemihyperplasia. Intellectual disability also has been noted in about 20% of affected individuals.

Treatment of hemifacial hyperplasia may include cosmetic and orthognathic surgery as well as appropriate orthodontic care. Periodic abdominal ultrasound examinations during childhood are important to screen for development of abdominal tumors.

■ **Figure 1.52**
Hemihyperplasia
Young girl showing enlargement and asymmetry of the right side of the face. (With appreciation to Dr. Ryan Colosi.)

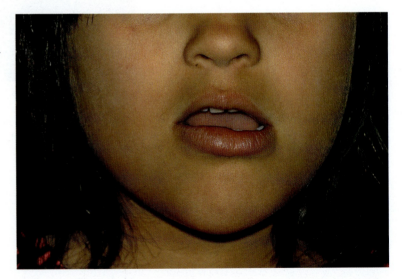

■ Figure **1.53**
Hemihyperplasia

Same patient as in Fig. 1.52 demonstrating enlargement of the lower lip on her right side. (With appreciation to Dr. Ryan Colosi.)

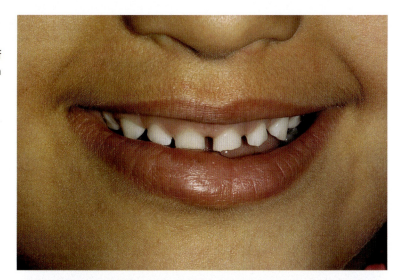

■ Figure **1.54**
Hemihyperplasia

Intraoral photograph of the same patient showing earlier development and eruption of the teeth on her right side. (With appreciation to Dr. Ryan Colosi.)

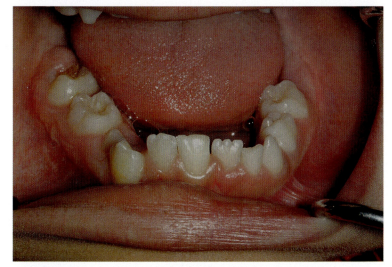

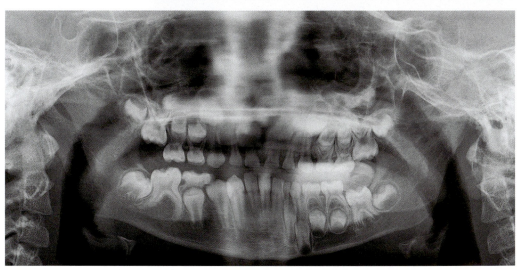

■ Figure **1.55**
Hemihyperplasia

Panoramic radiograph of the same patient showing early development of the right mandibular teeth. Note the large splayed roots of the right mandibular first molar. (With appreciation to Dr. Ryan Colosi.)

Segmental Odontomaxillary Dysplasia

Figs. **1.56 and 1.57**

Segmental odontomaxillary dysplasia is a rare and unusual developmental anomaly that results in unilateral enlargement of the maxillary alveolar bone and the overlying tissues. The cause is unknown. The condition typically is discovered during childhood because of a painless expansion of the posterior maxilla. Thickening of the overlying gingival soft tissues and mild facial asymmetry also may be present, which can make the condition mimic hemifacial hyperplasia. Radiographically, the affected bone exhibits a coarse, granular quality with thickened vertical trabeculae. Although this pattern sometimes is confused with fibrous dysplasia, classic ground-glass radiographic features are not present. Frequently one or both of the developing maxillary premolars will be missing, and the associated deciduous molars also may show various malformations. A few examples have been associated with hypertrichosis of the overlying facial skin.

After diagnosis, segmental odontomaxillary dysplasia usually remains relatively stable; any further enlargement typically will be proportional to the overall growth of the patient. Mild examples may not require any specific treatment, although surgery may be performed for aesthetic reasons or to aid in tooth eruption. Dental implants have been successfully placed to replace missing teeth.

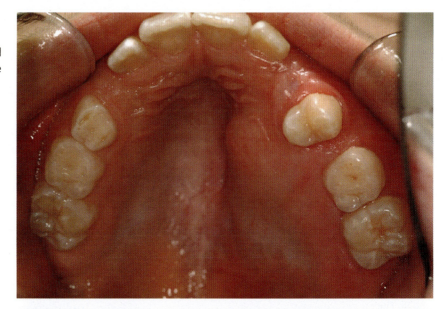

■ Figure 1.56
Segmental Odontomaxillary Dysplasia
Photograph of the maxillary arch showing marked expansion of the alveolar process on the right side of the image.

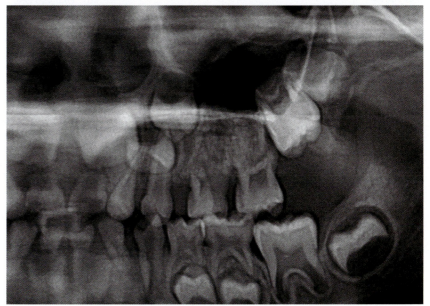

■ Figure 1.57
Segmental Odontomaxillary Dysplasia
Radiograph of the left maxillary arch in a 5-year-old boy showing a coarse quality of the alveolar bone with absence of the developing premolar teeth. (Courtesy Dr. Dan Cook.)

Bibliography

Cleft Lip, Cleft Palate, and Bifid Uvula

Carinci F, Pezzetti F, Scapoli L, et al. Recent developments in orofacial cleft genetics. *J Craniofac Surg.* 2003;14:130–143.

Eppley BL, van Aalst JA, Robey A, Havlik RJ, Sadove AM. The spectrum of orofacial clefting. *Plast Reconstr Surg.* 2005;115:101e–114e.

Hennekam RCM, Krantz ID, Allanson JE. Orofacial clefting syndromes: general aspects. In: *Gorlin's Syndromes of the Head and Neck.* 5th ed. New York: Oxford University Press.; 2010:943–972, [Chapter 21]. Note: They are the authors; the chapter was not contributed by someone else; it seems silly to indicate that they edited their own writing; Gorlin died in 2006 and was not an author if this edition.

Nanci A. Embryology of the head, face, and oral cavity. In: *Ten Cate's Oral Histology.* 8th ed. St. Louis: Elsevier.; 2013:26–47. Note: same logic.

Van Laer L, Dietz H, Loeys B. Loeys-Dietz syndrome. *Adv Exp Med Biol.* 2014;802:95–105.

Weinberg SM, Neiswanger K, Martin RA, et al. The Pittsburgh oral-facial cleft study: expanding the cleft phenotype. Background and justification. *Cleft Palate Craniofac J.* 2006;43:7–20.

Double Lip

Ali K. Ascher syndrome: a case report and review of the literature. *Oral Surg Oral Med Oral Pathol Oral Radiol Endod.* 2007;103:e26–e28.

Eski M, Nisanci M, Atkas A, Sengezer M. Congenital double lip: review of 5 cases. *Br J Oral Maxillofac Surg.* 2007;45:68–70.

Gomez-Duaso AJ, Seoane J, Vazquez-Garcia J, Arjona C. Ascher syndrome: report of two cases. *J Oral Maxillofac Surg.* 1997;55:88–90.

Palma MC, Taub DI. Recurrent double lip: literature review and report of a case. *Oral Surg Oral Med Oral Pathol Oral Radiol Endod.* 2009;107:e20–e23.

Commissural Lip Pits

Baker BR. Pits of the lip commissures in caucasoid males. *Oral Surg Oral Med Oral Pathol.* 1966;21:56–60.

Everett FG, Wescott WB. Commissural lip pits. *Oral Surg Oral Med Oral Pathol.* 1961;14:202–209.

Gorsky M, Buchner A, Cohen C. Commissural lip pits in Israeli Jews of different ethnic origin. *Community Dent Oral Epidemiol.* 1985;13:195–196.

Paramedian Lip Pits and Van Der Woude Syndrome

Hennekam RCM, Krantz ID, Allanson JE. Popliteal pterygium syndrome (facio-genito-popliteal syndrome). In: *Gorlin's Syndromes of the Head and Neck.* 5th ed. New York: Oxford University Press; 2010:862–865.

James O, Adeyemo WL, Emeka CI, et al. Van der Woude syndrome: a review of 11 cases seen at the Lagos University Teaching Hospital. *Afr J Paediatr Surg.* 2014;11:52–55.

Lam AK, David DJ, Townsend GC, Anderson PJ. Van der Woude syndrome: dentofacial features and implications for clinical practice. *Aust Dent J.* 2010;55:51–58.

Matsumoto N, Niikawa N. Kabuki make-up syndrome: a review. *Am J Med Genet C Semin Med Genet.* 2003;117:57–65.

Fordyce Granules

Daley TD. Pathology of intraoral sebaceous glands. *J Oral Pathol Med.* 1993;22:241–245.

Fordyce JA. A peculiar affection of the mucous membrane of the lips and oral cavity. *J Cutan Genito-Urin Dis.* 1896;14:413–419.

Halperin V, Kolas S, Jefferis KR, Huddleston SO, Robinson HB. The occurrence of Fordyce spots, benign migratory glossitis, median rhomboid glossitis, and fissured tongue in 2,478 dental patients. *Oral Surg Oral Med Oral Pathol.* 1953;6:1072–1077.

Sewerin I. The sebaceous glands in the vermilion border of the lips and in the oral mucosa of man. *Acta Odontol Scand.* 1975;33(suppl 68):13–226.

Leukoedema

Archard HO, Carlson KP, Stanley HR. Leukoedema of the human oral mucosa. *Oral Surg Oral Med Oral Pathol.* 1968;25:717–728.

Axéll T, Henricsson V. Leukoedema—an epidemiologic study with special reference to the influence of tobacco habits. *Community Dent Oral Epidemiol.* 1981;9:142–146.

Martin JL. Leukoedema: an epidemiological study in white and African Americans. *J Tenn Dent Assoc.* 1997;77:18–21.

Ankyloglossia

Brookes A, Bowley DM. Tongue tie: the evidence for frenotomy. *Early Hum Dev.* 2014;90:765–768.

Chinnadurai S, Francis DO, Epstein RA, et al. Treatment of ankyloglossia for reasons other than breastfeeding: a systematic review. *Pediatrics.* 2015;135:e1467–e1474.

Francis DO, Krishnaswami S, McPheeters M. Treatment of ankyloglossia and breastfeeding outcomes: a systematic review. *Pediatrics.* 2015;135:e1458–e1466.

Hong P, Lago D, Seargeant J, et al. Defining ankyloglossia: a case series of anterior and posterior tongue ties. *Int J Pediatr Otorhinolaryngol.* 2010;74:1003–1006.

Lingual Thyroid

Baughman RA. Lingual thyroid and lingual thyroglossal tract remnants: a clinical and histopathologic study with review of the literature. *Oral Surg Oral Med Oral Pathol.* 1972;34:781–799.

Carranza Leon BG, Turcu A, Bahn R, Dean DS. Lingual thyroid: 35-year experience at a tertiary care referral center. *Endocr Pract.* 2016;22:343–349.

Gu T, Jiang B, Wang N, et al. New insight into ectopic thyroid glands between the neck and maxillofacial region from a 42-case study. *BMC Endocr Disord.* 2015;15:70. doi:10.1186/s12902-015-0066-6.

Fissured Tongue

Bouquot JE, Gundlach KKH. Odd tongues: the prevalence of common tongue lesions in 23,616 white Americans over 35 years of age. *Quintessence Int.* 1986;17:719–730.

Eidelman E, Chosack A, Cohen T. Scrotal tongue and geographic tongue: polygenic and associated traits. *Oral Surg Oral Med Oral Pathol.* 1976;42:591–596.

Picciani BL, Souza TT, Santos VC, et al. Geographic tongue and fissured tongue in 348 patients with psoriasis: correlation with disease severity. *ScientificWorldJournal.* 2015;2015:564326. doi:10.1155/2015/564326.

Hairy Tongue

Gurvits GE, Tan A. Black hairy tongue syndrome. *World J Gastroenterol.* 2014;20:10845–10850.

Schlager E, St Claire C, Ashack K, Khachemoune A. Black hairy tongue: predisposing factors, diagnosis, and treatment. *Am J Clin Dermatol.* 2017;18(4):563–569. doi:10.1007/s40257-017-0268-y.

Thompson DF, Kessler TL. Drug-induced black hairy tongue. *Pharmacotherapy.* 2010;30:585–593.

Varicosities

Hedström L, Albrektsson M, Bergh H. Is there a connection between sublingual varices and hypertension? *BMC Oral Health.* 2015;15:78. doi:10.1186/s12903-015-0054-2.

Hedström L, Bergh H. Sublingual varices in relation to smoking and cardiovascular diseases. *Br J Oral Maxillofac Surg.* 2010;48:136–138.

Lazos JP, Piemonte ED, Panico RL. Oral varix: a review. *Gerodontology.* 2015;32:82–89.

Weathers DR, Fine RM. Thrombosed varix of oral cavity. *Arch Dermatol.* 1971;104:427–430.

Caliber-Persistent Artery

Awni S, Conn B. Caliber-persistent labial artery: a rarely recognized cause of lower lip swelling – report of 5 cases and review of the literature. *J Oral Maxillofac Surg.* 2016;74:1391–1395.

Lovas JG, Goodday RH. Clinical diagnosis of caliber-persistent labial artery of the lower lip. *Oral Surg Oral Med Oral Pathol.* 1993;76:480–483.

Lovas JGL, Rodu B, Hammond HL, Allen CM, Wysocki GP. Caliber-persistent labial artery: a common vascular anomaly. *Oral Surg Oral Med Oral Pathol Oral Radiol Endod.* 1998;86:308–312.

Coronoid Hyperplasia

McLoughlin PM, Hopper C, Bowley NB. Hyperplasia of the mandibular coronoid process: an analysis of 31 cases and a review of the literature. *J Oral Maxillofac Surg.* 1995;53:250–255.

Mulder CH, Kalaylova SI, Gortzak RA. Coronoid process hyperplasia: a systematic review of the literature from 1995. *Int J Oral Maxillofac Surg.* 2012;41:1483–1489.

Condylar Hyperplasia

Mouallem G, Vernex-Boukerma Z, Longis J, et al. Efficacy of proportional condylectomy in a treatment protocol for unilateral condylar hyperplasia: a review of 73 cases. *J Craniomaxillofac Surg.* 2017;45:1083–1093.

Rodrigues DB, Castro V. Condylar hyperplasia of the temporomandibular joint. Types, treatment, and surgical implications. *Oral Maxillofac Surg Clin North Am.* 2015;27:155–167.

Wolford CM, Movahed R, Perez DE. A classification system for conditions causing condylar hyperplasia. *J Oral Maxillofac Surg.* 2014;72:567–595.

Bifid Condyle

Nikolova SY, Toneva DH, Lazarov NE. Incidence of a bifid mandibular condyle in dry mandibles. *J Craniofac Surg.* 2017;28(8):2168–2173. doi:10.1097/SCS.0000000000003173.

Sala-Pérez S, Vázquez-Delgado E, Rodríguez-Baeza A, Gay-Escoda C. Bifid mandibular condyle. A disorder in its own right? *J Am Dent Assoc.* 2010;141:1076–1085.

Stefanou EP, Fanourakis IG, Vlastos K, Katerelou J. Bilateral bifid mandibular condyles. Report of four cases. *Dentomaxillofac Radiol.* 1998;27:186–188.

Exostoses, Torus Mandibularis, and Torus Palatinus

Auškalnis A, Bernhardt O. Putnienė E, et al. Oral bony outgrowths: prevalence and genetic factor influence. Study of twins. *Medicina.* 2015;51:228–232.

Bertazzo-Silveira E, Stuginski-Barbosa J, Porporatti AL, et al. Association between signs and symptoms of bruxism and presence of tori: a systematic review. *Clin Oral Investig.* 2017;21(9):2789–2799. doi:10.1007/s00784-017-2081-7.

Islam MN, Cohen DM, Waite MT, Bhattacharyya I. Three cases of subpontic osseous hyperplasia of the mandible: a report. *Quintessence Int.* 2010;41:299–302.

Morton TH Jr, Natkin E. Hyperostosis and fixed partial denture pontics: report of 16 patients and review of the literature. *J Prosthet Dent.* 1990;64:539–547.

Romanos GE, Sarmiento HL, Yunker M, Malmstrom H. Prevalence of torus mandibularis in Rochester, New York, region. *N Y State Dent J.* 2013;79:25–27.

Sonnier KE, Horning GM, Cohen ME. Palatal tubercles, palatal tori, and mandibular tori: prevalence and anatomical features in a U.S. population. *J Periodontol.* 1999;70:329–336.

Eagle Syndrome

Badhey A, Jategaonkar A, Kovacs AJ, et al. Eagle syndrome: a comprehensive review. *Clin Neurol Neurosurg.* 2017;159:34–38.

Colby CC, Del Gaudio JM. Stylohyoid complex syndrome. A new diagnostic classification. *Arch Otolaryngol Head Neck Surg.* 2011;137:248–252.

Elimairi I, Baur DA, Altay MA, Quereshy FA, Minisandram A. Eagle's syndrome. *Head Neck Pathol.* 2015;9:492–495.

Stafne Defect

Assaf AT, Solaty M, Zrnc TA, et al. Prevalence of Stafne's bone cavity – retrospective analysis of 14,005 panoramic views. *In Vivo.* 2014;28:1159–1164.

Buchner A, Carpenter WM, Merrell PW, Leider AS. Anterior lingual mandibular salivary gland defect. Evaluation of twenty-four cases. *Oral Surg Oral Med Oral Pathol.* 1991;71:131–136.

Shimizu M, Osa N, Okamura K, Yoshiura K. CT analysis of the Stafne's bone defects of the mandible. *Dentomaxillofac Radiol.* 2006;35:95–102.

Sisman Y, Miloglu O, Sekerci AE, et al. Radiographic evaluation on prevalence of Stafne bone defect: a study from two centres in Turkey. *Dentomaxillofac Radiol.* 2012;41:152–158.

Stafne EC. Bone cavities situated near the angle of the mandible. *J Am Dent Assoc.* 1942;29:1969–1972.

Epstein Pearls

Cataldo E, Berkman MD. Cysts of the oral mucosa in newborns. *Am J Dis Child.* 1968;116:44–48.

Haveri FT, Inamadar AC. A cross-sectional prospective study of cutaneous lesions in newborn. *ISRN Dermatol.* 2014;2014:360590. doi:10.1155/2014/360590.

Paula JDR, Dezan CC, Frossard WTG, Walter LR, Pinto LM. Oral and facial inclusion cysts in newborns. *J Clin Pediatr Dent.* 2006;31:127–129.

Nasopalatine Duct Cyst

Al-Shamiri HM, Al-Maweri SA, Alaizari NA, Alaizari NA, Tarakji B. Development of nasopalatine duct cyst in relation to dental implant placement. *N Am J Med Sci.* 2016;8:13–16.

Suter VGA, Sendi P, Reichart PA, Bornstein MM. The nasopalatine duct cyst: an analysis of the relation between clinical symptoms, cyst dimensions, and involvement of neighboring anatomical structures using cone beam computed tomography. *J Oral Maxillofac Surg.* 2011;69:2595–2603.

Swanson KS, Kaugars GE, Gunsolley JC. Nasopalatine duct cyst: an analysis of 334 cases. *J Oral Maxillofac Surg.* 1991;49:268–271.

Epidermoid Cyst and Pilar Cyst

Golden BA, Zide MF. Cutaneous cysts of the head and neck. *J Oral Maxillofac Surg.* 2005;63:1613–1619.

McGavran MH, Binnington B. Keratinous cysts of the skin. *Arch Dermatol.* 1966;94:499–508.

Morritt AN, Tiffin N, Brotherston TM. Squamous cell carcinoma arising in epidermoid cysts: report of four cases and review of the literature. *J Plast Reconstr Aesthet Surg.* 2012;65:1267–1269.

Rajayogeswaran V, Eveson JW. Epidermoid cyst of the buccal mucosa. *Oral Surg Oral Med Oral Pathol.* 1989;67:181–184.

Dermoid Cyst

Gordon PE, Faquin WC, Lahey E, Kaban LB. Floor-of-mouth dermoid cysts: report of 3 variants and a suggested change in terminology. *J Oral Maxillofac Surg.* 2013;71:1034–1041.

Kyriakidou E, Howe T, Veale B, Atkins S. Sublingual dermoid cysts: case report and review of the literature. *J Laryngol Otol.* 2015;129:1036–1039.

MacNeil SD, Moxham JP. Review of floor of mouth dysontogenic cysts. *Ann Otol Rhinol Laryngol.* 2010;119:165–173.

Thyroglossal Duct Cyst

Brousseau VJ, Solares CA, Xu M, Krakovitz P, Koltai PJ. Thyroglossal duct cysts: presentation and management in children versus adults. *Int J Pediatr Otorhinolaryngol.* 2003;67:1285–1290.

Rayess HM, Monk I, Svider PF, et al. Thyroglossal duct cyst carcinoma: a systematic review of clinical features and outcomes. *Otolaryngol Head Neck Surg.* 2017;156:794–802.

Thompson LD, Herrera HB, Lau SK. A clinicopathologic series of 685 thyroglossal duct remnant cysts. *Head Neck Pathol.* 2016;10:465–474.

Zhu Y-S, Lee C-T, Ou C-Y, et al. A 16-year experience in treating thyroglossal duct cysts with a "conservative" Sistrunk approach. *Eur Arch Otorhinolaryngol.* 2016;273:1019–1025.

Branchial Cleft Cyst

LaRiviere CA, Waldhausen JHT. Congenital cervical cysts, sinuses, and fistulae in pediatric surgery. *Surg Clin North Am.* 2012;92:583–597.

Muller S, Aiken A, Magliocca K, Chen AY. Second branchial cleft cyst. *Head Neck Pathol.* 2015;9:379–383.

Prosser JD, Myer CM III. Branchial cleft anomalies and thymic cysts. *Otolaryngol Clin North Am.* 2015;48:1–14.

Spinelli C, Rossi L, Strambi S, et al. Branchial cleft and pouch anomalies in childhood: a report of 50 surgical cases. *J Endocrinol Invest.* 2016;39:529–535.

Oral Lymphoepithelial Cyst

Buchner A, Hansen LS. Lymphoepithelial cysts of the oral cavity. *Oral Surg Oral Med Oral Pathol.* 1980;50:441–449.

Chaudhry AP, Yamane GM, Scharlock SE, SunderRaj M, Jain R. A clinico-pathological study of intraoral lymphoepithelial cysts. *J Oral Med.* 1984;39:79–84.

Yang X, Ow A, Zhang C-P, et al. Clinical analysis of 120 cases of intraoral lymphoepithelial cyst. *Oral Surg Oral Med Oral Pathol Oral Radiol.* 2012;113:448–452.

Progressive Hemifacial Atrophy

El-Kehdy J, Abbas O, Rubeiz N. A review of Parry-Romberg syndrome. *J Am Acad Dermatol.* 2012;67:769–784.

Tolkachjov SN, Patel NG, Tollefson MM. Progressive hemifacial atrophy: a review. *Orphanet J Rare Dis.* 2015;10:39. doi:10.1186/s13023-015-0250-9.

Wong M, Phillips CD, Hagiwara M, Shatzkes DR. Parry Romberg syndrome: 7 cases and literature review. *AJNR Am J Neuroradiol.* 2015;36:1355–1361.

Hemihyperplasia

Hennekam RCM, Krantz ID, Allanson JE. Hemihyperplasia. In: *Gorlin's Syndromes of the Head and Neck.* 5th ed. New York: Oxford University Press; 2010:477–480, [Chapter 21].

Horswell BB, Holmes AD, Barnett JS, Hookey SR. Primary hemihypertrophy of the face: review and report of two cases. *J Oral Maxillofac Surg.* 1987;45:217–222.

Hoyme HE, Seaver LH, Jones KL, et al. Isolated hemihyperplasia (hemihypertrophy): report of a prospective multicenter study of the incidence of neoplasia and review. *Am J Med Genet.* 1998;79:274–278.

Segmental Odontomaxillary Dysplasia

Danforth RA, Melrose RJ, Abrams AM, Handlers JP. Segmental odontomaxillary dysplasia. Report of eight cases and comparison with hemimaxillofacial dysplasia. *Oral Surg Oral Med Oral Pathol.* 1990;70:81–85.

Miles DA, Lovas JL, Cohen MM Jr. Hemimaxillofacial dysplasia: a newly recognized disorder of facial asymmetry, hypertrichosis of the facial skin, unilateral enlargement of the maxilla, and hypoplastic teeth in two patients. *Oral Surg Oral Med Oral Pathol.* 1987;64:445–448.

Packota GV, Pharoah MJ, Petrikowski CG. Radiographic features of segmental odontomaxillary dysplasia. A study of 12 cases. *Oral Surg Oral Med Oral Pathol Oral Radiol Endod.* 1996;82:577–584.

Whitt JC, Rokos JW, Dunlap CL, Barker BF. Segmental odontomaxillary dysplasia: report of a series of 5 cases with long-term follow-up. *Oral Surg Oral Med Oral Pathol Oral Radiol Endod.* 2011;112:e29–e47.

2

Pathology of Teeth

Environmental Defects of Enamel

Figs. **2.1 and 2.2**

Tooth enamel develops in three major stages: matrix deposition, initial mineralization, and final maturation. Ameloblasts are extremely sensitive to external influences, with more than 90 different factors known to be associated with disturbance in enamel formation. Although the causes are diverse, the most commonly reported factors include serious disease during the first 3 years of life, hypocalcemia, renal disorders, nutritional deficiencies, and viral infections associated with high fever.

Unlike bone, dental enamel cannot be remodeled. With knowledge of the timing of tooth formation, the site of defective enamel can be used to pinpoint the time of damage. The formation of the deciduous tooth crowns begins around the 14th week of pregnancy and continues until 12 months of age. The formation of the permanent tooth crowns is initiated at 6 months and continues to age 15.

The associated enamel disturbance may be quantitative, qualitative, or both. **Enamel hypoplasia** arises from failure of appropriate matrix deposition and presents as pits, grooves, or larger areas of missing enamel. In contrast, **enamel opacities** are areas of enamel hypomaturation in which the tooth presents with a normal size and shape but demonstrates an area of white, cream, yellow, or brown opacity.

The pattern of enamel disturbance tends to be bilaterally symmetric and involves only the portion of enamel that was developing at the time of the insult. Early environmental influences affect the anterior dentition and first molars, whereas damage later in tooth development alters the bicuspids and second molars. The enamel damage usually is associated with aesthetic rather than functional difficulties. Significantly altered anterior teeth may be repaired with composite resin restorations, labial veneers, or full crowns.

Turner Hypoplasia

Fig. **2.3**

Environmental enamel defects also may be isolated to a single permanent tooth when associated with a local rather than systemic influence. When seen in an incisor, the ameloblasts typically were damaged by a traumatic event that forced a deciduous incisor into the underlying developing permanent tooth. Much more frequently, localized developmental defects arise in bicuspids secondary to infection of an overlying deciduous molar. The enamel defects vary from focal areas of white or yellow hypomaturation to extensive hypoplasia that can involve the entire crown.

■ Figure **2.1**
Environmental Enamel Hypoplasia
Dentition demonstrating bilaterally symmetric enamel grooves affecting the anterior teeth.

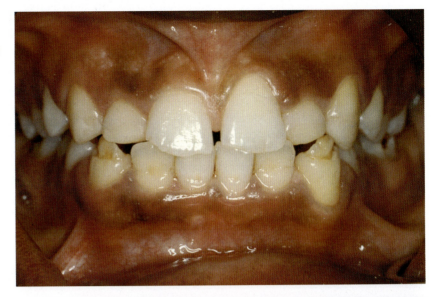

■ Figure **2.2**
Environmental Enamel Hypoplasia
Dentition demonstrating enamel grooves affecting both premolars and second molars in both arches.

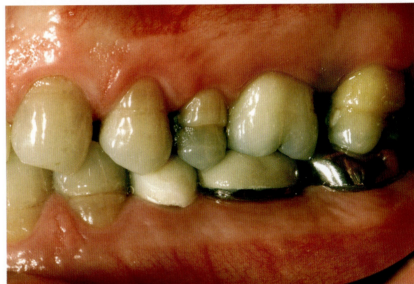

■ Figure **2.3**
Turner Hypoplasia
Maxillary central incisors demonstrating localized area of yellowish hypomaturation.

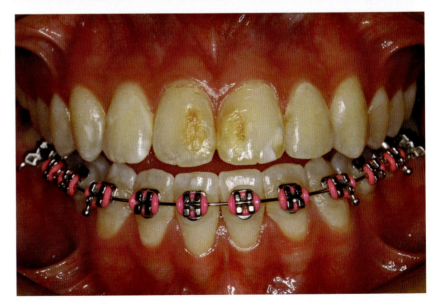

Dental Disturbances due to Antineoplastic Therapy

Fig. **2.4**

Antineoplastic therapy administered during childhood has been associated with alterations in tooth formation. The developing teeth are most sensitive to local radiation therapy, but less significant effects also can be seen in association with systemic chemotherapy. Radiation induces both quantitative and qualitative defects, whereas chemotherapy predominantly produces qualitative changes. The severity varies with the patient's age at treatment, the type of therapy, and the dose and field of radiation.

The alterations are seen primarily in children treated prior to the age of 12, with the most severe effects noted in children younger than 5 years. If exposure occurs prior to crown formation, then microdontia or hypodontia may occur. If exposure occurs during later stages of tooth development, then enamel hypomaturation, short pointed roots, and taurodontism may be seen.

Dental Fluorosis

Figs. **2.5 and 2.6**

Exposure to fluoride has been shown to be an effective agent for reduction in dental caries, but it also can be associated with enamel defects known as dental fluorosis. Healthcare advocates strive to determine the most appropriate level of fluoride exposure that will result in maximal caries reduction and minimal dental fluorosis.

In 1962 the US Public Health Service recommended fluoridation of the water supply nationwide, with concentrations varying by climate. Because of increased water consumption in warmer regions of the United States, the recommended concentration of fluoride in the nation's water supply varied from 0.7 to 1.2 mg/L. A recent increased prevalence of dental fluorosis has led to a reexamination of the recommended fluoride levels in the nation's water supply. Secondary to increased availability of fluoride from other sources, the US Public Health Service in 2015 recommended a single nationwide standard of 0.7 mg/L of fluoride in all community water supplies. Even in communities with fluoride levels maintained at 0.7 ppm, a Cochrane review revealed the prevalence of aesthetically obvious fluorosis to be approximately 12%.

Teeth with clinically evident fluorosis are caries resistant and demonstrate areas of white opaque enamel that may exhibit intermixed areas of yellow or brown discoloration. In severe fluorosis, irregular brownish depressed areas of defective surface enamel may be seen, which has been termed **mottled enamel**. Surface microabrasion of zones of yellow or brown discoloration often results in a permanent improvement of the enamel coloration. Elimination of the white lusterless enamel usually requires labial veneers or full crowns.

■ Figure **2.4**
Dental Disturbances due to Antineoplastic Therapy

Dentition demonstrating short pointed roots, hypodontia, microdontia, and areas of enamel hypoplasia in a patient who received radiation for a hematologic malignancy. (Courtesy Dr. Matthew D'Addario.)

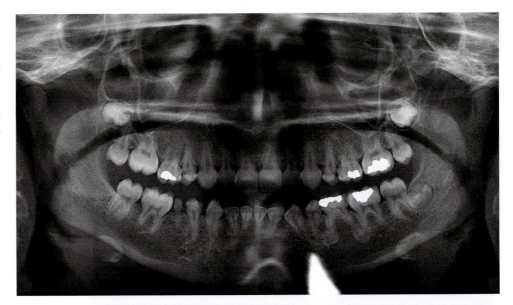

■ Figure **2.5**
Dental Fluorosis

Dentition demonstrating diffuse white hypomaturation with areas of brown staining and mottling.

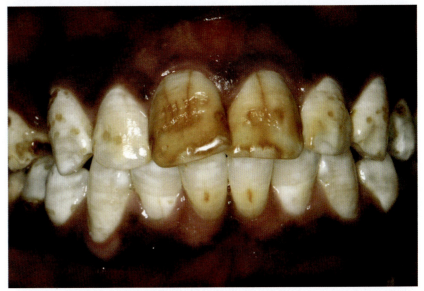

■ Figure **2.6**
Dental Fluorosis

Patient in mixed dentition demonstrating white hypomaturation of the permanent teeth and clinically normal deciduous teeth.

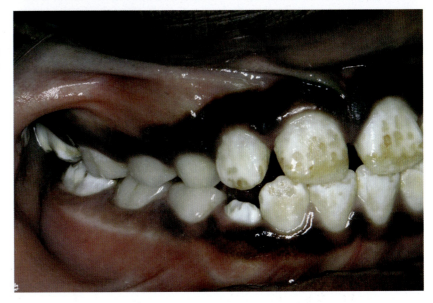

Tooth Wear

Tooth wear is a normal physiologic process that occurs with aging. When the extent of lost tooth structure results in symptoms, functional problems, or aesthetic concerns, the changes must be considered pathologic. Tooth surface loss occurs from attrition, abrasion, erosion, and possibly abfraction. Although these processes are discussed separately, the vast majority of pathologic tooth wear occurs from a combination of these influences.

Attrition

Fig. **2.7**

Attrition is tooth wear caused by tooth-to-tooth contact. Occlusal and incisal attrition presents as flattened wear facets on opposing teeth and arises from local forces of mastication often combined with abrasion related to the coarseness of the diet. Interproximal attrition also can be seen but is reduced in the modern population, most likely secondary to dietary changes since the agricultural revolution. Attrition affects both the deciduous and permanent dentitions, resulting in both a decreased height and length of both arches. The loss of tooth structure is slow and rarely results in dentin sensitivity or pulp exposure. Bruxism, premature contacts, and developmental abnormalities of tooth structure, such as amelogenesis imperfecta and dentinogenesis imperfecta, may accelerate the process.

Abrasion

Figs. **2.8 and 2.9**

Abrasion is the pathologic loss of tooth structure secondary to an external mechanical action. The most common pattern occurs on the facial surfaces of the teeth at the cementoenamel junction secondary to toothbrushing. This pattern of tooth wear increases with age, the degree of force applied, the frequency of brushing, and in association with an inappropriate toothbrushing technique (horizontal vs. vertical). Chewing abrasive materials such a smokeless tobacco can accelerate tooth wear, and inappropriate biting of items such as thread or fingernails also can be damaging. Habits such as chewing pencils, inappropriate use of floss or toothpicks, constant holding of pipe stems, opening bobby pins, or cracking nuts also can produce significant abrasion.

Toothbrush abrasion typically creates horizontal cervical notches that may be more advanced on prominent teeth. Damage associated with pipe smoking or chronic bobby pin use often creates V-shaped notches, whereas inappropriate use of floss or toothpicks results in loss of interdental tooth structure. Pulp exposure is not expected because of the slow progression of the process. Often, tertiary dentin can be seen filling the space previously occupied by the pulp.

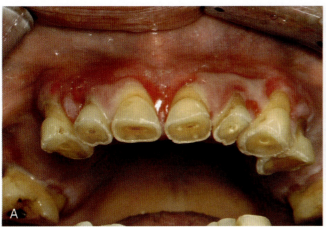
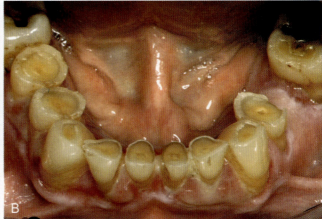

■ Figure **2.7**
Dental Attrition

(A) Patient demonstrating extensive loss of maxillary tooth height secondary to tooth wear. Note the tertiary dentin filling the canal secondary to pulpal recession. (B) Mandibular arch in the same patient.

■ Figure **2.8**
Dental Abrasion

Patient demonstrating extensive cervical notching secondary to inappropriate and overzealous toothbrushing. The anterior teeth are splinted with resin because of coronal instability.

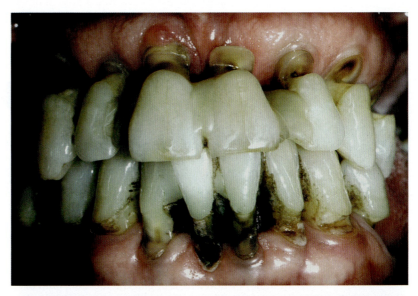

■ Figure **2.9**
Dental Abrasion

Dentition demonstrating extensive loss of vertical tooth height due to a combination of attrition and abrasion in a patient who chronically chewed tobacco. Note tertiary dentin filling the pulp canals.

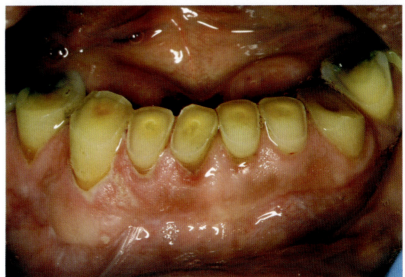

Erosion

Erosion is tooth wear caused by chemical action other than a bacterial process. Although saliva has significant buffering ability, this protection can be overwhelmed by poor salivary flow or excess acid. The source of the acid can be intrinsic secondary to prolonged or repeated exposure to stomach acid, or it can be extrinsic from exposure to food, drink, or environmental factors.

Because saliva has the ability to remineralize enamel following acid exposure, the loss of tooth structure also is thought to involve abrasion or attrition that removes enamel previously softened by an acid. Low salivary flow appears associated with an increased prevalence of erosion and may be secondary to medication-induced xerostomia, systemic diseases such as Sjögren syndrome, or dehydration from factors such as high levels of exercise or simply insufficient hydration. Consumption of carbonated soft drinks, natural fruit juices, and acidic snacks is associated with an increased prevalence of dental erosion, whereas drinking milk or eating yogurt appears to exert a protective effect.

Affected occlusal surfaces demonstrate cupping of cusp tips and flattening of the occlusal anatomy. In advanced cases the entire anatomy may be lost and replaced by a hollowed out occlusal surface. Erosion of smooth surfaces creates a flattened appearance that may evolve into concavities that usually are more wide than deep. Previously placed dental restorations may appear raised above the tooth surface because of loss of adjacent enamel and dentin, a presentation known as *perimolysis*. As seen in the other forms of tooth wear, pulpal exposure is not expected despite extensive loss of tooth structure.

Abfraction

Fig. **2.12**

Abfraction is a theory that suggests tooth damage may develop secondary to occlusal stresses and repeated tooth flexure, creating disruption of the enamel in the cervical region. Once damaged, these areas would be more susceptible to the effects of abrasion and erosion, resulting in wedge-shaped, noncarious cervical lesions. The existence of this condition is controversial. Some investigators have reported no convincing clinical evidence for this theory, with some clinical findings seemingly in conflict with the basic hypothesis.

Damage created by abfraction is confined to the facial surfaces in the cervical region. Although the cervical damage resembles that secondary to abrasion and erosion, the defects often are deeper and more narrow with sharper side walls. The process may affect a single tooth with adjacent teeth being unaffected, or it may be noted in a subgingival location, both of which would be unusual in teeth affected by abrasion or erosion.

Figure **2.10**
Dental Erosion
Maxillary central incisors demonstrating localized enamel defects secondary to chronic lemon sucking.

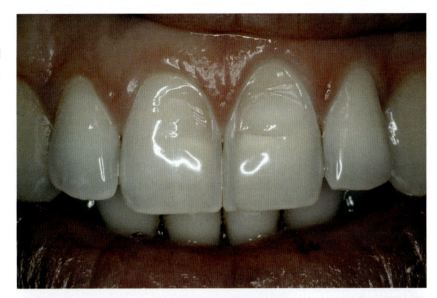

Figure **2.11**
Dental Erosion
Dentition demonstrating diffuse loss of coronal enamel and dentin. Note elevated rims of enamel surround central dentin concavities. This destruction resulted in complete loss of the buccal cusp in the depicted premolar tooth.

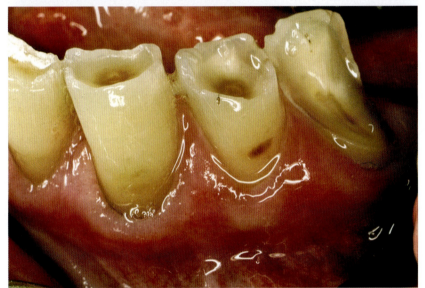

Figure **2.12**
Dental Abfraction
Mandibular premolar and molar demonstrating isolated area of cervical enamel loss.

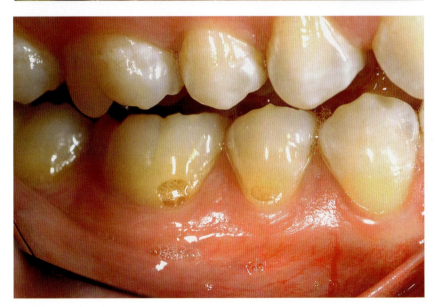

Internal Resorption

Fig. **2.13**

Internal resorption refers to loss of tooth structure on the dentinal walls of the pulp. This process is relatively uncommon and occurs when the predentin and odontoblastic layers are lost, with exposure of the mineralized dentin to dentinoclastic cells within the pulp. The resorption most commonly arises secondary to an inflammatory reaction triggered by trauma or bacterial invasion of the pulp. Once initiated, the process often continues until the pulp tissue is removed endodontically or becomes necrotic.

Radiographically, the area of resorption typically presents as a symmetric, oval to round radiolucent enlargement of the pulp canal. If diagnosed prior to perforation of the root, endodontic therapy usually is successful in eliminating the soft tissue responsible for the resorption. In some cases, periapical radiographs are insufficient to delineate the full extent of the process, with computed tomography proven to be superior in accurately outlining the area of destruction.

External Resorption

Figs. **2.14 and 2.15**

External resorption refers to a loss of tooth structure along the external surface of the root, secondary to destruction of the precementum and exposure of the adjacent mineralized cementum to cementoclasts within the periodontal ligament. In contrast to internal resorption, this process is very common, although it often is insignificant clinically. Localized pressure is a common cause, which may arise from orthodontic therapy, excessive occlusal forces, or adjacent impacted teeth, cysts, or tumors. Periodontal and periapical inflammatory disease also frequently are associated with external resorption. Avulsed teeth replaced after degeneration of the periodontal ligament may demonstrate progressive external resorption and subsequent ankylosis.

When compared with internal resorption, the area of tooth loss often creates a more irregular radiolucency. When resorptive defect is superimposed over the pulp, the original outline of the canal remains visible without the radiolucent pulpal expansion noted in internal resorption.

Although the resorption often stops after removal of an obvious trigger, many examples do not demonstrate an obvious cause, making successful intervention difficult. Resorption secondary to periodontitis or periapical inflammatory disease often ceases with elimination of any associated infection. Removal of the granulation tissue and restoration of the defect in areas of surgically accessible resorption have been successful in arresting the process.

■ Figure **2.13**
Internal Resorption

(A) Tooth demonstrating oval radiolucent expansion of the pulp canal. (B) Gross photograph of the same tooth exhibiting a radicular defect that perforated the lateral aspect of the root.

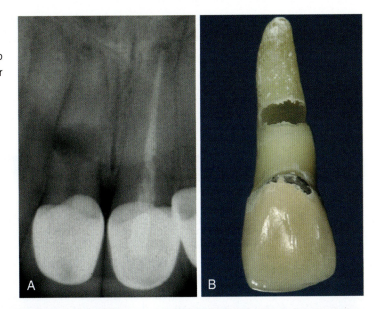

■ Figure **2.14**
External Resorption

(A) Mandibular cuspid demonstrating radiolucency of the root. Note the original outline of the pulp canal is retained. (B) Mandibular first premolar exhibiting oval radiolucency superimposed over the pulp canal (Courtesy Dr. Todd Barrett.)

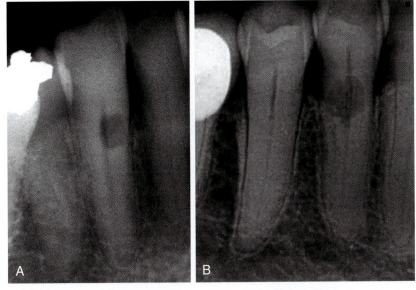

■ Figure **2.15**
External Resorption

(A) Anterior maxillary dentition demonstrating blunt, short roots. These alterations arose following orthodontic therapy. (B) Maxillary central incisor exhibiting extensive loss of root structure. This tooth was avulsed during a traumatic event, treated endodontically, and reimplanted.

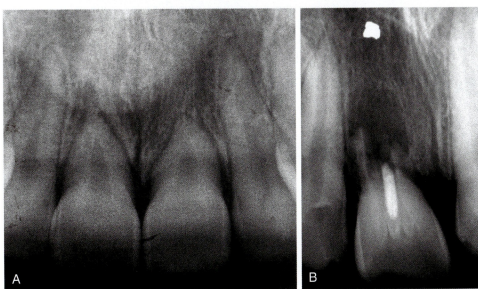

Discolorations of Teeth

The normal color of deciduous teeth is bluish white, whereas permanent teeth appear grayish white. Upon aging, the enamel often thins and the teeth become more yellow. More stark discolorations also can occur and may be extrinsic or intrinsic in origin.

Extrinsic Tooth Staining

Fig. **2.16**

Extrinsic discolorations of teeth arise from deposition of a surface stain that typically can be removed by professional cleaning with prophy paste. Common causes include stains from bacteria, tobacco products, foods, beverages (especially coffee and tea), systemic medications, and certain mouthwashes or toothpastes.

Plaque containing chromogenic bacteria may create green to orange areas of discoloration. Black to brown areas also may be seen secondary to formation of ferric sulfide when bacterial hydrogen sulfide combines with iron in the crevicular fluid. Stains from tobacco and beverages tend to demonstrate discoloration most frequently on the lingual and palatal surfaces. Stannous fluoride is used in many current toothpastes, and the stannous ion (tin) may combine with bacterial sulfides to create a black stain. Chronic use of chlorhexidine mouth rinse can result in a yellow-brown discoloration that is seen with an increased frequency in patients who also frequently consume tannin-containing beverages, such as tea and wine.

Intrinsic Tooth Staining

Figs. **2.17 and 2.18**

Intrinsic tooth discolorations may arise from developmental tooth abnormalities or an endogenous material that is incorporated into tooth structure during development. Because these do not represent surface stains, removal is not possible. Developmental discolorations include variants of amelogenesis imperfecta, dentinogenesis imperfecta, and dental fluorosis.

The development of deciduous tooth crowns extends from the 4th month of gestation to approximately the 12th month of life, whereas the crowns of the permanent teeth begin formation around birth with completion at approximately 8 years of age. During this time, stains can be permanently incorporated into the developing teeth from a variety of conditions (such as erythropoietic porphyria, alkaptonuria, hyperbilirubinemia) and medications (especially tetracycline and minocycline). In the majority of these situations, the discoloration affects only the portion of the tooth developing at the time the condition or medication was present. One exception is minocycline. This agent has the ability to stain dental pulp, which can result in a diffuse discoloration of teeth long after formation has been completed.

■ Figure **2.16**
Extrinsic Tooth Staining
Patient from Palau who chronically used betel quid and developed diffuse reddish-brown discoloration of the palatal surfaces of the teeth (Courtesy Dr. Lynn Wallace.)

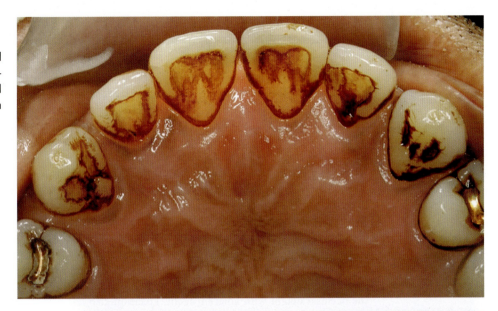

■ Figure **2.17**
Intrinsic Tooth Staining
Greenish discoloration of the incisal third of the deciduous dentition in a patient who had liver disease and hyperbilirubinemia as an infant. (Courtesy Dr. Ronnie Carr.)

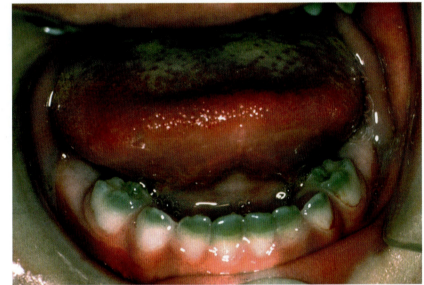

■ Figure **2.18**
Intrinsic Tooth Staining
Diffuse grayish dentition in a patient who used systemic tetracycline as a child.

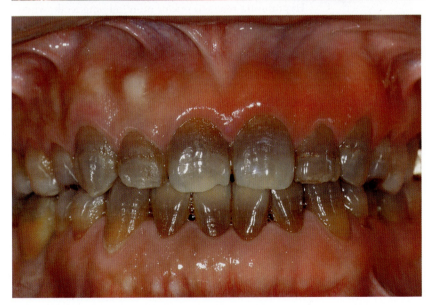

Fig. **2.19**

Emergence of teeth is a continuous process that compensates for tooth wear and does not cease after full eruption. **Ankylosis** refers to cessation of emergence that occurs secondary to fusion of the tooth with the alveolar bone. Many believe the periodontal ligament represents an anatomic barrier that separates the tooth from adjacent bone and helps prevent ankylosis. Although the cause of ankylosis is unknown, trauma or a genetically decreased periodontal ligament space may predispose to fusion between teeth and the alveolar ridge.

Although permanent teeth may be affected, the deciduous molars are associated most commonly with clinically significant ankylosis. In most cases the fusion is detected by infraocclusion of the affected tooth in which its occlusal plane is below that of adjacent teeth. Occasionally, percussion will demonstrate a sharp solid or metallic sound. Although the fusion often does not create obvious radiographic alterations, occasionally loss of the typical periodontal ligament space is noted.

In the vast majority of cases, ankylosis of deciduous molars resolves spontaneously as the underlying permanent bicuspids erupt. In cases with significantly delayed eruption, extraction of the ankylosed deciduous molar is indicated. In teeth without an underlying successor, a prosthetic buildup can be placed to equalize the occlusal height with adjacent teeth. Luxation also has been used in an attempt to break the osseous fusion and encourage redevelopment of an intact periodontal ligament.

Transposition

Fig. **2.20**

Dental transposition is a type of ectopic eruption in which two adjacent teeth interchange positions. The vast majority are unilateral and involve the maxillary cuspid. The most common pattern involves the cuspid and first premolar, with the cuspid and lateral incisor being the second most frequent interchange. Although an association with dental trauma during childhood has been suggested in some cases, significant evidence suggests involvement of genetic factors.

If caught during the early stages of eruption, surgical and orthodontic procedures can be performed to guide the teeth into their appropriate positions. If the transposition is well established, alignment of the teeth with subsequent restorative treatment to camouflage the altered positions is appropriate. Another option is removal of one or both affected teeth, with implant placement.

Hypodontia

Fig. **2.21**

Hypodontia refers to one or more missing teeth, whereas the term **oligodontia** is used when more than six teeth are missing. A total absence of teeth is known as **anodontia** and is seen primarily in association with ectodermal dysplasia. The dental lamina is extremely sensitive to external influences, and damage prior to tooth formation possibly can result in hypodontia. Local trauma, infection, radiation therapy, chemotherapy, medications, endocrine abnormalities, and severe intrauterine disturbances have been associated with missing teeth.

With more than 200 genes known to be involved in odontogenesis, genetics exert a strong influence on tooth numbers. Hypodontia may be an isolated finding, or it may be a component of various genetic syndromes that are inherited as autosomal dominant, autosomal recessive, or X-linked traits. At least 111 syndromes are known to be associated with hypodontia, with another 80 associated with oligodontia. Mutations in five genes *(AXIN2, MSX1, PAX9, EDA, WNT10A)* have been confirmed to be associated with isolated hypodontia, and another 79 gene mutations have been found in association with a wide variety of syndromes that may include hypodontia as a feature. Of significant interest is *AXIN2* because of its association with both hypodontia and carcinoma of the colon. Other investigators also have suggested an association between hypodontia and other forms of human cancer, but these correlations are less strong. It must be stressed that in the majority of the cases of hypodontia, the involved genes have yet to be discovered.

Hypodontia is uncommon in the deciduous dentition. The most commonly missing teeth are the third molars, mandibular second molars, maxillary permanent lateral incisors, and maxillary second premolars. In contrast, the least commonly missing permanent teeth are the maxillary central incisors, the maxillary and mandibular first molars, and the mandibular canines. Hypodontia demonstrates a female predominance, with affected individuals demonstrating teeth that generally are smaller than normal and often have a more simplified shape.

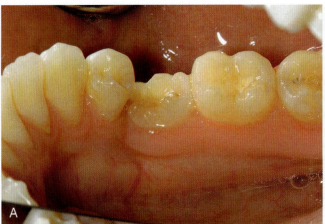
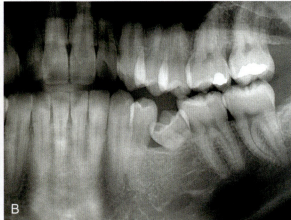

■ Figure **2.19**
Ankylosis
(A) Mandibular second deciduous molar with occlusal plane below the adjacent teeth. (B) Radiograph of the same patient reveals significant radicular resorption and no underlying second premolar. (With appreciation to Dr. Jordan Brown.)

■ Figure **2.20**
Dental Transposition
Rotated maxillary first premolar demonstrating eruption between the lateral and cuspid.

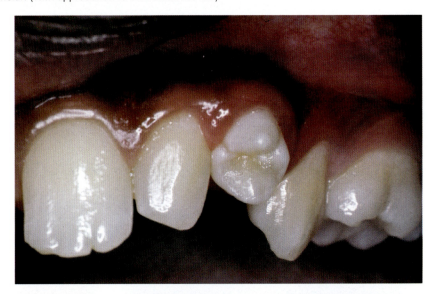

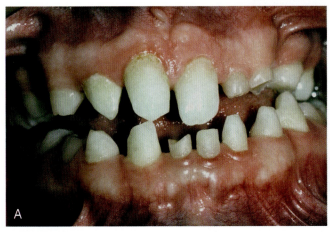
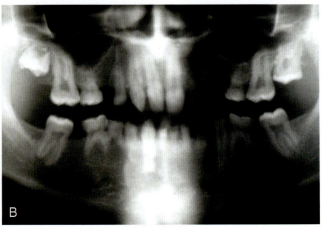

■ Figure **2.21**
Oligodontia
(A) Patient demonstrating numerous missing teeth and retained deciduous teeth. (B) Panoramic radiograph of the same patient.

Figs. **2.22–2.24**

Hyperdontia refers to an excess number of teeth beyond the expected 20 deciduous and 32 permanent teeth. The additional teeth are termed **supernumerary** and demonstrate a male and maxillary predominance. Supernumerary teeth are five times more common in the permanent dentition than in the deciduous dentition. Affected patients often demonstrate teeth that are larger in size with a more complex anatomy.

The additional teeth may be single or multiple; unilateral or bilateral; and in one or both jaws. The most common supernumerary tooth arises in the midline of the anterior maxilla and is known as a **mesiodens**. Following the mesiodens in order of decreasing frequency are maxillary fourth molars, maxillary lateral incisors, mandibular fourth molars, and mandibular premolars. In contrast to single-tooth hyperdontia, the most common site for multiple supernumerary teeth is the mandibular premolar region. A supernumerary tooth lingual or buccal to a molar is termed a **paramolar**, whereas one located distal to a third molar is known as a **distodens** or **distomolar**. Although the vast majority of supernumerary teeth are nonsyndromic, at least 20 syndromes demonstrate an association with hyperdontia, with cleidocranial dysplasia and Gardner syndrome being the most frequently mentioned.

Many supernumerary teeth are asymptomatic and discovered incidentally during imaging obtained for other indications. However, complications are not rare and include delayed or ectopic eruption of adjacent teeth, root resorption of adjacent teeth, crowding, malocclusion, objectionable diastema, and development of a significant pericoronal cyst or tumor. Although disagreement exists related to early or late removal of problematic supernumerary teeth, investigators have suggested the optimal time for removal of a mesiodens is approximately 6 to 7 years of age, after which the prevalence of complications appears to increase. Prior to surgical removal, cone beam computed tomography has been shown to be beneficial in precisely defining the location of the tooth and its proximity to vital anatomic structures such as the nasal floor and nasopalatine canal.

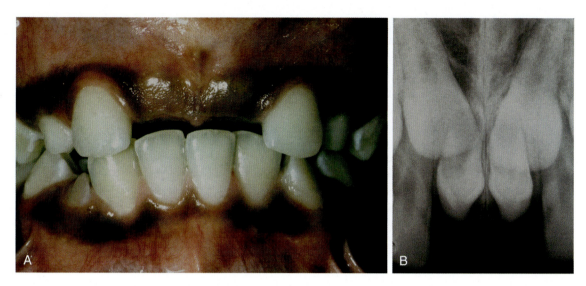

■ Figure **2.22**
Hyperdontia (Mesiodens)
(A) Patient presenting with failure of eruption of the maxillary central incisors. (B) Radiograph of the same patient demonstrating bilateral supernumerary teeth superimposed on the central incisors.

■ Figure **2.23**
Hyperdontia
Patient demonstrating two lateral incisors of the right maxillary quadrant.

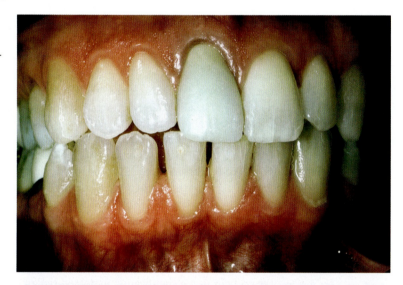

■ Figure **2.24**
Hyperdontia
Patient exhibiting multiple bilateral supernumerary mandibular premolars.

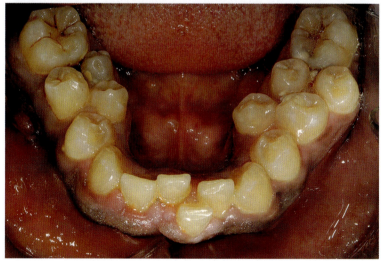

Natal Teeth

Fig. **2.25**

Eruption of the deciduous dentition begins at approximately 6 months of age. Teeth evident at birth are known as **natal teeth**, whereas those erupting within the first 30 days of life have been termed **neonatal teeth**. The vast majority represent prematurely erupted deciduous teeth rather than supernumerary teeth, with the anterior mandibular incisors being affected most frequently.

During breast-feeding, natal mandibular incisors have been associated with traumatic ulcerations of the ventral tongue termed **Riga-Fede disease**. Management includes smoothing of the sharp incisal edges, covering the incisal edges with composite resin, or use of a protective mouthguard during feeding. Extraction of the tooth is recommended only if it is radiographically proven to be a supernumerary tooth or if extreme mobility is noted. Although aspiration of a mobile tooth is a concern, this complication has never been reported even though natal teeth are not rare. If possible, surgical removal should be delayed because early tooth mobility frequently resolves within a month, thereby eliminating the need for extraction. In addition, delaying extraction negates the need for administration of vitamin K to reduce surgery-related bleeding. Although occasionally performed by medical staff without significant oral health training, this procedure is performed best by a dental professional who should ensure that all radicular remnants are curetted thoroughly at the time of crown removal.

Microdontia and Macrodontia

Figs. **2.26 and 2.27**

Microdontia refers to teeth that are smaller than normal, whereas **macrodontia** (**megadontia**) relates to teeth that are larger than normal. There is a direct correlation between microdontia and hypodontia, along with a similar association between macrodontia and hyperdontia. Missing teeth demonstrate a strong female predominance, with affected individuals exhibiting teeth that are incrementally smaller than normal and often with a more simplified shape. In contrast, supernumerary teeth exhibit a male predominance, with teeth that are larger than normal and often exhibit a more complex anatomy. In spite of these associations, the decreased/increased tooth size is subtle.

Generalized marked microdontia or macrodontia is rare and usually is noted in association with pituitary dysfunction. In contrast, isolated microdontia is not uncommon and most often involves the maxillary lateral incisors (so-called peg laterals) or third molars. Localized macrodontia is less common and can be difficult to separate from gemination or fusion. Hereditary and environmental influences appear active in hypodontia/microdontia and hyperdontia/macrodontia. In studies of monozygotic twins, strong concordance of hypodontia/microdontia is not present. In spite of this, if one twin demonstrates hypodontia/microdontia, the co-twin is at a significantly increased risk of showing this same trait (13-fold in one study).

■ Figure **2.25**
Natal Tooth
Newborn demonstrating prematurely erupted mandibular left central incisor adjacent to eruption cyst associated with the right central incisor. (With appreciation to Dr. Matthew Tillman.)

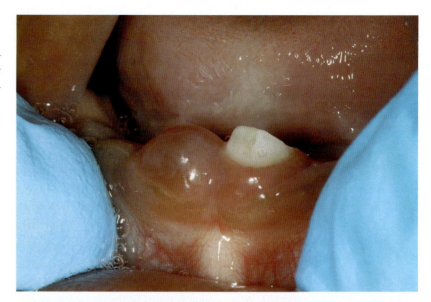

■ Figure **2.26**
Microdontia
Patient demonstrating small peg-shaped right maxillary lateral incisor.

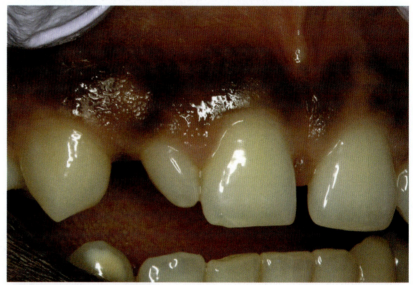

■ Figure **2.27**
Macrodontia
Patient demonstrating enlarged left maxillary central incisor. (Courtesy Dr. Peter Fam.)

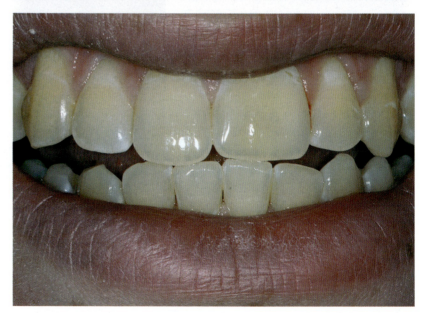

Figs. 2.28–2.31

Double teeth are two teeth joined together or one enlarged tooth that shows an incomplete attempt to divide into two teeth. **Gemination** occurs when a single tooth bud attempts to divide, resulting in a bifid, grooved, or enlarged crown. The process begins at the incisal edge but ceases prior to complete division of the tooth. The affected tooth typically is associated with a common root and pulp canal. **Fusion** occurs when two normally separated teeth are joined by dentin. Fused teeth may share a root and pulp canal or demonstrate separated roots. **Concrescence** is noted when two fully formed teeth are united by cementum without confluence of the dentin. This union may develop during or after initial completion of root formation.

Classically, gemination appears as a single enlarged or double tooth in which the tooth count is normal when the anomalous tooth is counted as one. In contrast, the tooth count in fusion reveals a missing tooth when the anomalous tooth is counted as one. Like most definitions, exceptions do occur. Fusion with a supernumerary tooth is suspected when a bifid crown is associated with two separated roots but the tooth count is normal when the anomalous tooth is counted as one.

Gemination and fusion can involve either dentition, with the incisors and canines most commonly affected. When fusion is noted in the deciduous dentition, the majority of patients will demonstrate lack of formation of the associated succedaneous tooth. Gemination demonstrates a maxillary predominance, whereas fusion occurs more frequently in the mandible. Bilateral examples are uncommon. Concrescence is noted more frequently in the posterior maxilla because of the frequent approximation of the apices of the second and third molars.

Gemination and fusion can create aesthetic concerns, malocclusion, an enlarged diastema, and predisposition to caries and periodontal disease. The therapeutic options must be individualized to the patient's needs and include reshaping and restoration of the altered crown; hemisection into two separate teeth; or extraction with replacement by a partial denture, fixed bridge, or implant. Many cases of concrescence require no therapy, although some may be associated with delayed eruption or extraction difficulties.

■ **Figure 2.28**
Gemination
Bilaterally enlarged maxillary central incisors exhibiting a groove in the midline of each tooth. Unrelated spongiotic gingival hyperplasia also is noted in association with the partially erupted right maxillary lateral incisor.

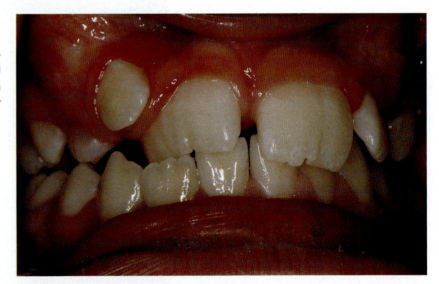

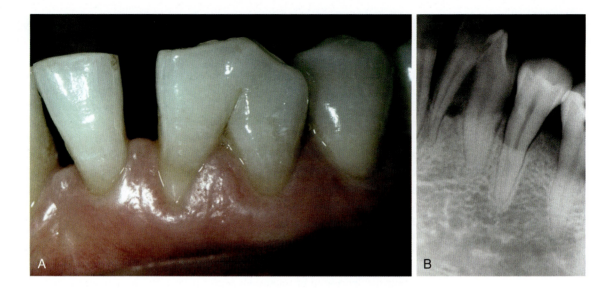

■ Figure 2.29
Fusion

(A) Facial view of mandibular right lateral incisor attached to the crown of the adjacent cuspid. (B) Radiograph of the same teeth.

■ Figure 2.30
Fusion

Enlarged mandibular right central incisor in a patient who also is missing the lateral incisor in that quadrant.

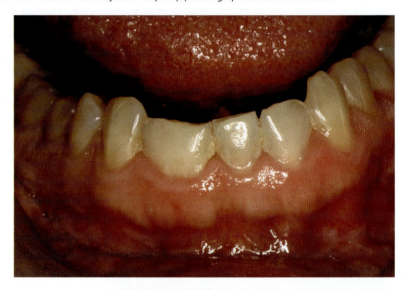

■ Figure 2.31
Concrescence

Maxillary second and third molar demonstrating radicular attachment. Upon histopathologic examination, the teeth shared cementum but not dentin.

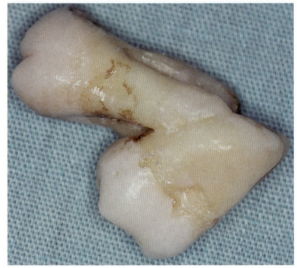

Talon Cusp

Fig. **2.32**

A **talon cusp** is an accessory cusp of an anterior tooth that is located most often on the palatal surface and extends at least half way from the cementoenamel junction to the incisal edge. There is a male predominance, with the vast majority occurring in the maxillary permanent teeth. The maxillary lateral is the most commonly affected permanent tooth, whereas the central incisor is the most frequently involved deciduous tooth. Facial talon cusps are uncommon. An increased prevalence has been seen in a number of syndromes including Rubinstein-Taybi, Ellis-van Creveld, Sturge-Weber, Mohr, incontinentia pigmenti achromians, and Berardinelli-Seip.

The cusp consists of enamel and dentin that may contain a central pulp horn. Developmental grooves that are prone to caries may be present where the cusp joins the palatal surface. In addition to caries along these grooves, the cusp also is associated with occlusal interferences, displacement of the affected tooth, irritation of the adjacent soft tissues, and an increased prevalence of periodontal and pulpal disease. Any evident developmental groove should be restored with a resin-modified glass ionomer. Cusps creating occlusal problems can be removed incrementally at 6- to 8-week intervals and coated with a fluoride varnish to allow for deposition of reparative dentin in an effort to maintain pulpal vitality.

Dens Evaginatus and Shovel-Shaped Incisors

Figs. **2.33 and 2.34**

Dens evaginatus is an accessory cusp that originates from the central groove or lingual ridge of the buccal cusp of a premolar or molar tooth. The mandibular premolar is affected most frequently, and the condition usually is bilateral. The finding is rare in whites; it is discovered most often in Asians, the Inuit, and Native Americans. As would be expected, dens evaginatus has been associated with occlusal problems, cuspal fracture, and pulpal pathosis. Removal of the cusp while maintaining pulpal vitality is difficult but has been achieved by slow periodic grinding and removal of all opposing occlusal interferences. Another option is placement of resin reinforcement around the cusp until pulpal recession has occurred, thereby increasing the possibility of maintaining vitality during removal.

Dens evaginatus often is associated with **shovel-shaped incisors**. Once again, this variation in dental anatomy is unusual in whites but common in Asians, the Inuit, and Native Americans. Affected incisors demonstrate prominent lateral margins that create a hollowed lingual surface similar to the scoop of a shovel. Not uncommonly, the marginal ridges converge on a deep cingulum pit that is prone to caries and should be restored to prevent loss of vitality.

■ Figure **2.32**
Talon Cusp
Right maxillary lateral incisor demonstrating a palatal elevation of tooth structure extending halfway from the cingulum to the incisal edge.

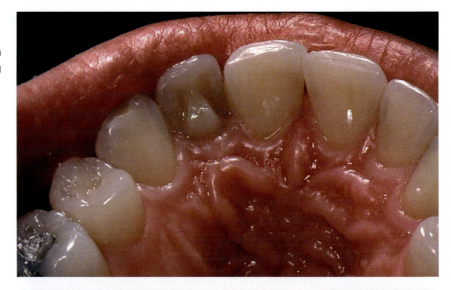

■ Figure **2.33**
Dens Evaginatus
Left mandibular first premolar demonstrating accessory cusp located in the central groove. (Courtesy Dr. Josh Raleigh.)

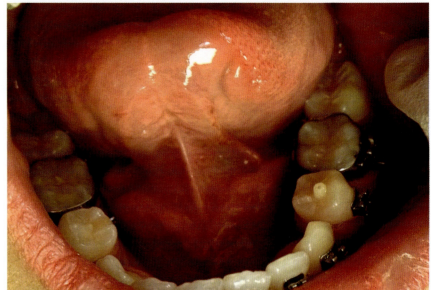

■ Figure **2.34**
Shovel-Shaped Incisors
Palatal surfaces of the maxillary central incisors demonstrating prominent marginal ridges and hollowed lingual surface.

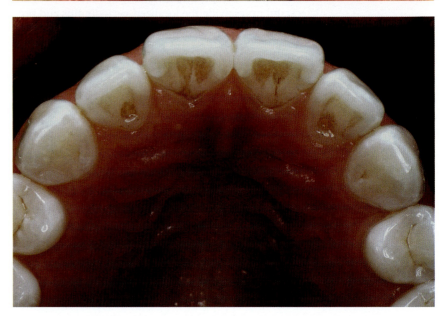

Dens Invaginatus

Figs. **2.35 and 2.36**

Dens invaginatus is a tooth with a surface invagination lined by enamel. According to the classic description of coronal dens invaginatus by Oehlers, the invagination may be confined to the crown (type I), extend past the cementoenamel junction (type II), or parallel the pulp and exit along the lateral or apical aspect of the root (type III). Type III can be confusing because of the potential for interradicular abscess formation in association with a vital tooth. In addition, an extremely rare radicular variant has been documented in which the enamel invagination arises from the cementum surface and extends into the underlying radicular dentin. Dens invaginatus exhibits a strong maxillary predominance, with the lateral incisor most commonly affected. Bilateral involvement is common. Involvement of mandibular teeth, premolars, and molars occurs infrequently.

Ideally, the invagination should be restored to prevent loss of pulpal vitality. Frequently, however, periapical inflammatory disease secondary to pulpal necrosis leads to discovery of the anomaly. Cone beam computed tomography is superior to periapical and panoramic radiographs for identifying the invaginations and demonstrating the complex pulpal anatomy of the distorted tooth. Although conventional endodontic therapy is successful in the majority of cases, some teeth are extremely distorted and may require extraction.

Enamel Pearls

Fig. **2.37**

Enamel pearls (enamelomas) are ectopic exophytic globules of enamel located on the root surface. Most commonly, the lesion is composed of a ball of enamel with a dentin core, but it may consist entirely of enamel or also contain dental pulp. The majority are discovered on the mesial or distal surfaces of molars, with a predilection for the furcation or the groove between incompletely separated roots. There may be multiple affected teeth or multiple pearls on a single tooth, and the finding demonstrates a strong maxillary predominance. Involvement of premolars, canines, and incisors is uncommon. Rare examples may be encased in the radicular dentin or found separate from the teeth within the alveolar bone.

The enamel pearl prevents connective tissue attachment of the root with the adjacent periodontium, provides a niche for bacterial colonization, and complicates cleansing of the site once exposed to the oral cavity. An association with progressive localized periodontitis can occur, necessitating extraction in many cases. Surgical therapy with removal of the enamel pearl, scaling, root planning, and osteoplasty have been successful in resolving the localized periodontitis and preventing loss of the affected tooth.

■ Figure **2.35**
Dens Invaginatus

Periapical radiograph of right maxillary lateral incisor demonstrating incisal invagination lined by radiopaque enamel.

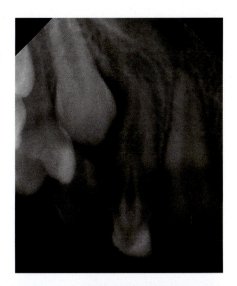

■ Figure **2.36**
Dens Invaginatus

(A) Deformed right maxillary lateral incisor. (B) Radiograph of the same tooth exhibiting a channel lined by radiopaque enamel. The channel parallels the pulp and extends from the incisal edge to an exit along the lateral aspect of the root.

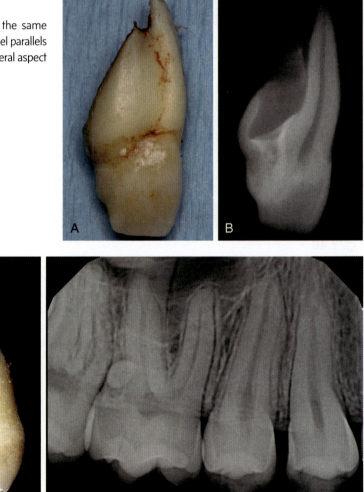

■ Figure **2.37**
Enamel Pearl

(A) Maxillary molar exhibiting exophytic mass of enamel located at the bifurcation of fused roots. (B) Radiograph of a different maxillary molar exhibiting a radiopaque mass of ectopic enamel attached to the distal root of the first molar. (Courtesy Drs. James Lemon and Mary Ellis.)

Cervical Enamel Extension

Fig. **2.38**

Cervical enamel extensions are not exophytic globules but represent sessile fingerlike tracts of enamel from the cementoenamel junction toward the bifurcation of a molar. This creates an isosceles triangle-like extension of enamel with the base toward the coronal enamel and the leading point directed at the bifurcation. Cervical enamel extensions are not rare and demonstrate a slight mandibular predominance. Although any molar may be affected, the third molars are affected much less frequently.

Because the enamel prevents normal connective tissue attachment, the process can be associated with localized loss of periodontal attachment with furcation involvement. In addition, these enamel extensions have been associated with a clinically and radiographically distinctive inflammatory odontogenic cyst known as the **buccal bifurcation cyst**, although the association remains controversial. Flattening or removing the enamel with an excisional new attachment procedure and furcationplasty has been successful in preventing further loss of periodontal attachment.

Taurodontism

Fig. **2.39**

Taurodontism is an apical extension of the pulp chamber that increases its apico-occlusal height and displaces the radicular bifurcation closer to the apex of a molar tooth. Taurodontism may be unilateral or bilateral and predominantly involves the permanent dentition. This dental anomaly may occur as an isolated finding or in association with greater than 20 syndromes. Patients with hypodontia or cleft lip and/or cleft palate demonstrate an increased prevalence of taurodontism. Although the alteration can complicate endodontic therapy, taurodonts require no specific therapy.

Hypercementosis

Fig. **2.40**

Hypercementosis is a nonneoplastic deposition of excessive cementum. Most frequently, there is a uniform deposition with a drumstick-like thickening of the apical third of the root. Less commonly and less well known are small focal knots or projections of excess cementum on the lateral or interradicular root surfaces. Diffuse hypercementosis may be associated with various syndromes and systemic diseases, such as Paget disease of bone, acromegaly, thyroid goiter, calcinosis, arthritis, and rheumatic fever. Isolated hypercementosis may be related to local factors such as periradicular inflammation, occlusal trauma, impaction, loss of antagonistic teeth, and dilaceration. Although teeth demonstrating hypercementosis require no specific therapy, the thickened root occasionally may create problems during extraction and may require sectioning to aid in removal.

■ Figure **2.38**
Cervical Enamel Extension

(A) Extracted mandibular molar with associated buccal bifurcation cyst. (B) Facial view of the same tooth demonstrating a white, opaque line of enamel extending into the bifurcation.

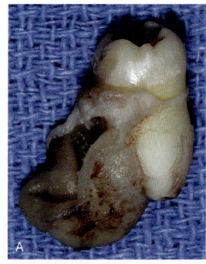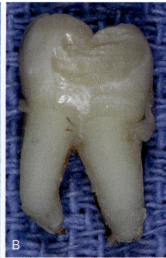

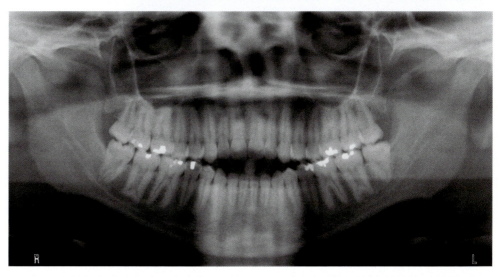

■ Figure **2.39**
Taurodontism

Panoramic radiograph demonstrating alteration of multiple molars in all four quadrants. These molars exhibit enlarged pulp chambers and root bifurcations that approximate the apex. (Courtesy Dr. Sarah Marks Leach.)

■ Figure **2.40**
Hypercementosis

Left maxillary premolar demonstrating radiopaque clublike thickening of the radicular portion of the tooth (Courtesy Dr. Eddie White.)

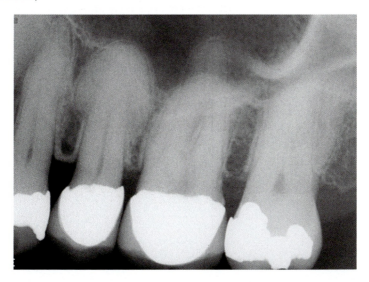

Dilaceration

Fig. **2.41**

Dilaceration is an abnormal bend in the root or crown of a tooth. Although the root is affected most frequently, the bend may occur anywhere along the length of the tooth and has been noted in various teeth throughout the dentition. Although many examples appear idiopathic, others arise in association with significant trauma during tooth development, such as avulsion or intrusion of an overlying deciduous tooth. An adjacent anatomic structure, cyst, or tumor also may induce an abnormal angulation in a developing tooth. Dilaceration usually is diagnosed radiographically, but the change often is subtle when the bend occurs in a facial or lingual direction.

Minor dilaceration requires no therapy. Dilaceration of a deciduous tooth can alter its resorption and delay eruption of the underlying permanent tooth, occasionally mandating extraction of the bent tooth. Severe dilacerations also can prevent eruption of the affected tooth and create endodontic or extraction difficulties.

Supernumerary Roots

Fig. **2.42**

Supernumerary roots refer to teeth with a greater than normal number of roots. Although any tooth in either dentition may be affected, the permanent molars of both arches followed by the mandibular canines and premolars are involved most frequently.

As would be expected, supernumerary roots can create problems during endodontic therapy and exodontia. Although some examples are obvious on periapical radiographs, many are subtle and difficult to identify. All extracted teeth should be examined closely to ensure small supernumerary roots did not separate during removal. In addition, a thorough search for all accessory canals during endodontic therapy increases the chance of success. When questions arise, cone beam computed tomography has been shown to be superior for demonstrating the number of roots and the complex anatomy of their pulp canals.

Syndrome-Associated Enamel Defects

Fig. **2.43**

Development of enamel involves thousands of genes and their associated protein products. It is not surprising that certain molecular alterations result in enamel disturbances along with other systemic manifestations. More than 80 syndromes are known to demonstrate associated enamel defects.

One excellent and well-known example is **tricho-dento-osseous syndrome**, an autosomal dominant disorder that arises secondary to alteration of the *DLX3* gene. Affected patients present with osteosclerosis (most often in the base of the skull and the mastoid), infantile kinky hair, and brittle nails. The dental phenotype includes enamel hypomaturation/hypoplasia (diffuse creamy enamel with pits) or enamel hypoplasia/hypomaturation (generalized thin enamel that also is creamy and opaque) combined with taurodontism.

■ Figure **2.41**
Dilaceration
Maxillary central incisor demonstrating abnormal curvature of its root.

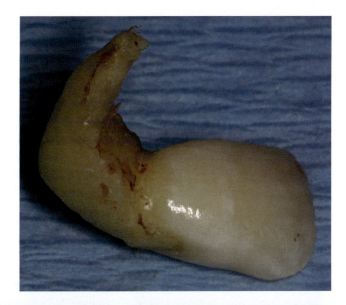

■ Figure **2.42**
Supernumerary Roots
(A) Gross photograph of mandibular molar exhibiting third accessory root. (B) Radiograph of same tooth exhibiting the accessory root.

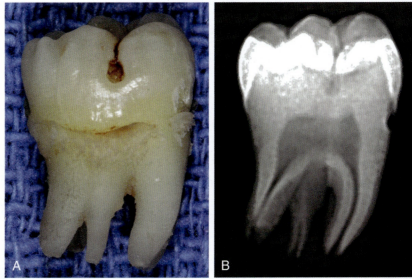

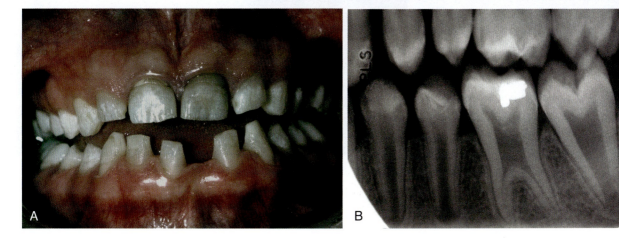

■ Figure **2.43**
Tricho-Dento-Osseous Syndrome
(A) Dentition demonstrating small, widely spaced teeth with white hypomature enamel (hypoplasia-hypomaturation). (B) Radiograph of same patient demonstrating thin enamel and taurodontism.

Figs. **2.44–2.47**

Amelogenesis imperfecta refers to genetic alterations in enamel formation unrelated to a systemic disorder or syndrome. The inheritance patterns include autosomal dominant, autosomal recessive, and X-linked. Phenotypic classification remains popular and includes hypoplastic (localized pitted, generalized pitted, generalized thin), hypomaturation (diffuse creamy, diffuse pigmented, snow capped), hypocalcification, and hypomaturation combined with hypoplasia and taurodontism. Numerous weaknesses in this system have become evident as the associated genetic alterations have been defined. Although all of the involved loci are not known, 10 genes have been associated definitively with amelogenesis imperfecta and allow for molecular diagnosis in the majority of the cases. In spite of this, molecular diagnosis also demonstrates numerous weaknesses, and many believe the most appropriate system must include the mode of inheritance, phenotype, and gene mutation with its associated protein function.

Amelogenesis imperfecta can be associated with significant aesthetic concerns, dental sensitivity, loss of vertical dimension with an increased frequency of caries, anterior open bite, delayed eruption, tooth impaction, and associated gingivitis/periodontitis. Mild variants often can be approached satisfactorily with facial veneers, whereas more severe cases require full coverage as soon as practical. Although many clinicians avoid crown placement in young individuals, studies have demonstrated positive results when following a multisession pattern that allows for the full eruption of the teeth (incisors first followed by premolars and cuspids). Although sensitivity often is a problem associated with conventional crown placement in younger patients, those with amelogenesis imperfecta usually report diminished sensitivity after crown placement, not more. Another option includes using milled acetal resin overlays until eruption is complete.

■ Figure **2.44**
Amelogenesis Imperfecta, Generalized Pitted Hypoplastic Variant
Dentition demonstrating diffuse pitting of coronal enamel.

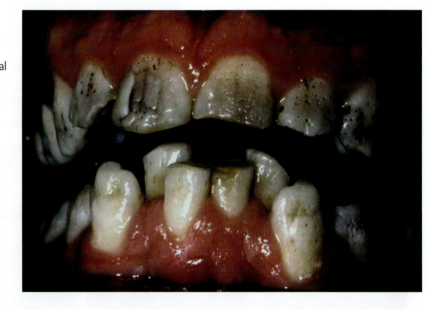

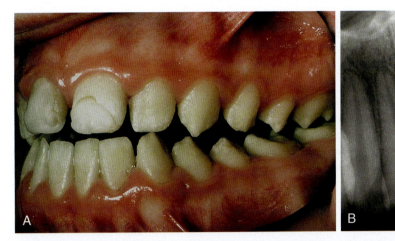

■ Figure **2.45**
Amelogenesis Imperfecta, Generalized Thin Hypoplastic Variant
(A) Dentition demonstrating small, yellowish teeth with open contacts in a patient with anterior open bite. (B) Periapical radiograph of same patient demonstrating absence of enamel and areas of composite restoration.

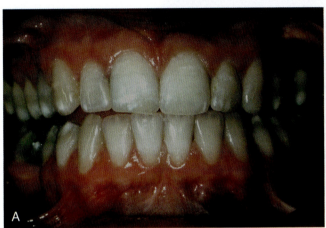

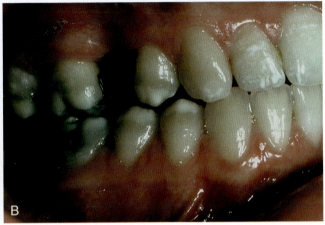

■ Figure **2.46**
Amelogenesis Imperfecta, Snow-Capped Hypomaturation Variant
(A) Facial view of dentition demonstrating white, opaque enamel restricted to the incisal and apical third of the teeth. (B) Buccal view of the posterior dentition in the same patient.

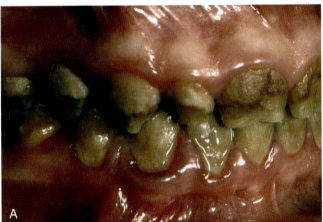

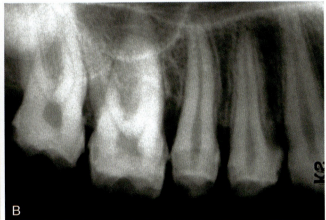

■ Figure **2.47**
Amelogenesis Imperfecta, Hypocalcification Variant
(A) Dentition demonstrating brown-to-orange, crumbly enamel. (B) Periapical radiograph demonstrating enamel with decreased opacity and irregular loss due to rigors of mastication.

Figs. **2.48–2.50**

Dentinogenesis imperfecta (DGI) is an autosomal dominant abnormality of dentin in the absence of a systemic disease and associated with alteration of the dentin sialophosphoprotein *(DSPP)* gene. Dentin matrix is 90% collagen and 10% noncollagenous proteins. The majority of the noncollagenous proteins are produced under control of the *DSPP* gene. Disruption of either collagen or noncollagenous protein formation can result in a clinically obvious dentin disorder.

The widely used Shields classification includes two forms of dentin dysplasia (DD I and DD II) and three patterns of dentinogenesis imperfecta (DGI I, DGI II, DGI III). However, with advances in the genetics of tooth formation, the Shields classification is becoming obsolete. DD I (discussed later) does not appear to be associated with *DSPP* or a gene that controls collagen formation. DGI I is associated with the systemic disease, osteogenesis imperfecta, and is caused by genetic mutations that affect formation of collagen, not dentin protein. This disorder should be termed *osteogenesis imperfecta with opalescent teeth* and is an entity distinct from DGI. The remaining disorders in the Shields classification, DD II, DGI II, and DGI III, appear related to variations of the *DSPP* gene and are proposed to represent varying degrees of severity of the same disease, dentinogenesis imperfecta.

Classically, DGI presents with blue-to-brown translucent teeth that radiographically present with bulbous crowns, cervical constrictions, thin roots, and early obliteration of pulp chambers and canals. Although the enamel is normal, it often is lost prematurely because of an altered enamel-dentin junction.

In the moderate (old Shields DGI II) and severe (old Shields DGI III) variants of DGI, both dentitions demonstrate the features described previously, with the primary difference being the presence of shell teeth in those patients with severe disease. **Shell teeth** demonstrate enamel with normal thickness and roots with thin dentinal walls surrounding enlarged pulps. In the mild pattern (Shields DD II), the deciduous teeth resemble the other two variants, but the permanent teeth are normal, clinically. Radiographically, the permanent teeth are distinctive and demonstrate dramatically enlarged thistle tube-shaped pulp chambers that develop pulp stones over time.

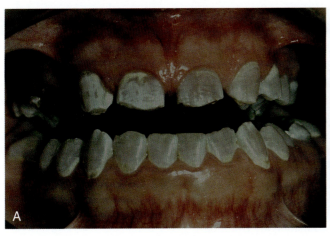
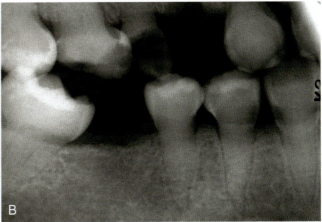

■ Figure **2.48**
Dentinogenesis Imperfecta, Moderate Form
(A) Permanent dentition demonstrating diffuse grayish translucence. (B) Radiograph of same patient demonstrating bulbous crowns, cervical constrictions, and thin roots.

■ Figure **2.49**
Dentinogenesis Imperfecta, Severe Form
Periapical radiograph demonstrating shell teeth with enlarged pulp canals and thin radicular dentin. Prior to eruption these teeth demonstrated normal thickness of enamel, but the enamel was lost prior to the radiograph. (Courtesy Dr. Robin Wilson.)

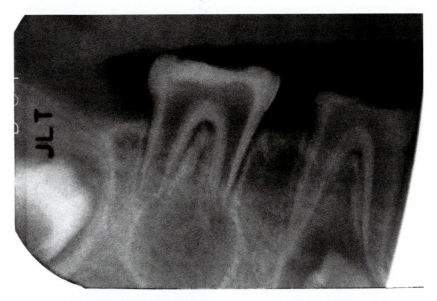

■ Figure **2.50**
Dentinogenesis Imperfecta, Mild Form (Dentin Dysplasia, Type II)
(A) Periapical radiograph demonstrating mandibular incisors exhibiting thistle tube-shaped pulp chambers. (B) Periapical radiograph of different patient with posterior dentition demonstrating thistle tube-shaped pulp chambers with pulp stones. These permanent teeth were normal clinically. (Courtesy Dr. James Zettler.)

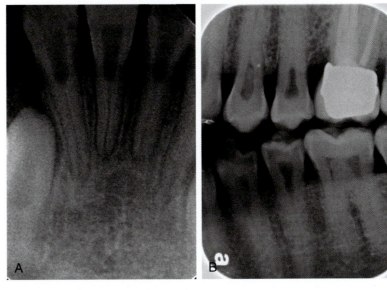

Dentin Dysplasia, Type 1

Figs. **2.51 and 2.52**

Dentin dysplasia, type I is a rare autosomal dominant disorder of dentin not associated with a systemic disease. Affected patients demonstrate teeth with normal-appearing crowns associated with failure of root formation or dramatically shortened roots. When root formation is noted, root canals typically are absent with only a thin crescent of pulp noted at the junction between the crown and the root. Typically in molar teeth, the bifurcation close to the apex. An unusual variation exhibiting root canals with midroot bulges associated with large pulp stones has been described, but there is concern this pattern often is due to a systemic disease such as hyperphosphatemic familial tumoral calcinosis.

Dentin dysplasia, type I diffusely involves both dentitions, with the deciduous teeth often revealing more severe manifestations. Because of dentinal clefts that extend to the dentinoenamel junction, loss of pulpal vitality with associated periapical inflammatory disease often is noted without significant caries or trauma. Tooth mobility and premature exfoliation are common.

Regional Odontodysplasia

Fig. **2.53**

Regional odontodysplasia is a nonhereditary and localized dental malformation that typically affects several contiguous teeth. Although a number of causative factors have been proposed, the pathogenesis has yet to be determined. The process demonstrates a strong maxillary predominance and typically affects both dentitions or only the permanent teeth. Although the malformation usually is limited to a single quadrant, bilateral involvement or ipsilateral alterations in both arches may be seen. Diffuse involvement is extremely rare, as is an unaffected tooth intermixed within a quadrant of altered teeth.

Although many affected teeth demonstrate delayed eruption, once exposed, the teeth are yellow to brown with a rough surface. Radiographically, the affected dentition has been coined **ghost teeth** because of the wispy image created by their large pulps surrounded by extremely thin layers of enamel and dentin. Short roots and open apices are common. Frequent signs and symptoms include failure of eruption, early exfoliation, and associated abscess formation.

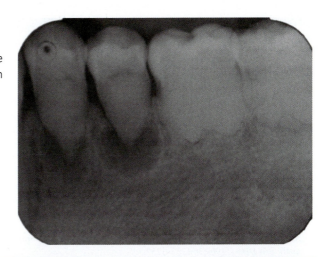

■ Figure **2.51**
Dentin Dysplasia, Type I
Periapical radiograph of posterior dentition demonstrating short roots, absence of root canals, and a small crescent-shaped pulp chamber. Note the bifurcation adjacent to the apex in the molar teeth. (Courtesy Dr. Michael Quinn.)

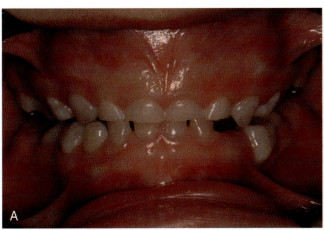

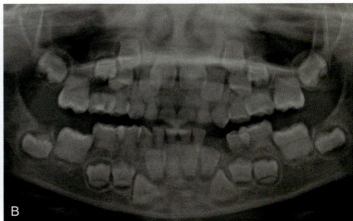

■ Figure **2.52**
Dentin Dysplasia, Type I
(A) Patient with clinically normal appearing deciduous dentition. (B) Panoramic radiograph of the same patient. Note short roots, no pulp canals, and crescent-shaped pulp chambers. (Courtesy Dr. Thomas Ison.)

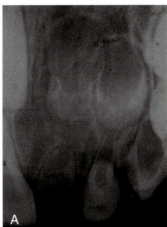

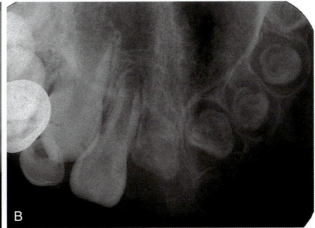

■ Figure **2.53**
Regional Odontodysplasia
(A) Periapical radiograph of the left maxillary anterior teeth. Both the deciduous and permanent dentition demonstrate enlarged pulps associated with paper-thin enamel and dentin. All other teeth in both arches are not affected. (Courtesy Dr. Gregory Dimmich.) (B) Occlusal radiograph of different patient demonstrating similar alterations, also involving the maxilla on the left side. (Courtesy Dr. Román Carlos.)

Bibliography

Environmental Defects of Enamel

Brook AH, Smith JM. Environmental causes of enamel defects. *Ciba Found Symp.* 1997;205:212–225.

Suckling GW. Developmental defects of enamel – historical and present day perspective of their pathogenesis. *Adv Dent Res.* 1989;3:87–94.

Wong HM, Peng S-M, Wen YF, et al. Risk factors of development defects of enamel – A prospective cohort study. *PLoS ONE.* 2014;9:e109351.

Turner Hypoplasia

Andreasen JO, Sundström B, Ravn JJ. The effect of traumatic injuries to primary teeth on their permanent successors. 1. A clinical and histologic study of 117 injured permanent teeth. *Scand J Dent Res.* 1971;79: 219–283.

Turner JG. Injury to the teeth of succession by abscess of the temporary teeth. *Brit Dent J.* 1909;30:1233–1237.

Von Arx T. Developmental disturbances of permanent teeth following trauma to the primary dentition. *Aust Dent J.* 1993;38:1–10.

Dental Disturbances due to Antineoplastic Therapy

Gawade PL, Hudson MM, Kaste SC, et al. A systematic review of dental late effects in survivors of childhood cancer. *Pediatr Blood Cancer.* 2014;61:407–416.

Holtta L, Levy SM, Warren JJ, et al. Long-term adverse effects on dentition in children with poor-risk and autologous stem cell transplantation with or without total body radiation. *Bone Marrow Transplant.* 2002;29: 121–127.

Näsman M, Björk O, Söderhäll S, et al. Disturbances in the oral cavity in pediatric long-term survivors after different forms of antineoplastic therapy. *Pediatr Dent.* 1994;16:217–223.

Dental Fluorosis

Iheozor-Ejiofor Z, Worthington HV, Walsh T, et al. Water fluoridation for the prevention of dental caries. *Cochrane Database Syst Rev.* 2015;(6):CD010856, doi:10.1002/14651858.CD010856.pub2.

O'Mullane DM, Baez RJ, Jones S, et al. Fluoride and oral health. *Community Dent Health.* 2016;33:69–99.

U.S. Department of Health and Human Services Federal Panel on Community Water Fluoridation. U.S. Public Health Service recommendations for fluoride concentration in drinking water for the prevention of dental caries. *Public Health Rep.* 2015;130:318–331.

Tooth Wear

Bartlett DW, Shah P. A critical review of non-carious cervical (wear) lesions and the role of abfraction, erosion, and abrasion. *J Dent Res.* 2006;85:306–312.

Carvalho TS, Colon P, Ganss C, et al. Erosive tooth wear – diagnosis and management. *Swiss Dent J.* 2016;126:342–346.

Grippo JO, Simring M, Coleman TA. Abfraction, abrasion, biocorrosion, and the enigma of noncarious cervical lesions: a 20-year perspective. *J Esthet Restor Dent.* 2012;24:10–25.

Kontaxopoulou I, Alam S. Risk assessment for tooth wear. *Prim Dent J.* 2015;4:25–29.

Litonjua LA, Andreana S, Patra AK, et al. An assessment of stress analyses in the theory of abfraction. *Biomed Mater Eng.* 2004;14:311–321.

Salas MMS, Nascimento GG, Vargas-Ferreira F, et al. Diet influenced tooth erosion prevalence in children and adolescents: results of a meta-analysis and meta-regression. *J Dent.* 2015;43:865–875.

Sarig R, Hershkovitz I, Shvalb N, et al. Proximal attrition facets: morphometric, demographic, and aging characteristics. *Eur J Oral Sci.* 2014;122:271–278.

Shellis RP, Addy M. The interactions between attrition, abrasion and erosion in tooth wear. *Monogr Oral Sci.* 2014;25:32–45.

Young WG, Khan F. Sites of dental erosion are saliva-dependent. *J Oral Rehabil.* 2002;29:35–43.

Young WG. Tooth wear: diet analysis and advice. *Int Dent J.* 2005;55:68–72.

Yule PL, Barclay SC. Worn down by toothwear? Aetiology, diagnosis and management revisited. *Dent Update.* 2015;42:525–532.

Tooth Resorption

Aziz K, Hoover T, Sidhu G. Understanding root resorption with diagnostic imaging. *CDA J.* 2014;42:159–164.

Bakland LK. Root resorption. *Dent Clin North Am.* 1992;36:491–507.

Gartner AH, Mack T, Somerlott RG, et al. Differential diagnosis of internal and external resorption. *J Endod.* 1976;2:329–334.

Germain L. Tooth resorption: the "black hole" of dentistry. *Dent Today.* 2015;34:78–83.

Tronstad L. Root resorption – etiology, terminology and clinical manifestations. *Endod Dent Traumatol.* 1988;4:241–252.

Discolorations of Teeth

Dayan D, Heifferman A, Gorski M, et al. Tooth discoloration – extrinsic and intrinsic factors. *Quintessence Int.* 1983;14:195–199.

Eisenberg E, Bernick SM. Anomalies of the teeth with stains and discolorations. *J Prev Dent.* 1975;2:7–20.

Giunta JL, Tsamtsouris A. Stains and discolorations of teeth: review and case reports. *J Pedod.* 1978;2:175–182.

Ankylosis

de Moura MS, Pontes AS, Brito MHSF, et al. Restorative management of severely ankylosed primary molars. *J Dent Child.* 2015;82:41–46.

Douglass J, Tinanoff N. The etiology, prevalence, and sequelae of infraocclusion of primary molars. *J Dent Child.* 1991;58:481–483.

Ekim SL, Hatibovic-Kofman S. A treatment decision-making model for infraoccluded primary molars. *Int J Paediatr Dent.* 2001;11:340–346.

Dental Transposition

Danielsen JC, Karimian K, Ciarlantini R, et al. Unilateral and bilateral dental transposition in the maxilla – dental and skeletal findings in 63 individuals. *Eur Arch Paediatr Dent.* 2015;16:467–476.

Lorente T, Lorente C, Murry PG, et al. Surgical and orthodontic management of maxillary canine-lateral incisor transpositions. *Am J Orthod Dentofacial Orthop.* 2016;150:876–885.

Peck L, Peck S, Attia Y. Maxillary canine-first premolar transpositions, associated dental anomalies and genetic basis. *Angle Orthod.* 1993;63:99–109.

Peck S, Peck L. Classification of maxillary tooth transpositions. *Am J Orthod Dentofacial Orthop.* 1995;107:505–517.

Hypodontia

Khalaf K, Miskelly J, Voge E, et al. Prevalence of hypodontia and associated factors: a systemic review and meta-analysis. *J Orthod.* 2014;41:299–316.

Lammi L, Arte S, Somer M, et al. Mutations in AXIN2 cause familial tooth agenesis and predispose to colorectal cancer. *Am J Hum Genet.* 2004;74:1043–1050.

Longtin R. Chew on this: mutation may be responsible for tooth loss, colon cancer. *J Natl Cancer Inst.* 2004;96:987–989.

Nieminen P. Genetic basis of tooth agenesis. *J Exp Zool B Mol Dev Evol.* 2009;312B:320–342.

Pani SC. The genetic basis of tooth agenesis: basic concepts and genes involved. *J Indian Soc Pedod Prev Dent.* 2011;29:84–89.

Yin W, Bian Z. The gene network underlying hypodontia. *J Dent Res.* 2015;94:878–885.

Hyperdontia

Bereket C, Çakir-Özkan N, Sener I, et al. Analyses of 100 supernumerary teeth in a nonsyndromic Turkish population: a retrospective multicenter study. *Niger J Clin Pract.* 2015;18:731–738.

Bodin I, Julin P, Thomsson M. Hyperdontia. I. Frequency and distribution of supernumerary teeth among 21,609 patients. *Dentomaxillofac Radiol.* 1978;7:15–17.

Brook AH, Jernvall J, Smith RN, et al. The dentition: the outcomes of morphogenesis leading to variations in tooth number, size, and shape. *Aust Dent J.* 2014;59(suppl 1):131–142.

Cassetta M, Altieri F, Giansanti M, et al. Morphological and topographical characteristics of posterior supernumerary molar teeth: an epidemiological study on 25, 186 subjects. *Med Oral Patol Oral Cir Bucal.* 2014;19:e545–e549.

Mossaz J, Kloukos D, Pandis N, et al. Morphologic characteristics, location, and associated complications of maxillary and mandibular supernumerary teeth as evaluated using cone beam computed tomography. *Eur J Orthod.* 2014;36:708–718.

Omer RS, Anthonappa RP, King NM. Determination of the optimum time for surgical removal of unerupted anterior supernumerary teeth. *Pediatr Dent.* 2010;32:14–20.

Rajab LD, Hamdan MAM. Supernumerary teeth: review of the literature and a survey of 152 cases. *Int J Pediatr Dent.* 2002;12:244–254.

Natal Teeth

Baldiwala M, Nayak R. Conservative management of Riga-Fede disease. *J Dent Child.* 2014;81:103–106.

Kana A, Markou I, Arhakis A, et al. Natal and neonatal teeth: a systemic review of prevalence and management. *Eur J Paediatr Dent.* 2013;14:27–32.

Khandelwal V, Nayak UA, Nayak PA, et al. Management of an infant having natal teeth. *BMJ Case Rep.* 2013;doi:10.11366/bcr-2013-010049.

Moura LFAD, Moura MS, Lima MDM, et al. Natal and neonatal teeth: a review of 23 cases. *J Dent Child.* 2014;81:107–111.

Microdontia and Macrodontia

Brook AH, Jernvall J, Smith RN, et al. The dentition: the outcomes of morphogenesis leading to variations in tooth number, size, and shape. *Aust Dent J.* 2014;59(suppl 1):131–142.

Jeong KH, Kim D, Song Y-M, et al. Epidemiology and genetics of hypodontia and microdontia: a study of twin families. *Angle Orthod.* 2015;85:980–985.

Kyriazidou A, Haider D, Mason C, et al. Case report: macrodont mandibular second premolars a hereditary dental anomaly. *Eur Arch Paediatr Dent.* 2013;14:411–416.

Pereira L, Assunção PA, Salazar SLA, et al. Uncommon true isolated macrodontia of a maxillary tooth. *J Contemp Dent Pract.* 2014;15:116–118.

Double Teeth

Brook AH, Winter GB. Double teeth: a retrospective study of "geminated" and "fused" teeth in children. *Br Dent J.* 1970;129:123–130.

Finkelstein T, Shapira Y, Bechor N, et al. Fused and geminated permanent maxillary central incisors: prevalence, treatment options, and outcome in orthodontic patients. *J Dent Child.* 2015;82:147–152.

Neves FS, Rovaris K, Oliveira ML, et al. Concrescence. Assessment of case by periapical radiography, cone beam computed tomography, and micro-computed tomography. *N Y State Dent J.* 2014;80:21–23.

Prabhu RV, Chatra L, Shenai P, et al. Bilateral fusion in primary mandibular teeth. *Indian J Dent Res.* 2013;24:277–278.

Ruprecht A, Batniji S, El-Neweihi E. Double teeth: the incidence of germination and fusion. *J Pedod.* 1985;9:332–337.

Smail-Ferguson V, Terradot J, Bolla MM, et al. Management of non-syndromic double tooth affecting permanent maxillary central incisors: a systematic review. *BMJ Case Rep.* 2016;doi:10.1136/bcr-2016-215482.

Talon Cusp

Dankner E, Harari D, Rotstein I. Dens evaginatus of anterior teeth. Literature review and radiographic survey of 15,000 teeth. *Oral Surg Oral Med Oral Pathol Oral Radiol Endod.* 1996;81:472–476.

Davis PJ, Brook AH. The presentation of talon cusp: diagnosis, clinical features, associations and possible aetiology. *Br Dent J.* 1986;160:84–88.

Manuja N, Chaudhary S, Nagpal R, et al. Bilateral dens evaninatus (talon cusp) in permanent maxillary lateral incisors: a rare developmental dental anomaly with great clinical significance. *BMJ Case Rep.* 2013;doi:10.1136/bcr-2013-009184.

Mellor JK, Ripa LW. Talon cups: a clinically significant anomaly. *Oral Surg Oral Med Oral Pathol.* 1970;29:225–228.

Dens Evaginatus and Shovel-Shaped Incisors

Gaynor WN. Dens evaginatus – how does it present and how should it be managed? *N Z Dent J.* 2002;98:104–107.

Levitan ME, Himel VT. Dens evaginatus: literature review, pathophysiology, and comprehensive treatment regimen. *J Endod.* 2006;32:1–9.

Saini TS, Kharat DU, Mokeem S. Prevalence of shovel-shaped incisors in Saudi Arabian dental patients. *Oral Surg Oral Med Oral Pathol.* 1990;70:540–544.

Dens Invaginatus

Capar ID, Ertas H, Arslan H, et al. A retrospective comparative study of cone-beam computed tomography versus rendered panoramic images in identifying the presence, types, and characteristics of dens invaginatus in a Turkish population. *J Endod.* 2015;41:473–478.

Macho AZ, Ferreiroa A, Rico-Romano C, et al. Diagnosis and endodontic treatment of type II dens invaginatus by using cone-beam computed tomography and splint guides for cavity access. *J Am Dent Assoc.* 2015;146:266–270.

Oehlers FAC. Dens invaginatus (dilated composite odontome). I. Variations of the invagination process and associated anterior crown forms. *Oral Surg Oral Med Oral Pathol.* 1957;10:1204–1218.

Oehlers FAC. Dens invaginatus (dilated composite odontome). II. Associated posterior crown forms and pathogenesis. *Oral Surg Oral Med Oral Pathol.* 1957;10:1302–13116.

Oehlers FAC. The radicular variant of dens invaginatus. *Oral Surg Oral Med Oral Pathol.* 1958;11:1251–1260.

Enamel Pearls

Cavanha AO. Enamel pearls. *Oral Surg Oral Med Oral Pathol.* 1965;19: 373–382.

Lòpez SP, Warren RN, Bromage TG, et al. Treatment of an unusual non-tooth related enamel pearl (EP) and 3 teeth-related EPs with localized periodontal disease without teeth extractions: a case report. *Compend Contin Educ Dent.* 2015;36:592–599.

Risnes S, Segura JJ, Casado A, et al. Enamel pearls and cervical enamel projections in 2 maxillary molars with localized periodontal disease. Case report and histologic study. *Oral Surg Oral Med Oral Pathol Oral Radiol Endod.* 2000;89:493–497.

Romeo U, Palaia G, Botti R, et al. Enamel pearls as a predisposing factor to localized periodontitis. *Quintessence Int.* 2011;42:69–71.

Cervical Enamel Extension

Fowler CB, Brannon RB. The paradental cyst: a clinicopathologic study of six new cases and review of the literature. *J Oral Maxillofac Surg.* 1989;47:243–248.

Hou G-L, Tsai C-C. Cervical enamel projection and intermediate bifurcational ridge correlated with molar furcation involvement. *J Periodontol.* 1997;68:687–693.

Pompura JR, Sándor GKB, Stoneman DW. The buccal bifurcation cyst: a prospective study of treatment outcomes in 44 sites. *Oral Surg Oral Med Oral Pathol Oral Radiol Endod.* 1997;83:215–221.

Taurodontism

Hashova JE, Gill DS, Figueiredo JAP, et al. Taurodontism – a review. *Dent Update.* 2009;36:235–243.

Jafarzadeh H, Azarpazhooh A, Mayhall JT. Taurodontism: a review of the condition and endodontic treatment challenges. *Int Endod J.* 2008;41: 375–388.

Melo Filho MR, dos Santos LAN, Barbosa Martelli DR, et al. Taurodontism in patients with nonsyndromic cleft lip and palate in a Brazilian population: a case control evaluation with panoramic radiographs. *Oral Surg Oral Med Oral Pathol Oral Radiol Endod.* 2015;120:744–750.

Hypercementosis

Abbot F. Hyperostosis of roots of teeth. *Dent Cosmos.* 1886;28:665–683.

d'Incau E, Couture C, Crépeau N, et al. Determination and validation of criteria to define hypercementosis in two medieval samples from France (Sains-en-Gohelle, AD 7th-17th century; Jau-Dignac-et-Loirac, AD 7th-8th century). *Arch Oral Biol.* 2015;60:293–303.

Gardner BS, Goldstein H. The significance of hypercementosis. *Dent Cosmos.* 1931;73:1065–1069.

Leider AS, Garbarino VE. Generalized hypercementosis. *Oral Surg Oral Med Oral Pathol.* 1987;63:375–380.

Dilaceration

Jafarzadeh H, Abbott PV. Dilaceration: review of an endodontic challenge. *J Endod.* 2007;33:1025–1030.

Ligh RQ. Coronal dilacerations. *Oral Surg Oral Med Oral Pathol.* 1981;51:567.

Topouzelis N, Tsaousoglou P, Pisoka V, et al. Dilaceration of maxillary central incisor: a literature review. *Dent Traumatol.* 2010;26:427–433.

Supernumerary Roots

Kannan SK, Suganya, Santharam H. Supernumerary roots. *Indian J Dent Res.* 2002;13:116–119.

Chauhan R, Singh S. Endodontic treatment of mandibular molars with atypical root canal anatomy: report of 4 cases. *Gen Dent.* 2015;63:67–70.

Syndromic Enamel Defects and Amelogenesis Imperfecta

Aldred MJ, Savarirayan R, Crawford PJM. Amelogenesis imperfecta: a classification and catalogue for the 21st century. *Oral Dis.* 2003;9:19–23.

Lundgren GP, Vestlund GIM, Trulsson M, et al. A randomized controlled trial of crown therapy in young individuals with amelogenesis imperfecta. *J Dent Res.* 2015;94:1041–1047.

Wilson OL, Bradshaw JP, Marks MK. Amelogenesis imperfecta, facial esthetics and Snap-on Smile®. *J Tenn Dent Assoc.* 2015;95:18–21.

Witkop CJ Jr. Amelogenesis imperfecta, dentinogenesis imperfecta and dentin dysplasia revisited: problems in classification. *J Oral Pathol.* 1988;17:547–553.

Wright JT, Carrion IA, Morris C. The molecular basis of hereditary enamel defects in humans. *J Dent Res.* 2015;94:52–61.

DSPP-Associated Dentin Disorders

Barron MJ, McDonnell ST, MacKie I, et al. Hereditary dentine disorders: dentinogenesis imperfecta and dentine dysplasia. *Orphanet J Rare Dis.* 2008;3:31.

Dean JA, Hartsfield JK Jr, Wright JT, et al. Dentin dysplasia, type II linkage to chromosome 4q. *J Craniofac Genet Dev Biol.* 1997;17:172–177.

de Dure-Molla M, Fournier BP, Berdal A. Isolated dentinogenesis imperfecta and dentin dysplasia: revision of the classification. *Eur J Hum Genet.* 2015;23:445–451.

MacDougall M. Refined mapping of the human dentin sialophosphoprotein (DSPP) gene within the critical dentinogenesis imperfecta type II and dentin dysplasia type II loci. *Eur J Oral Sci.* 1998;106(suppl 1):227–233.

McKnight DA, Simmer JP, Hart PS, et al. Overlapping DSPP mutations cause DD and DGI. *J Dent Res.* 2008;87:1108–1111.

Shields ED, Bixler D, El-Kafrawy AM. A proposed classification for heritable human dentine defects with a description of a new entity. *Arch Oral Biol.* 1973;18:543–553.

Dentin Dysplasia, Type I

O'Carroll MK, Duncan WK, Perkins TM. Dentin dysplasia: review of the literature and a proposed subclassification based on radiographic findings. *Oral Surg Oral Med Oral Pathol.* 1991;72:119–125.

Ranta H, Lukinmaa P-L, Waltimo J. Heritable dentin defects: nosology, pathology, and treatment. *Am J Med Genet.* 1993;45:193–200.

Vieira AR, Lee M, Vairo F, et al. Root anomalies and dentin dysplasia in autosomal recessive hyperphosphatemic familial tumoral calcinosis. *Oral Surg Oral Med Oral Pathol Oral Radiol.* 2015;120:e235–e239.

Regional Odontodysplasia

Al-Tuwirqi A, Lambie D, Seow WK. Regional odontodysplasia: literature review and report of unusual case located in the mandible. *Pediatr Dent.* 2014;36:62–67.

Crawford PJM, Aldred MJ. Regional odontodysplasia: a bibliography. *J Oral Pathol Med.* 1989;18:251–263.

Kahn MA, Hinson RL. Regional odontodysplasia. Case report with etiologic and treatment considerations. *Oral Surg Oral Med Oral Pathol Oral Radiol Endod.* 1991;72:462–467.

Tervonon SA, Stratmann U, Mokrys K, et al. Regional odontodysplasia: a review of the literature and report of four cases. *Clin Oral Invest.* 2004;8:45–51.

3

Pulp and Periapical Disease

Fig. **3.1**

Pulp stones are discrete calcifications that form within the pulp chamber. They may lie free within the pulp, adhere to the chamber wall, or become embedded in dentin. It is believed that the calcification initially forms around a central nidus of collagen fibrils, ground substance, or necrotic cell remnants. Subsequently, concentric rings of calcification are deposited around the central nidus. Pulp stones that become sufficiently large (i.e., greater than approximately 200 μm in maximum diameter) may be detected incidentally on bitewing or periapical radiographs. The true prevalence of pulp stones is difficult to ascertain because radiographic analysis may not detect small stones that would be evident microscopically. However, a recent retrospective study of adult patients examined by cone-beam computed tomography (CBCT) found pulp stones in approximately 32% of individuals and 10% of teeth, with the maxillary and mandibular molars most frequently affected. In addition, an increased prevalence of pulp stones has been reported in association with aging and local irritation (e.g., attrition, abrasion, erosion, caries, periodontitis, dental restorations, orthodontic tooth movement, dental injury). An association with certain hereditary or systemic conditions (e.g., dentin dysplasia types Id and II, pulpal dysplasia, Ehlers-Danlos syndrome, end-stage renal disease) has been noted as well. Although most pulp stones are not clinically significant, large ones may make endodontic treatment difficult.

Hyperplastic Pulpitis

Fig. **3.2**

Hyperplastic pulpitis (or a "pulp polyp") represents an inflammatory enlargement of the pulp that typically develops in the teeth of young patients with large pulpal exposures. Trauma and/or caries may result in extensive coronal defects that lack a dentinal roof; such defects may become occupied by a polypoid growth of hyperplastic granulation tissue extruding from the pulp chamber. The deciduous and permanent molars are the most frequently involved teeth. Patients may be asymptomatic or feel pressure when biting. The absence of a pulp chamber roof and the presence of open root apices may reduce intrapulpal pressure, maintain the microcirculation, and decrease the likelihood of pulpal necrosis. Nevertheless, because the inflammation is irreversible, tooth extraction or endodontic therapy is required.

Palatal Abscess

Fig. **3.3**

A **palatal abscess** represents a localized, suppurative swelling typically caused by underlying odontogenic infection. In general, the location of dental abscesses is influenced by the position of the tooth root apices, the thickness of the surrounding bone, and the presence of adjacent muscle attachments or other anatomic structures. Although most abscesses arising from maxillary dental infection form on the buccal aspect, palatal abscesses also are possible—especially when the infection originates from the maxillary lateral incisors or the palatal roots of maxillary molars/premolars. The lesion may be tender to palpation, and the infected tooth is nonvital. Treatment includes incision and drainage of the abscess as well as endodontic therapy or extraction of the infected tooth.

■ Figure **3.1**
Pulp Stones

Molar teeth exhibiting radiopacities within their pulp chambers.

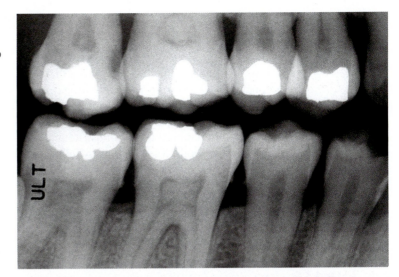

■ Figure **3.2**
Hyperplastic Pulpitis

This mandibular molar has a large pulpal exposure with hyperplastic granulation tissue extruding from the pulp chamber. (Courtesy Dr. David Davidson.)

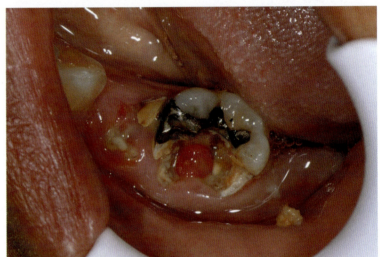

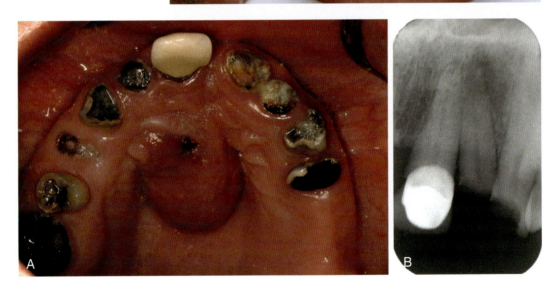

■ Figure **3.3**
Palatal Abscess

(A) Suppurative swelling of the palate resulting from odontogenic infection. (B) Source of infection appeared to be a nonvital maxillary lateral incisor with a periapical radiolucency; several other infected maxillary teeth in this patient may have contributed to abscess formation as well.

Parulis

Fig. **3.4**

A **parulis** (or "gum boil") appears as a mass of granulation tissue on the gingiva/alveolar mucosa at the opening of a sinus tract. The lesion usually is caused by underlying odontogenic or periodontal infection. The mass typically appears erythematous or yellowish; in some cases, a punctate opening (stoma) may be evident, from which pus can be expressed. Patency and drainage may alleviate the patient's pain or discomfort. Radiographic evaluation following insertion of a gutta-percha point into the sinus tract may aid in locating the infected tooth. Management includes establishing drainage and treating the underlying source of infection (i.e., nonvital tooth or infected periodontal pocket).

Cutaneous Sinus

Figs. **3.5 and 3.6**

Cutaneous sinuses in the cervicofacial region often are related to underlying odontogenic infection; however, various other causes (e.g., periodontal infection, skin infection, osteomyelitis, mycobacterial infection of the cervical lymph nodes, parotid abscess) also are possible. In cases arising from odontogenic infection, the exudate perforates the cortical bone and drains through a sinus tract, terminating at the skin surface. The mandibular teeth represent the source of infection more often than the maxillary teeth. Accordingly, common sites for cutaneous sinus formation include the skin overlying the inferior border of the mandible and the chin, although other locations also are possible. Clinically, the opening of a cutaneous sinus may appear as a dimple, nodule, ulcer, or abscess. Purulent drainage may or may not be evident. Insertion of a gutta-percha point or other radiopaque material may aid in tracing the source of infection. Because many patients are asymptomatic and the sinus may extend a considerable distance from the offending infected tooth, there is the potential for confusion with localized skin lesions (such as epidermoid cysts, furuncles, or skin cancers). Addressing the underlying odontogenic infection by tooth extraction or endodontic therapy with antibiotic treatment typically results in resolution of the lesion.

■ Figure **3.4**
Parulis

Exophytic, yellowish mass of granulation tissue on the alveolar mucosa at the opening of a sinus tract.

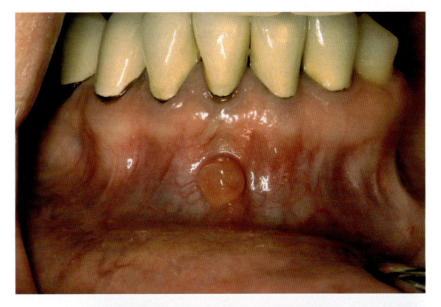

■ Figure **3.5**
Cutaneous Sinus

This patient had an underlying mandibular odontogenic infection that led to formation of a sinus tract, terminating on the skin surface as an erythematous nodule.

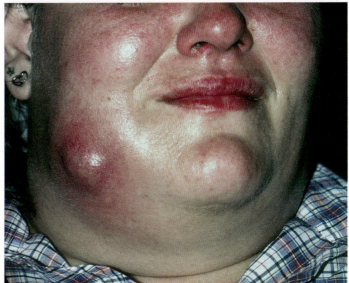

■ Figure **3.6**
Cutaneous Sinus

The skin overlying the inferior border of the mandible is a common site for cutaneous sinus formation. In this case, the opening of the sinus tract appeared as a dimple.

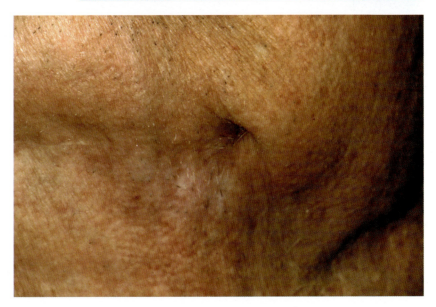

Periapical Granuloma (Dental Granuloma)

Figs. **3.7 and 3.8**

A **periapical granuloma** is a mass of inflamed granulation tissue that forms around the apex of a tooth with pulpal necrosis. Radiographic examination shows a periapical radiolucency of variable size with well- to ill-defined borders and loss of the adjacent lamina dura. There may or may not be a radiopaque rim. The patient may be asymptomatic or complain of pain, and at times the involved tooth exhibits percussion sensitivity. Treatment consists of endodontic therapy or tooth extraction, with clinical and radiographic follow-up to monitor for resolution of the lesion. As seen in Fig. 3.7, sometimes a periapical radiolucency does not resolve after nonsurgical root canal therapy. In such cases, it is important to evaluate potential causes for lesion persistence (e.g., missed accessory root canals, inflammatory response to foreign material, bacterial infection, a cyst or tumor mimicking periapical inflammatory disease); nonsurgical retreatment, apicoectomy, or extraction may be considered. If apicoectomy or extraction is performed, submission of the periapical tissue for microscopic diagnosis is recommended.

Periapical Scar

Fig. **3.9**

After extraction or endodontic therapy for a tooth with periapical inflammatory disease, the bony defect sometimes becomes filled with scar tissue rather than bone. **Periapical scar** formation tends to occur when both the buccal and lingual cortical plates are lost (due to inflammation and/or surgical treatment). If a clinician has surgical access and anticipates that periapical scar formation is likely, then guided tissue regeneration with membrane barriers and bone grafting may be considered to enhance periapical wound healing and prevent the ingrowth of fibroblasts. The dense fibrous connective tissue that comprises a periapical scar appears radiolucent. The lesion can be mistaken for a persistent periapical granuloma or cyst, which may prompt biopsy for microscopic diagnosis. Once a definitive diagnosis has been established, no further treatment is necessary.

■ Figure **3.7**
Periapical Granuloma

Periapical radiolucency associated with the mesial root apex of an endodontically treated mandibular molar. There is loss of the lamina dura in the area of the lesion. (Courtesy Dr. Michael Piepenbring.)

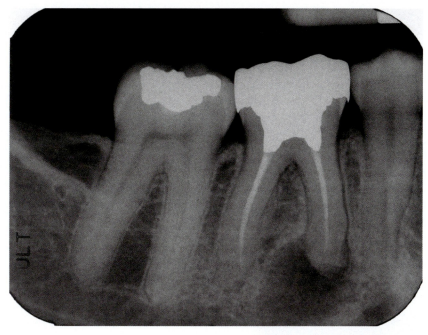

■ Figure **3.8**
Periapical Granuloma

Well-defined radiolucency at the apex of a maxillary lateral incisor.

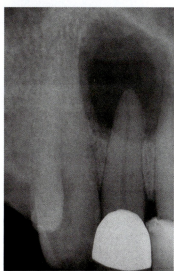

■ Figure **3.9**
Periapical Scar

Radiolucency representing scar tissue that formed after extraction of a maxillary lateral incisor with periapical inflammatory disease. Loss of both the buccal and lingual cortical plates can predispose to scar formation.

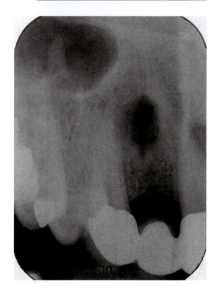

Periapical Cyst (Radicular Cyst; Apical Periodontal Cyst)

Figs. **3.10 and 3.11**

The **periapical cyst** exhibits the same clinical and radiographic features as the periapical granuloma (i.e., variably sized radiolucency at the apex of a nonvital tooth). Some investigators have noted a greater tendency for periapical cysts to be larger, to cause root displacement, or to exhibit well-defined radiographic borders compared to periapical granulomas. Nevertheless, histopathologic examination is the only reliable method for distinguishing between these lesions. Whereas a periapical granuloma comrprises inflamed granulation tissue, a periapical cyst represents an epithelium-lined cavity with an inflamed fibrovascular connective tissue wall. The cyst lining is usually stratified squamous, although pseudostratified columnar epithelium also is possible. The epithelium generally is thought to arise from the rests of Malassez, although an origin from the maxillary sinus lining, crevicular lining, or sinus tract lining also is possible. The growth of periapical cysts traditionally has been hypothesized to be related to increased osmotic pressure caused by necrotic cellular debris within the cyst lumen; however, complex epithelial-stromal interactions mediated by inflammatory cytokines also appear to play an important role. The term *lateral radicular cyst* may be used for such an inflammatory cyst that occurs along the lateral root surface (see Fig. 3.10B).

In practice, microscopic distinction between a periapical cyst and a periapical granuloma is not necessary to render appropriate treatment. Based on a presumptive clinical/radiographic diagnosis of periapical inflammatory disease, both lesion types are treated by tooth extraction or endodontic therapy. Alternative treatment options for large lesions include decompression, marsupialization, or fenestration combined with biopsy and endodontic therapy. Periodic clinical and radiographic follow-up is recommended to monitor for disease resolution.

Residual Periapical Cyst

Fig. **3.12**

When a tooth is extracted without removal of an associated periapical cyst, the remaining lesion is termed a **residual periapical cyst** (residual radicular cyst, residual cyst). Radiographic examination shows a round to oval radiolucency of variable size in the previous extraction site. In some cases, dystrophic calcification of degenerating cellular debris within the cyst lumen appears as a central radiopacity. Surgical removal with histopathologic examination for diagnostic confirmation is indicated.

■ Figure **3.10**
Periapical Cyst

(A) Radiolucency associated with the apex of a maxillary lateral incisor that had been treated endodontically. (Courtesy Dr. Michael Piepenbring.) (B) The term *lateral radicular cyst* may be used for an inflammatory cyst that forms between the roots of teeth, as seen in this example between the roots of the maxillary lateral incisor and canine. (Courtesy Dr. William Dunlap.)

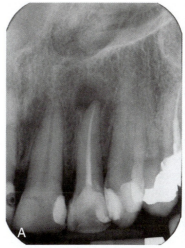
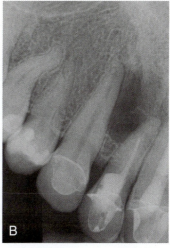

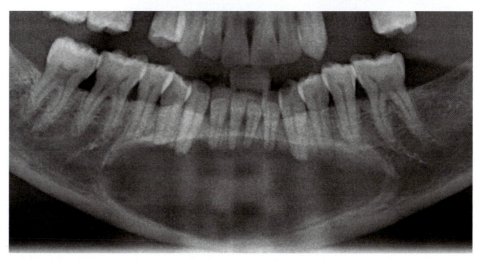

■ Figure **3.11**
Periapical Cyst

This radiolucency is an especially large periapical cyst involving much of the mandible. (Courtesy Dr. Jay Sikes.)

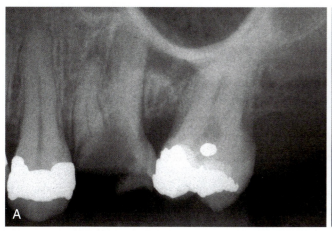
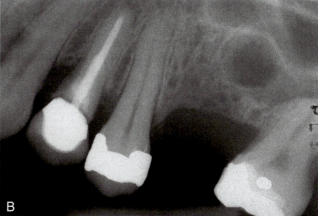

■ Figure **3.12**
Residual Periapical Cyst

(A) Grossly carious molar with a periapical radiolucency adjacent to the floor of the maxillary sinus. (B) Although the tooth has been extracted, a well-circumscribed residual periapical cyst can still be seen beneath the sinus.

Ludwig Angina

Fig. **3.13**

Ludwig angina is a rapidly spreading and potentially fatal infection of the sublingual, submandibular, and submental spaces bilaterally. It represents an aggressive form of *cellulitis* (diffuse spread of infection through fascial planes of soft tissue) and typically results from infection of the mandibular molars. In addition, some reported cases have arisen secondary to nonodontogenic infections (e.g., related to peritonsillar abscess, mandibular fracture, soft tissue trauma, lymphadenitis, submandibular sialadenitis). Predisposing factors include diabetes mellitus and immunosuppression. As seen here, affected individuals usually present with massive neck swelling. In addition, the tongue exhibits firm, board-like swelling with associated elevation, protrusion, and possible airway compromise. Additional signs and symptoms include pain, fever, chills, dysphagia, dysphonia, dyspnea, and trismus. Upon entry into the submandibular space, the infection may spread to the lateral pharyngeal space, retropharyngeal space, and mediastinum. In addition to respiratory obstruction and mediastinitis, potential life-threatening complications include necrotizing fasciitis, sepsis with multiorgan failure, pneumonia, empyema, pericarditis, and epidural abscess. Bacterial cultures typically show a mixture of aerobic and anaerobic species. Management includes airway maintenance, intravenous antibiotics, incision and drainage, elimination of the underlying focus of infection, fluid management, and nutritional support.

Acute Osteomyelitis

Fig. **3.14**

Osteomyelitis is an inflammatory process of bone that spreads through the medullary cavity. Typically, the process begins as an infection in the medullary bone, which then spreads into the cortical and periosteal bone. Accumulation of pus and edema within the medullary cavity and beneath the periosteum compromises the blood supply, resulting in ischemia, necrosis, and bone sequestration.

Osteomyelitis of the jaws usually is caused by odontogenic infection, although other etiologic factors include traumatic jaw fracture, vascular insufficiency, necrotizing ulcerative gingivitis, and noma. Predisposing factors include diabetes mellitus, immunosuppression, malnutrition, and radiation therapy. Because of its limited blood supply and denser cortical bone, the mandible is affected more often than the maxilla.

Acute osteomyelitis is typically suppurative (pus-forming) and generally defined, albeit arbitrarily, as occurring within 1 month of the onset of symptoms. Clinical findings include intense pain, indurated swelling, paresthesia or anesthesia of the inferior alveolar nerve, cervical lymphadenopathy, and fever. Over time, fistula formation, necrotic bone exfoliation, and tooth mobility may develop. In the early stages, findings on plain radiographs may be unremarkable. However, as the disease progresses, an ill-defined radiolucency and loss of trabecular architecture become evident. Other possible findings include widening of the periodontal ligament, loss of the lamina dura, and loss of circumscription of the inferior alveolar canal/mental foramen. With disease progression, periosteal thickening and sequestration (opacification representing necrotic bone fragments) may be noted. Additional imaging modalities include computed tomography, magnetic resonance imaging, and scintigraphy. Management includes drainage, débridement, elimination of the source of infection, antibiotics (guided by culture and sensitivity testing), supportive care, and surgical reconstruction. Early diagnosis and prompt treatment are important for achieving favorable patient outcomes.

Chronic Osteomyelitis

Fig. **3.15**

The chronic phase of osteomyelitis generally is defined as a diffuse, medullary bone infection that persists longer than 1 month after the onset of symptoms. However, some forms of **chronic osteomyelitis** apparently arise *de novo* without an acute phase. Chronic osteomyelitis may be suppurative or nonsuppurative. Within the jaws, it usually results from long-standing odontogenic infection, inadequately treated fracture, or postextraction complications. Clinical findings include deep pain, indurated swelling, paresthesia or anesthesia of the inferior alveolar nerve, cervical lymphadenopathy, fever, malaise, and anorexia. As the infection progresses, fistula formation, necrotic bone exfoliation, tooth mobility, trismus, malocclusion, and pathologic fracture may develop. Plain radiography typically exhibits an ill-defined, patchy mixed radiolucency/radiopacity. New periosteal bone formation, cortical expansion or erosion, sequestra, and involucra (new bone enveloping nonvital bone) also may be evident. Further evaluation typically includes computed tomography as well, at times supplemented by magnetic resonance imaging or scintigraphy.

■ Figure **3.13**
Ludwig Angina

(A) Prominent submental and neck swelling with associated erythema. (B) Swelling resolved after treatment, including incision and drainage (drain shown here), eliminating the underlying source of infection, intravenous antibiotics, fluid management, and nutritional support.

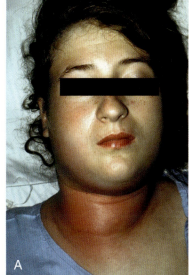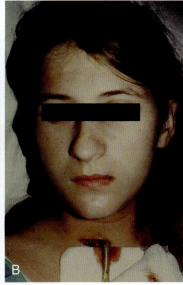

■ Figure **3.14**
Acute Osteomyelitis With Sequestra

Ill-defined radiolucency with associated opacities in the mandible.

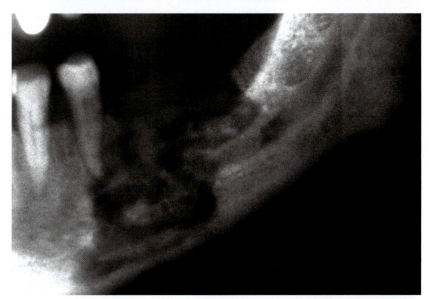

■ Figure **3.15**
Chronic Osteomyelitis

Ill-defined radiolucency in the posterior mandible after tooth extraction.

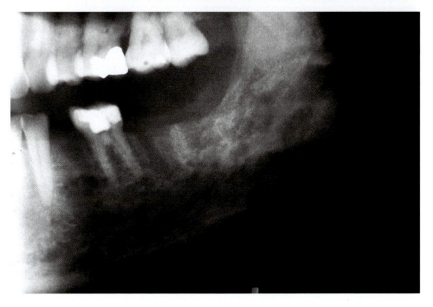

Microscopic examination shows chronically or subacutely inflamed granulation tissue occupying the intertrabecular areas of the bone. In addition, portions of nonvital bone (sequestra) and pockets of abscess formation may be noted. Treatment involves surgical removal of all infected tissue down to vital, bleeding bone; management of the underlying source of infection; antibiotics (typically over an extended period and guided by culture and sensitivity testing); supportive care; and surgical reconstruction. Hyperbaric oxygen therapy may be considered for refractory cases.

Sclerosing Osteomyelitis

Fig. **3.16**

Some cases of chronic osteomyelitis stimulate sclerosis of the surrounding bone. This sclerosis may be localized or diffuse. Within the jaws, several subtypes of chronic osteomyelitis have been described, which are characterized by varying degrees of sclerosis, rarefaction, and/or periosteal hyperplasia. These subtypes include diffuse sclerosing osteomyelitis, focal sclerosing osteomyelitis (condensing osteitis), proliferative periostitis, primary chronic osteomyelitis, and secondary chronic osteomyelitis. In addition, some authors use the term *diffuse sclerosing osteomyelitis* descriptively in reference to the radiographic appearance of several disease subtypes. The differential diagnosis for diffuse sclerosis of the jaws also includes florid cemento-osseous dysplasia; however, this condition is primarily a fibro-osseous condition, with infection and osteomyelitis sometimes developing secondarily in late stages of the disease.

Condensing Osteitis

Fig. **3.17**

Condensing osteitis (focal sclerosing osteomyelitis, focal sclerosing osteitis) presents as a localized area of bone sclerosis that forms in response to a low-grade inflammatory stimulus. The inflammation usually arises from a tooth with pulpitis (caused by a large carious lesion or deep restoration) or pulpal necrosis. The condition occurs over a broad age range, with a predilection for young patients and the premolar/molar region of the mandible. Clinically, no expansion is evident. Radiographic examination shows an area of opacification surrounding the apex of the inflamed tooth. No radiolucent rim is evident; this feature aids in distinction from focal cemento-osseous dysplasia. In addition, there may be concurrent widening of the periodontal ligament. Treatment requires elimination of the underlying odontogenic infection, usually by extraction or endodontic therapy. Following appropriate treatment, there is usually partial or total resolution of the lesion over time.

Proliferative Periostitis

Fig. **3.18**

Proliferative periostitis (periostitis ossificans or so-called "Garrè's osteomyelitis") represents a periosteal reaction to the presence of inflammation. This condition exhibits a marked predilection for children and young adults. Gnathic cases often are caused by underlying odontogenic infection, especially originating from a mandibular molar. In addition, the condition may arise in association with traumatic jaw fracture, tooth extraction, periodontal disease, inflamed cysts, third molar pericoronitis, dental follicles, developing unerupted teeth, and neoplasms (e.g., Langerhans cell histiocytosis, Ewing sarcoma, osteosarcoma). Radiographic examination shows an area of cortical bone thickening produced by parallel layers of new periosteal bone formation. Although not always evident, the classic "onion-skinning" pattern may be best demonstrated by occlusal radiographs. Other possible radiographic findings include cortical consolidation with fine, radiating trabeculae or coarse trabeculae. The original cortex and contour of the bone may or may not be evident. Clinically, the patient exhibits a bony, hard swelling that may be asymptomatic or tender. Treatment involves addressing the underlying inflammatory stimulus. Infected teeth typically require extraction or endodontic therapy. Over time, bone remodeling gradually produces a normal bone contour. If no infection is evident, then biopsy should be performed to rule out underlying neoplasia or other conditions.

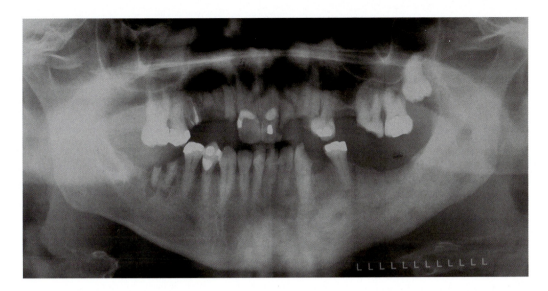

■ Figure **3.16**
Sclerosing Osteomyelitis
Diffuse opacification of the anterior and left posterior mandible.

■ Figure **3.17**
Condensing Osteitis
Periapical opacification in association with a nonvital mandibular first molar.

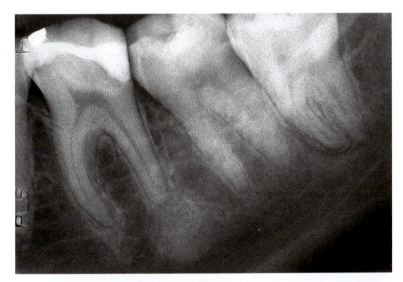

■ Figure **3.18**
Proliferative Periostitis
New periosteal bone formation *(arrow)* along the inferior border of the right posterior mandible. The underlying inflammatory stimulus was infection of the right mandibular first molar.

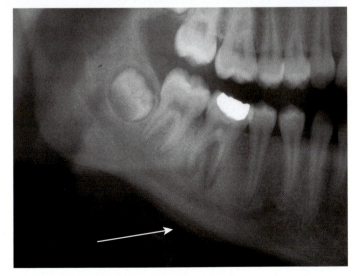

Bibliography

Pulp Stones

da Silva EJ, Prado MC, Queiroz PM, et al. Assessing pulp stones by cone-beam computed tomography. *Clin Oral Investig.* 2016;Dec 9, [Epub ahead of print].

Goga R, Chandler NP, Oginni AO. Pulp stones: a review. *Int Endod J.* 2008;41:457–468.

Hyperplastic Pulpitis

Calişkan MK, Oztop F, Calişkan G. Histological evaluation of teeth with hyperplastic pulpitis caused by trauma or caries: case reports. *Int Endod J.* 2003;36:64–70.

Levin LG, Law AS, Holland GR. Identify and define all diagnostic terms for pulpal health and disease states. *J Endod.* 2009;35:1645–1657.

Palatal Abscess

Standring S. Oral cavity. In: *Gray's Anatomy. The Anatomical Basis of Clinical Practice.* 41th ed. St. Louis: Elsevier; 2016:507–533.e1, [Chapter 31].

Tronstad L. The apical periodontium. In: *Clinical Endodontics: A Textbook.* 2nd ed. Stuttgart: Thieme; 2003:31–64, [Chapter 2].

Parulis

Neville BW, Damm DD, Allen CM, Chi AC. Periapical abscess. In: *Oral and Maxillofacial Pathology.* 4th ed. St. Louis: Elsevier; 2016:123–126.

Cutaneous Sinus

Giménez-García R, Martinez-Vera F, Fuentes-Vera L. Cutaneous sinus tracts of odontogenic origin: two case reports. *J Am Board Fam Med.* 2015;28:838–840.

Kishore Kumar RV, Devireddy SK, Gali RS, et al. Cutaneous sinuses of cervicofacial region: a clinical study of 200 cases. *J Maxillofac Oral Surg.* 2012;11:411–415.

Lee EY, Kang JY, Kim KW, et al. Clinical characteristics of odontogenic cutaneous fistulas. *Ann Dermatol.* 2016;28:417–421.

Periapical Inflammatory Disease (Periapical Granuloma, Periapical Scar, Periapical Cyst, Residual Periapical Cyst)

Bernardi L, Visioli F, Nör C, et al. Radicular cyst: an update of the biological factors related to lining epithelium. *J Endod.* 2015;41:1951–1961.

Carrillo C, Penarrocha M, Ortega B, et al. Correlation of radiographic size and the presence of radiopaque lamina with histological findings in 70 periapical lesions. *J Oral Maxillofac Surg.* 2008;66:1600–1605.

Gao L, Wang XL, Li SM, et al. Decompression as a treatment for odontogenic cystic lesions of the jaw. *J Oral Maxillofac Surg.* 2014;72:327–333.

García CC, Sempere FV, Diago MP, et al. The post-endodontic periapical lesion: histologic and etiopathogenic aspects. *Med Oral Patol Oral Cir Bucal.* 2007;12:E585–E590.

Lin LM, Huang GTJ. Pathobiology of apical periodontitis. In: *Cohen's Pathways of the Pulp.* 11th ed. St. Louis: Elsevier; 2016:630–659, [Chapter 15].

Lin LM, Ricucci D, Lin J, et al. Nonsurgical root canal therapy of large cyst-like inflammatory periapical lesions and inflammatory apical cysts. *J Endod.* 2009;35:607–615.

Peñarrocha M, Carrillo C, Peñarrocha M, et al. Symptoms before periapical surgery related to histologic diagnosis and postoperative healing at 12 months for 178 periapical lesions. *J Oral Maxillofac Surg.* 2011;69:e31–e37.

Pitcher B, Alaqla A, Noujeim M, et al. Binary decision trees for preoperative periapical cyst screening using cone-beam computed tomography. *J Endod.* 2017;43:383–388.

Santos Soares SM, Brito-Júnior M, de Souza FK, et al. Management of cyst-like periapical lesions by orthograde decompression and long-term calcium hydroxide/chlorhexidine intracanal dressing: a case series. *J Endod.* 2016;42:1135–1141.

Tavares DP, Rodrigues JT, Dos Santos TC, et al. Clinical and radiological analysis of a series of periapical cysts and periapical granulomas diagnosed in a Brazilian population. *J Clin Exp Dent.* 2017;9:e129–e135.

Ludwig Angina

Botha A, Jacobs F, Postma C. Retrospective analysis of etiology and comorbid diseases associated with Ludwig's angina. *Ann Maxillofac Surg.* 2015;5:168–173.

Jaworsky D, Reynolds S, Chow AW. Extracranial head and neck infections. *Crit Care Clin.* 2013;29:443–446.

Lin HW, O'Neill A, Cunningham MJ. Ludwig's angina in the pediatric population. *Clin Pediatr (Phila).* 2009;48:583–587.

Osteomyelitis (Acute Osteomyelitis, Chronic Osteomyelitis, and Sclerosing Osteomyelitis)

Baltensperger M, Eyrich GK. Osteomyelitis of the jaws: definition and classification. In: Baltensperger M, Eyrich GK, eds. *Osteomyelitis of the Jaws.* Berlin: Springer-Verlag; 2009:5–56, [Chapter 2].

Dym H, Zeidan J. Microbiology of acute and chronic osteomyelitis and antibiotic treatment. *Dent Clin North Am.* 2017;61:271–282.

Koorbusch GF, Deatherage JR, Curé JK. How can we diagnose and treat osteomyelitis of the jaws as early as possible? *Oral Maxillofac Surg Clin North Am.* 2011;23:557–567.

Condensing Osteitis

Eliasson S, Halvarsson C, Ljungheimer C. Periapical condensing osteitis and endodontic treatment. *Oral Surg Oral Med Oral Pathol.* 1984;57:195–199.

Eversole LR, Stone CE, Strub D. Focal sclerosing osteomyelitis/focal periapical osteopetrosis: radiographic patterns. *Oral Surg Oral Med Oral Pathol.* 1984;58:456–460.

Green TL, Walton RE, Clark JM, et al. Histologic examination of condensing osteitis in cadaver specimens. *J Endod.* 2013;39:977–979.

Proliferative Periostitis

Kannan SK, Sandhya G, Selvarani R. Periostitis ossificans (Garrè's osteomyelitis) radiographic study of two cases. *Int J Paediatr Dent.* 2006;16:59–64.

Kawai T, Hiranuma H, Kishino M, et al. Gross periostitis ossificans in mandibular osteomyelitis. Review of the English literature and radiographic variation. *Oral Surg Oral Med Oral Pathol Oral Radiol Endod.* 1998;86:376–381.

Kawai T, Murakami S, Sakuda M, Fuchihata H. Radiographic investigation of mandibular periostitis ossificans in 55 cases. *Oral Surg Oral Med Oral Pathol Oral Radiol Endod.* 1996;82:704–712.

4

Periodontal Pathology

Gingivitis is a general term that refers to inflammation of the gingivae. The condition is prevalent worldwide. Most cases of gingivitis are plaque-related, although several non–plaque-related forms also are recognized. Plaque-related gingivitis typically develops when poor oral hygiene results in accumulation of dental plaque and calculus. In addition, the clinical presentation of plaque-related gingivitis can be modified by various systemic factors, such as endocrine influences (e.g., puberty, menstrual cycle, pregnancy, diabetes mellitus); medications (e.g., phenytoin, calcium channel blockers, cyclosporine, oral contraceptives); hematologic disorders; and malnutrition (e.g., vitamin C deficiency). Furthermore, local factors that may contribute to gingivitis include trauma, dental crowding, tooth fracture, dental prostheses/appliances, defective dental restorations, and mouth breathing. Studies also suggest that the host response plays an important role in the etiopathogenesis of gingivitis.

Gingival inflammation can be acute or chronic, and it can be either localized or generalized. In some cases, the inflammation may be confined to the gingival margin *(marginal gingivitis)* or interdental papillae *(papillary gingivitis)*, whereas in other cases there may be diffuse involvement of the gingival margin, attached gingiva, and interdental papillae *(diffuse gingivitis)*. Clinical features of gingivitis include erythema, swelling, bleeding on gentle probing, blunting of the interdental papillae, boggy to firm consistency, and loss of stippling.

Management typically includes professionally administered plaque control, oral hygiene reinforcement, and addressing modifiable systemic or local factors. Twice daily tooth brushing and once daily interdental cleaning (with an interdental brush or dental floss) are recommended, and adjunctive chemical plaque control agents (such as chlorhexidine or essential oil-containing mouthwash) may be beneficial.

Localized Juvenile Spongiotic Gingival Hyperplasia (Localized Juvenile Spongiotic Gingivitis, Juvenile Spongiotic Gingivitis)

Fig. **4.3**

Initially described in 2007, **localized juvenile spongiotic gingival hyperplasia** represents a type of inflammatory gingival hyperplasia with distinctive clinicopathologic features. The etiology is unknown, although some investigators have suggested that the condition results from exteriorization of the junctional or sulcular epithelium, with secondary changes caused by local irritating factors (such as mouth breathing). Notably, the alteration does not appear to be plaque-related and does not respond to improved oral hygiene.

Clinically, the condition typically appears as a bright red, slightly raised lesion on the facial gingiva of a young patient. The majority of reported cases have occurred in children and adolescents (average age: 12 years, range: 5 to 39 years), with a female-to-male ratio of 1.3 : 1. There is a strong predilection for the anterior maxillary gingiva. The alteration generally involves the attached gingiva and free gingival margin overlying a tooth root, although some examples primarily involve the interdental papilla. Most patients exhibit a solitary, localized lesion measuring 2 to 10 mm in diameter; however, multifocal or more diffuse involvement also is possible. The surface may appear velvety, granular, pebbly, or papillary. The lesion is usually painless but may bleed easily upon manipulation. In one study, 15% of affected patients had orthodontic brackets, although this finding could be coincidental.

Most reported cases have been treated by conservative excision, with a recurrence rate of 6% to 25%. Isolated examples have been managed by laser treatment or cryotherapy. The paucity of cases occurring in adults suggests that spontaneous resolution is likely, albeit after an unpredictable time period.

■ Figure **4.1**
Gingivitis
Diffuse inflammation of the maxillary and mandibular gingivae.

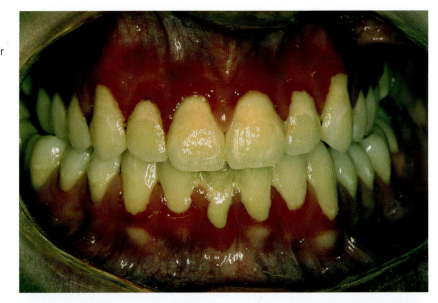

■ Figure **4.2**
Gingivitis
Inflammation of the marginal gingiva.

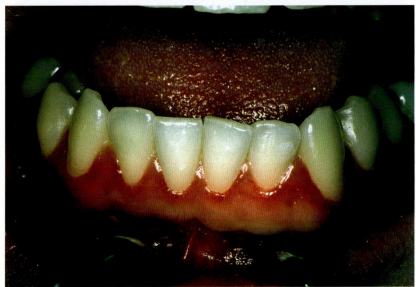

■ Figure **4.3**
Localized Juvenile Spongiotic Gingival Hyperplasia
Bright red alteration of the anterior maxillary gingiva in a young patient who was receiving orthodontic treatment. (Courtesy Dr. Drane Oliphant.)

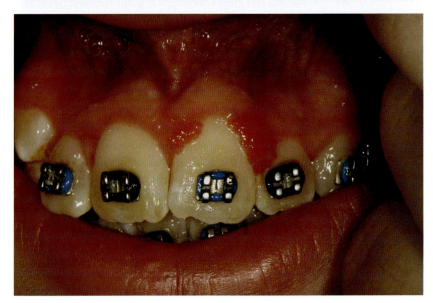

Necrotizing ulcerative gingivitis (Vincent infection, trench mouth, acute necrotizing ulcerative gingivitis) is a distinctive type of gingivitis, characterized by rapid onset of gingival pain, interproximal gingival necrosis, and bleeding. This condition belongs to a group of necrotizing diseases, which also includes necrotizing ulcerative periodontitis, necrotizing stomatitis, and noma. The prevalence of necrotizing ulcerative gingivitis has varied over time, with particularly high rates noted among military populations during the First and Second World Wars. Predisposing factors include smoking, poor oral hygiene, stress, malnutrition, inadequate sleep, preceding illness (e.g., measles), and immunosuppression (e.g., human immunodeficiency virus infection). The microbial profile is complex, with high levels of spirochetes, fusiform bacteria, and *Prevotella intermedia.*

Necrotizing ulcerative gingivitis may occur at any age. However, in the United States and Europe, the disease tends to occur in young to middle-aged adults. In contrast, in developing countries, young children suffering from malnutrition are often affected. Patients typically complain of intense pain. Clinical examination shows marked inflammation, edema, and hemorrhage of the interdental and marginal gingivae. In the early stages, there only may be ulceration of the tip of the interdental papillae; however, with progression, the papillae become overtly blunted, with characteristic "punched-out" or crater-like necrosis covered by a gray-tan pseudomembrane. Other findings may include a fetid odor, cervical lymphadenopathy, fever, and malaise.

In the acute phase, patients typically are treated by débridement under local anesthesia. Rinsing with chlorhexidine, warm saltwater, or diluted hydrogen peroxide may be beneficial; also, adjunctive systemic antibiotics (such as metronidazole or amoxicillin) may be prescribed, particularly if the patient is immunocompromised or exhibits systemic signs of infection (i.e., fever, malaise, lymphadenopathy). Supportive care includes analgesics, rest, fluid intake, and a soft nutritious diet. Oral hygiene instruction and tobacco counseling also should be provided. There is often dramatic resolution within a few days of receiving appropriate treatment. Once the acute inflammation has subsided, management typically includes additional débridement, more comprehensive evaluation of periodontal and systemic health, and periodontal maintenance.

Plasma Cell Gingivitis

Fig. **4.6**

Plasma cell gingivitis (atypical gingivostomatitis) is an unusual form of gingivitis, characterized by rapid onset and a diffuse inflammatory infiltrate predominantly composed of plasma cells. Although the etiology is poorly understood, many cases appear to represent a hypersensitivity reaction. Potential stimuli include flavoring agents in chewing gum or candy, herbal toothpaste, certain spices (such as pepper or cardamom), and khat. The condition generally is not considered to be plaque-related, although some authors have suggested the possibility of an allergic response to bacteria. Patients typically complain of soreness, pain, or burning. Clinical examination usually shows diffuse, bright red swelling of the entire free and attached gingivae. There is often a sharp line of demarcation along the mucogingival junction. On occasion, involvement of additional sites (such as the vestibules, palate, lips, and tongue) may be evident as well. Management involves identification and removal of allergenic stimuli. A complete history (including a review of foods, beverages, oral hygiene products, tobacco, gum/candy, medications), systematic elimination of potential allergens, and/or allergy testing may be helpful. If no underlying cause is identified, then topical or systemic corticosteroids may be administered; however, response to such treatment is variable. In addition, inconsistent results have been reported with conventional plaque control measures (such as scaling, oral hygiene instruction, and chlorhexidine mouth rinse) or topical fusidic acid.

■ Figure **4.4**
Necrotizing Ulcerative Gingivitis
Inflamed, hemorrhagic gingiva with blunting of the interdental papillae.

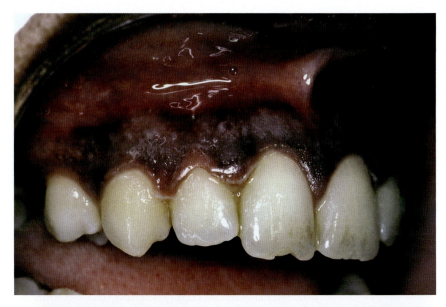

■ Figure **4.5**
Necrotizing Ulcerative Gingivitis
Extensive inflammation and necrosis of the mandibular gingiva.

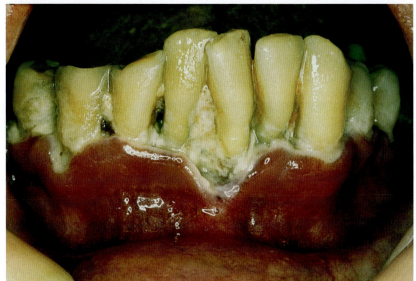

■ Figure **4.6**
Plasma Cell Gingivitis
Diffuse, bright red swelling of the free and attached gingivae in both arches. (Courtesy Dr. Michael Quinn.)

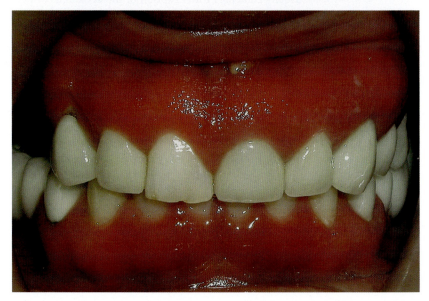

Fig. **4.7**

Foreign body gingivitis refers to gingival inflammation that develops in response to foreign material. During oral hygiene or restorative procedures, there may be damage to the sulcular epithelium, which allows the introduction of foreign matter (e.g., amalgam dust, polishing paste, polishing disk fragments, diatomaceous earth in toothpaste) into the gingival tissues. Patients often complain of pain, swelling, and tenderness; bleeding and tooth sensitivity also may be noted. The lesions may be solitary or multifocal, and they may occur on the marginal gingiva, attached gingiva, and/or interdental papillae. The involved mucosa typically appears red or red-white. Edema, granular surface change, ulceration, and/or atrophy also may be evident. The clinical appearance and histopathologic findings can resemble lichen planus; however, the presence of localized, nonmigrating lesions of the gingiva and the lack of concurrent extragingival involvement would favor foreign body gingivitis over lichen planus. Persistence despite conventional periodontal therapy and improved oral hygiene often prompts biopsy. Histopathologic examination may show granulomatous inflammation, interface mucositis (at times mimicking lichen planus), or a nonspecific mixed inflammatory infiltrate. Depending on particle size, foreign material may or may not be evident on light microscopic examination. Topical corticosteroid application may provide symptomatic relief, although many lesions require surgical excision in order to achieve complete resolution. Gingival grafting using a healthy donor site may be considered to repair the surgical defect. As a preventive measure, clinicians should exercise caution when performing procedures that could introduce foreign material into the adjacent soft tissue.

Figs. **4.8 and 4.9**

Gingival fibromatosis is a rare condition in which accumulation of extracellular matrix components causes slowly progressive enlargement of the gingiva. It may be either hereditary or idiopathic, with hereditary examples occurring as an isolated finding or as part of a syndrome (e.g., multiple hamartoma syndrome, Cross syndrome, Murray-Puretic-Drescher syndrome, Rutherfurd syndrome, Zimmermann-Laband syndrome). Extraoral features that can be noted in association with hereditary gingival fibromatosis include hypertrichosis, epilepsy, intellectual disability, and sensorineural hearing loss. Clinically, gingival fibromatosis may be generalized or localized to one or more quadrants; localized examples often involve the maxillary tuberosities or the facial gingivae in the mandibular molar regions. The onset of enlargement usually coincides with eruption of the deciduous or permanent dentition. With progression, the gingival tissue may cover all or part of the tooth crowns and displace teeth. Sequelae may include diastema formation, cross bite, open bite, open-lip posture, over-retained deciduous teeth, and delayed eruption of permanent teeth. The patient may develop problems with mastication, speech, or aesthetics. The gingiva typically is firm, normal in color, nonhemorrhagic, and smooth or finely stippled. However, it may appear erythematous if there is superimposed inflammation due to plaque accumulation. Usually, there is involvement of the free and attached gingivae without extension beyond the mucogingival junction.

Clinical management includes professional prophylaxis and oral hygiene reinforcement in order to minimize exacerbation by plaque-related gingival inflammation. For severe cases, surgical removal of excess gingival tissue may be performed; in addition, because there is a high risk for recurrence in tooth-bearing areas, gingivectomy may be combined with selective tooth extraction. Some clinicians prefer to delay surgery until after the permanent teeth have erupted in order to reduce the risk of recurrence. In addition, orthodontic and prosthodontic treatment may be needed, and genetic counseling is indicated for hereditary cases.

■ Figure **4.7**
Foreign Body Gingivitis
Localized, erythematous swelling of the marginal gingiva in response to foreign material. (Courtesy Dr. Neal Lemmerman.)

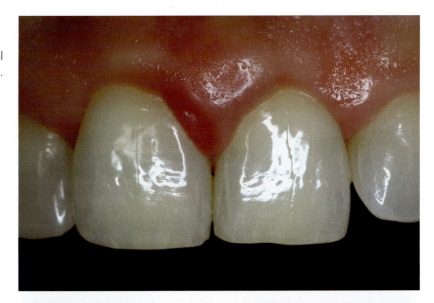

■ Figure **4.8**
Gingival Fibromatosis
Marked enlargement of the maxillary gingiva.

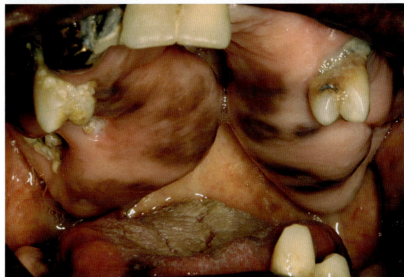

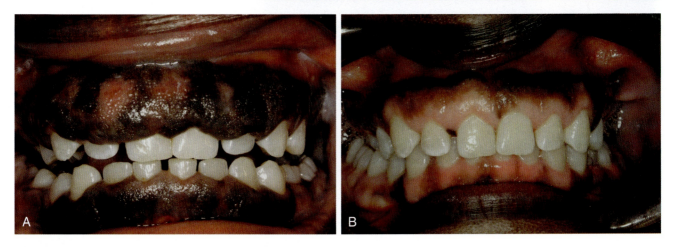

■ Figure **4.9**
Gingival Fibromatosis
(A) Diffuse enlargement of the maxillary and mandibular gingivae, with partial coverage of the tooth crowns. (B) Same patient in image A after professional plaque/calculus removal and gingivectomy. (Courtesy Dr. Lynn Wallace.)

Figs. **4.10–4.12**

Gingival overgrowth may be an adverse effect of various systemic medications. It is best recognized in association with phenytoin, cyclosporine, and nifedipine, although associations with other anticonvulsants, immunosuppressants, and calcium channel blockers have been noted as well. Also, some studies have implicated oral contraceptives and antibiotics. Proposed underlying mechanisms are related to disrupted cellular calcium gradients, altered fibroblast function, elevated proinflammatory cytokines, and reduced matrix metalloproteinases; the end result is increased extracellular matrix (rather than true cellular hyperplasia or hypertrophy). Poor plaque control appears to be an important cofactor. In addition, genetic factors likely play a role, as evidenced by increased or decreased susceptibility in association with certain histo-compatibility leukocyte antigen (HLA) types and other genetic polymorphisms.

Many cases of **drug-induced gingival overgrowth** develop within the first 1 to 3 months of starting drug treatment; in addition, a second peak has been described after 12 months of treatment. The gingival enlargement often begins in the interdental papillae, especially in the anterior and facial segments. With progression, there may be more diffuse gingival overgrowth, with envelopment of part or all of the adjacent tooth crowns. The tissue exhibits varying degrees of fibrosis and inflammation, and the mucosal surface may appear lobulated, smooth, granular, pebbly, or papillary. Some patients experience problems with speech, mastication, and aesthetics. Discontinuation of the offending medication or substitution of another suitable drug may cease progression and, possibly, induce some regression. Plaque control (i.e., with professional cleaning, frequent recall visits, oral hygiene reinforcement, and chlorhexidine rinse) also is beneficial. Some studies have noted improvement of cyclosporine-associated gingival overgrowth after a short course of azithromycin, and other studies have suggested that folic acid may be helpful for the prevention and treatment of drug-induced gingival overgrowth. However, further research is needed. Surgical removal of excess gingival tissue may be considered for severe or refractory cases.

■ Figure **4.10**
Drug-Induced Gingival Overgrowth

Diffuse, fibrotic gingival enlargement with partial coverage of the tooth crowns in a patient taking phenytoin for seizures.

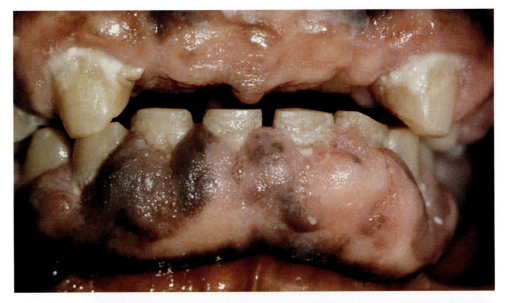

■ Figure **4.11**
Drug-Induced Gingival Overgrowth

Fibrotic and erythematous enlargement of the gingivae with areas of nodularity in a patient taking amlodipine (a calcium channel blocker).

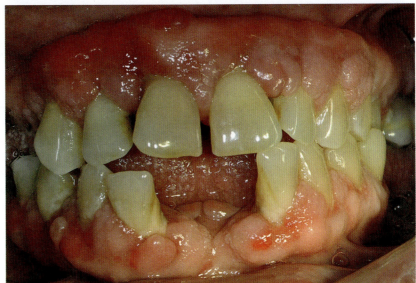

■ Figure **4.12**
Drug-Induced Gingival Overgrowth

Dramatic overgrowth of the maxillary and mandibular gingivae in a renal transplant patient who was taking both cyclosporine and amlodipine. The mucosal surface appears pebbly in many areas. (With appreciation to Dr. Graham Lee.)

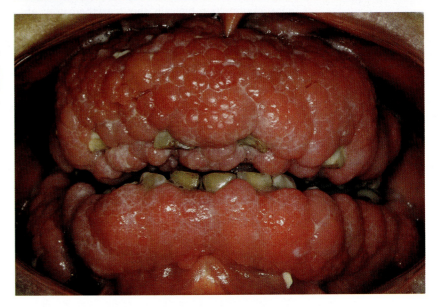

Fig. **4.13**

Periodontitis refers to inflammation of the supporting tissues of the teeth, with accompanying loss of the periodontal ligament attachment and bony support. It is characterized by deep periodontal pocket formation and/or gingival recession. With progression, there is the potential for tooth mobility and tooth loss. The prevalence of periodontitis is difficult to determine because of varying case definitions; however, according to the Centers for Disease Control and Prevention, nearly half of adults in the United States aged 30 years or older have periodontitis. The prevalence increases with age and is greater among males than females. Major risk factors include smoking, genetic predisposition, systemic diseases (e.g., diabetes), and low socioeconomic status. The disease appears to result from a complex interplay between bacterial infection and the host response, often modified by behavioral factors.

In general, periodontitis can be categorized according to extent (localized or generalized) and severity (mild, moderate, or severe). Major types of periodontitis include the following: chronic periodontitis, aggressive periodontitis, periodontitis as a manifestation of systemic diseases, necrotizing ulcerative periodontitis, abscesses of the periodontium, and periodontitis associated with endodontic lesions. Treatment depends on the disease type but generally includes addressing modifiable risk factors, nonsurgical or surgical root débridement, oral hygiene reinforcement, and periodontal maintenance therapy. Additional management may include guided tissue regeneration and local or systemic antibiotics.

Periodontal Abscess

Fig. **4.14**

A **periodontal abscess** is a localized, purulent infection arising in the tissues surrounding a periodontal pocket. The infection causes rapid destruction of the adjacent alveolar bone and periodontal ligament. According to some studies, periodontal abscesses comprise 7% to 14% of dental emergencies. The lesion most often occurs within the context of preexisting periodontitis—either as an acute exacerbation of untreated chronic periodontitis or over the course of treatment for chronic periodontitis. For example, calculus dislodged by scaling may be introduced into the adjacent tissues, or inadequate scaling may reduce inflammation enough to cause occlusion of the gingival margin while calculus remains in deeper portions of the pocket. Other contributory factors include changes in the subgingival flora (e.g., secondary to systemic antibiotic therapy) and decreased host resistance. In addition, some periodontal abscesses arise in the absence of periodontitis as a result of foreign body impaction, local trauma, cemental tears, external root resorption, or anatomic dental anomalies (e.g., dens invaginatus, enamel pearls).

Patients with periodontal abscesses can have mild to severe pain. Other findings may include tenderness on palpation, tooth sensitivity, tooth mobility or extrusion, foul taste, lymphadenopathy, fever, and malaise. Clinical examination typically shows erythematous gingival swelling along the lateral aspect of the root, with associated bleeding on probing. Pus may be expressed from the sulcus upon probing or palpation, or pus may drain from the opening of a sinus tract. Radiographic examination may or may not demonstrate bone loss.

Treatment involves establishing drainage by débriding the pocket (to remove any plaque, calculus, or foreign material) and/or incising the abscess. Management also may include irrigation of the pocket and limited occlusal adjustment. Systemic antibiotics are indicated if the patient exhibits fever or other systemic signs of infection. Supportive care includes analgesics, warm saline rinses, and soft diet. After resolution of the acute infection, any underlying chronic periodontitis should be addressed.

Pericoronitis

Fig. **4.15**

Pericoronitis refers to inflammation of the soft tissue surrounding the crown of a partially erupted or impacted tooth. The mandibular third molar region is most commonly affected. Typically, the condition results from impaction of bacteria and food debris beneath the gingival flap (operculum) overlying the tooth crown. Other potential contributory factors include trauma from the opposing teeth, preceding illness (e.g., upper respiratory tract infection), and stress.

The inflammation may be acute or chronic. Chronic pericoronitis often produces no or only mild symptoms, whereas acute pericoronitis usually causes pain, tenderness, and difficulty eating. The inflamed tissues appear erythematous and swollen. With abscess formation, there can be foul, purulent discharge. Trismus, fever, cervical lymphadenopathy, leukocytosis, and malaise also may be evident. Treatment of

■ Figure **4.13**
Periodontitis

Severe bone loss in association with a mandibular molar.

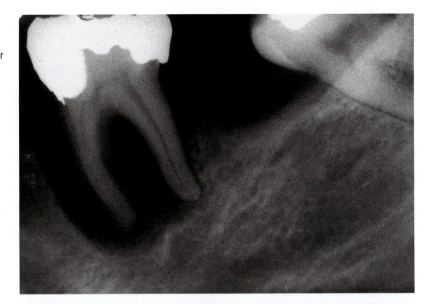

■ Figure **4.14**
Periodontal Abscess

Erythematous, nodular swelling with purulent drainage. (With appreciation to Dr. Kevin Riker.)

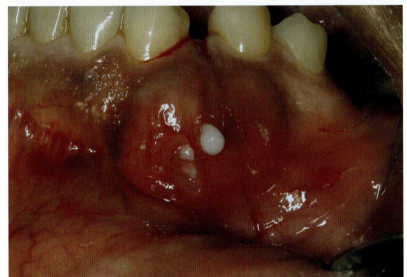

■ Figure **4.15**
Pericoronitis

Erythematous swelling of the soft tissue on the distal-occlusal aspect of an incompletely erupted mandibular third molar.

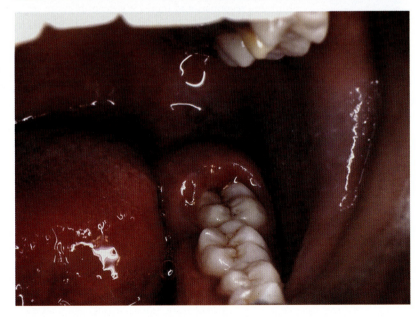

acute pericoronitis includes débridement, abscess drainage, irrigation, and analgesics; if the patient has fever or other systemic signs of infection, then antibiotics may be prescribed. Once the infection is controlled, tooth extraction may be considered. Alternatively, if maintenance of the tooth is desired, then surgical removal of the gingival flap overlying the tooth crown may be performed.

Aggressive Periodontitis

Fig. **4.16**

Aggressive periodontitis represents a group of destructive periodontal diseases characterized by rapid progression. By definition, it is not associated with clinically evident systemic disease. At onset, affected individuals are typically young (<25 years old) and appear otherwise healthy; a familial aggregation of patients suggests underlying genetic factors. Abnormal host immune responses (e.g., neutrophil dysfunction, macrophage hyperresponsiveness) also have been implicated. The microbial profile is heterogeneous and poorly understood; however, in some populations, the JP2 clone of *Aggregatibacter actinomycetemcomitans* appears to play an important role in disease development. Some investigators hypothesize that among genetically susceptible individuals, certain microbial triggers may induce an altered host response, disruption of tissue homeostasis, and microbial imbalance.

Aggressive periodontitis can be localized or generalized. *Localized aggressive periodontitis* is characterized by circumpubertal onset and attachment loss localized to the first molars and incisors (with involvement of no more than two teeth other than the first molars and incisors). There may be a relatively low amount of plaque accumulation despite severe periodontal destruction. Radiographic examination typically shows significant bilateral, symmetric bone loss in the permanent first molar and incisor regions. The bone loss often exhibits a vertical pattern in the first molar region and a horizontal pattern in the incisor region. Over time, the disease may self-arrest, although a subset of individuals can go on to develop *generalized aggressive periodontitis*. The generalized form involves the periodontium of most or all of the permanent dentition; by definition, there should be interproximal attachment loss affecting at least three teeth other than the first molars and incisors. Management of aggressive periodontitis typically includes surgical or nonsurgical root débridement, systemic antibiotics, and frequent maintenance visits.

Papillon-Lefèvre Syndrome

Figs. **4.17 and 4.18**

Papillon-Lefèvre syndrome is a rare, autosomal recessive disorder that is mainly characterized by oral and cutaneous manifestations. Most patients exhibit mutations in the *cathepsin C (CTSC)* gene, located on chromosome 11q14-q21. *CTSC* mutations may alter the growth and development of skin, impair the immune response, and increase susceptibility to infection.

Affected individuals exhibit severe periodontitis in both the deciduous and permanent dentitions. As the deciduous teeth erupt, the gingiva becomes very inflamed, swollen, and boggy. Rapid periodontal destruction ensues, with radiographic examination showing severe alveolar bone loss and teeth that appear to be "floating in air." Most patients exhibit complete loss of the deciduous dentition by 4 to 5 years of age; during this edentulous period, the gingiva returns to a normal state of health. However, aggressive periodontitis reappears with eruption of the permanent teeth, and most patients are edentulous by 15 years of age.

Cutaneous manifestations typically become evident in the first 4 years of life. The most salient finding is palmar and plantar keratosis. Hyperkeratosis also may be evident on the elbows, knees, external malleoli, tibial tuberosities, and dorsal surfaces of the digits. The skin lesions appear as white, yellow, red, or brown plaques with associated crusts, cracks, and fissures. The fissured, thickened plantar skin may cause walking difficulty. Nail dystrophy and superimposed skin infections also may develop. Other possible findings include impaired somatic development, calcification of the falx cerebri and choroid plexus, and hepatic abscesses.

Optimal management requires a multidisciplinary approach, including specialists in pediatric dentistry, periodontics, prosthodontics, dermatology, and pediatric medicine. Early diagnosis and treatment may improve patient outcomes. For management of periodontitis, conventional treatment (scaling, root planning, chlorhexidine rinse, and oral hygiene maintenance) may be combined with systemic antibiotics and extraction of severely affected teeth. Alternatively, some investigators advocate extraction of all deciduous teeth to eliminate periodontal pathogens, followed by antibiotic administration to prevent periodontitis in the permanent dentition. The skin lesions may be treated with systemic retinoids, emollients, topical corticosteroids, or keratolytic agents.

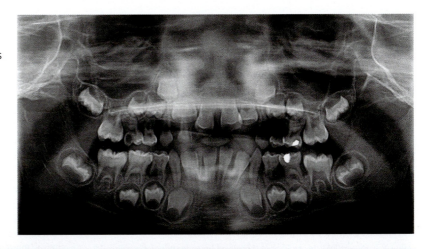

■ Figure **4.16**
Aggressive Periodontitis
Loss of bone support in the molar and incisor regions of a young patient. (Courtesy Dr. Erwin Turner.)

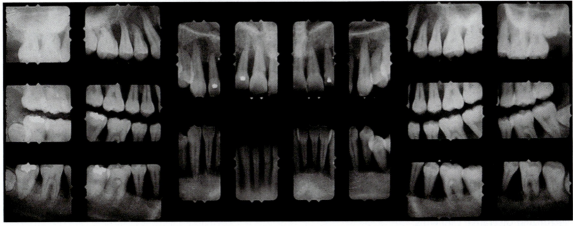

■ Figure **4.17**
Papillon-Lefèvre Syndrome
Severe, generalized bone loss, with some teeth appearing to "float in air." (Courtesy Dr. Román Carlos.)

■ Figure **4.18**
Papillon-Lefèvre Syndrome
Plantar keratosis of both feet. (Courtesy Dr. Román Carlos.)

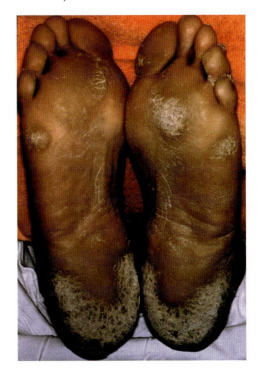

Bibliography

Gingivitis

Armitage G. Development of a classification system for periodontal diseases and conditions. *Ann Periodontol.* 1999;4:1–6.

Chapple IL, Van der Weijden F, Doerfer C, et al. Primary prevention of periodontitis: managing gingivitis. *J Clin Periodontol.* 2015;42(suppl 16): S71–S76.

Fiorellini JP, Stathopoulou PG. Clinical features of gingivitis. In: *Carranza's Clinical Periodontology.* 12th ed. St. Louis: Elsevier Saunders; 2015:224–231, [Chapter 15].

Serrano J, Escribano M, Roldán S, et al. Efficacy of adjunctive anti-plaque chemical agents in managing gingivitis: a systematic review and meta-analysis. *J Clin Periodontol.* 2015;42:S106–S138.

Localized Juvenile Spongiotic Gingival Hyperplasia

Allon I, Lammert KM, Iwase R, et al. Localized juvenile spongiotic gingival hyperplasia possibly originates from the junctional gingival epithelium-an immunohistochemical study. *Histopathology.* 2016;68:549–555.

Chang JY, Kessler HP, Wright JM. Localized juvenile spongiotic gingival hyperplasia. *Oral Surg Oral Med Oral Pathol Oral Radiol Endod.* 2008;106:411–418.

Darling MR, Daley TD, Wilson A, et al. Juvenile spongiotic gingivitis. *J Periodontol.* 2007;78:1235–1240.

Kalogirou EM, Chatzidimitriou K, Tosios KI, et al. Localized juvenile spongiotic gingival hyperplasia: report of two cases. *J Clin Pediatr Dent.* 2017;41:228–231.

Nogueira VK, Fernandes D, Navarro CM, et al. Cryotherapy for localized juvenile spongiotic gingival hyperplasia: preliminary findings on two cases. *Int J Paediatr Dent.* 2017;27:231–235.

Solomon LW, Trahan WR, Snow JE. Localized juvenile spongiotic gingival hyperplasia: a report of 3 cases. *Pediatr Dent.* 2013;35:360–363.

Necrotizing Ulcerative Gingivitis

American Academy of Periodontology. Parameter on acute periodontal diseases. *J Periodontol.* 2000;71(suppl 5):863–866.

Dufty J, Gkranias N, Petrie A, et al. Prevalence and treatment of necrotizing ulcerative gingivitis (NUG) in the British Armed Forces: a case-control study. *Clin Oral Investig.* 2017;21:1935–1944.

Rowland RW. Necrotizing ulcerative gingivitis. *Ann Periodontol.* 1999;4: 65–73, 78.

Atout RN, Todescan S. Managing patients with necrotizing ulcerative gingivitis. *J Can Dent Assoc.* 2013;79:d46.

Plasma Cell Gingivitis

Anil S. Plasma cell gingivitis among herbal toothpaste users: a report of three cases. *J Contemp Dent Pract.* 2007;8:60–66.

Arduino PG, D'Aiuto F, Cavallito C, et al. Professional oral hygiene as a therapeutic option for pediatric patients with plasma cell gingivitis: preliminary results of a prospective case series. *J Periodontol.* 2011;82:1670–1675.

Hedin CA, Karpe B, Larsson A. Plasma-cell gingivitis in children and adults. A clinical and histological description. *Swed Dent J.* 1994;18:117–124.

Jadwat Y, Meyerov R, Lemmer J, et al. Plasma cell gingivitis: does it exist? Report of a case and review of the literature. *SADJ.* 2008;63:394–395.

Kerr DA, McClatchey KD, Regezi JA. Idiopathic gingivostomatitis. Cheilitis, glossitis, gingivitis syndrome; atypical gingivostomatitis, plasma-cell gingivitis, plasmacytosis of gingiva. *Oral Surg Oral Med Oral Pathol.* 1971;32:402–423.

Makkar A, Tewari S, Kishor K, et al. An unusual clinical presentation of plasma cell gingivitis related to "acacia" containing herbal toothpaste. *J Indian Soc Periodontol.* 2013;17:527–530.

Marker P, Krogdahl A. Plasma cell gingivitis apparently related to the use of khat: report of a case. *Br Dent J.* 2002;192:311–313.

Foreign Body Gingivitis

Gordon SC, Daley TD. Foreign body gingivitis: clinical and microscopic features of 61 cases. *Oral Surg Oral Med Oral Pathol Oral Radiol Endod.* 1997;83:562–570.

Gordon SC, Daley TD. Foreign body gingivitis: identification of the foreign material by energy-dispersive x-ray microanalysis. *Oral Surg Oral Med Oral Pathol Oral Radiol Endod.* 1997;83:571–576.

Gravitis K, Daley TD, Lochhead MA. Management of patients with foreign body gingivitis: report of 2 cases with histologic findings. *J Can Dent Assoc.* 2005;71:105–109.

Koh RU, Ko E, Oh TJ, Edwards PC. Foreign body gingivitis. *J Mich Dent Assoc.* 2015;97:44–47.

Koppang HS, Roushan A, Srafilzadeh A, et al. Foreign body gingival lesions: distribution, morphology, identification by X-ray energy dispersive analysis and possible origin of foreign material. *J Oral Pathol Med.* 2007;36:161–172.

Gingival Fibromatosis

DeAngelo S, Murphy J, Claman L, et al. Hereditary gingival fibromatosis–a review. *Compend Contin Educ Dent.* 2007;28:138–143, quiz 144, 152.

Gawron K, Łazarz-Bartyzel K, Potempa J, et al. Gingival fibromatosis: clinical, molecular and therapeutic issues. *Orphanet J Rare Dis.* 2016;11:9.

Häkkinen L, Csiszar A. Hereditary gingival fibromatosis: characteristics and novel putative pathogenic mechanisms. *J Dent Res.* 2007;86:25–34.

Hennekam RCM, Krantz ID, Allanson JE. Syndromes with gingival/ periodontal components. In: *Gorlin's Syndromes of the Head and Neck.* 5th ed. Oxford: Oxford University Press; 2010:1210–1224, [Chapter 27].

Ko YC, Farr JB, Yoon A, Philipone E. Idiopathic Gingival Fibromatosis: Case Report and Review of the Literature. *Am J Dermatopathol.* 2016;38:e68–e71.

Poulopoulos A, Kittas D, Sarigelou A. Current concepts on gingival fibromatosis-related syndromes. *J Investig Clin Dent.* 2011;2:156–161.

Drug-Induced Gingival Overgrowth

Bondon-Guitton E, Bagheri H, Montastruc JL. Drug-induced gingival overgrowth: a study in the French Pharmacovigilance Database. *J Clin Periodontol.* 2012;39:513–518.

Brown RS, Arany PR. Mechanism of drug-induced gingival overgrowth revisited: a unifying hypothesis. *Oral Dis.* 2015;21:e51–e61.

Dongari-Bagtzoglou A, Research, Science and Therapy Committee, American Academy of Periodontology. Drug-associated gingival enlargement. *J Periodontol.* 2004;75:1424–1431.

Eggerath J, English H, Leichter JW. Drug-associated gingival enlargement: case report and review of aetiology, management and evidence-based outcomes of treatment. *J N Z Soc Periodontol.* 2005;88:7–14.

Hatahira H, Abe J, Hane Y, et al. Drug-induced gingival hyperplasia: a retrospective study using spontaneous reporting system databases. *J Pharm Health Care Sci.* 2017;3:19.

Rafiee RM. DIGO: drug-induced gingival overgrowth. Part I: clinical features and pharmacology. *J West Soc Periodontol Periodontal Abstr.* 2010;58(3):67–70.

Rafiee RM. DIGO: drug-induced gingival overgrowth. Part II: molecular mechanism. *J West Soc Periodontol Periodontal Abstr.* 2010;58:99–101.

Periodontitis

American Academy of Periodontology Task Force. Report on the update to the 1999 classification of periodontal diseases and conditions. *J Periodontol.* 2015;86:835–838.

Armitage GC. Development of a classification system for periodontal diseases and conditions. *Ann Periodontol.* 1999;4:1–6.

Burt B, Research, Science and Therapy Committee of the American Academy of Periodontology. Position paper: epidemiology of periodontal diseases. *J Periodontol.* 2005;76:1406–1419.

Eke PI, Dye BA, Wei L, et al. Update on prevalence of periodontitis in adults in the United States: NHANES 2009 to 2012. *J Periodontol.* 2015;86:611–622.

Periodontal Abscess

American Academy of Periodontology. Parameter on acute periodontal diseases. *J Periodontol.* 2000;71(suppl 5):863–866.

Herrera D, Alonso B, de Arriba L, et al. Acute periodontal lesions. *Periodontol 2000.* 2014;65:149–177.

Herrera D, Roldán S, González I, et al. The periodontal abscess (I). Clinical and microbiological findings. *J Clin Periodontol.* 2000;27:387–394.

Herrera D, Roldán S, Sanz M. The periodontal abscess: a review. *J Clin Periodontol.* 2000;27:377–386.

Jaramillo A, Arce RM, Herrera D, et al. Clinical and microbiological characterization of periodontal abscesses. *J Clin Periodontol.* 2005;32:1213–1218.

Marquez IC. How do I manage a patient with periodontal abscess? *J Can Dent Assoc.* 2013;79:d8.

Pericoronitis

Bradshaw S, Faulk J, Blakey GH, et al. Quality of life outcomes after third molar removal in subjects with minor symptoms of pericoronitis. *J Oral Maxillofac Surg.* 2012;70:2494–2500.

Folayan MO, Ozeigbe EO, Onyejaeka N, et al. Non-third molar related pericoronitis in a sub-urban Nigeria population of children. *Niger J Clin Pract.* 2014;17:18–22.

Magraw CB, Golden B, Phillips C, et al. Pain with pericoronitis affects quality of life. *J Oral Maxillofac Surg.* 2015;73:7–12.

Neville BW, Damm DD, Allen CM, et al. Pericoronitis. In: *Oral and Maxillofacial Pathology.* 4th ed. St. Louis: Elsevier; 2016:156–157.

Aggressive Periodontitis

Albandar JM. Aggressive and acute periodontal diseases. *Periodontol 2000.* 2014;65:7–12.

Albandar JM. Aggressive periodontitis: case definition and diagnostic criteria. *Periodontol 2000.* 2014;65:13–26.

American Academy of Periodontology. Parameter on aggressive periodontitis. *J Periodontol.* 2000;71(suppl 5):867–869.

Califano JV, Research, Science and Therapy Committee American Academy of Periodontology. Position paper: periodontal diseases of children and adolescents. *J Periodontol.* 2003;74:1696–1704.

Könönen E, Müller HP. Microbiology of aggressive periodontitis. *Periodontol 2000.* 2014;65:46–78.

Nibali L. Aggressive periodontitis: microbes and host response, who to blame? *Virulence.* 2015;6:223–228.

Sgolastra F, Petrucci A, Gatto R, et al. Effectiveness of systemic amoxicillin/metronidazole as an adjunctive therapy to full-mouth scaling and root planing in the treatment of aggressive periodontitis: a systematic review and meta-analysis. *J Periodontol.* 2012;83:731–743.

Papillon-Lefèvre Syndrome

Hennekam RCM, Krantz ID, Allanson JE. Hyperkeratosis palmoplantaris and periodontoclasia in childhood (Papillon-Lefèvre syndrome and Haim-Munk syndrome). In: *Gorlin's Syndromes of the Head and Neck.* 5th ed. Oxford: Oxford University Press; 2010:1219–1222.

Papillon MM, Lefèvre P. Deux cas de keratoderma palmaire et plantaire symmetrique familiale (maladie de Meleda) chez le frere et la soeur: coexistence dans les deux cas d'alterations dentaires graves. *Bull Soc Fr Dermatol Syph.* 1924;31:82–87.

Pimentel SP, Kolbe MF, Pereira RS, et al. Papillon-Lefèvre syndrome in 2 siblings: case report after 11-year follow-up. *Pediatr Dent.* 2012;34:e231–e236.

Sreeramulu B, Shyam ND, Ajay P, et al. Papillon-Lefèvre syndrome: clinical presentation and management options. *Clin Cosmet Investig Dent.* 2015;7:75–81.

5

Bacterial Infections

Fig. **5.1**

Tonsillitis refers to inflammation of the tonsils. The tonsils form a ring of lymphoid tissue *(Waldeyer ring)* in the pharynx, consisting of the palatine tonsils, adenoids, lingual tonsils, and tubal tonsils. However, by convention, the terms "tonsillitis" and "tonsils" often are used when specifically referring to the palatine tonsils, which are located between the palatoglossal and palatopharyngeal folds in the lateral walls of the oropharynx.

Tonsillitis can be acute or chronic. Acute tonsillitis primarily affects pediatric patients and may be caused by various pathogens (e.g., *Streptococcus pyogenes*, *Haemophilus influenzae*, adenovirus, influenza virus, parainfluenza virus, enteroviruses, Epstein-Barr virus, herpes simplex virus). There is typically a sudden onset of sore throat. Other possible findings include dysphagia, tonsillar hyperplasia, cervical lymphadenopathy, halitosis, fever, and headache. With acute viral infection, there may be cough, coryza, and conjunctivitis. In addition, children with acute tonsillitis sometimes experience abdominal pain and vomiting. Clinical examination typically shows swelling and erythema of the palatine tonsils, at times accompanied by pus or a yellow-white exudate. Potential complications include airway obstruction and peritonsillar or parapharyngeal abscess formation. With streptococcal infection, further potential sequelae include scarlet fever, rheumatic fever, and glomerulonephritis. Patients with chronic tonsillitis may develop cervical lymphadenopathy and tonsilloliths (see next section).

Rapid antigen testing or cultures may aid in the diagnosis of streptococcal infection, which usually is treated with antibiotics (e.g., penicillin) and supportive therapy. Acute viral tonsillitis is managed by supportive therapy (i.e., rest, fluids, warm salt water gargle, topical anesthetics, single-dose dexamethasone, acetaminophen, and/or ibuprofen). Chronic tonsillitis may respond to broad-spectrum antibiotic therapy. Tonsillectomy may be considered for patients with recurrent, persistent, or severe disease.

Figs. **5.2 and 5.3**

A **tonsillolith** represents a calcified nidus of debris within the tonsils. Bacteria, desquamated epithelial cells, food debris, and other matter frequently become impacted within the *tonsillar crypts* (or tonsillar surface invaginations). If this impacted matter (or "tonsillar plug") undergoes calcification, a tonsillolith forms. Tonsilloliths are quite common; using computed tomography (CT), investigators have detected these calcifications in 15% to 46% of individuals.

Tonsilloliths have been reported over a broad age range, with a mean of approximately 46 years. They may be unilateral or bilateral. Most tonsilloliths are relatively small and asymptomatic. However, patients with larger tonsilloliths may complain of halitosis, foul taste, a foreign body–like sensation, dysphagia, odynophagia, sore throat, irritable cough, or otalgia. Rare complications include abscess formation and aspiration pneumonia. Upon clinical examination, a yellow-white, hard mass may be evident. Tonsilloliths may be noted incidentally during radiographic examination performed for other reasons. On panoramic radiographs, they may appear as radiopacities superimposed on the midportion of the ascending ramus of the mandible; radiographs (such as CT images) taken from various angles may help to avoid confusion with intraosseous pathology. CT scans are more sensitive than plain radiographs for demonstrating tonsilloliths and may help to rule out other entities in the differential diagnosis (e.g., elongated styloid process, prominent hamulus, calcified stylohyoid ligament, prominent maxillary tuberosity, idiopathic osteosclerosis, phleboliths, sialoliths of the parotid glands, calcified intraparotid lymph nodes).

Asymptomatic tonsilloliths require no treatment. Some patients may be able to remove them simply by gargling with warm salt water. For symptomatic cases, enucleation of superficial stones or tonsillectomy for deep-seated, larger stones may be performed.

■ Figure **5.1**
Tonsillitis

Markedly enlarged palatine tonsils that meet in the midline. (Courtesy Rachel Huffman.)

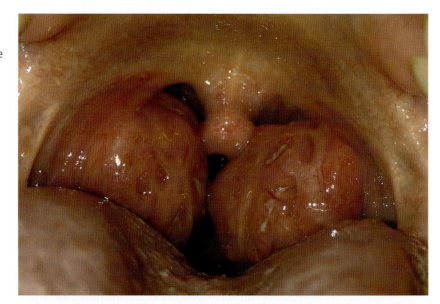

■ Figure **5.2**
Tonsilloliths

Enlarged palatine tonsil with prominent crypts exhibiting focal yellowish-white calcifications.

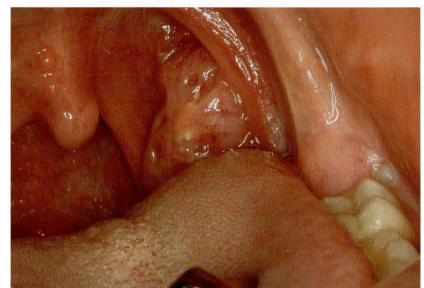

■ Figure **5.3**
Tonsilloliths

Panoramic radiograph showing radiopacities superimposed on the right and left posterior mandible. (Courtesy Dr. Fred Howard.)

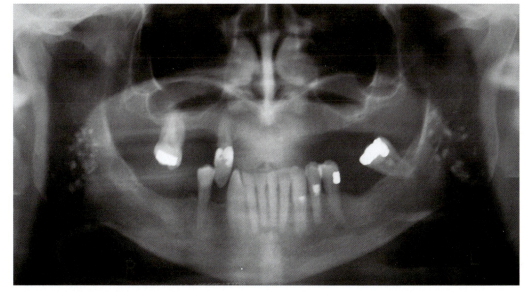

Fig. **5.4**

Impetigo is a superficial skin infection primarily caused by *Staphylococcus aureus* and/or *Streptococcus pyogenes*. Predisposing factors include trauma, preexisting dermatitis, insect bites, poor hygiene, hot and humid climates, crowded living conditions, diabetes, and human immunodeficiency virus infection. Impetigo tends to arise in pediatric patients and exhibits two major clinical patterns: nonbullous and bullous. The nonbullous form comprises approximately 70% of cases and most frequently involves the extremities and face. The lesions initially appear as red macules with associated vesicle formation. The vesicles readily rupture and become covered by an amber or honey-colored crust. Such lesions involving the perioral skin may mimic herpes labialis. However, nonbullous impetigo is typically pruritic, whereas herpes labialis tends to be more painful. Bullous impetigo most often involves the trunk, extremities, intertriginous areas, and face. It is characterized by large, flaccid blisters filled with clear or purulent fluid. These blisters usually rupture to form a brown, lacquer-like crust.

For limited nonbullous disease, topical antibiotics (e.g., mupirocin, fusidic acid, retapamulin) are effective. Patients with bullous or extensive nonbullous disease typically receive systemic antibiotic therapy (e.g., amoxicillin/clavulanate, cephalexin, dicloxacillin). If infection with methicillin-resistant *S. aureus* is suspected, trimethoprim/sulfamethoxazole, clindamycin, or a tetracycline is recommended, pending culture and sensitivity results. Preventive measures include avoiding contact with infected individuals and practicing proper hygiene (e.g., handwashing, cleaning minor skin injuries with soap and water, regular bathing, no sharing of clothing or towels). Impetigo is generally self-limiting. However, in rare cases, there may be serious complications (e.g., cellulitis, lymphangitis, septicemia, poststreptococcal glomerulonephritis).

Figs. **5.5 and 5.6**

Tuberculosis is an infectious disease caused by *Mycobacterium tuberculosis* complex. The annual worldwide incidence of tuberculosis has been declining for over a decade; nevertheless, the World Health Organization estimates that in 2015 there were more than 10 million new cases and 1.8 million deaths from the disease. The greatest disease burden is seen in parts of Asia and Africa. Although approximately a third of the world population is infected with *M. tuberculosis,* only approximately 12% of exposed, immune-sensitized individuals develop active disease. Major risk factors for tuberculosis include human immunodeficiency virus infection, diabetes, malnutrition, smoking, alcohol abuse, poverty, and overcrowding.

Tuberculosis is transmitted by aerosolized respiratory droplets. Upon inhalation of the organisms, primary infection typically develops in the lungs, where a localized fibrocalcified nodule may form. In most individuals, primary infection is asymptomatic and is cleared by innate or adaptive immune mechanisms. However, in some cases, viable organisms persist in macrophages within pulmonary nodules or draining lymph nodes. In addition, patients with a decreased immune response can exhibit active, symptomatic primary infection. After a variable latency period or, less frequently, immediately following primary infection, a subset of individuals may go on to develop secondary infection. During this phase, the infection may spread to the lung apices or may become more widely disseminated in the lungs and other organs. Characteristic clinical features of active pulmonary tuberculosis include cough, hemoptysis, fever, night sweats, fatigue, and weight loss.

Although tuberculosis primarily affects the lungs, nearly any anatomic site may be involved. Extrapulmonary disease most often develops in the lymph nodes, pleura, bones/joints, and genitourinary tract. In the United States, approximately 20% of annually recorded tuberculosis cases represent extrapulmonary disease without concurrent pulmonary involvement.

In the head and neck region, the most common manifestation of tuberculosis is cervical lymphadenitis. Occasionally, calcifications within the infected cervical lymph nodes can be detected radiographically. Lesions also may develop in the larynx, middle ear, nasal cavity, nasopharynx, maxillary sinus, parotid glands, tonsils, facial skin, and oral cavity.

Oral involvement has been noted in only approximately 0.5% to 1.5% of patients with tuberculosis. Some patients exhibit a solitary chronic ulcer, particularly on the tongue. The ulcer may or may not be painful and sometimes is accompanied by cervical lymphadenopathy. Other potential oral findings in tuberculosis include nonhealing extraction sockets, diffuse gingivitis with associated nodular or papillary proliferation, osteomyelitis of the jaws, and periapical inflammatory lesions. Most oral tubercular lesions represent secondary infection in patients with primary pulmonary disease; it is unclear whether these lesions result from hematogenous spread, lymphatic spread, or exposure to infected sputum. In very rare

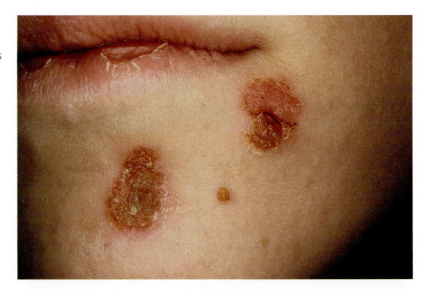

■ Figure **5.4**
Impetigo
Perioral skin exhibiting amber crusts on an erythematous base.

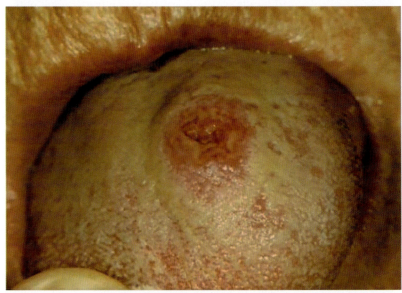

■ Figure **5.5**
Tuberculosis
Solitary, chronic ulcer on the dorsal tongue.

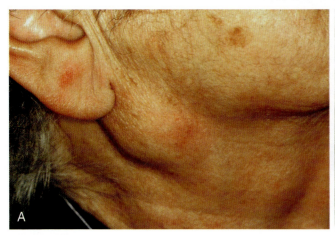
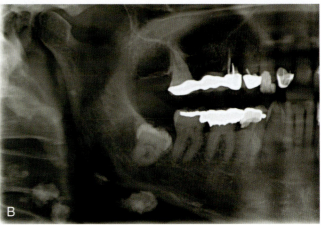

■ Figure **5.6**
Tuberculosis
(A) Enlarged cervical lymph node near the angle of the mandible. (Courtesy Dr. Román Carlos.) (B) Panoramic radiograph showing calcified cervical lymph nodes in the right neck. (Courtesy Dr. Louis M. Beto.)

cases, primary oral tuberculosis without pulmonary involvement also has been reported, especially among younger individuals.

Active tuberculosis is treated by multidrug therapy (typically including isoniazid, rifampicin, pyrazinamide, and ethambutol) administered over several months. Patient compliance is important to prevent development of multidrug-resistant mycobacterial strains.

Leprosy (Hansen Disease)

Figs. 5.7 and 5.8

Leprosy (Hansen disease) is a chronic infectious disease caused by *Mycobacterium leprae*. According to the World Health Organization, the global registered prevalence of leprosy is approximately 0.18 cases per 10,000 people, which represents a dramatic decrease over the past several decades. Nevertheless, the disease remains highly endemic in certain regions, including parts of India, Brazil, Indonesia, and Africa. In the United States, fewer than 200 new cases of leprosy are reported annually; most of these cases are noted in immigrants, although some are attributed to overseas travel or exposure to infected armadillos. The exact mechanism of transmission remains uncertain. However, the primary route of disease entry and elimination appears to be the upper respiratory tract. Only a small subset of exposed individuals develops clinically evident disease, apparently as a result of the host's immune status, genetic influences, and other factors.

Leprosy mainly affects the skin and peripheral nerves, but involvement of the mucous membranes and internal organs is also possible. There are two major clinical disease patterns (*tuberculoid* and *lepromatous*), as well as various borderline variants. In tuberculoid leprosy, the host exhibits a high degree of cell-mediated immunity and delayed hypersensitivity to the bacteria. Typical clinical findings include a small number of hypopigmented skin lesions, which may be associated with a localized decrease in nerve sensation. In lepromatous leprosy, the host is anergic and exhibits more severe disease. Characteristic findings include numerous erythematous, maculopapular to nodular skin lesions; a distorted facial appearance (*leonine facies*); hair loss (often including the eyebrows and eyelashes); nasal stuffiness; collapsed or depressed nasal bridge; painful neuropathy; loss of sensory and/or motor nerve function; chronic skin ulcers; and claw-like hands. Facial nerve involvement may interfere with speech and mastication.

Oral lesions are found predominantly in lepromatous leprosy. The reported prevalence of oral lesions in leprosy ranges from 0% to nearly 60%; this variation may reflect difficulty in distinguishing between nonspecific versus leprosy-specific alterations. Some authors have suggested that the frequency of oral lesions has been decreasing over time because of improvements in the diagnosis and treatment of leprosy. Frequently involved subsites include the hard and soft palate, anterior maxillary gingiva, and tongue. Oral findings include red-yellow papules or nodules, ulceration, necrosis, and macrocheilia (diffuse lip enlargement). In addition, scarring may cause mucosal hypopigmentation, fissured or depapillated tongue, retraction of the uvula, and microstomia. Maxillofacial bone involvement can cause atrophy of the anterior nasal spine, resorption of the anterior maxillary alveolar ridge, and subsequent tooth loss. In children, maxillary involvement also may be associated with shortened tooth roots and enamel hypoplasia. Furthermore, dental pulp infection can cause tooth necrosis and internal resorption.

Standard therapy for leprosy consists of a multidrug regimen (dapsone and rifampin, with or without clofazimine). Patients with maxillary alveolar destruction may require prosthetic rehabilitation. Occupational therapy may be beneficial for patients with hand deformities that make it difficult to perform oral hygiene procedures and other fine motor functions.

Noma

Fig. 5.9

Noma is an opportunistic bacterial infection characterized by rapidly progressive necrosis of the orofacial tissues. It represents the most severe part of a spectrum of necrotizing oral and maxillofacial diseases. The microbial profile is complex, and no specific causative microorganism has been established. However, some investigators believe that *Fusobacterium necrophorum* and *Prevotella intermedia* are key pathogens. Major risk factors include malnutrition, poverty, poor sanitation and oral hygiene, recent illness (e.g., measles, diarrhea, malaria), malignancy, and human immunodeficiency virus infection.

Noma exhibits a marked predilection for young children living in extreme poverty in sub-Saharan Africa. However, the infection can be found worldwide and also can arise in adolescents and adults. The disease initially may appear as gingival inflammation and ulceration. The condition then rapidly spreads to cause inflammation, necrosis, and destruction of other sites, such as the jaw bones, buccal mucosa, overlying facial skin, upper lip, nose, and infraorbital rim. The necrotic tissues usually appear blue-black

Figure **5.7**
Leprosy

Erythematous facial skin nodules in lepromatous leprosy.

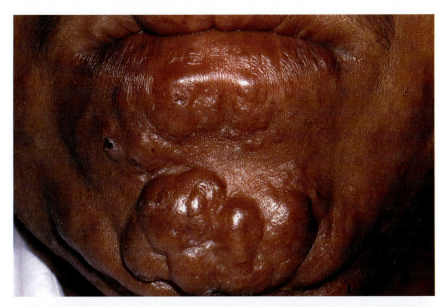

Figure **5.8**
Leprosy

Foot with chronic skin ulcers and neuropathy in a patient with lepromatous leprosy.

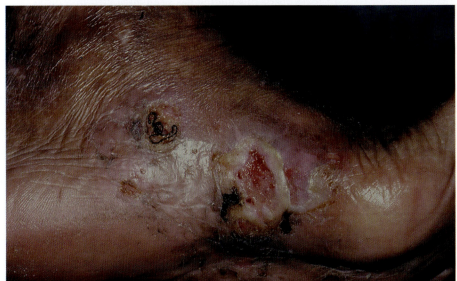

Figure **5.9**
Noma

Grayish-black, necrotic tissue in the oral cavity of an immunocompromised patient. The patient was receiving chemotherapy for lymphoma.

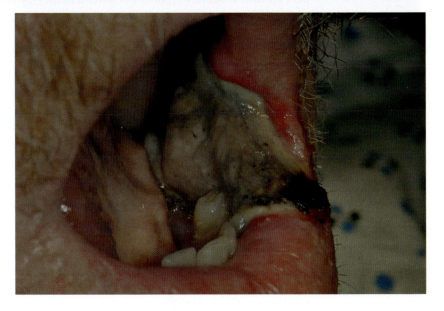

with well-demarcated borders and a fetid odor. Patients also often exhibit pain, tooth loss, fever, tachycardia, increased respiratory rate, anemia, leukocytosis, and anorexia. Major sequelae include scarring, trismus, speech and eating problems, facial disfigurement, and psychological trauma.

Management during the acute phase consists of antibiotics, local wound care, correction of dehydration and electrolyte imbalance, nutrition, and treatment of any underlying systemic diseases. During the healing phase, physiotherapy should be initiated to reduce scarring. In the long term, surgical reconstruction can be performed but is often difficult. Because many patients with noma in developing countries receive no treatment, the overall mortality is high (approximately 85%).

Syphilis

Figs. **5.10–5.12**

Syphilis is an infectious disease caused by the spirochete *Treponema pallidum.* The disease is spread mainly by sexual contact, although transmission via the placenta (see the following section "Congenital Syphilis"), infected blood products, or contaminated needles also is possible. Syphilis was common for centuries but became much less prevalent in the 1940s with the introduction of penicillin. Nevertheless, worldwide more than 5 million cases of syphilis are diagnosed annually, particularly in low- and middle-income countries. In North America and Western Europe, there has been a resurgence in syphilis over the past 10 to 15 years; this finding has been attributed to a disproportionate increase in infection among men who have sex with men, many of whom are coinfected with human immunodeficiency virus.

The clinical manifestations of syphilis are diverse, and the disease generally can be divided into primary, secondary, and tertiary stages. Oral lesions may occur in any of these three stages but most frequently are noted during the secondary stage. **Primary syphilis** develops within 3 to 90 days after exposure and is characterized by a painless ulcer, or *chancre,* at the site of inoculation. The ulcer typically exhibits an indurated margin and may be accompanied by regional lymphadenopathy. Spontaneous resolution usually occurs within 5 weeks. Although chancres predominantly arise in the anogenital region, approximately 4% of cases involve the oral mucosa. In particular, oral examples often occur on the upper lip in men and the lower lip in women. Subsequently, **secondary syphilis** develops in up to 90% of untreated patients with primary disease and results from dissemination via blood or lymphatic vessels. A common initial manifestation of secondary syphilis is an asymptomatic, maculopapular skin rash. Patients also may exhibit fever, malaise, fatigue, weight loss, and generalized reactive lymphadenopathy. In the oral cavity and oropharynx, secondary syphilis may appear as a grayish white *mucous patch,* which exhibits a predilection for the soft palate, tonsillar pillars, tongue, and buccal mucosa/vestibules. These lesions may be solitary or multifocal and are often painful. In some cases, elevated mucous patches (termed *split papules*) may develop bilaterally at the oral commissures. In the anogenital region or oral cavity, secondary syphilis also can cause warty or papillary nodules (termed *condyloma lata*). Approximately two thirds of untreated patients with secondary syphilis will enter a latency period of 1 to 30 years, which may be followed by tertiary disease. **Tertiary syphilis** can cause serious neurologic and cardiovascular complications. Some patients also develop a granulomatous lesion known as a *gumma.* In the oral cavity, gummas exhibit a predilection for the hard palate, although the tongue, lips, and other sites also may be affected. The lesion often begins as a swelling, which then ulcerates, undergoes necrosis, and ultimately may cause palatal perforation. Some patients with tertiary syphilis also exhibit atrophic glossitis. Interestingly, investigators have suggested an association between tertiary syphilis and squamous cell carcinoma of the dorsal tongue; however, it is unclear whether these cancers have resulted from carcinogenic agents (such as arsenic) formerly used to treat syphilis or other cofactors (e.g., tobacco, alcohol, malnutrition).

Diagnostic testing for syphilis typically includes serologic evaluation. However, some serologic tests may be negative during the first several weeks of infection or during later disease stages (including latency and tertiary syphilis). Thus direct visualization of *T. pallidum* (e.g., smear examined by direct immunofluorescence, incisional biopsy examined by immunohistochemistry, fresh exudate examined by dark-field microscopy) can be particularly helpful during early primary disease, when the organisms are numerous but antibodies are not detectable. For patients diagnosed with syphilis, additional testing to rule out concurrent human immunodeficiency virus infection should be considered.

The mainstay of therapy for syphilis is penicillin. Long-acting, intramuscular benzathine penicillin G is preferred for most cases, although neurosyphilis may require intravenous penicillin G or other alternative regimens. Furthermore, any recent sexual partners should be notified of their disease risk and offered preventive antibiotic therapy.

■ Figure 5.10
Primary Syphilis
Chancre presenting as an erythematous, ulcerated mass on the anterior buccal mucosa and upper labial mucosa. (Courtesy Dr. Benjamin Martinez.)

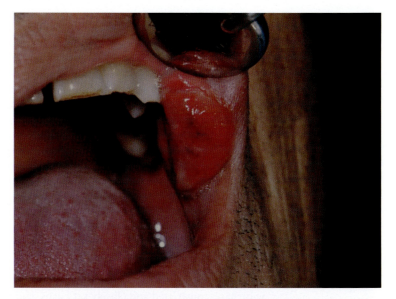

■ Figure 5.11
Secondary Syphilis
Mucous patch presenting as a white plaque on the palate.

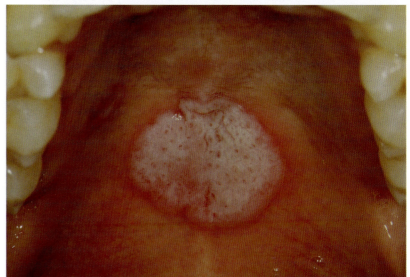

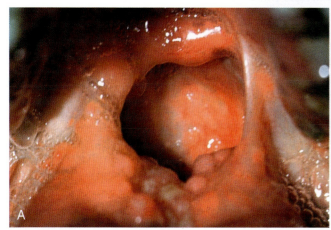

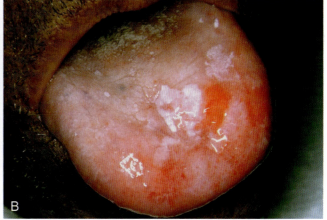

■ Figure 5.12
Tertiary Syphilis
(A) Gumma with palatal perforation. (With appreciation to Dr. Emmett Costich.) (B) Squamous cell carcinoma appearing as an irregular, white-red plaque on the dorsal tongue within a background of atrophic glossitis. (With appreciation to Dr. Emmett Costich.)

Congenital Syphilis

Fig. **5.13**

Congenital syphilis occurs via vertical transmission (i.e., from infected mother to fetus) of *Treponema pallidum*. The organism can cross the placenta after the 16th week of intrauterine life, and the timing of infection correlates with various types of developmental defects that may result. Congenital syphilis is associated with substantial morbidity and mortality. Investigators have estimated that syphilis accounts for more than 500,000 adverse pregnancy outcomes per year globally, including early fetal deaths, stillbirths, neonatal deaths, prematurity, and low birth weight. Among infected infants who survive the neonatal period, it may take several weeks before clinical features of syphilis become evident. In the early stages, there may be a diffuse maculopapular rash, rhinitis, "sabre shins" (anterior bowing of the tibias), hepatosplenomegaly, and neurologic abnormalities. Potential orofacial manifestations include frontal bossing, saddle nose deformity, short maxilla, high-arched palate, perioral fissures or scars *(rhagades)*, atrophic glossitis, and dental defects. The dental defects tend to be most pronounced in teeth that calcify during the first year of life (i.e., the permanent incisors and permanent first molars). *Hutchinson incisors* exhibit "screwdriver-shaped" incisal edges often with central notches and "barrel-shaped" crowns with widening in the middle third and constriction in the incisal third. *Moon molars* are small and dome shaped with a wide base, constricted and closely set cusps, and missing occlusal grooves. *Mulberry* (or *Fournier) molars* exhibit numerous globular occlusal projections that are surrounded at the base by deep grooves of hypoplastic enamel. In later stages, patients may exhibit *Hutchinson triad* (dental defects, ocular interstitial keratitis, and eighth nerve deafness); gummas; and intellectual deterioration. All pregnant women should be screened for syphilis during early prenatal care. Recommended treatment (e.g., parenteral benzathine penicillin G) during pregnancy usually cures the mother and protects the developing fetus.

Actinomycosis

Fig. **5.14**

Actinomycosis represents infection caused by gram-positive, anaerobic or microaerophilic bacilli in the *Actinomyces* genus. Among the various isolated pathogenic species, *Actinomyces israelii* is the most prevalent. Actinomycetes can be part of the normal oral, oropharyngeal, gastrointestinal, and genital flora. However, in some cases they invade tissues and cause symptomatic infection. Approximately 55% of these infections occur in the cervicofacial region, with a predilection for the mandible and the buccal, submental, and submandibular soft tissues. Predisposing factors for cervicofacial actinomycosis include trauma (e.g., tooth extraction, soft tissue injury), odontogenic or periodontal infection, poor oral hygiene, diabetes mellitus, immunosuppression, local tissue damage by a neoplasm or irradiation, and malnutrition. The infection may be acute or chronic and tends to spread rapidly without regard for typical fascial planes and lymphatic routes. Clinical findings may include abscess formation, indurated ("wooden") fibrosis, cutaneous sinus formation, tonsillar hyperplasia, osteomyelitis of the jaws, and trismus. Some lesions exhibit purulent or serous discharge with *sulfur granules* (small, yellow "grains" representing bacterial colonies). Pain may be minimal or absent, especially in chronic cases. Fever, malaise, and fatigue may be noted with acute infection. Cultures can aid in diagnosis but may be complicated by strict anaerobic incubation requirements over an extended period, overgrowth of other associated bacteria, and prior antimicrobial therapy. Histopathologic examination may show colonies of filamentous bacteria surrounded by neutrophils. Although such bacterial colonies are not entirely specific for *Actinomyces*, they help to suggest the diagnosis when occurring in the appropriate clinical context. For patients with chronic cervicofacial actinomycosis, treatment typically consists of prolonged, high doses of antibiotics (such as penicillin G) combined with abscess drainage, excision or marsupialization of sinus tracts, débridement of necrotic bone, and addressing any underlying odontogenic or periodontal infection.

Cat-Scratch Disease

Fig. **5.15**

Cat-scratch disease is a bacterial infection predominantly caused by *Bartonella henselae*. This organism can be transmitted to humans via a bite or scratch by an infected cat or via a bite by an infected flea. The disease exhibits a worldwide distribution and a predilection for young individuals. In the United States, one large-scale study reported an estimated annual incidence of 4.7 per 100,000 persons younger than 65 years, with a peak among patients 5 to 9 years of age. Cat-scratch disease typically begins as a cutaneous vesicle or papule that develops at the site of inoculation and heals in approximately 1 to 3 weeks. Around

■ Figure **5.13**
Congenital Syphilis

Hutchinson incisors: occlusal radiograph showing unerupted permanent central incisors with notched incisal edges. (The patient presented to the clinic because of a traumatic fracture of the overlying primary central incisor.) (Courtesy Dr. Cindy Hipp.)

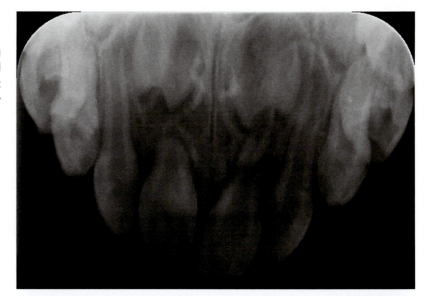

■ Figure **5.14**
Actinomycosis

Draining sinus tract with surrounding erythema at the right angle of the mandible. (Courtesy Dr. Jon Pike.)

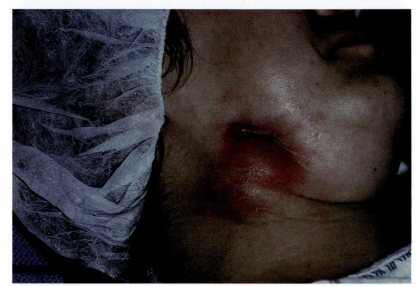

■ Figure **5.15**
Cat-Scratch Disease

Young patient with unilateral cervical lymphadenopathy.

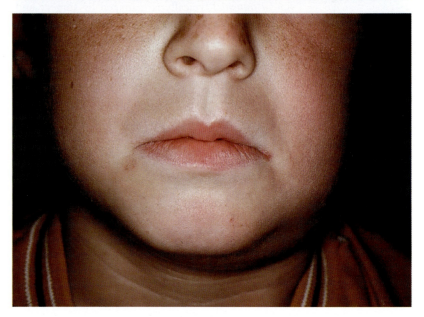

the time that this initial lesion heals, approximately 85% to 90% of patients develop chronic, ipsilateral lymphadenopathy in the head and neck, axillary, inguinal, or other regions. The enlarged lymph nodes are painful and tender, and suppuration may be evident in some cases. Fever, malaise, myalgia, arthralgia, and anorexia may also be noted. Infrequently, there may be serious disease complications, such as hepatosplenomegaly, endocarditis, and meningoencephalitis. Diagnosis is aided by serologic testing. Cultures are not recommended because the causative organism is difficult to cultivate. In most cases, cat-scratch disease is self-limiting and resolves within a few months. Supportive therapy typically includes analgesics, local heat, and aspiration of any suppuration. For patients with prolonged or severe disease, antibiotic therapy (e.g., azithromycin, erythromycin, doxycycline, gentamicin) is indicated.

Sinusitis

Fig. **5.16**

Sinusitis refers to inflammation of the paranasal sinuses. It is quite common, with approximately 12% of adults in the United States reporting this diagnosis over a 12-month period. The inflammation can be caused by bacteria (e.g., *Streptococcus pneumoniae, Haemophilus influenzae, Moraxella catarrhalis)*, viruses, fungi, allergies, and pollutants. In some cases, maxillary sinusitis may develop from an endodontic or a periodontal infection of an adjacent maxillary tooth; in addition, tooth extraction, implant placement, and other sources of trauma can lead to maxillary sinus inflammation. Furthermore, mechanical obstruction (e.g., nasal polyps), mucociliary dysfunction, and immunosuppression may be cofactors in the development of sinusitis.

Clinically, sinusitis may be classified as acute, subacute, or chronic. Common findings include nasal obstruction and congestion, facial pain or pressure, and purulent rhinorrhea. Additional symptoms may include headache, cough, fever, hyposmia, ear fullness, and halitosis. Sometimes sinusitis can cause a maxillary toothache, which prompts the patient to seek dental evaluation. Although sinusitis often is diagnosed clinically, endoscopy and imaging studies can aid in the evaluation of chronic or complicated acute sinusitis. Radiographic examination may show air-fluid levels, mucosal thickening, diffuse opacification, and bone thickening/remodeling.

Treatment for sinusitis depends on the cause. Most cases of acute sinusitis are viral and will resolve spontaneously; these cases can be managed by supportive measures (e.g., steam inhalation, vasoconstrictors, saline irrigation). Antibiotics typically are reserved for patients with acute sinusitis who develop persistent, severe, or worsening symptoms suggestive of bacterial infection. For patients with chronic sinusitis refractory to medical treatment, surgery may be considered. Sinusitis caused by allergy to *Aspergillus* spp. *(allergic fungal sinusitis)* typically is managed by surgery and corticosteroids. Invasive fungal sinusitis—usually seen in immunocompromised patients—requires aggressive therapy, such as intravenous amphotericin B and surgical débridement.

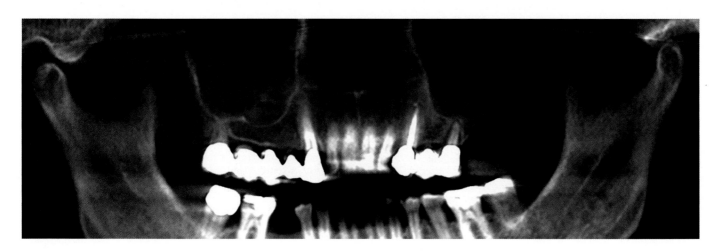

■ Figure **5.16**
Sinusitis
Radiograph showing opacification of the right maxillary sinus.

Bibliography

Tonsillitis

Bird JH, Biggs TC, King EV. Controversies in the management of acute tonsillitis: an evidence-based review. *Clin Otolaryngol.* 2014;39: 368–374.

Burton MJ, Glasziou PP, Chong LY, et al. Tonsillectomy or adenotonsillectomy versus non-surgical treatment for chronic/recurrent acute tonsillitis. *Cochrane Database Syst Rev.* 2014;(11):CD001802.

Georgalas CC, Tolley NS, Narula PA. Tonsillitis. *BMJ Clin Evid.* 2014;2014:0503.

Tagliareni JM, Clarkson EI. Tonsillitis, peritonsillar and lateral pharyngeal abscesses. *Oral Maxillofac Surg Clin North Am.* 2012;24:197–204, viii.

Windfuhr JP, Toepfner N, Steffen G, et al. Clinical practice guideline: tonsillitis I. Diagnostics and nonsurgical management. *Eur Arch Otorhinolaryngol.* 2016;273:973–987.

Windfuhr JP, Toepfner N, Steffen G, et al. Clinical practice guideline: tonsillitis II. Surgical management. *Eur Arch Otorhinolaryngol.* 2016;273: 989–1009.

Tonsilloliths

Caldas MP, Neves EG, Manzi FR, et al. Tonsillolith–report of an unusual case. *Br Dent J.* 2007;202:265–267.

Fauroux MA, Mas C, Tramini P, et al. Prevalence of palatine tonsilloliths: a retrospective study on 150 consecutive CT examinations. *Dentomaxillofac Radiol.* 2013;42:20120429.

Oda M, Kito S, Tanaka T, et al. Prevalence and imaging characteristics of detectable tonsilloliths on 482 pairs of consecutive CT and panoramic radiographs. *BMC Oral Health.* 2013;13:54.

Ram S, Siar CH, Ismail SM, et al. Pseudo bilateral tonsilloliths: a case report and review of the literature. *Oral Surg Oral Med Oral Pathol Oral Radiol Endod.* 2004;98:110–114.

Impetigo

Bangert S, Levy M, Hebert AA. Bacterial resistance and impetigo treatment trends: a review. *Pediatr Dermatol.* 2012;29:243–248.

Hartman-Adams H, Banvard C, Juckett G. Impetigo: diagnosis and treatment. *Am Fam Physician.* 2014;90:229–235.

Koning S, van der Sande R, Verhagen AP, et al. Interventions for impetigo. *Cochrane Database Syst Rev.* 2012;(1):CD003261.

Yeoh DK, Bowen AC, Carapetis JR. Impetigo and scabies - Disease burden and modern treatment strategies. *J Infect.* 2016;72 Suppl:S61–S67.

Tuberculosis

Bansal R, Jain A, Mittal S. Orofacial tuberculosis: clinical manifestations, diagnosis and management. *J Family Med Prim Care.* 2015;4: 335–341.

Centers for Disease Control and Prevention (CDC). Reported Tuberculosis in the United States, 2015, Atlanta, GA; 2016. United States Department of Health and Human Services. Available at: https://www.cdc.gov/tb/statistics/reports/2015/pdfs/2015_Surveillance_Report_FullReport.pdf. Accessed September 27, 2017.

Dheda K, Barry CE 3rd, Maartens G. Tuberculosis. *Lancet.* 2016;387:1211–1226.

Jain P, Jain I. Oral manifestations of tuberculosis: step towards early diagnosis. *J Clin Diagn Res.* 2014;8:ZE18–ZE21.

Krawiecka E, Szponar E. Tuberculosis of the oral cavity: an uncommon but still a live issue. *Postepy Dermatol Alergol.* 2015;32:302–306.

World Health Organization. Global Tuberculosis Report 2014, Geneva; 2014. World Health Organization. Available at: http://apps.who.int/iris/bitstream/10665/250441/1/9789241565394-eng.pdf?ua=1. Accessed August 25, 2017.

Leprosy

National Hansen's Disease Program. A Summary of Hansen's Disease in the United States-2015, Rockville, MD; 2015. U.S. Department of Health and Human Services Health Resources and Services Administration. Available at: https://www.hrsa.gov/hansensdisease/pdfs/hansens2015report.pdf. Accessed August 26, 2017.

Pooja VK, Vanishree M, Ravikumar S, et al. Evaluation of the orofacial lesions in treated leprosy patients. *J Oral Maxillofac Pathol.* 2014;18:386–389.

Rodrigues GA, Qualio NP, de Macedo LD, et al. The oral cavity in leprosy: what clinicians need to know. *Oral Dis.* 2017;23:749–756.

Taheri JB, Mortazavi H, Moshfeghi M, et al. Oro-facial manifestations of 100 leprosy patients. *Med Oral Patol Oral Cir Bucal.* 2012;17:e728–e732.

World Health Organization. Global leprosy update, 2015: time for action, accountability and inclusion. *Wkly Epidemiol Rec.* 2015;91:405–420.

World Health Organization. Leprosy Fact Sheet, Geneva; 2017. World Health Organization. Available at: http://www.who.int/mediacentre/factsheets/fs101/en/. Accessed August 26, 2017.

Noma

Baratti-Mayer D, Gayet-Ageron A, Hugonnet S, et al; Geneva Study Group on Noma (GESNOMA). Risk factors for noma disease: a 6-year, prospective, matched case-control study in Niger. *Lancet Glob Health.* 2013;1:e87–e96.

Enwonwu CO, Falkler WA Jr, Phillips RS. Noma (cancrum oris). *Lancet.* 2006;368:147–156, 368.

Feller L, Altini M, Chandran R, et al. Noma (cancrum oris) in the South African context. *J Oral Pathol Med.* 2014;43:1–6.

Srour ML, Marck K, Baratti-Mayer D. Noma: overview of a neglected disease and human rights violation. *Am J Trop Med Hyg.* 2017;96: 268–274.

Syphilis

Compilato D, Amato S, Campisi G. Resurgence of syphilis: a diagnosis based on unusual oral mucosa lesions. *Oral Surg Oral Med Oral Pathol Oral Radiol Endod.* 2009;108:e45–e49.

de Voux A, Kidd S, Grey JA, et al. State-specific rates of primary and secondary syphilis among men who have sex with men - United States, 2015. *MMWR Morb Mortal Wkly Rep.* 2017;66:349–354.

Ficarra G, Carlos R. Syphilis: the renaissance of an old disease with oral implications. *Head Neck Pathol.* 2009;3:195–206.

Hertel M, Matter D, Schmidt-Westhausen AM, et al. Oral syphilis: a series of 5 cases. *J Oral Maxillofac Surg.* 2014;72:338–345.

Hook EW 3rd. Syphilis. *Lancet.* 2017;389:1550–1557.

Kelner N, Rabelo GD, da Cruz Perez DE, et al. Analysis of nonspecific oral mucosal and dermal lesions suggestive of syphilis: a report of 6 cases. *Oral Surg Oral Med Oral Pathol Oral Radiol.* 2014;117:1–7.

Leuci S, Martina S, Adamo D, et al. Oral syphilis: a retrospective analysis of 12 cases and a review of the literature. *Oral Dis.* 2013;19:738–746.

Morshed MG, Singh AE. Current trends in the serologic diagnosis of syphilis. *Clin Vaccine Immunol.* 2015;22:137–147.

Pires FR, da Silva PJ, Natal RF, et al. Clinicopathologic features, microvessel density, and immunohistochemical expression of ICAM-1 and VEGF in 15 cases of secondary syphilis with oral manifestations. *Oral Surg Oral Med Oral Pathol Oral Radiol.* 2016;121:274–281.

Seibt CE, Munerato MC. Secondary syphilis in the oral cavity and the role of the dental surgeon in STD prevention, diagnosis and treatment: a case series study. *Braz J Infect Dis.* 2016;20:393–398.

Congenital Syphilis

Hutchinson J. Clinical lecture on heredito-syphilitic struma: and on the teeth as a means of diagnosis. *Br Med J.* 1861;1:515–517.

Newman L, Kamb M, Hawkes S, et al. Global estimates of syphilis in pregnancy and associated adverse outcomes: analysis of multinational antenatal surveillance data. *PLoS Med.* 2013;10:e1001396.

Nissanka-Jayasuriya EH, Odell EW, Phillips C. Dental stigmata of congenital syphilis: a historic review with present day relevance. *Head Neck Pathol.* 2016;10:327–331.

Actinomycosis

Boyanova L, Kolarov R, Mateva L, et al. Actinomycosis: a frequently forgotten disease. *Future Microbiol.* 2015;10:613–628.

Kolm I, Aceto L, Hombach M, et al. Cervicofacial actinomycosis: a long forgotten infectious complication of immunosuppression - report of a case and review of the literature. *Dermatol Online J.* 2014;20: 22640.

Moghimi M, Salentijn E, Debets-Ossenkop Y, et al. Treatment of cervicofacial actinomycosis: a report of 19 cases and review of literature. *Med Oral Patol Oral Cir Bucal.* 2013;18:e627–e632.

Valour F, Sénéchal A, Dupieux C, et al. Actinomycosis: etiology, clinical features, diagnosis, treatment, and management. *Infect Drug Resist.* 2014;7:183–197.

Cat-Scratch Disease

Klotz SA, Ianas V, Elliott SP. Cat-scratch Disease. *Am Fam Physician.* 2011;83:152–155.

Lindeboom JA. Pediatric cervicofacial lymphadenitis caused by *Bartonella henselae. Oral Surg Oral Med Oral Pathol Oral Radiol.* 2015;120:469–473.

Nelson CA, Saha S, Mead PS. Cat-scratch disease in the United States, 2005-2013. *Emerg Infect Dis.* 2016;22:1741–1746.

Prutsky G, Domecq JP, Mori L, et al. Treatment outcomes of human bartonellosis: a systematic review and meta-analysis. *Int J Infect Dis.* 2013;17:e811–e819.

Sinusitis

Blackwell DL, Villarroel MA. Tables of Summary Health Statistics for U.S. Adults: 2015 National Health Interview Survey. Hyattsville, MD, National Center for Health Statistics; 2016. Available at: http://www.cdc.gov/nchs/nhis/SHS/tables.htm. Accessed September 20, 2017.

Chow AW, Benninger MS, Brook I, et al. Infectious Diseases Society of America. IDSA clinical practice guideline for acute bacterial rhinosinusitis in children and adults. *Clin Infect Dis.* 2012;54:e72–e112.

Head K, Chong LY, Piromchai P, et al. Systemic and topical antibiotics for chronic rhinosinusitis. *Cochrane Database Syst Rev.* 2016;(4):CD011994.

Patel NA, Ferguson BJ. Odontogenic sinusitis: an ancient but under-appreciated cause of maxillary sinusitis. *Curr Opin Otolaryngol Head Neck Surg.* 2012;20:24–28.

Vidal F, Coutinho TM, Carvalho Ferreira D, et al. Odontogenic sinusitis: a comprehensive review. *Acta Odontol Scand.* 2017;6:1–11.

6

Fungal and Protozoal Infections

Figs. 6.1–6.4

Candidiasis is the most common type of oral fungal infection. *Candida albicans* is the predominant pathogen, although various other *Candida* species have also been implicated. *Candida* can be part of the normal oral microflora; however, various factors may contribute to the development of clinically evident infection. Such factors include immunosuppression (e.g., caused by human immunodeficiency virus infection, malignancy, chemotherapy, radiotherapy, corticosteroids, biologic agents), endocrine disorders (e.g., diabetes), extremes of age, xerostomia, broad-spectrum antibiotic therapy, and nutritional deficiencies.

Pseudomembranous candidiasis ("thrush") is the best-recognized clinical pattern of oral candidal infection. It is characterized by white to yellow-white, "curd-like" plaques that represent tangled masses of fungal organisms, desquamated epithelial cells, and debris. The lesions may occur on the palate, buccal mucosa, tongue, or other sites. The white plaques can be wiped away (e.g., by using a wooden blade or gauze), and the underlying mucosa may appear normal to erythematous. The ability to wipe away the lesions aids in distinction from leukoplakia. Some patients with pseudomembranous candidiasis are asymptomatic, whereas others complain of burning, pain, and/or a salty to bitter taste. In individuals with poorly controlled human immunodeficiency virus infection, the clinical presentation can be severe, with painful, widespread lesions involving the oral cavity, oropharynx, and esophagus. In such cases the patient may have considerable difficulty eating and drinking.

Management of oral candidiasis typically consists of prescribing antifungal medication and addressing underlying predisposing factors. For patients with mild disease, topical agents (e.g., clotrimazole troches, nystatin suspension [preferably without sucrose], miconazole buccal tablets) are often sufficient. For patients with more severe involvement, refractory disease, or immunosuppression, systemic agents (e.g., fluconazole) or alternative topical agents (e.g., itraconazole solution, posaconazole solution) should be considered. In patients with human immunodeficiency virus infection, oral candidiasis may indicate progression of immunodeficiency and thus warrants prompt referral for institution of effective combined antiretroviral therapy.

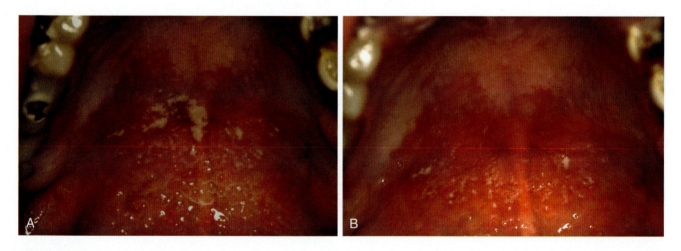

■ Figure **6.1**
Pseudomembranous Candidiasis
(A) Palatal mucosa showing white, irregular plaques on an erythematous base. (B) Same patient from A after the white plaques were wiped away with a wooden blade.

■ Figure **6.2**
Pseudomembranous Candidiasis
Irregular, yellowish white, "curd-like" plaques involving the maxillary vestibule.

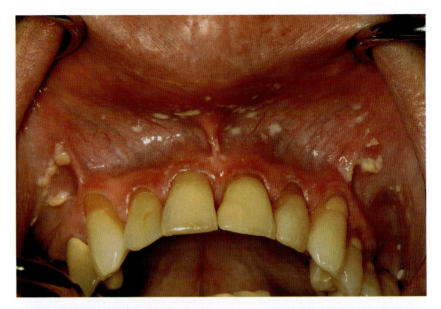

■ Figure **6.3**
Pseudomembranous Candidiasis
Diffuse white, irregular plaques on an erythematous base. The patient developed candidiasis as a complication of topical clobetasol therapy for benign mucous membrane pemphigoid.

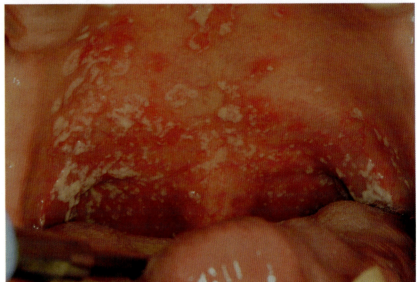

■ Figure **6.4**
Pseudomembranous Candidiasis
Same patient from Fig. 6.3 after treatment with clotrimazole troches.

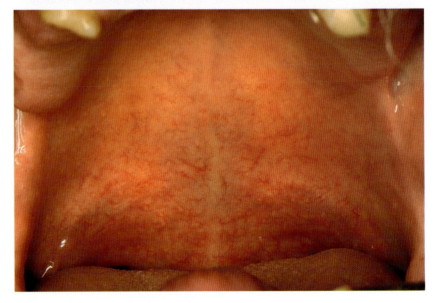

Figs. **6.5 and 6.6**

Many cases of oral candidiasis exhibit mucosal erythema with minimal to no white changes. Symptoms may be absent or mild to severe. The distribution of lesions can range from localized to diffuse or multifocal.

In one clinical subtype of **erythematous candidiasis** known as *acute atrophic candidiasis* ("antibiotic sore mouth"), broad-spectrum antibiotic therapy or other factors may induce a sudden onset of mucosal erythema with an associated burning or scalding sensation. The dorsal tongue, palate, or other sites may be affected. Dorsal tongue lesions also usually exhibit loss of filiform papillae, which results in a smooth or "bald" appearance.

In other instances, erythematous candidiasis may exhibit a more chronic course (typically >4 weeks) with no or relatively minor symptoms. Distinctive clinical presentations of chronic erythematous candidiasis are discussed separately (see the following sections regarding median rhomboid glossitis, angular cheilitis, and denture stomatitis). The term *chronic multifocal candidiasis* may be used when there are two or more chronic, erythematous lesions. Many such cases occur in older male tobacco smokers.

Median Rhomboid Glossitis

Fig. **6.7**

Median rhomboid glossitis (central papillary atrophy) appears as a well-demarcated zone of erythema in the dorsal midline region of the tongue, slightly anterior to the circumvallate papillae. The lesion is typically asymptomatic and has a somewhat symmetric, rhomboidal, or elliptical shape. Most examples demonstrate a smooth, atrophic, and flat surface, although at times the surface may be lobulated or exophytic. Some studies have noted a predilection among middle-aged, male tobacco users. Occasionally, median rhomboid glossitis can occur in association with a "kissing" candidal lesion on the palate. The etiology of median rhomboid glossitis is controversial. In the past, the lesion was thought to represent a developmental anomaly resulting from failure of the lateral processes of the tongue to cover the tuberculum impar. However, this theory has been disputed because the condition typically is not seen in childhood. Because *Candida albicans* can be found in greater than 80% of cases, many investigators regard this lesion as a subtype of erythematous candidiasis. Furthermore, some authorities hypothesize that the decreased microvasculature in the midline area of the tongue predisposes to central papillary atrophy with aging and secondary candidiasis. Other possible contributory factors include dental prostheses, tobacco use, and microtrauma (e.g., from mastication and swallowing). Antifungal therapy (e.g., clotrimazole troches, fluconazole tablets) typically induces complete or partial resolution of the lesion.

■ Figure **6.5**
Erythematous Candidiasis
Diffuse palatal erythema in a patient who developed candidiasis secondary to adalimumab therapy for psoriatic arthritis.

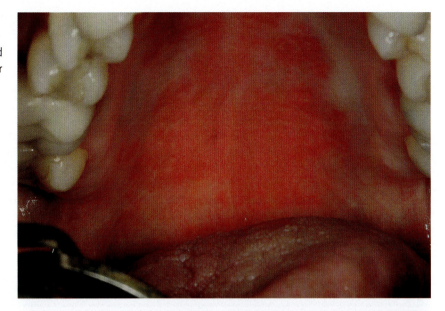

■ Figure **6.6**
Erythematous Candidiasis
(A) Erythema in the midline region of the dorsal tongue. (B) Same patient after antifungal therapy.

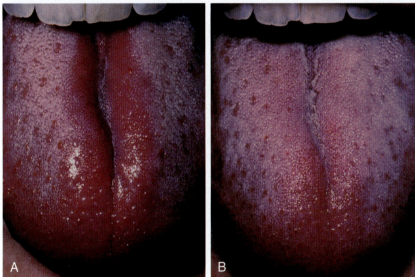

■ Figure **6.7**
Median Rhomboid Glossitis
Erythematous, atrophic, and roughly symmetric lesion involving the midline region of the dorsal tongue, just anterior to the circumvallate papillae.

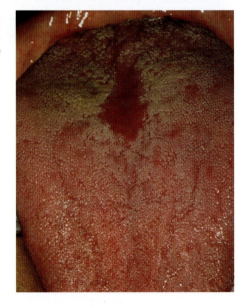

Chronic Hyperplastic Candidiasis

Fig. **6.8**

Chronic hyperplastic candidiasis ("candidal leukoplakia") is an uncommon form of oral candidiasis characterized by a white plaque that cannot be removed by scraping. Many affected patients are middle-aged to older adult males. Potential cofactors include tobacco use, nutritional deficiency, and host immune system defects. The condition exhibits a predilection for the anterior buccal mucosa, although the tongue, palate, or other sites also may be involved. Some examples exhibit a finely "speckled," red and white appearance, which should alert the clinician of an increased risk for underlying epithelial dysplasia. The etiopathogenesis of chronic hyperplastic candidiasis is controversial. Some investigators have proposed that candidal organisms can induce a hyperkeratotic lesion, whereas others believe that the lesion represents a preexisting leukoplakia with superimposed candidiasis. In practice, for any lesion presumed to represent chronic hyperplastic candidiasis, it is important to monitor for resolution after an appropriate course of antifungal therapy. If the lesion persists, then biopsy is recommended to rule out epithelial dysplasia or squamous cell carcinoma.

Angular Cheilitis

Fig. **6.9**

Angular cheilitis (perlèche) is a condition characterized by erythema, fissures, scaling, and/or crusting at the corners of the mouth. It may occur as an isolated finding or as a component of chronic multifocal candidiasis. Microbiologic studies suggest that the condition is caused by *Candida albicans* and/or *Staphylococcus aureus*. Additional contributory factors may include loss of vertical dimension of occlusion (which creates a favorable environment for microbial overgrowth due to accentuation of the commissural folds with salivary pooling), prosthodontic or orthodontic appliances (which may harbor fungal organisms), nutritional deficiencies (e.g., iron or vitamin B complex deficiency), local irritation (e.g., from chewing on objects, thumb sucking, lip licking or picking, flossing), and medications (e.g., isotretinoin, indinavir, sorafenib). In addition, more general risk factors for candidiasis were discussed previously (see the section "Pseudomembranous Candidiasis").

Clinically, angular cheilitis may affect one or both corners of the mouth. The patient may complain of soreness, pain, burning, or pruritus. The condition can last anywhere from a few days to several years, and alternating periods of relapse and remission are common in chronic cases. Management typically includes topical medication (e.g., nystatin/triamcinolone acetonide cream or ointment, hydrocortisone/iodoquinol cream) for the corners of the mouth, appropriate antifungal therapy for any concurrent intraoral candidiasis, and addressing underlying contributory factors.

Denture Stomatitis

Fig. **6.10**

Denture stomatitis (chronic atrophic candidiasis) is an inflammatory condition characterized by erythema localized to denture-bearing areas of the palate and alveolar ridges. Epidemiologic studies have noted this condition in approximately 15% to 70% of removable denture wearers. Although denture stomatitis often is classified as a form of erythematous candidiasis, its exact etiopathogenesis is uncertain. Some studies suggest that it represents an inflammatory response to *Candida* within the denture base rather than a true fungal infection. In general, fungal/bacterial biofilms and poor denture hygiene are considered to be important factors—many patients admit to wearing their removable prostheses continuously, with only periodic removal for cleaning. Other proposed factors include trauma or excessive pressure on the mucosa from dentures, allergy to denture materials, impaired immune response, and impaired salivary flow or function. Clinically, most patients are asymptomatic, although pain, burning, or itching is possible. Intraoral examination may show pinpoint hyperemic macules or more generalized erythema. The erythema often exhibits a distinct border corresponding to the outline of the denture base. The condition is found more often with maxillary than mandibular dentures. Management typically includes denture disinfection, with or without antifungal treatment of the mucosa; patient education (i.e., denture and oral hygiene instruction, overnight removal of dentures); and adjustment or redesign/refabrication of dentures that fit poorly or exert excessive tissue pressure. Various denture disinfection methods (e.g., sodium hypochlorite [for non–metal-containing dentures only], chlorhexidine, nystatin, hydrogen peroxide) have been reported, but further research is needed.

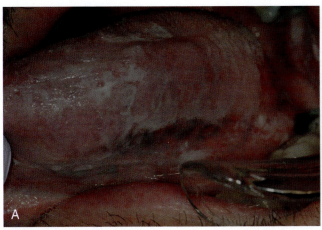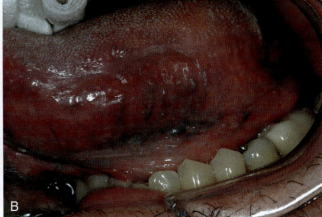

■ Figure 6.8
Hyperplastic Candidiasis
(A) Left tongue showing a white lesion that could not be wiped away with gauze. (B) Same patient from A after antifungal therapy.

■ Figure 6.9
Angular Cheilitis
Erythema and fissures involving the skin at the corners of the mouth.

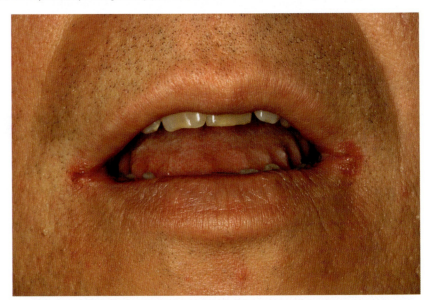

■ Figure 6.10
Denture Stomatitis
Erythema involving areas of the maxillary alveolar mucosa that came into contact with the base of a denture.

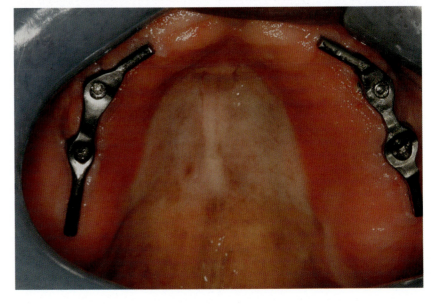

Figs. **6.11 and 6.12**

Histoplasmosis is a deep fungal infection caused by *Histoplasma capsulatum*. The disease is found worldwide and represents the most common endemic mycosis in North America, Central America, and parts of South America. In the United States, highly endemic regions include the Mississippi and Ohio River Valley basins. The infection typically results from inhalation of airborne spores from disrupted soil, often enriched with bird or bat excrement.

Most infected individuals are asymptomatic or develop mild, self-limited illness. However, severe pulmonary disease and, at times, extrapulmonary dissemination may develop—especially with immunosuppression, extremes of age, or exposure to a large inoculum. Notably, disseminated histoplasmosis is considered an acquired immunodeficiency syndrome (AIDS)-defining illness. Major sites for dissemination include the liver, spleen, gastrointestinal tract, skin, adrenal glands, and central nervous system.

Oral lesions usually occur within the setting of progressive disseminated disease, although primary inoculation of the oral mucosa is possible. Frequently involved subsites include the tongue, palate, and buccal mucosa. Clinical examination may show a solitary, chronic ulcer with a rolled margin. In other cases, there is a plaque or nodule, with a granular, erythematous, or white surface. Pain is a variable finding. Many oral lesions mimic squamous cell carcinoma.

Treatment for histoplasmosis depends on disease severity/extent and host factors. Disseminated histoplasmosis is usually fatal without treatment; management includes antifungal therapy (e.g., liposomal amphotericin B followed by itraconazole) and addressing underlying causes of immunodeficiency.

Fig. **6.13**

Blastomycosis is a fungal disease caused by *Blastomyces dermatitidis*. In North America, the infection is endemic in regions surrounding the Ohio and Mississippi Rivers, Great Lakes, and Saint Lawrence Seaway. Infection typically occurs via inhalation of spores aerosolized by disruption of moist soil enriched with decomposing vegetation. Many infected patients exhibit no or mild symptoms, whereas others develop more severe disease. The condition exhibits a marked male predilection and mainly affects the lungs, although dissemination to extrapulmonary sites (especially the skin, bones/joints, and genitourinary tract) is possible.

Rare cases of head and neck involvement usually result from extrapulmonary dissemination, although primary inoculation is possible. The most frequently reported subsites include the facial skin, larynx, and oral cavity. Skin lesions may appear as plaques, pustules, or nodules, with associated ulceration, a warty surface, crusting, and/or exudate. Laryngeal disease can produce exophytic vocal cord masses and chronic, progressive hoarseness. Within the oral cavity, the tongue, buccal mucosa, or other sites may be involved. The patient may exhibit a gradually enlarging ulcer with a rolled border or an erythematous nodule with a granular to warty surface. Rarely, oral mucosal infection can spread to the underlying jawbones. Treatment depends on disease severity/extent and host factors. Patients with disseminated extrapulmonary blastomycosis typically receive systemic antifungal therapy (e.g., amphotericin B, itraconazole).

■ Figure **6.11**
Histoplasmosis
Diffuse, irregular ulcerative changes of the anterior mandibular gingiva.

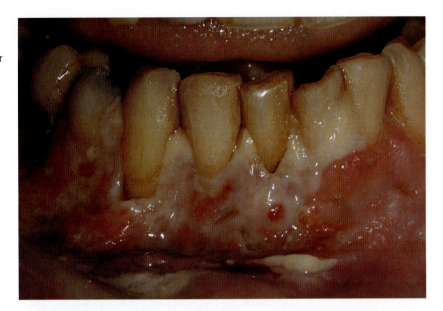

■ Figure **6.12**
Histoplasmosis
Chronic ulcer on the right lateral tongue in an immunosuppressed patient taking prednisone, azathioprine, and methotrexate for polymyositis. After biopsy and diagnosis, the patient began antifungal therapy with amphotericin B, but she subsequently died from disseminated infection, multiorgan failure, and cardiac arrest.

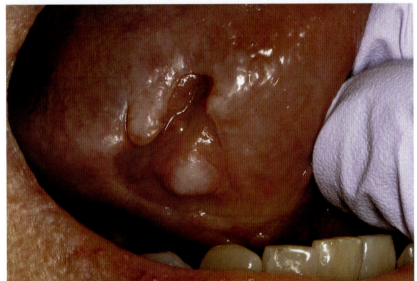

■ Figure **6.13**
Blastomycosis
Erythematous mass on the mandibular gingiva with associated ulceration. (Courtesy Dr. Ashleigh Briody.)

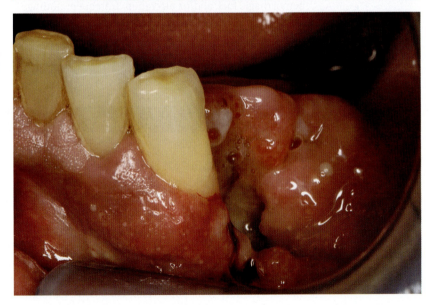

Coccidioidomycosis

Fig. **6.14**

Coccidioidomycosis is a disease caused by inhalation of spores of the soil-dwelling fungi *Coccidiodes immitis* and *Coccidiodes posadasii*. It is confined to the Western Hemisphere and is highly endemic in desert regions of the southwestern United States. Most infected individuals exhibit no symptoms or self-limited, influenza-like symptoms (e.g., fatigue, cough, chest pain, myalgias, headache). However, chronic pulmonary disease and extrapulmonary dissemination are possible. Major risk factors for dissemination include immunosuppression, old age, Filipino or African descent, and pregnancy. The most common sites for disseminated lesions include the skin, bones/joints, and meninges.

Spread of infection to the head and neck region is also possible. Lesions on the facial skin may appear as verrucous plaques, subcutaneous abscesses, papules, nodules, or pustules. In particular, such lesions often arise in the nasolabial fold area. Other possible head and neck findings include cervical lymphadenopathy; laryngeal granulomas with possible airway obstruction; peritonsillar, retropharyngeal, thyroid, or parotid abscess formation; noduloulcerative eruptions of the external ear and preauricular skin; and otitis media with extension of infection into adjacent structures. Oral involvement is extremely rare and may present as an ulcerated tongue nodule, erythematous granular mucosal mass, or osteomyelitis of the jaws.

Treatment for coccidioidomycosis depends on disease severity/extent and host factors. Patients with debilitating disease, extensive pulmonary involvement, significant comorbidities, or extrapulmonary dissemination typically receive systemic antifungal therapy (e.g., fluconazole, itraconazole, amphotericin B).

Paracoccidioidomycosis

Fig. **6.15**

Endemic in parts of Latin and Central America, **paracoccidioidomycosis** (South American blastomycosis) is a deep fungal disease caused by *Paracoccidioides brasiliensis* and *Paracoccidioides lutzii*. Approximately 80% of registered cases occur in Brazil, where the estimated incidence is 0.7 to 3.7 cases per 100,000 inhabitants per year. Infection occurs primarily via inhalation of airborne spores. However, only approximately 2% of infected individuals develop active disease.

Major clinical patterns of active disease include the following: (1) *acute/subacute*: mainly affects individuals younger than 30 years, develops within weeks to months after initial infection, and often involves the reticuloendothelial system; (2) *chronic*: comprises the majority of cases, exhibits a marked predilection among adult male agricultural workers, develops months to years after initial infection, and mainly affects the lungs, lymph nodes, oral mucosa, skin, and larynx.

Oral lesions may be solitary or multifocal and can involve the gingiva, palate, lips, buccal mucosa, tongue, or other sites. The mucosa typically exhibits erythema, a granular (or "mulberry-like") surface, hemorrhagic foci, and/or ulceration. Infrequent findings include palatal perforation, diffuse lip enlargement (*macrocheilia*), alveolar bone destruction, and tooth loss. In addition, the skin around the mouth and nose may exhibit ulceration, erythema, crusting, and/or hemorrhagic foci.

Clinical management depends on disease severity/extent and host factors. Mild to moderate disease may be treated with itraconazole or sulfamethoxazole-trimethoprim, whereas severe disease typically requires amphotericin B.

Mucormycosis

Fig. **6.16**

Mucormycosis (formerly known as *zygomycosis* or *phycomycosis*) is an opportunistic infection caused by saprophytic fungi within the subphylum Mucormycotina. Major pathogens within this group include *Rhizopus, Lichtheimia, Mucor, Rhizomucor,* and *Cunninghamella* species. The organisms are distributed worldwide and can cause aggressive, life-threatening disease, marked by a tendency for angioinvasion and tissue necrosis. Risk factors include uncontrolled diabetes mellitus (often with ketoacidosis), hematologic malignancy, solid organ or hematopoietic stem cell transplantation, prolonged neutropenia, systemic corticosteroid therapy, human immunodeficiency virus infection, iron overload, major trauma, and intravenous drug abuse. Infection typically develops via inhalation of fungal spores. Major clinical disease patterns include rhinocerebral, pulmonary, cutaneous, disseminated, and others.

In rhinocerebral mucormycosis, infection begins in the paranasal sinuses and often spreads rapidly into adjacent structures, such as the palate, cavernous sinus, orbits, and cranium. Clinically, the patient may experience nasal obstruction, bloody nasal discharge, facial pain, headache, cellulitis, cranial nerve

■ Figure **6.14**
Coccidioidomycosis

Erythematous, granular lesion on the dorsal tongue. (Courtesy Dr. German Trujillo.)

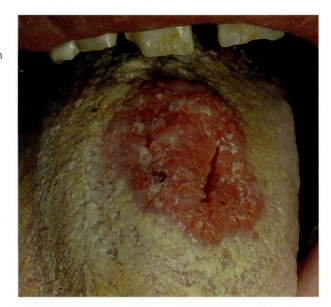

■ Figure **6.15**
Paracoccidioidomycosis

Erythematous, granular lesions involving the lower labial mucosa and anterior mandibular buccal gingiva. (Courtesy Drs. Vera and Ney Araújo.)

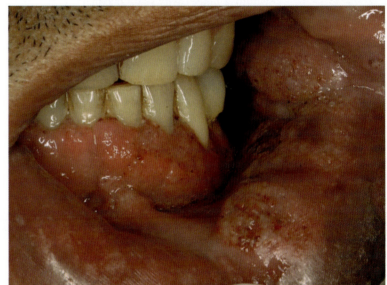

■ Figure **6.16**
Mucormycosis

Palatal ulceration with dark areas of tissue necrosis. (Courtesy Dr. Matt Dillard.)

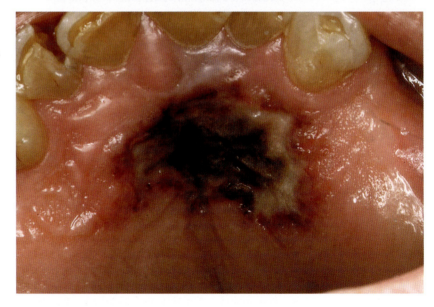

palsies, proptosis, visual disturbance, and seizures. During the early stages of disease, intraoral examination may show swelling of the palate and/or maxillary alveolar process due to antral involvement. If left untreated, the patient subsequently can develop palatal ulceration, an oronasal fistula, frank oral/sinonasal necrosis with black eschar formation, and massive tissue destruction. Prompt diagnosis and treatment are crucial for patient survival. Clinical management typically includes surgical débridement, lipid formulations of amphotericin B, and addressing underlying risk factors.

Aspergillosis

Fig. **6.17**

Among the most common fungal diseases in humans, aspergillosis is second only to candidiasis. Major pathogenic species include *Aspergillus fumigatus* and *Aspergillus flavus*. These saprobic organisms are found worldwide in soil, decaying organic matter, or water. In most cases, the fungal spores enter the host via inhalation, although contamination of skin wounds or water systems is possible. In addition, some disease outbreaks are nosocomial. Only a minority of exposed individuals develop symptomatic disease.

Aspergillosis exhibits a broad spectrum of clinical manifestations, ranging from noninvasive disease (e.g., fungus ball, allergy) in immunocompetent hosts to life-threatening, invasive disease in immuno-compromised individuals. A **fungus ball** (mycetoma, aspergilloma) represents a mass of fungal organisms within a body cavity (e.g., maxillary sinus, sphenoid sinus, area of the lungs previously damaged by bronchiectasis). Patients with sinonasal fungus balls may have nonspecific complaints (e.g., purulent nasal discharge, chronic nasal obstruction, facial pain, postnasal drip) or no symptoms. Radiographic examination may show sinus opacification with focal calcifications. The surrounding bone can exhibit thickening, sclerosis, erosion, or remodeling. **Allergic fungal sinusitis** is caused by immunoglobulin E (IgE)-mediated hypersensitivity to fungal antigens. The patient may complain of sinonasal congestion, rhinorrhea, and headache. Additional findings can include nasal polyposis, peripheral eosinophilia, and a history of asthma. Treatment typically consists of surgical débridement and corticosteroids.

In some cases, aspergillosis develops after dental procedures (e.g., tooth extraction, endodontic therapy) involving the posterior maxillary region. The tissue damage apparently predisposes to the development of a sinus fungus ball or, possibly, invasive infection. Clinical examination may show gingival ulceration and palatal swelling with a gray to violaceous hue. Management typically consists of surgical débridement and—if there is invasive disease—voriconazole.

Leishmaniasis

Fig. **6.18**

Leishmaniasis represents a spectrum of protozoal diseases caused by more than 20 *Leishmania* species. The parasites are transmitted via phlebotomine sandfly bites. According to the World Health Organization, approximately 700,000 to 1 million new cases occur annually, with endemic regions identified in more than 90 reporting countries. Risk factors include malnutrition, poverty, poor sanitation, population displacement/migration, deforestation, and immunosuppression (e.g., human immunodeficiency virus infection, organ transplantation).

Leishmaniasis exhibits three major clinical patterns: *visceral* ("kala-azar," life-threatening systemic infection), *cutaneous* (the most common form), and *mucocutaneous* (causing skin disease, as well as significant destruction of the nose, oral cavity, pharynx, and larynx). **Cutaneous leishmaniasis** typically develops several weeks after the patient is bitten, appearing as painless, erythematous papules or nodules with depressed, ulcerated centers. The lesions heal spontaneously within several months but can cause severe scarring. In **mucocutaneous leishmaniasis**, there can be widespread skin lesions, and mucosal involvement may develop after several months to years. Nasal findings can include epistaxis, rhinorrhea, and septal perforation. Oral lesions often stem from progression of nasal disease, although isolated oral involvement also is possible. The lips may exhibit generalized swelling, a localized nodule, crusting, or scaling. Intraorally, there may be mucosal erythema, nodules, papules, plaques, granular or cobblestone surface changes, swelling, ulceration, and necrosis. The palate, tongue, buccal mucosa, gingiva, or other sites may be involved. Palatal necrosis may lead to oronasal fistula formation.

Treatment depends on disease extent/severity, host factors, and *Leishmania* species. In the United States, the Food and Drug Administration has approved intravenous liposomal amphotericin B for visceral leishmaniasis and oral miltefosine for visceral, cutaneous, and mucocutaneous disease. Pentavalent antimonial compounds are less expensive and widely used alternatives. Small, isolated oral lesions may be excised.

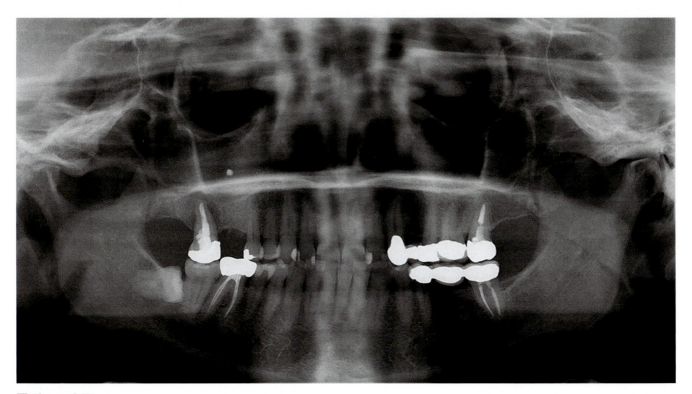

■ Figure **6.17**
Aspergillosis
Diffuse opacification of the right maxillary sinus in a patient with a fungus ball. The small focus of brightly radiopaque material within the sinus could represent some root canal filling material. (Courtesy Dr. Jay Sikes.)

■ Figure **6.18**
Leishmaniasis
Ulcerated, erythematous swelling on the right dorsal tongue. (Courtesy Dr. José Bagan.)

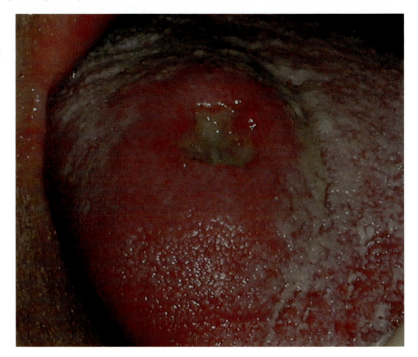

Bibliography

Pseudomembranous Candidiasis and Erythematous Candidiasis

Gaitán-Cepeda LA, Martínez-González M, Ceballos-Salobreña A. Oral candidosis as a clinical marker of immune failure in patients with HIV/AIDS on HAART. *AIDS Patient Care STDS.* 2005;19:70–77.

Millsop JW, Fazel N. Oral candidiasis. *Clin Dermatol.* 2016;34:487–494.

Pappas PG, Kauffman CA, Andes DR, et al. Clinical practice guideline for the management of candidiasis: 2016 update by the Infectious Diseases Society of America. *Clin Infect Dis.* 2016;62:e1–e50.

Patil S, Rao RS, Majumdar B, et al. Clinical appearance of oral Candida infection and therapeutic strategies. *Front Microbiol.* 2015;6:1391.

Sharon V, Fazel N. Oral candidiasis and angular cheilitis. *Dermatol Ther.* 2010;23:230–242.

Telles DR, Karki N, Marshall MW. Oral fungal infections: diagnosis and management. *Dent Clin North Am.* 2017;61:319–349.

Median Rhomboid Glossitis

Goregen M, Miloglu O, Buyukkurt MC, et al. Median rhomboid glossitis: a clinical and microbiological study. *Eur J Dent.* 2011;5:367–372.

Lago-Méndez L, Blanco-Carrión A, Diniz-Freitas M, et al. Rhomboid glossitis in atypical location: case report and differential diagnosis. *Med Oral Patol Oral Cir Bucal.* 2005;10:123–127.

Manfredi M, Polonelli L, Aguirre-Urizar JM, et al. Urban legends series: oral candidosis. *Oral Dis.* 2013;19:245–261.

Chronic Hyperplastic Candidiasis

Shah N, Ray JG, Kundu S, et al. Surgical management of chronic hyperplastic candidiasis refractory to systemic antifungal treatment. *J Lab Physicians.* 2017;9:136–139.

Sitheeque MA, Samaranayake LP. Chronic hyperplastic candidosis/candidiasis (candidal leukoplakia). *Crit Rev Oral Biol Med.* 2003;14:253–267.

Angular Cheilitis

Cross D, Eide ML, Kotinas A. The clinical features of angular cheilitis occurring during orthodontic treatment: a multi-centre observational study. *J Orthod.* 2010;37:80–86.

Park KK, Brodell RT, Helms SE. Angular cheilitis, part 1: local etiologies. *Cutis.* 2011;87:289–295.

Park KK, Brodell RT, Helms SE. Angular cheilitis, part 2: nutritional, systemic, and drug-related causes and treatment. *Cutis.* 2011;88:27–32.

Denture Stomatitis

de Souza RF, de Freitas Oliveira Paranhos H, Lovato da Silva CH, et al. Interventions for cleaning dentures in adults. *Cochrane Database Syst Rev.* 2009;(4):CD007395.

Emami E, de Grandmont P, Rompré PH, et al. Favoring trauma as an etiological factor in denture stomatitis. *J Dent Res.* 2008;87:440–444.

Emami E, Kabawat M, Rompre PH, et al. Linking evidence to treatment for denture stomatitis: a meta-analysis of randomized controlled trials. *J Dent.* 2014;42:99–106.

Gendreau L, Loewy ZG. Epidemiology and etiology of denture stomatitis. *J Prosthodont.* 2011;20:251–260.

Hilgert JB, Giordani JM, de Souza RF, et al. Interventions for the management of denture stomatitis: a systematic review and meta-analysis. *J Am Geriatr Soc.* 2016;64:2539–2545.

Histoplasmosis

Akin L, Herford AS, Cicciù M. Oral presentation of disseminated histoplasmosis: a case report and literature review. *J Oral Maxillofac Surg.* 2011;69:535–541.

Klein IP, Martins MA, Martins MD, et al. Diagnosis of HIV infection on the basis of histoplasmosis-related oral ulceration. *Spec Care Dentist.* 2016;36:99–103.

Wheat LJ, Azar MM, Bahr NC, et al. Histoplasmosis. *Infect Dis Clin North Am.* 2016;30:207–227.

Blastomycosis

Castillo CG, Kauffman CA, Miceli MH. Blastomycosis. *Infect Dis Clin North Am.* 2016;30:247–264.

Chapman SW, Dismukes WE, Proia LA, et al; Infectious Diseases Society of America. Clinical practice guidelines for the management of blastomycosis: 2008 update by the Infectious Diseases Society of America. *Clin Infect Dis.* 2008;46:1801–1812.

Kruse AL, Zwahlen RA, Bredell MG, et al. Primary blastomycosis of oral cavity. *J Craniofac Surg.* 2010;21:121–123.

Rucci J, Eisinger G, Miranda-Gomez G, et al. Blastomycosis of the head and neck. *Am J Otolaryngol.* 2014;35:390–395.

Coccidioidomycosis

Arnold MG, Arnold JC, Bloom DC, et al. Head and neck manifestations of disseminated coccidioidomycosis. *Laryngoscope.* 2004;114:747–752.

Cooksey GS, Nguyen A, Knutson K, et al. Notes from the field: increase in coccidioidomycosis — California, 2016. *MMWR Morb Mortal Wkly Rep.* 2017;66:833–834.

Galgiani JN, Ampel NM, Blair JE, et al. 2016 Infectious Diseases Society of America (IDSA) clinical practice guideline for the treatment of coccidioidomycosis. *Clin Infect Dis.* 2016;63:e112–e146.

Galgiani JN, Ampel NM, Blair JE, et al. Infectious diseases society of America: coccidioidomycosis. *Clin Infect Dis.* 2005;41:1217–1223.

Mendez LA, Flores SA, Martinez R, et al. Ulcerated lesion of the tongue as manifestation of systemic coccidioidomycosis. *Case Rep Med.* 2017;2017:1489501.

Rodriguez RA, Konia T. Coccidioidomycosis of the tongue. *Arch Pathol Lab Med.* 2005;129:e4–e6.

Tang CG, Nuyen BA, Puligandla B, et al. The coccidioidomycosis conundrum: a rare parotid mass. *Perm J.* 2014;18:86–88.

Paracoccidioidomycosis

Abreu e Silva MÀ, Salum FG, Figueiredo MA, et al. Important aspects of oral paracoccidioidomycosis – a literature review. *Mycoses.* 2013;56:189–199.

Almeida OP, Jacks J Jr, Scully C. Paracoccidioidomycosis of the mouth: an emerging deep mycosis. *Crit Rev Oral Biol Med.* 2003;14:377–383.

Bicalho RN, Santo MF, de Aguiar MC, et al. Oral paracoccidioidomycosis: a retrospective study of 62 Brazilian patients. *Oral Dis.* 2001;7:56–60.

Marques SA. Paracoccidioidomycosis. *Clin Dermatol.* 2012;30:610–615.

Martinez R. Epidemiology of paracoccidioidomycosis. *Rev Inst Med Trop Sao Paulo.* 2015;57(suppl 19):11–20.

Shikanai-Yasuda MA, Mendes RP, Colombo AL, et al. Brazilian guidelines for the clinical management of paracoccidioidomycosis. *Rev Soc Bras Med Trop.* 2017;50(5):715–740. doi:10.1590/0037-8682-0230-2017. [Epub ahead of print July 20, 2017].

Mucormycosis

Barrak HA. Hard palate perforation due to mucormycosis: report of four cases. *J Laryngol Otol.* 2007;121:1099–1102.

Binder U, Maurer E, Lass-Flörl C. Mucormycosis – from the pathogens to the disease. *Clin Microbiol Infect.* 2014;20(suppl 6):60–66.

Miceli MH, Kauffman CA. Treatment options for mucormycosis. *Curr Treat Options Infect Dis.* 2015;7:142–154.

Petrikkos G, Skiada A, Lortholary O, et al. Epidemiology and clinical manifestations of mucormycosis. *Clin Infect Dis.* 2012;54(suppl 1): S23–S34.

Prasad K, Lalitha RM, Reddy EK, et al. Role of early diagnosis and multimodal treatment in rhinocerebral mucormycosis: experience of 4 cases. *J Oral Maxillofac Surg.* 2012;70:354–362.

Reddy SS, Rakesh N, Chauhan P, et al. Rhinocerebral mucormycosis among diabetic patients: an emerging trend. *Mycopathologia.* 2015;180:389–396.

Aspergillosis

Aït-Mansour A, Pezzettigotta S, Genty E, et al. Evaluation of the prevalence and specificities of asymptomatic paranasal sinus aspergillosis: retrospective study of 59 cases. *Eur Ann Otorhinolaryngol Head Neck Dis.* 2015;132:19–23.

Grosjean P, Weber R. Fungus balls of the paranasal sinuses: a review. *Eur Arch Otorhinolaryngol.* 2007;264:461–470.

Ni Mhurchu E, Ospina J, Janjua AS, et al. Fungal rhinosinusitis: a radiological review with intraoperative correlation. *Can Assoc Radiol J.* 2017;68:178–186.

Pasqualotto AC, Denning DW. Post-operative aspergillosis. *Clin Microbiol Infect*. 2006;12:1060–1076.

Walsh TJ, Anaissie EJ, Denning DW, et al. Infectious diseases society of America: treatment of aspergillosis: clinical practice guidelines of the infectious diseases society of America. *Clin Infect Dis*. 2008;46:327–360.

Leishmaniasis

Almeida TF, da Silveira EM, Dos Santos CR, et al. Exclusive primary lesion of oral leishmaniasis with immunohistochemical diagnosis. *Head Neck Pathol*. 2016;10:533–537.

Aronson N, Herwaldt BL, Libman M, et al. Diagnosis and treatment of leishmaniasis: clinical practice guidelines by the Infectious Diseases Society of America (IDSA) and the American Society of Tropical Medicine and Hygiene (ASTMH). *Am J Trop Med Hyg*. 2017;96:24–45.

Mignogna MD, Celentano A, Leuci S, et al. Mucosal leishmaniasis with primary oral involvement: a case series and a review of the literature. *Oral Dis*. 2015;21:e70–e78.

Mohammadpour I, Motazedian MH, Handjani F, et al. Lip leishmaniasis: a case series with molecular identification and literature review. *BMC Infect Dis*. 2017;17:96.

Nadler C, Enk CD, Leon GT, et al. Diagnosis and management of oral leishmaniasis–case series and literature review. *J Oral Maxillofac Surg*. 2014;72:927–934.

World Health Organization. Leishmaniasis Fact Sheet. Geneva; 2017. World Health Organization. Available at: http://www.who.int/mediacentre/factsheets/fs375/en/. Accessed November 8, 2017.

Yeşilova Y, Aksoy M, Sürücü HA, et al. Lip leishmaniasis: clinical characteristics of 621 patients. *Int J Crit Illn Inj Sci*. 2015;5:265–266.

7

Viral Infections

Figs. **7.1–7.4**

Acute herpetic gingivostomatitis represents the most common symptomatic form of primary oral herpes simplex virus (HSV) infection. More than 90% of cases are caused by HSV type 1 (HSV-1). This virus is found worldwide and is spread predominantly via infected saliva or contact with active perioral lesions. In the United States, the estimated HSV-1 seroprevalence is greater than 50% among individuals 14 to 49 years old. The infection is acquired most often during childhood and adolescence. Although many people who develop primary HSV-1 infection are asymptomatic, some individuals exhibit clinically evident disease.

Acute herpetic gingivostomatitis occurs most frequently in patients between the ages of 6 months and 5 years. There is typically an abrupt onset of signs and symptoms, such as fever, chills, malaise, headache, irritability, anorexia, and cervical lymphadenopathy. After a variable prodrome period, the oral lesions initially appear as numerous small, pinpoint vesicles on an erythematous base. Subsequently, the vesicles readily rupture to form coalescing ulcers covered by a yellowish fibrinopurulent membrane. In all cases, the gingiva exhibits painful swelling and erythema; in addition, characteristic "punched-out" erosions may be evident along the midfacial free gingival margin. Lesions also can involve other oral sites, such as the labial mucosa, lip vermilion, buccal mucosa, and tongue. Typically, the lesions heal within 1 to 2 weeks. However, in rare cases, the patient may develop serious complications, such as esophagitis, keratoconjunctivitis, pneumonitis, and meningoencephalitis.

Management considerations for acute herpetic gingivostomatitis include antiviral medication, palliative therapy, and maintenance of fluids and electrolytes. Antiviral agents (e.g., acyclovir suspension or capsules, valacyclovir tablets) may be beneficial if initiated early—ideally during the first 3 days of symptomatic infection. Pain can be controlled with topical anesthetic agents (e.g., dyclonine hydrochloride spray, tetracaine hydrochloride lollipops), nonsteroidal antiinflammatory drugs, and popsicles. Because many patients have difficulty drinking, it is important to monitor for severe dehydration, which may necessitate hospitalization and parenteral fluids. In addition, in order to prevent autoinoculation or disease spread to others, the patient should be instructed to avoid contact with active lesions.

■ Figure **7.1**
Acute Herpetic Gingivostomatitis
Erythema and ulceration of the lower lip.

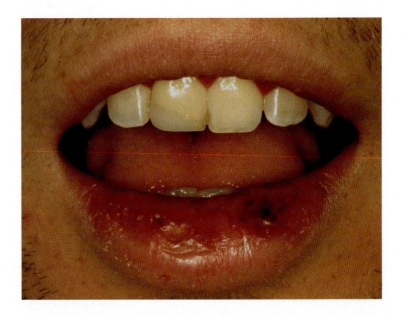

■ Figure **7.2**
Acute Herpetic Gingivostomatitis
Ulcers on the dorsal tongue.

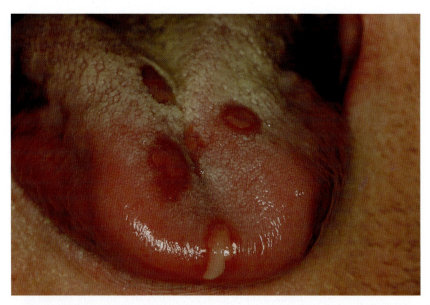

■ Figure **7.3**
Acute Herpetic Gingivostomatitis
Maxillary facial gingiva with erythema and focal marginal erosions. (Courtesy Dr. Gina Rotkvich.)

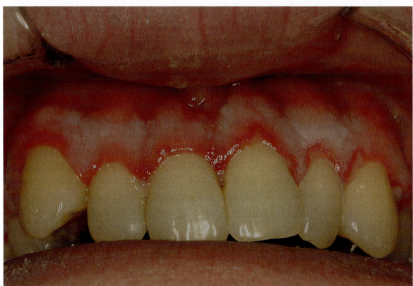

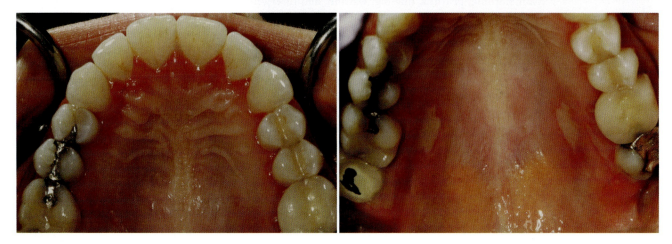

■ Figure **7.4**
Acute Herpetic Gingivostomatitis
Erythema and ulceration of the maxillary lingual gingiva and palate.

Fig. **7.5**

Herpetic whitlow refers to primary or recurrent herpes simplex virus (HSV) infection of the hands or, rarely, the feet. It is seen most often in children less than 10 years old and adults between 20 and 30 years. The condition typically results from autoinoculation in children with orofacial HSV type 1 (HSV-1) infection, autoinoculation in adults with genital HSV type 2 (HSV-2) infection, or occupational exposure of healthcare workers to patients with active lesions or infected saliva. Before the implementation of universal precautions, dental and medical personnel were among the most commonly affected individuals. Clinically, patients with herpetic whitlow may complain of prodromal tingling, pruritus, or burning; fever, regional lymphadenopathy, and lymphadenitis also may be noted infrequently. Subsequently, lesions typically develop on the fingers or thumbs—especially the palmar aspect of the fingertips (pulp spaces) and, occasionally, the sides or periungual areas of the digits. The involved skin exhibits erythema, swelling, and vesicles. The vesicles often coalesce to form a large blister *(bulla)*, which subsequently ruptures to form ulceration and crusting. The fluid within the blister is usually clear at first but may become turbid after a few days; frank suppuration is not typically present unless there is superimposed bacterial infection. In immunocompetent patients, resolution usually occurs within 3 to 4 weeks. Most patients are treated with systemic antiviral medication (e.g., acyclovir). A dry dressing should be applied in order to prevent disease transmission. Incision and drainage is not recommended because of the risk for inducing viremia or secondary bacterial infection. Other potential sequelae of herpetic whitlow include nail loss and hypoesthesia. The recurrence rate is approximately 20%.

Herpes Labialis

Figs. **7.6 and 7.7**

After primary infection, herpes simplex virus type 1 (HSV-1) can establish latency in the trigeminal or other sensory ganglia. Reactivation of the virus may be stimulated by various factors (e.g., old age, ultraviolet light, stress, extreme temperatures, respiratory illness, menstruation, trauma, malignancy) to produce recurrent infection. The most common clinical pattern of recurrent HSV-1 infection is **herpes labialis** ("cold sore" or "fever blister"), which involves the lip vermilion and skin adjacent to the lips. In the United States, approximately 20% to 45% of the adult population has a history of herpes labialis, and about 100 million episodes occur annually among immunocompetent individuals.

Clinically, up to 60% of patients with herpes labialis experience a brief prodrome, characterized by pain, burning, pruritus, tingling, warmth, and/or erythema. Subsequently, there is typically an eruption of multiple small, erythematous papules, which evolve into clusters of fluid-filled vesicles. Within a couple of days, the vesicles rupture and crust. Periodic hemorrhage may occur when the crusted lesions are stretched.

In immunocompetent individuals, herpes labialis is self-limited and typically resolves within 7 to 10 days. Nevertheless, patients often seek treatment because the condition is painful and unsightly. Unfortunately, once the lesions have appeared, the initiation of antiviral therapy does not provide any benefit. However, if begun promptly during the prodrome, antiviral medication (e.g., acyclovir capsules or cream, penciclovir cream, valacyclovir tablets) may produce a modest reduction in the duration of lesions. Also, there is some evidence showing that oral antiviral agents may help to prevent herpes labialis, although the clinical benefit appears to be small. Various alternative methods (e.g., laser therapy, immunotherapy, photodynamic therapy) for the treatment or prevention of herpes labialis have been reported, but further studies are needed.

■ Figure **7.5**
Herpetic Whitlow
Ulcerated blister on the skin of a finger.

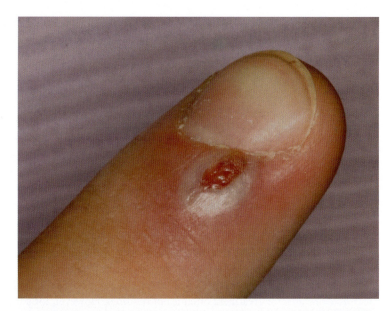

■ Figure **7.6**
Herpes Labialis
Multiple vesicles involving the skin adjacent to the lower lip.

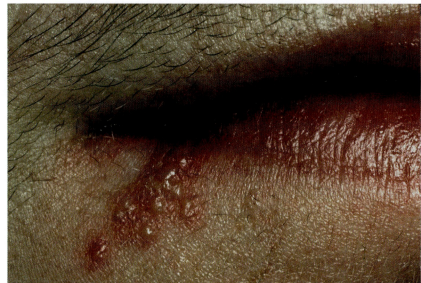

■ Figure **7.7**
Herpes Labialis
Multiple vesicles involving the lip vermilion and adjacent skin.

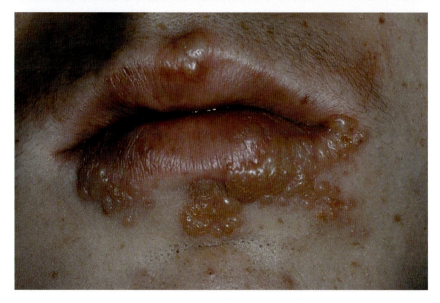

Recurrent Intraoral Herpes

Figs. **7.8 and 7.9**

Although the most common clinical manifestation of recurrent herpes simplex virus type 1 (HSV-1) infection is herpes labialis, intraoral lesions also are possible. Potential triggers for recurrent intraoral herpes include preceding dental procedures or other sources of trauma. In immunocompetent individuals, recurrent intraoral herpes typically involves the keratinized mucosa bound to bone (i.e., the mucosa of the hard palate and attached gingiva), at times with spread to the adjacent unattached mucosa. This predilection for the fixed, keratinized mucosa aids in distinguishing recurrent intraoral herpes from recurrent aphthous stomatitis. Also, in rare examples, a patient may have recurrent intraoral herpes and herpes labialis simultaneously.

Clinically, recurrent intraoral herpes tends to be less painful than herpes labialis. The patient may experience no symptoms or relatively mild discomfort, burning, or pain. Initially, there is an eruption of multiple small vesicles, which readily rupture to form punctate, erythematous ulcers. These punctate ulcers often enlarge and coalesce to form broader areas of ulceration with irregular borders. The ulceration may be covered by a yellowish fibrinopurulent membrane and exhibit surrounding erythema. The lesions usually heal within 7 to 10 days. Because the lesions typically are self-limited and cause minimal to no symptoms, treatment often is not required. However, for patients with more significant symptoms, chlorhexidine rinse and/or acyclovir may be prescribed.

Chronic Intraoral Herpes

Fig. **7.10**

Although most herpetic lesions are acute and self-limited, unusual cases of chronic intraoral herpes are possible. Such chronic lesions tend to occur in immunocompromised individuals, such as organ transplant recipients, patients with human immunodeficiency virus (HIV) infection, individuals receiving chemotherapy or radiation therapy, and patients receiving immunosuppressive therapy for autoimmune diseases. The lesions can cause severe pain, making it difficult for the patient to eat and swallow. In contrast to the relatively small lesions typically seen on the keratinized mucosa in immunocompetent individuals with recurrent intraoral herpes, the lesions that develop in immunocompromised patients tend to be larger, with an approximately even distribution between the keratinized and nonkeratinized mucosa. Clinical examination typically shows one or more areas of erosion, ulceration, or superficial necrosis, often with raised, yellowish, and circinate borders. Because of the atypical clinical presentation, the diagnosis may not be readily apparent. For example, chronic ulcers on the nonkeratinized mucosa may be confused with major aphthous stomatitis; in addition, malignancy and cytomegalovirus or other chronic infections may be considered in the differential diagnosis. Procedures that may aid in diagnosis include exfoliative cytology and incisional biopsy, which may be submitted for light microscopic examination, *in situ* hybridization, immunohistochemistry, or direct immunofluorescence. Immunocompromised hosts with recurrent intraoral herpes simplex virus (HSV) infection typically are treated with systemic antiviral therapy (e.g., oral or intravenous acyclovir). In addition, prophylactic antiviral therapy may be considered for patients with severe immunosuppression.

Recurrent Intraoral Herpes

Multiple punctate ulcers on the mandibular attached gingiva.

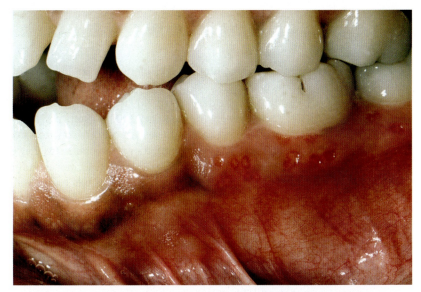

■ Figure **7.9**
Recurrent Intraoral Herpes

Multiple punctate ulcers on the hard palate.

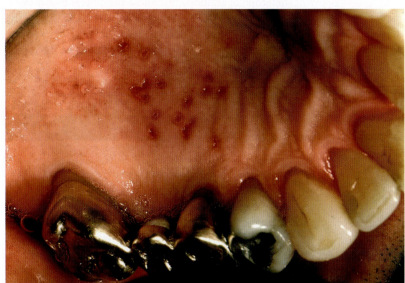

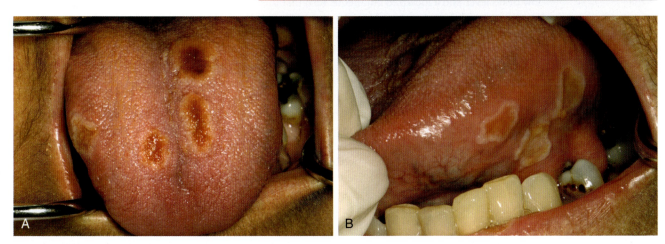

■ Figure **7.10**
Chronic Intraoral Herpes

(A) Dorsal and (B) ventrolateral tongue exhibiting multiple erosions and ulcers with slightly raised, yellowish borders. The patient was on immunosuppressive therapy for two autoimmune disorders.

Infectious Mononucleosis

Fig. **7.11**

Infectious mononucleosis ("mono") is a condition closely associated with primary Epstein-Barr virus (EBV) infection. Although EBV infection may be detected in greater than 95% of adults worldwide, clinically evident disease develops in only a subset. In the United States, the incidence of infectious mononucleosis is approximately five cases per 1000 persons per year, with a peak among individuals 15 to 24 years old. Transmission mainly occurs via exposure to contaminated saliva (e.g., from kissing, sharing straws or cutlery).

Initially, patients with infectious mononucleosis may experience malaise, fatigue, headache, and low-grade fever. As the condition progresses, typical clinical findings include pharyngitis, fever up to 104°F, markedly enlarged and tender lymph nodes, and bilateral tonsillar enlargement. The tonsillar surfaces may exhibit a white, yellowish, or gray exudate. Oral findings may include necrotizing ulcerative gingivitis and transient palatal petechiae. Other possible clinical manifestations include periorbital edema, rash, splenomegaly, hepatomegaly, and jaundice. Although most findings resolve within about 1 month, fatigue and cervical lymphadenopathy can persist for several additional weeks to months. Potential complications include hemolytic anemia, thrombocytopenia, facial nerve palsy, meningoencephalitis, splenic rupture, and upper airway obstruction. The diagnosis may be made by correlation of the clinical findings with a positive heterophile antibody test and a peripheral blood smear showing atypical lymphocytosis. The mainstay of treatment for infectious mononucleosis is supportive care (i.e., acetaminophen or nonsteroidal anti-inflammatory drugs, fluids, nutrition). Also, sports participation should be avoided for at least 3 weeks after onset of symptoms in order to prevent the rare possibility of splenic rupture.

Varicella (Chickenpox)

Figs. **7.12 and 7.13**

Varicella (chickenpox) is an acute disease caused by primary infection with the varicella-zoster virus (VZV). The disease is highly contagious and is transmitted via direct contact with active lesions or inhalation of aerosolized droplets. Since the implementation of the varicella vaccination in 1996, there have been dramatic declines in the annual incidence of the disease in the United States.

Because of high vaccination rates, more than half of new varicella cases in the United States currently represent breakthrough infection (i.e., infection with wild-type VZV occurring in a previously immunized patient). Such cases tend to be relatively mild and resolve within about 4 to 6 days. The patient may exhibit low or no fever and a localized cutaneous rash that includes a small number of maculopapular lesions and few to no vesicles.

In contrast, in unvaccinated individuals, varicella typically causes a generalized, pruritic skin rash, often accompanied or preceded by fever and malaise. The rash initially appears on the head and then spreads to involve the trunk and extremities. The lesions initially appear as erythematous macules, which subsequently evolve into papules, vesicles, pustules, and crusts. Over several days, there may be successive crops of hundreds of lesions in various stages of development.

Lesions also may involve the oral/oropharyngeal mucosa and perioral skin. Sometimes such lesions precede the skin lesions. Frequently involved oral subsites include the vermilion border, palate, and buccal mucosa. Initially, there may be white, opaque vesicles with surrounding erythema; subsequently, the vesicles rupture to form small white, yellow-white, or brown ulcers with erythematous halos. The ulcers are usually asymptomatic or slightly painful. Depending on disease severity, the number of oral lesions may vary from 1 to 30.

Varicella usually is mild and self-limited in otherwise healthy children. However, adults, infants, and immunocompromised individuals are at increased risk for severe disease and serious complications (e.g., secondary bacterial skin infection, viral or bacterial pneumonia, cerebellar ataxia, encephalitis, aseptic meningitis). Therefore, compliance with immunization protocols is advised. Immunocompetent children with uncomplicated varicella typically receive supportive care (e.g., acetaminophen, warm baking soda/oatmeal baths, calamine lotion, diphenhydramine). Children with varicella should not be administered aspirin because of the risk for developing Reye syndrome; also, nonsteroidal anti-inflammatory drugs are contraindicated because of the risk for severe skin and soft tissue complications. Antiviral therapy (e.g., acyclovir—ideally initiated within 24 hours after the appearance of the rash) generally is reserved for patients at increased risk for severe disease complications.

■ Figure **7.11**
Infectious Mononucleosis
Multiple petechiae on the soft palate.

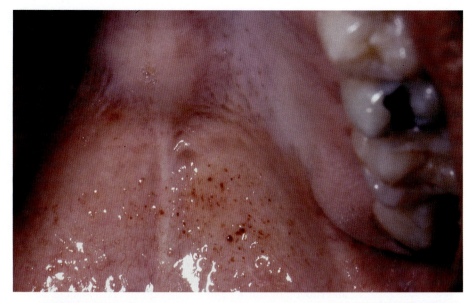

■ Figure **7.12**
Varicella
Skin rash on the neck with erythema, vesicles, and crusting.

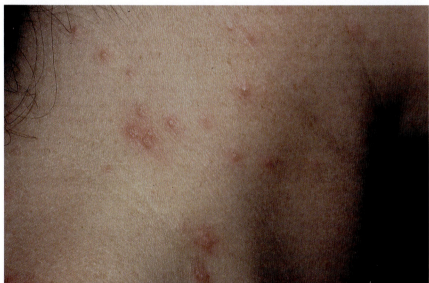

■ Figure **7.13**
Varicella
White, opaque vesicle at the base of the uvula.
(With appreciation to Tristan Neville.)

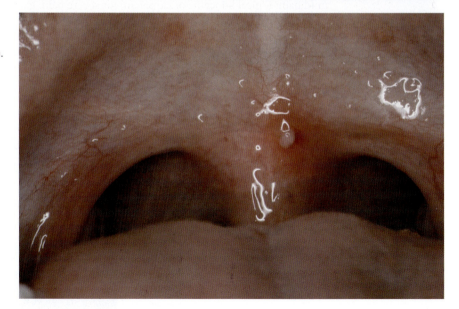

Figs. 7.14–7.17

After primary infection, varicella-zoster virus (VZV) establishes latency in the regional nerve ganglia. Upon reactivation, the virus can cause recurrent disease, which is termed **herpes zoster** (shingles). Factors associated with reactivation include aging, human immunodeficiency virus (HIV) infection, malignancy, cytotoxic or immunosuppressive drug therapy, radiation therapy, stress, and dental manipulation. In the United States, there are approximately 1 million episodes of herpes zoster per year, and the disease occurs during the lifetime of about one in three individuals.

Clinically, herpes zoster usually causes pain and an acute rash along the distribution of the affected sensory nerve (dermatome). The dermatomes of the trunk and trigeminal nerve are involved most often. With trigeminal nerve involvement, the oral cavity and/or skin can be affected. *Ramsay Hunt syndrome* is a clinical variant caused by VZV reactivation in the geniculate ganglion with involvement of cranial nerves VII and VIII. In addition to skin lesions of the external auditory canal, these patients often develop unilateral facial nerve paralysis, hearing loss, and vertigo. Initially, greater than 90% of patients with herpes zoster experience prodromal pain and paresthesia, at times accompanied by fever, malaise, and headache. The patient may complain of a burning, boring, prickly, or knifelike sensation. Subsequently, there is typically an eruption of vesicles and pustules on an erythematous base. After several days, the blisters rupture to form ulcers, often with cutaneous crusts. Intraoral lesions may appear as a unilateral eruption on the palate, buccal mucosa, or tongue; the lesions characteristically extend to the midline. In addition, sometimes teeth in the affected area can develop pulpitis, pulpal necrosis, or root resorption. In rare cases, tooth mobility and tooth loss may result from gnathic osteonecrosis (during or after the rash). In otherwise healthy individuals, the lesions of the acute phase heal within about 2 to 3 weeks. However, after resolution of the rash, approximately 15% of patients develop chronic pain (termed *postherpetic neuralgia*), which, at times, can be debilitating. Older age has been associated with increased risk and severity of postherpetic neuralgia.

Severe complications of herpes zoster are rare but possible, especially among immunocompromised individuals. Such complications may include viremia, pneumonia, hepatitis, encephalitis, and disseminated intravascular coagulopathy. In addition, ocular involvement can cause blindness; importantly, patients with cutaneous lesions on the tip of the nose should be evaluated by an ophthalmologist; such lesions indicate involvement of the nasociliary branch of the trigeminal nerve and an increased risk for ocular infection. Furthermore, in very rare cases, patients with herpes zoster involving the trigeminal nerve may develop an ischemic stroke syndrome (known as *granulomatous angiitis*).

Treatment considerations for herpes zoster include supportive care (e.g., diphenhydramine, nonaspirin antipyretics, keeping the skin lesions clean and covered); antiviral medication (e.g., acyclovir, valacyclovir, famciclovir), preferably initiated within 72 hours after the rash appears; and pain management (e.g., for mild pain: topical lidocaine or capsaicin; for severe pain: gabapentin, pregabalin, tricyclic antidepressants, desipramine, opioids). In addition, vaccination is effective in reducing the incidence of herpes zoster and postherpetic neuralgia. In the United States, the Advisory Committee on Immunization Practices (ACIP) recently decided to recommend the preferential use of a new recombinant herpes zoster subunit (HZ/su) vaccine over the live herpes zoster vaccine for adults 50 years and older.

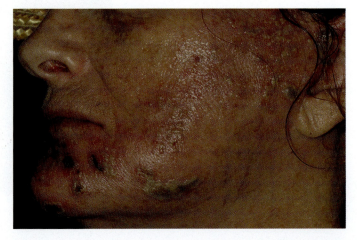

■ Figure **7.14**
Herpes Zoster
Facial skin rash with vesicles, ulceration, and crusting. Note the dermatomal distribution.

■ Figure **7.15**
Herpes Zoster

Same patient as seen in Fig. 7.14 with ulcers involving the left tongue and left lower lip vermilion. The lesions extend to the midline. The patient subsequently was diagnosed with underlying human immunodeficiency virus infection.

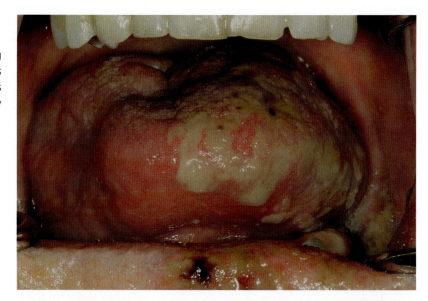

■ Figure **7.16**
Herpes Zoster (Ramsay Hunt Syndrome)

Same patient as depicted in Figs. 7.14 and 7.15 with a previous outbreak of herpes zoster several years earlier. This time the eruption involved the right side of the face with associated facial nerve paralysis and hearing loss. When the patient was asked to smile, the muscles of the right face did not respond.

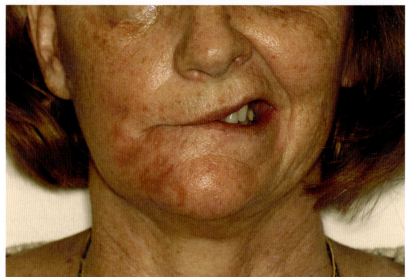

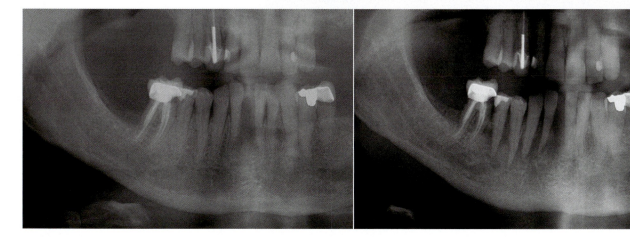

■ Figure **7.17**
Herpes Zoster

Radiographs of the same patient from Fig. 7.16, showing right mandibular osteonecrosis and severe alveolar bone loss that developed over a 5-month period. (With appreciation to Dr. Michael Tabor.)

Fig. **7.18**

Herpangina is a clinical disease pattern caused by various enterovirus serotypes, especially coxsackievirus A1 to A6, A8, A10, and A22. These viruses are transmitted via the fecal-oral route, saliva, or respiratory droplets. Although many infected individuals are asymptomatic, clinically evident disease is possible. Herpangina most frequently develops in infants and children. The patient typically experiences an acute onset of fever and sore throat, at times accompanied by anorexia, vomiting, diarrhea, and abdominal pain. Clinical examination exhibits an enanthem, mainly involving the soft palate, tonsillar pillars, and uvula. The lesions initially appear as erythematous macules, which subsequently evolve into vesicles that readily rupture to form shallow ulcers. The ulcers typically measure about 2 to 4 mm in diameter and are surrounded by intense erythema. The total number of lesions is usually small (approximately two to six). Most patients develop self-limited disease, with fever lasting several days and the oropharyngeal lesions healing within 10 days. Clinical management includes supportive care (i.e., nonaspirin antipyretics, fluid maintenance). In rare cases, patients may develop severe disease complications necessitating hospitalization. Preventive measures should be undertaken, including handwashing and disinfecting surfaces, especially in childcare settings.

Hand-Foot-and-Mouth Disease

Figs. **7.19 and 7.20**

Hand-foot-and-mouth disease is the best-known clinical presentation of enterovirus infection. Major serotypes associated with this condition include coxsackie virus A16, A6, and A10, as well as enterovirus 71. The disease occurs worldwide, with major outbreaks noted in the Asia–Pacific region over the past few decades. Most patients who develop hand-foot-and-mouth disease are younger than 10 years old, and epidemics often arise in schools and daycare facilities. In temperate regions, outbreaks tend to happen in the summer or early autumn. Disease transmission occurs via the fecal-oral route, saliva, or respiratory secretions.

Early clinical manifestations of hand-foot-and-mouth disease include fever, malaise, poor appetite, and sore throat. Subsequently, within a couple of days, the patient typically develops an oral enanthem; frequently involved subsites include the buccal mucosa, labial mucosa, and tongue. The oral lesions appear as zones of erythema, which then evolve into vesicles that rupture to form painful ulcers. In addition, the patient usually develops a skin rash. Classically, the exanthem involves the palms, soles, and digits; however, more widespread or, at times, perioral skin involvement also may be seen. The cutaneous lesions tend to be painful and may appear as small erythematous macules that evolve into vesicles or papules. The enanthem and exanthem usually resolve within about 7 to 10 days. However, some patients develop nail changes (e.g., horizontal grooves or ridges known as *Beau's lines*, nail shedding) several weeks later.

Most cases of hand-foot-and-mouth disease are mild and managed by supportive measures (i.e., nonaspirin antipyretics and analgesics, maintaining adequate hydration and nutrition). However, there is the potential for serious complications (such as severe dehydration, meningitis, paralysis, brainstem encephalitis, neurogenic pulmonary edema, cerebellar ataxia) and death. In particular, significant morbidity and mortality has been reported in Asian outbreaks of the enterovirus 71 infection. Patients with severe disease may receive intravenous immunoglobulin therapy, although further research is needed. Preventive measures for hand-foot-and-mouth disease include handwashing, disinfecting surfaces and objects, and keeping sick children out of school or daycare.

■ Figure **7.18**

Herpangina

Ulcers, vesicles, and erythema involving the soft palate and uvula.

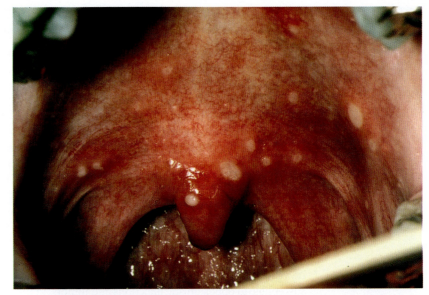

■ Figure **7.19**

Hand-Foot-and-Mouth Disease

Vesicles on the dorsal tongue. (Courtesy Dr. Nathan Wilson.)

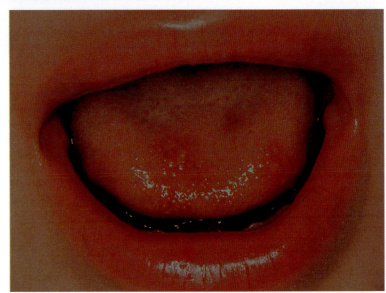

■ Figure **7.20**

Hand-Foot-and-Mouth Disease

Vesicles and focal ulceration on the skin of the toes. (Courtesy Dr. Nathan Wilson.)

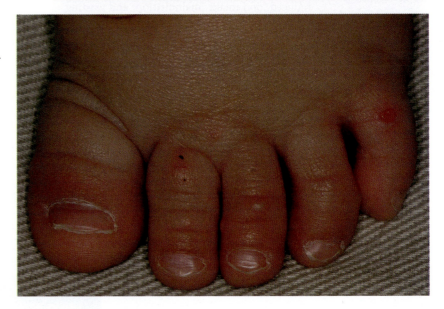

Human Immunodeficiency Virus and Acquired Immunodeficiency Syndrome

The **human immunodeficiency virus (HIV)** is a single-stranded ribonucleic acid (RNA) retrovirus that causes **acquired immunodeficiency syndrome (AIDS)**. Over the past several decades, significant advances in our understanding of HIV/AIDS etiopathogenesis have led to improved treatment and prevention. Nevertheless, the infection remains a major global health problem. In 2016 there were approximately 37 million people living with HIV worldwide. The virus is transmitted most often via sexual contact (both heterosexual and male-to-male) or shared injection paraphernalia among injection drug users. Other possible modes of transmission include from mother to infant during pregnancy, birth, or breastfeeding; occupational exposure to contaminated needles/sharp objects; and contaminated blood, blood products, or organ/tissue transplants. The virus primarily targets CD4+ T-lymphocytes, although other CD4+ cells (e.g., dendritic cells and macrophages) can be infected as well. During the early stages of infection, there is an acute burst of viremia, with dissemination and formation of a lymphoid viral reservoir. Subsequently, chronic (latent) infection is established, with low levels of viral replication. In an untreated patient, latency can last many years before progression to AIDS. An HIV-infected patient is diagnosed with AIDS (stage 3 disease) if the CD4+ T-lymphocyte count falls below a certain threshold (<200 cells/mm^3 for patients ≥6 years old) or if there is an AIDS-defining opportunistic illness. Immunosuppression renders the patient susceptible to opportunistic infections and tumors. In the following subsections, various oral manifestations of HIV/AIDS are presented.

HIV-Associated Oral Candidiasis

Figs. **7.21–7.24**

Candidiasis is the most common oral manifestation of HIV infection. In some cases, oral candidiasis is a presenting sign that leads to an initial diagnosis of HIV infection. In addition, the development of oral candidiasis may be a harbinger of progression to AIDS. With the advent of combined antiretroviral therapy, most studies have noted an overall decline in the prevalence of oral candidiasis among HIV-infected patients. Nevertheless, HIV-associated oral candidiasis still occurs with some frequency, and it can be a clinical sign of antiretroviral treatment failure.

Any of the various clinical patterns of oral candidiasis (e.g., pseudomembranous, erythematous, hyperplastic, angular cheilitis) can be seen within the setting of HIV infection. Interestingly, some investigators have reported an increase in the erythematous variant and a decrease in the pseudomembranous and hyperplastic variants when comparing HIV-infected patient cohorts before and after the introduction of widespread combined antiretroviral therapy. Particularly in individuals with profound immunosuppression, the clinical presentation can be severe. There may be diffuse involvement of the oral cavity as well as the oropharynx and esophagus. The patient may experience pain, burning, and dysgeusia, which can lead to reduced food intake, malnutrition, and wasting.

HIV-associated oral candidiasis is treated with antifungal medication (e.g., for mild disease: clotrimazole troches, miconazole mucoadhesive buccal tablets; for moderate to severe disease: fluconazole; for fluconazole-refractory disease: itraconazole solution, posoconazole suspension, voriconazole). In addition, the initiation or optimization of combined antiretroviral therapy is important for addressing underlying HIV infection and for reducing the risk of recurrence of candidiasis.

■ Figure **7.21**
HIV-Associated Oral Candidiasis
Pseudomembranous candidiasis with white plaques on the right tongue.

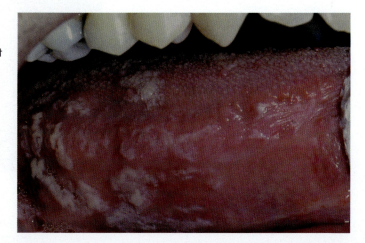

■ Figure **7.22**
HIV-Associated Oral Candidiasis
Pseudomembranous candidiasis with extensive white plaques on the palate and alveolar mucosa.

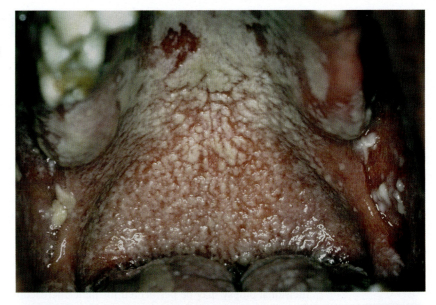

■ Figure **7.23**
HIV-Associated Oral Candidiasis
Diffuse erythema of the hard palate.

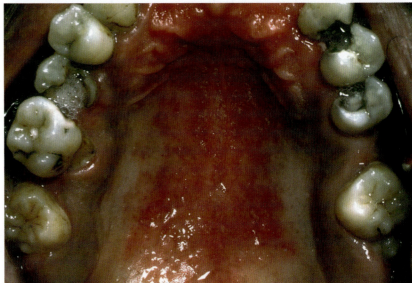

■ Figure **7.24**
HIV-Associated Oral Candidiasis
Angular cheilitis with erythema, fissures, and crusting at the left corner of the mouth.

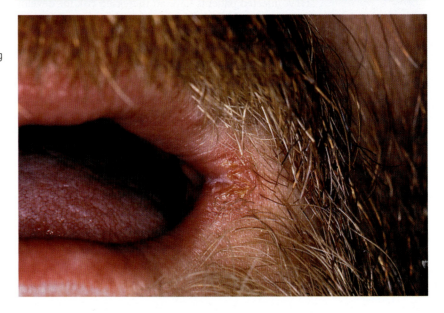

Figs. 7.25 and 7.26

Oral hairy leukoplakia is a condition caused by Epstein-Barr virus (EBV) and strongly associated with HIV infection. Importantly, the development of oral hairy leukoplakia in an HIV-infected individual is considered a clinical marker of severe immunosuppression and advanced HIV disease. In addition, the condition can occur in patients with other causes of immunosuppression (e.g., organ transplantation, systemic or inhaled corticosteroids, malignancy). In very rare cases, oral hairy leukoplakia also has been reported in older individuals, apparently due to immune senescence.

Clinical examination shows a white, corrugated plaque involving one or both sides of the lateral tongue. Sometimes the lesion can spread to the dorsal tongue, and rare examples may arise in other sites (e.g., buccal mucosa, oropharynx). The plaque cannot be wiped away, and the surface often exhibits vertical striations or a shaggy appearance. Most patients are asymptomatic, although superimposed candidiasis may cause discomfort or a burning sensation. In a patient with known HIV infection, a strong presumptive diagnosis often is made based on the clinical findings. However, other conditions that can be considered in the clinical differential diagnosis include morsicatio linguarum, frictional hyperkeratosis, cinnamon stomatitis, hyperplastic candidiasis, and conventional leukoplakia. If the diagnosis is uncertain, then an incisional biopsy may be performed for light microscopic examination and demonstration of EBV (e.g., by *in situ* hybridization or immunohistochemistry).

The clinical importance of oral hairy leukoplakia is that it usually indicates significant underlying immunosuppression. A thorough history and examination should be performed in order to assess for HIV infection or other causes of immunosuppression. In a patient with known HIV infection, the development of oral hairy leukoplakia may indicate the progression of HIV disease and/or the development of antiretroviral drug resistance; thus, the assessment of drug compliance and the optimization of combined antiretroviral therapy are advised.

Oral hairy leukoplakia is a benign condition, and in most cases it does not require direct treatment. However, some patients may request treatment because of aesthetic concerns or mild symptoms. Anti-herpesviral agents (e.g., acyclovir, valacyclovir) or topical retinoids can induce resolution, but the lesion often returns upon discontinuation of therapy.

HIV and Human Papillomavirus–Related Lesions

Fig. 7.27

HIV–infected patients have an increased risk for developing various types of oral human papillomavirus (HPV)–related lesions. For example, benign oral HPV-related lesions ("oral warts") occur in up to 5% of HIV-positive individuals compared to 0.5% of the general population. Such benign lesions include squamous papilloma, verruca vulgaris, condyloma acuminatum, and multifocal epithelial hyperplasia. In addition, HIV-infected individuals exhibit an increased risk for HPV-related oropharyngeal squamous cell carcinoma.

Oral HPV infection has been detected more frequently among HIV-positive (16% to 40%) than HIV-negative individuals (4% to 25%). This increased frequency may be related to traditional risk factors (e.g., oral sexual activity) as well as HIV-related immunosuppression. Although the majority of oral HPV infections clear within 1 to 2 years, persistence has been associated with older age, male gender, and current cigarette smoking. Interestingly, unlike most HIV-associated lesions, oral warts have increased in frequency since the introduction of combined antiretroviral therapy. Some investigators have proposed that these lesions may be induced by an immune reconstitution inflammatory syndrome.

Within the setting of HIV infection, oral warts are often multifocal. They may develop on the labial mucosa, tongue, buccal mucosa, gingiva, or other sites. The lesions can be white or pink, with a rough, warty, or cauliflower-like surface. Most cases are treated by surgical excision; microscopic examination and clinical follow-up are warranted because of the potential for the development of dysplasia or carcinoma.

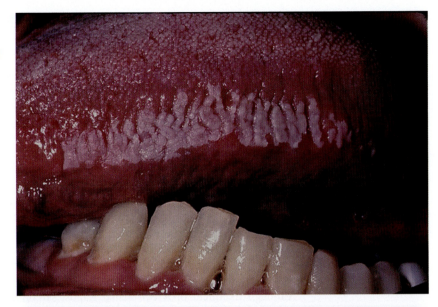

■ Figure 7.25

HIV-Associated Oral Hairy Leukoplakia

White plaque with vertical striations on the left lateral border of the tongue.

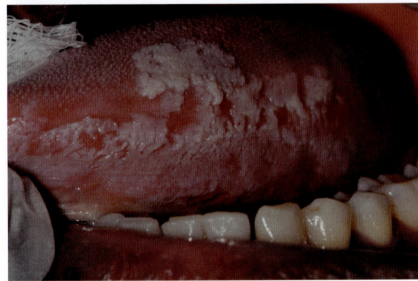

■ Figure 7.26

HIV-Associated Oral Hairy Leukoplakia

Extensive white plaque on the left tongue.

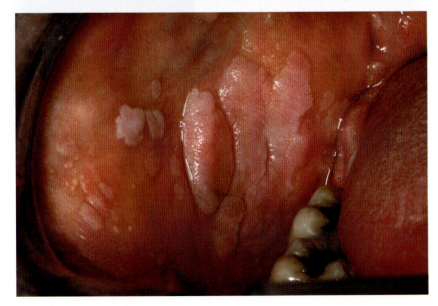

■ Figure 7.27

HIV and Human Papillomavirus–Related Lesions

Right buccal mucosa showing multiple raised, pink-white lesions with rough surfaces.

Figs. **7.28–7.31**

Kaposi sarcoma is a vascular malignancy caused by human herpesvirus 8 (HHV-8, Kaposi sarcoma–associated herpesvirus [KSHV]). It is considered an AIDS-defining cancer, and most cases of Kaposi sarcoma in the United States are AIDS-related. At the height of the HIV epidemic in the early 1990s, the age-adjusted annual incidence of Kaposi sarcoma in the United States peaked at around 4.7 cases per 100,000 persons. However, with advances in combined antiretroviral therapy, the annual incidence has been declining and currently is estimated at 0.6 cases per 100,000 persons. Among HIV-infected individuals in Western countries, Kaposi sarcoma exhibits a predilection for adult male homosexuals.

Oral lesions are noted at some point in about 70% of patients with AIDS-related Kaposi sarcoma, and in some cases, oral lesions represent the initial site of involvement. Frequently involved subsites include the palate, gingiva, and tongue. A given patient may exhibit one or more oral lesions. Initially, the lesions may appear as purplish, blue, or erythematous brown macules that subsequently develop into plaques and nodules. Pain, bleeding, and ulceration also may be noted. Progressive lesions on the palate or gingiva can lead to the destruction of underlying bone and the loosening of teeth. In addition, extensive oral lesions may cause rapidly progressive facial lymphedema.

Although treatment of AIDS-related Kaposi sarcoma depends on clinical staging, the mainstay of therapy is initiation or optimization of combined antiretroviral therapy. Oral lesions often regress with such therapy, although unusual cases of exacerbation due to an immune reconstitution inflammatory syndrome have been reported. For patients with advanced disease, systemic chemotherapy can be administered as well.

■ Figure **7.28**
AIDS-Related Kaposi Sarcoma
Purplish lesion on the skin of the chin.

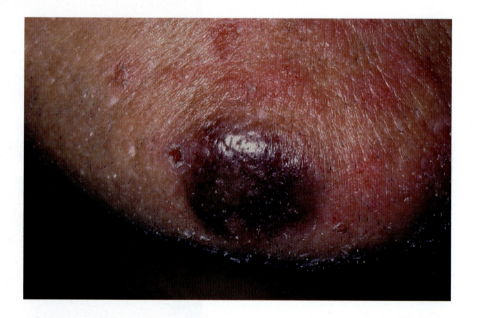

■ Figure **7.29**
AIDS-Related Kaposi Sarcoma
Purplish lesion involving the anterior maxillary frenum area.

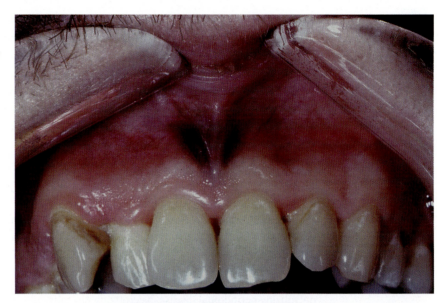

■ Figure **7.30**
AIDS-Related Kaposi Sarcoma
Purplish lesion involving the left posterior palate and palatal gingiva. Note the adjacent pseudomembranous candidiasis.

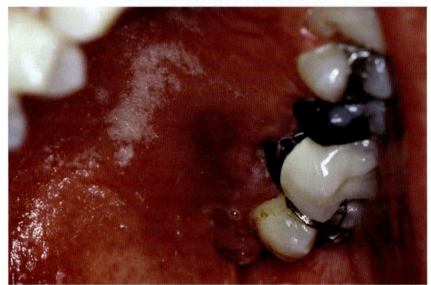

■ Figure **7.31**
AIDS-Related Kaposi Sarcoma
Purplish blue lesion on the palate with associated nodularity.

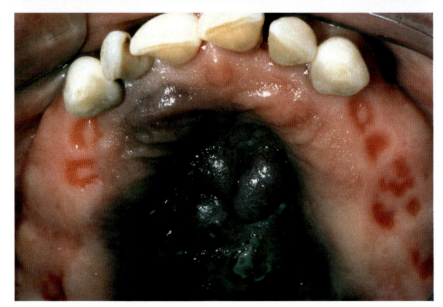

Figs. **7.32–7.34**

There is a strong association between HIV infection and certain unusual patterns of periodontal disease, including *linear gingival erythema*, *necrotizing ulcerative gingivitis*, and *necrotizing ulcerative periodontitis*. According to some studies, necrotizing ulcerative gingivitis can develop in HIV-infected patients with CD4+ T-lymphocyte counts less than 500 cells/mm^3, whereas linear gingival erythema and necrotizing ulcerative periodontitis typically occur in those with CD4+ T-lymphocyte counts less than 200 cells/mm^3. The frequency of these conditions among HIV-infected patients has decreased significantly with the introduction of combined antiretroviral therapy.

Clinically, linear gingival erythema appears as a distinct linear band of erythema along the free gingival margin. In some cases, punctate or more diffuse erythema also may be noted on the gingiva and alveolar mucosa. The etiopathogenesis of linear gingival erythema is uncertain, although some investigators hypothesize that the condition results from subgingival colonization and tissue invasion by *Candida* species. Treatment may include débridement, povidone-iodine irrigation, chlorhexidine mouth rinse, and/or antifungal therapy. Also, the clinician should ensure that the patient is receiving appropriate combined antiretroviral therapy.

Necrotizing ulcerative gingivitis and necrotizing ulcerative periodontitis are considered subtypes of necrotizing periodontal disease. Necrotizing ulcerative gingivitis is characterized by a rapid onset of gingival pain and bleeding with ulceration and crater-like necrosis of the interdental papillae. Fetid odor, fever, malaise, and cervical lymphadenopathy also may be present. In necrotizing ulcerative periodontitis, gingival ulceration and necrosis are accompanied by rapidly progressive periodontal attachment loss. In some cases, these necrotizing periodontal diseases may progress to cause more extensive destruction of the oral tissues *(necrotizing stomatitis)*. Management of necrotizing periodontal disease in HIV-positive patients typically includes débridement, topical and systemic antimicrobial therapy, pain management, long-term periodontal maintenance, and the initiation or optimization of combined antiretroviral therapy. In terms of prevention, some investigators have reported that trimethoprim/sulfamethoxazole (typically prescribed for prevention of *Pneumocystis jiroveci* pneumonia in HIV patients) may protect against necrotizing ulcerative gingivitis, although further studies are needed.

In addition to localized gingival erythema and necrotizing periodontal disease, patients with HIV infection may develop conventional chronic periodontitis. However, the reported prevalence of chronic periodontitis among HIV-infected individuals has been variable, and the impact of combined antiretroviral therapy on chronic periodontitis in HIV-positive patients requires further research. Nevertheless, it is advisable for patients with HIV infection to receive regular preventive oral health care, including professional prophylaxis and oral hygiene reinforcement.

Figure **7.32**
HIV-Associated Periodontal Disease
Necrotizing ulcerative gingivitis with multiple "punched-out" interdental papillae on the mandibular facial gingiva.

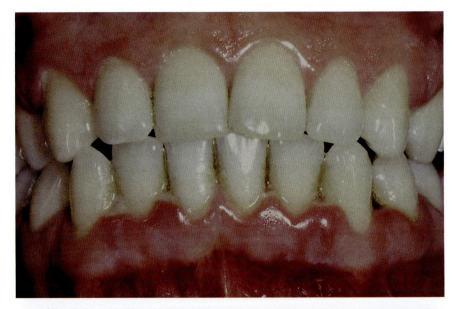

Figure **7.33**
HIV-Associated Periodontal Disease
Necrotizing ulcerative gingivitis with extensive areas of necrosis.

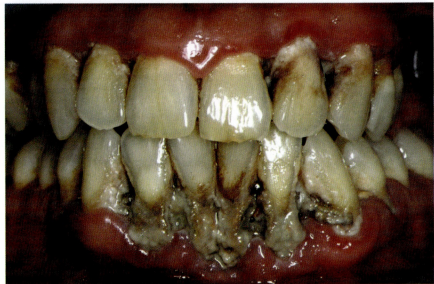

Figure **7.34**
HIV-Associated Periodontal Disease
Necrotizing ulcerative periodontitis with marked attachment loss and loss of several maxillary anterior teeth.

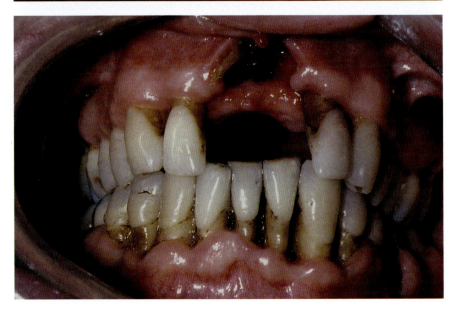

HIV-Associated Lymphadenopathy

Fig. 7.35

Lymphadenopathy is a common finding in HIV-infected patients and can occur during any stage of HIV disease. Various lymph node groups can be involved, including the cervical and periparotid lymph nodes. Lymph node enlargement may result from the direct effects of HIV as well as from opportunistic infections (e.g., mycobacterial infection, deep fungal infection, toxoplasmosis, bacillary angiomatosis); lymphoproliferative disorders (e.g., human herpesvirus 8 [HHV-8]–*associated multicentric Castleman disease)*; or malignancies (e.g., lymphoma, Kaposi sarcoma). Approximately 3 to 6 weeks after initial HIV infection, some patients develop an *acute retroviral syndrome*. This condition presents as a self-limited, infectious mononucleosis-like illness characterized by fever, pharyngitis, and cervical lymphadenopathy. In other cases, HIV-infected patients may develop *persistent generalized lymphadenopathy* (defined as extra-inguinal lymphadenopathy persisting ≥3 months and involving ≥2 noncontiguous lymph node groups). This condition often is accompanied by fever, malaise, weight loss, and headache. The most commonly involved sites include the cervical, submandibular, occipital, and axillary lymph nodes. In addition, some HIV-positive patients develop enlargement of the periparotid lymph nodes, which is often bilateral and characterized by cystic changes (termed *cystic lymphoid hyperplasia, benign lymphoepithelial lesion,* or *HIV-related salivary gland disease*). Fine-needle aspiration may aid in the diagnosis of enlarged lymph nodes in the head and neck region. Treatment depends on the specific diagnosis. HIV-associated reactive lymphadenopathy may improve with the administration of combined antiretroviral therapy, although the virus often persists within lymphoid tissue despite an undetectable viral load in the peripheral blood.

HIV-Associated Aphthous Stomatitis

Fig. 7.36

Aphthous stomatitis tends to be more severe in HIV-infected patients compared to otherwise healthy individuals. Within the setting of HIV infection, the ulcers may recur with increased frequency, reach a relatively large size, and exhibit a chronic course. In addition, the lesions can be very painful, making it difficult for the patient to eat and drink. Although all three major clinical subtypes (minor, major, herpetiform) of aphthae can be seen, up to two-thirds of affected patients exhibit the herpetiform and major variants. In particular, some investigators have noted that major aphthae tend to develop in AIDS patients with very low CD4+ T-lymphocyte counts (often <100 cells/mm^3) and high viral loads. In general, biopsy of persistent oral ulceration should be considered in order to rule out other conditions (e.g., herpes simplex virus [HSV] or cytomegalovirus infection, deep fungal infection, malignancy). Clinical management includes the initiation or optimization of combined antiretroviral therapy. Pain may be managed with topical anesthetics, coating agents, and systemic analgesics. In addition, depending on the severity of the aphthae, topical corticosteroids (e.g., dexamethasone solution, fluocinonide gel, clobetasol gel, augmented beta-methasone gel), intralesional corticosteroid injections, and/or systemic medications (e.g., corticosteroids, dapsone, thalidomide) may be administered. However, immunosuppressive and immunomodulatory agents should be used with caution because of the risk for inducing worsened immune status, increased viral load, and adverse side effects.

HIV-Associated Histoplasmosis

Fig. 7.37

Histoplasmosis is a deep fungal infection caused by *Histoplasma capsulatum*. Although histoplasmosis primarily affects the lungs, HIV-infected individuals with low CD4+ T-lymphocyte counts (<150/ mm^3) are at increased risk for disseminated disease. According to the Centers for Disease Control and Prevention's HIV surveillance case definition, disseminated or extrapulmonary histoplasmosis is an AIDS-defining opportunistic illness. In the United States, the frequency of disseminated histoplasmosis has declined with the advent of combined antiretroviral therapy. Nevertheless, the condition continues to cause significant morbidity and mortality in resource-limited, endemic regions.

In HIV-associated histoplasmosis, oral lesions typically result from extrapulmonary dissemination, although primary oral involvement is possible. Frequently involved subsites include the tongue, gingiva, palate, and buccal mucosa. The lesions can be painful and may be solitary, multifocal, or diffuse. Clinical examination often shows an ulcer with a rolled, indurated margin. Other examples may appear as a nodule, plaque, or mucosal erythema with granular surface change. Signs of systemic infection may include weight loss, fever, cough, and hepatosplenomegaly.

■ Figure **7.35**
HIV-Associated Lymphadenopathy
Enlarged left cervical lymph nodes.

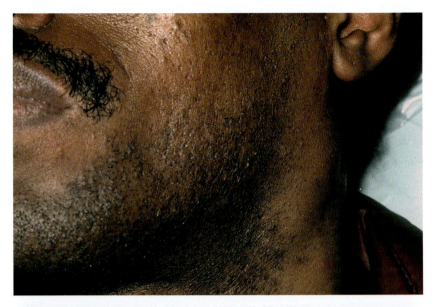

■ Figure **7.36**
HIV-Associated Aphthous Stomatitis
Ulceration with surrounding erythema in the maxillary labial frenum area.

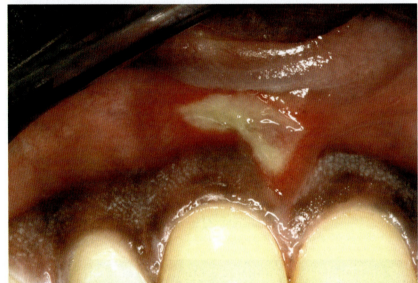

■ Figure **7.37**
HIV-Associated Histoplasmosis
Extensive lesion on the palate exhibiting erythema with granular surface change and ulceration.

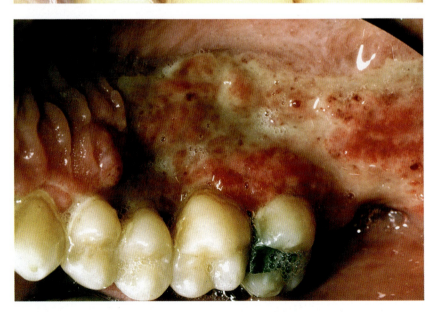

Management of HIV-associated disseminated histoplasmosis typically includes systemic antifungal medication (e.g., itraconazole, liposomal amphotericin B) as well as combined antiretroviral therapy. The condition is usually fatal without treatment, and prompt treatment is crucial for patient survival. In addition, prophylactic itraconazole is recommended for HIV-infected patients with CD4+ T-lymphocyte counts less than $150/mm^3$ in endemic regions where the incidence of histoplasmosis is great.

HIV-Associated Lymphoma

Fig. **7.38**

Lymphoma represents the most common type of malignancy among HIV-infected individuals in developed countries. Some investigators have estimated that, compared to the general population, HIV-infected patients exhibit a relative risk of 60 to 200 for non-Hodgkin lymphoma and 8 to 10 for Hodgkin lymphoma. In particular, non-Hodgkin lymphoma represents the most common cause of cancer-related death among HIV-infected individuals in the United States.

Major subtypes of non-Hodgkin lymphoma found within the setting of HIV infection include Burkitt lymphoma, diffuse large B-cell lymphoma, plasmablastic lymphoma, and primary effusion lymphoma (and its solid variants). The etiopathogenesis of the latter has been linked to human herpesvirus 8 (HHV-8) infection, whereas the other types may develop in association with Epstein-Barr virus (EBV) infection. Interestingly, plasmablastic lymphoma initially was described within the oral cavity of HIV-positive individuals, although unusual cases arising in other sites and/or HIV-negative patients have been reported also. In addition, according to the Centers for Disease Control and Prevention's HIV surveillance case definition, certain non-Hodgkin lymphomas (i.e., Burkitt lymphoma, immunoblastic lymphoma, primary brain lymphoma) are AIDS-defining opportunistic illnesses.

Primary oral involvement has been noted in only about 4% of AIDS-related non-Hodgkin lymphomas. Frequently involved subsites include the palate, gingiva, and tongue. The lesion may appear as an erythematous, rapidly enlarging mucosal mass, with or without ulceration. In addition, some examples arise within the jawbones; radiographic examination may show an ill-defined radiolucency, widening of the periodontal ligament, and/or loss of the lamina dura.

Management for patients with HIV-associated lymphoma typically includes combination chemotherapy in conjunction with combined antiretroviral therapy. The prognosis varies by lymphoma type. However, with advances in antiretroviral therapy, clinical outcomes have been improving and, in many cases, are now comparable to those seen in non-HIV-infected populations.

HIV and Oral/Head and Neck Squamous Cell Carcinoma

Fig. **7.39**

Although the most common head and neck malignancies arising in AIDS patients are Kaposi sarcoma and non-Hodgkin lymphoma, an increased risk for head and neck squamous cell carcinoma also has been noted in patients with HIV/AIDS. In general, over the past few decades since the introduction of combined antiretroviral therapy, patients with HIV infection have been living longer, with a decreased frequency of AIDS-defining cancers and an increased frequency of various non-AIDS–defining cancers. According to several large-scale studies, the risk for head and neck squamous cell carcinoma is approximately 1.5 to 4 times higher among HIV-infected individuals compared to the general population. In addition, an analysis of epidemiologic data from the United States in 2010 found an approximately 50% excess of oral cavity/ pharyngeal cancer among HIV-infected individuals compared to the general population. Head and neck tumor development appears to result from HIV-related immunosuppression as well as conventional risk factors (e.g., tobacco use, heavy alcohol consumption, ultraviolet light [for lower lip vermilion tumors], human papillomavirus (HPV) [especially for oropharyngeal tumors], and Epstein-Barr virus (EBV) [especially for nasopharyngeal tumors]). The tumors may arise in various head and neck mucosal sites, including the oral cavity, oropharynx, larynx, and conjunctiva. Several studies have reported that patients with HIV who develop squamous cell carcinomas of the oral cavity or head and neck region tend to exhibit a younger mean age and more advanced tumor stage at presentation compared to those without HIV.

The clinical appearance of oral squamous cell carcinoma is similar among HIV-infected and non-HIV–infected patients. The lesion may appear as a red and/or white plaque or mass, at times with ulceration. Frequently involved subsites include the tongue, floor of the mouth, buccal mucosa, gingiva, and lip. Depending on the clinical stage, treatment may include surgical resection, radiation therapy, and/or chemotherapy.

HIV-Associated Lymphoma

Erythematous, nodular mass on the right maxillary gingiva.

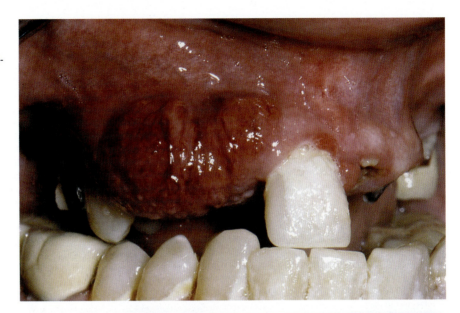

■ Figure **7.39**
HIV and Oral/Head and Neck Squamous Cell Carcinoma

Red and white mass involving the left posterior ventrolateral tongue.

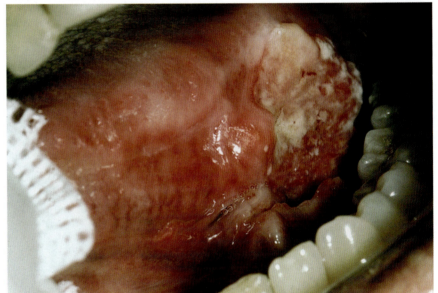

Bibliography

Primary Herpetic Gingivostomatitis

Allareddy V, Elangovan S. Characteristics of hospitalizations attributed to herpetic gingivostomatitis: analysis of nationwide inpatient sample. *Oral Surg Oral Med Oral Pathol Oral Radiol*. 2014;117:471–476.

Bradley H, Markowitz LE, Gibson T. Seroprevalence of herpes simplex virus types 1 and 2–United States, 1999-2010. *J Infect Dis*. 2014;209:325–333.

Kolokotronis A, Doumas S. Herpes simplex virus infection, with particular reference to the progression and complications of primary herpetic gingivostomatitis. *Clin Microbiol Infect*. 2006;12:202–211.

Usatine RP, Tinitigan R. Nongenital herpes simplex virus. *Am Fam Physician*. 2010;82:1075–1082.

Herpetic Whitlow

Adışen E, Önder M. Acral manifestations of viral infections. *Clin Dermatol*. 2017;35:40–49.

Browning WD, McCarthy JP. A case series: herpes simplex virus as an occupational hazard. *J Esthet Restor Dent*. 2012;24:61–66.

Rubright JH, Shafritz AB. The herpetic whitlow. *J Hand Surg Am*. 2011;36:340–342.

Wu IB, Schwartz RA. Herpetic whitlow. *Cutis*. 2007;79:193–196.

Herpes Labialis

Chi CC, Wang SH, Delamere FM, et al. Interventions for prevention of herpes simplex labialis (cold sores on the lips). *Cochrane Database Syst Rev*. 2015;(8):CD010095.

Honarmand M, Farhadmollashahi L, Vosoughirahbar E. Comparing the effect of diode laser against acyclovir cream for the treatment of herpes labialis. *J Clin Exp Dent*. 2017;9:e729–e732.

Opstelten W, Neven AK, Eekhof J. Treatment and prevention of herpes labialis. *Can Fam Physician*. 2008;54:1683–1687.

Palli MA, McTavish H, Kimball A, et al. Immunotherapy of recurrent herpes labialis with squaric acid. *JAMA Dermatol*. 2017;153:828–829.

Rahimi H, Mara T, Costella J, et al. Effectiveness of antiviral agents for the prevention of recurrent herpes labialis: a systematic review and meta-analysis. *Oral Surg Oral Med Oral Pathol Oral Radiol*. 2012;113:618–627.

Tubridy E, Kelsberg G, St Anna L. Clinical Inquiry: Which drugs are most effective for recurrent herpes labialis? *J Fam Pract*. 2014;63:104–105.

Worrall G. Herpes labialis. *BMJ Clin Evid*. 2009;2009:1704.

Recurrent Intraoral Herpes

Eisen D. The clinical characteristics of intraoral herpes simplex virus infection in 52 immunocompetent patients. *Oral Surg Oral Med Oral Pathol Oral Radiol Endod*. 1998;86:432–437.

Tovaru S, Parlatescu I, Tovaru M, et al. Recurrent intraoral HSV-1 infection: a retrospective study of 58 immunocompetent patients from Eastern Europe. *Med Oral Patol Oral Cir Bucal*. 2011;16:e163–e169.

Chronic Intraoral Herpes

Eisen D. The clinical characteristics of intraoral herpes simplex virus infection in 52 immunocompetent patients. *Oral Surg Oral Med Oral Pathol Oral Radiol Endod*. 1998;86:432–437.

Villa A, Treister NS. Intraoral herpes simplex virus infection in a patient with common variable immunodeficiency. *Oral Surg Oral Med Oral Pathol Oral Radiol*. 2013;116:e277–e279.

Infectious Mononucleosis

Balfour HH Jr, Dunmire SK, Hogquist KA. Infectious mononucleosis. *Clin Transl Immunology*. 2015;4:e33.

Dunmire SK, Hogquist KA, Balfour HH. Infectious mononucleosis. *Curr Top Microbiol Immunol*. 2015;390(Pt 1):211–240.

Luzuriaga K, Sullivan JL. Infectious mononucleosis. *N Engl J Med*. 2010;362:1993–2000.

Vouloumanou EK, Rafailidis PI, Falagas ME. Current diagnosis and management of infectious mononucleosis. *Curr Opin Hematol*. 2012;19:14–20.

Womack J, Jimenez M. Common questions about infectious mononucleosis. *Am Fam Physician*. 2015;91:372–376.

Varicella (Chickenpox)

Centers for Disease Control and Prevention. Chapter 22 Varicella. In: Hamborsky J, Kroger A, Wolfe S, eds. *Epidemiology and Prevention of Vaccine-Preventable Diseases*. 13th ed. Washington DC: Public Health Foundation; 2015:353–376. Available at: https://www.cdc.gov/vaccines/pubs/pinkbook/varicella.html. Accessed December 1, 2017.

Kolokotronis A, Louloudiadis K, Fotiou G, et al. Oral manifestations of infections of infections due to varicella zoster virus in otherwise healthy children. *J Clin Pediatr Dent*. 2001;25:107–112.

Lopez AS, Zhang J, Marin M. Epidemiology of varicella during the 2-dose varicella vaccination program - United States, 2005-2014. *MMWR Morb Mortal Wkly Rep*. 2016;65:902–905.

Mustafa MB, Arduino PG, Porter SR. Varicella zoster virus: review of its management. *J Oral Pathol Med*. 2009;38:673–688.

Herpes Zoster (Shingles)

American Academy of Family Physicians. ACIP recommends new herpes zoster subunit vaccine. In *AAFP News*. October 31, 2017. Available at: http://www.aafp.org/news/health-of-the-public/20171031acipmeeting.html. Accessed December 4, 2017.

Centers for Disease Control and Prevention. Chapter 22 Varicella. In: Hamborsky J, Kroger A, Wolfe S, eds. *Epidemiology and Prevention of Vaccine-Preventable Diseases*. 13th ed. Washington DC: Public Health Foundation; 2015:353–376. Available at: https://www.cdc.gov/vaccines/pubs/pinkbook/varicella.html. Accessed December 1, 2017.

Gan EY, Tian EA, Tey HL. Management of herpes zoster and post-herpetic neuralgia. *Am J Clin Dermatol*. 2013;14:77–85.

Harpaz R, Ortega-Sanchez IR, Seward JF, Advisory Committee on Immunization Practices (ACIP) Centers for Disease Control and Prevention (CDC). Prevention of herpes zoster: recommendations of the Advisory Committee on Immunization Practices (ACIP). *MMWR Recomm Rep*. 2008;57(RR–5):1–30.

Lambade P, Lambade D, Saha TK, et al. Maxillary osteonecrosis and spontaneous teeth exfoliation following herpes zoster. *Oral Maxillofac Surg*. 2012;16:369–372.

Herpangina

Chen SP, Huang YC, Li WC, et al. Comparison of clinical features between coxsackievirus A2 and enterovirus 71 during the enterovirus outbreak in Taiwan, 2008: a children's hospital experience. *J Microbiol Immunol Infect*. 2010;43:99–104.

Lo SH, Huang YC, Huang CG, et al. Clinical and epidemiologic features of Coxsackievirus A6 infection in children in northern Taiwan between 2004 and 2009. *J Microbiol Immunol Infect*. 2011;44:252–257.

Hand-Foot-and-Mouth Disease

Centers for Disease Control and Prevention (CDC). Notes from the field: severe hand, foot, and mouth disease associated with coxsackievirus A6 - Alabama, Connecticut, California, and Nevada, November 2011-February 2012. *MMWR Morb Mortal Wkly Rep*. 2012;61:213–214.

Hubiche T, Schuffenecker I, Boralevi F, et al. Clinical Research Group of the French Society of Pediatric Dermatology Groupe de Recherche Clinique de la Société Française de Dermatologie Pédiatrique: Dermatological spectrum of hand, foot and mouth disease from classical to generalized exanthema. *Pediatr Infect Dis J*. 2014;33:e92–e98.

Nassef C, Ziemer C, Morrell DS. Hand-foot-and-mouth disease: a new look at a classic viral rash. *Curr Opin Pediatr*. 2015;27:486–491.

Repass GL, Palmer WC, Stancampiano FF. Hand, foot, and mouth disease: identifying and managing an acute viral syndrome. *Cleve Clin J Med*. 2014;81:537–543.

Human Immunodeficiency Virus and Acquired Immunodeficiency Syndrome

Centers for Disease Control and Prevention (CDC). Revised surveillance case definition for HIV infection–United States, 2014. *MMWR Recomm Rep*. 2014;63:1–10.

Joint United Nations Programme on HIV/AIDS (UNAIDS). UNAIDS Data 2017. Geneva; 2017. Joint United Nations Programme on HIV/AIDS. Available at: http://www.unaids.org/sites/default/files/media_asset/20170720_Data_book_2017_en.pdf. Accessed December 30, 2017.

HIV-Associated Oral Candidiasis

Ceballos-Salobreña A, Gaitaín-Cepeda L, Ceballos-García L, et al. The effect of antiretroviral therapy on the prevalence of HIV-associated oral candidiasis in a Spanish cohort. *Oral Surg Oral Med Oral Pathol Oral Radiol Endod.* 2004;97:345–350.

de Almeida VL, Lima IFP, Ziegelmann PK, et al. Impact of highly active antiretroviral therapy on the prevalence of oral lesions in HIV-positive patients: a systematic review and meta-analysis. *Int J Oral Maxillofac Surg.* 2017;46:1497–1504.

Patuwo C, Young K, Lin M, et al. The changing role of HIV-associated oral candidiasis in the era of HAART. *J Calif Dent Assoc.* 2015;43: 87–92.

Pienaar ED, Young T, Holmes H. Interventions for the prevention and management of oropharyngeal candidiasis associated with HIV infection in adults and children. *Cochrane Database Syst Rev.* 2010;(11):CD003940.

Pappas PG, Kauffman CA, Andes DR, et al. Clinical practice guideline for the management of candidiasis: 2016 update by the Infectious Diseases Society of America. *Clin Infect Dis.* 2016;62:e1–e50.

HIV-Associated Oral Hairy Leukoplakia

Chambers AE, Conn B, Pemberton M. Twenty-first-century oral hairy leukoplakia–a non-HIV-associated entity. *Oral Surg Oral Med Oral Pathol Oral Radiol.* 2015;119:326–332.

Greenspan JS, Greenspan D, Webster-Cyriaque J. Hairy leukoplakia; lessons learned: 30-plus years. *Oral Dis.* 2016;22(suppl 1):120–127.

Vale DA, Martins FM, Silva PH, et al. Retrospective analysis of the clinical behavior of oral hairy leukoplakia in 215 HIV-seropositive patients. *Braz Oral Res.* 2016;30:e118.

HIV and Human Papillomavirus–Related Lesions

Anaya-Saavedra G, Flores-Moreno B, García-Carrancá A, et al. HPV oral lesions in HIV-infected patients: the impact of long-term HAART. *J Oral Pathol Med.* 2013;42:443–449.

Batavia AS, Secours R, Espinosa P, et al. Diagnosis of HIV-associated oral lesions in relation to early versus delayed antiretroviral therapy: results from the CIPRA HT001 Trial. *PLoS One.* 2016;11:e0150656.

Beachler DC, Sugar EA, Margolick JB, et al. Risk factors for acquisition and clearance of oral human papillomavirus infection among HIV-infected and HIV-uninfected adults. *Am J Epidemiol.* 2015;181:40–53.

Beachler DC, Weber KM, Margolick JB, et al. Risk factors for oral HPV infection among a high prevalence population of HIV-positive and at-risk HIV-negative adults. *Cancer Epidemiol Biomarkers Prev.* 2012;21: 122–133.

Cameron JE, Mercante D, O'Brien M, et al. The impact of highly active antiretroviral therapy and immunodeficiency on human papillomavirus infection of the oral cavity of human immunodeficiency virus-seropositive adults. *Sex Transm Dis.* 2005;32:703–709.

Feller L, Khammissa RA, Wood NH, et al. HPV-associated oral warts. *SADJ.* 2011;66:82–85.

AIDS-Related Kaposi Sarcoma

Fatahzadeh M, Schwartz RA. Oral Kaposi's sarcoma: a review and update. *Int J Dermatol.* 2013;52:666–672.

Gbabe OF, Okwundu CI, Dedicoat M, et al. Treatment of severe or progressive Kaposi's sarcoma in HIV-infected adults. *Cochrane Database Syst Rev.* 2014;(8):CD003256.

Gonçalves PH, Uldrick TS, Yarchoan R. HIV-associated Kaposi sarcoma and related diseases. *AIDS.* 2017;31:1903–1916.

Howlader N, Noone AM, Krapcho M, et al, eds. *SEER Cancer Statistics Review, 1975-2014.* Bethesda, MD: National Cancer Institute; 2017. Available at: https://seer.cancer.gov/csr/1975_2014/. Accessed December 9, 2017.

National Comprehensive Care Network. NCCN Clinical Practice Guidelines in Oncology (NCCN Guidelines): AIDS-related Kaposi Sarcoma Version 1.2018, Fort Washington, PA; 2017. National Comprehensive Care Network. Available at: https://www.nccn.org/professionals/physician_gls/pdf/kaposi.pdf. Accessed December 9, 2017.

Pantanowitz L, Khammissa RA, Lemmer J, et al. Oral HIV-associated Kaposi sarcoma. *J Oral Pathol Med.* 2013;42:201–207.

HIV-Associated Periodontal Disease

Gonçalves LS, Gonçalves BM, Fontes TV. Periodontal disease in HIV-infected adults in the HAART era: clinical, immunological, and microbiological aspects. *Arch Oral Biol.* 2013;58: 1385–1396.

Patton LL. Current strategies for prevention of oral manifestations of human immunodeficiency virus. *Oral Surg Oral Med Oral Pathol Oral Radiol.* 2016;121:29–38.

Portela MB, Souza IP, Abreu CM, et al. Effect of serine-type protease of *Candida* spp. isolated from linear gingival erythema of HIV-positive children: critical factors in the colonization. *J Oral Pathol Med.* 2010;39:753–760.

Ryder MI, Nittayananta W, Coogan M, et al. Periodontal disease in HIV/AIDS. *Periodontol 2000.* 2012;60:78–97.

HIV-Associated Lymphadenopathy

Barrionuevo-Cornejo C, Dueñas-Hancco D. Lymphadenopathies in human immunodeficiency virus infection. *Semin Diagn Pathol.* 2017 Dec 6. pii: S0740-2570(17)30150-8. doi:10.1053/j.semdp.2017.12.001. [Epub ahead of print].

Chadburn A, Abdul-Nabi AM, Teruya BS, et al. Lymphoid proliferations associated with human immunodeficiency virus infection. *Arch Pathol Lab Med.* 2013;137:360–370.

Ferry JA. Human immunodeficiency virus-associated lymphadenopathy. In: Kradin RL, ed. *Diagnostic Pathology of Infectious Disease.* 2nd ed. St. Louis: Elsevier; 2018:327–328.

HIV-Associated Aphthous Stomatitis

Kerr AR, Ship JA. Management strategies for HIV-associated aphthous stomatitis. *Am J Clin Dermatol.* 2003;4:669–680.

Kuteyi T, Okwundu CI. Topical treatments for HIV-related oral ulcers. *Cochrane Database Syst Rev.* 2012;(1):CD007975.

Miziara ID, Araujo Filho BC, Weber R. AIDS and recurrent aphthous stomatitis. *Braz J Otorhinolaryngol.* 2000;71:517–520.

HIV-Associated Histoplasmosis

Centers for Disease Control and Prevention. Revised surveillance case definition for HIV infection–United States, 2014. *MMWR Recomm Rep.* 2014;63(RR–03):1–10.

Economopoulou P, Laskaris G, Kittas C. Oral histoplasmosis as an indicator of HIV infection. *Oral Surg Oral Med Oral Pathol Oral Radiol Endod.* 1998;86:203–206.

Ferreira OG, Cardoso SV, Borges AS, et al. Oral histoplasmosis in Brazil. *Oral Surg Oral Med Oral Pathol Oral Radiol Endod.* 2002;93: 654–659.

Martin-Iguacel R, Kurtzhals J, Jouvion G, et al. Progressive disseminated histoplasmosis in the HIV population in Europe in the HAART era. Case report and literature review. *Infection.* 2014;42:611–620.

Wheat LJ, Freifeld AG, Kleiman MB, et al. Infectious Diseases Society of America: clinical practice guidelines for the management of patients with histoplasmosis: 2007 update by the Infectious Diseases Society of America. *Clin Infect Dis.* 2007;45:807–825.

HIV-Associated Lymphoma

Centers for Disease Control and Prevention. Revised surveillance case definition for HIV infection–United States, 2014. *MMWR Recomm Rep.* 2014;63(RR–03):1–10.

Cesarman E. Pathology of lymphoma in HIV. *Curr Opin Oncol.* 2013;25: 487–494.

Gloghini A, Dolcetti R, Carbone A. Lymphomas occurring specifically in HIV-infected patients: from pathogenesis to pathology. *Semin Cancer Biol.* 2013;23:457–467.

Grogg KL, Miller RF, Dogan A. HIV infection and lymphoma. *J Clin Pathol.* 2007;60:1365–1372.

Harmon CM, Smith LB. Plasmablastic lymphoma: a review of clinicopathologic features and differential diagnosis. *Arch Pathol Lab Med.* 2016;140:1074–1078.

Kaplan LD. HIV-associated lymphoma. *Best Pract Res Clin Haematol.* 2012;25:101–117.

HIV and Oral/Head and Neck Squamous Cell Carcinoma

Beachler DC, Abraham AG, Silverberg MJ, et al; North American AIDS Cohort Collaboration on Research and Design (NA-ACCORD) of IeDEA. Incidence and risk factors of HPV-related and HPV-unrelated head and neck squamous cell carcinoma in HIV-infected individuals. *Oral Oncol.* 2014;50:1169–1176.

Butt FM, Chindia ML, Rana F. Oral squamous cell carcinoma in human immunodeficiency virus positive patients: clinicopathological audit. *J Laryngol Otol.* 2012;126:276–278.

Chaturvedi AK, Madeleine MM, Biggar RJ, et al. Risk of human papillomavirus-associated cancers among persons with AIDS. *J Natl Cancer Inst.* 2009;101:1120–1130.

Purgina B, Pantanowitz L, Seethala RR. A review of carcinomas arising in the head and neck region in HIV-Positive patients. *Patholog Res Int.* 2011;2011:469150.

Robbins HA, Pfeiffer RM, Shiels MS, et al. Excess cancers among HIV-infected people in the United States. *J Natl Cancer Inst.* 2015;107:dju503.

Wang CC, Palefsky JM. Human papillomavirus-related oropharyngeal cancer in the HIV-infected population. *Oral Dis.* 2016;22(suppl 1): 98–106.

8

Physical and Chemical Injuries

Linea Alba

Fig. **8.1**

Linea alba (or "white line") represents a linear zone of hyperkeratosis that is commonly found on the buccal mucosa at the level of the occlusal plane. This alteration is caused by frictional irritation, pressure, or sucking trauma from the adjacent teeth. The condition has been reported over a broad age range and is often bilateral. The white line typically is restricted to areas of the buccal mucosa that are adjacent to teeth. The alteration may extend anywhere from the posterior buccal mucosa to the commissure, although many patients exhibit more prominent changes posteriorly. The linear zone of hyperkeratosis is slightly elevated and, in some examples, may appear scalloped. In most cases, the characteristic clinical presentation allows for a strong presumptive diagnosis of linea alba without biopsy. No treatment is needed.

Morsicatio

Figs. **8.2 and 8.3**

Morsicatio (also known as "morsicatio mucosae oris") refers to biting or nibbling of the oral mucosa. Common sites for habitual nibbling include the tongue *(morsicatio linguarum)*, buccal mucosa *(morsicatio buccarum)*, and labial mucosa *(morsicatio labiorum)*. In particular, the lateral border of the tongue, anterior buccal mucosa at the level of the occlusal plane, and lower labial mucosa are favored subsites. The patient may or may not be aware of a nibbling habit, and some investigators have suggested an association with stress or psychological disorders. The chronically traumatized mucosa develops a white to red-white plaque with a rough, ragged, or macerated appearance. Sometimes the patient can remove thread-like shreds of keratin from the surface. Accompanying ulceration or erosion also is possible. The characteristic clinical presentation typically is sufficient for a strong presumptive diagnosis, although biopsy may be performed if there is uncertainty. Microscopic examination shows a thickened, shredded keratin layer with overlying bacterial colonization. No specific treatment is needed, although cessation of the nibbling habit will induce resolution of the lesion. Some investigators have recommended fabrication of a removable prosthesis to help prevent cheek biting.

Linea Alba

White, linear zone of hyperkeratosis on the buccal mucosa at the level of the occlusal plane.

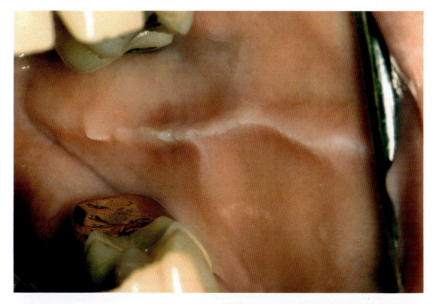

■ Figure **8.2**
Morsicatio Buccarum

White, ragged plaque involving the left buccal mucosa.

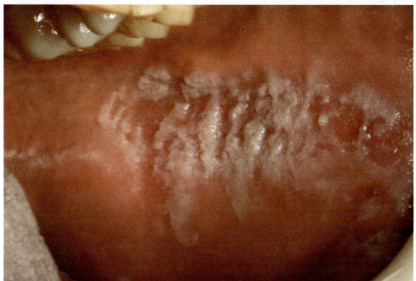

■ Figure **8.3**
Morsicatio Linguarum

White, ragged plaque involving the right lateral tongue.

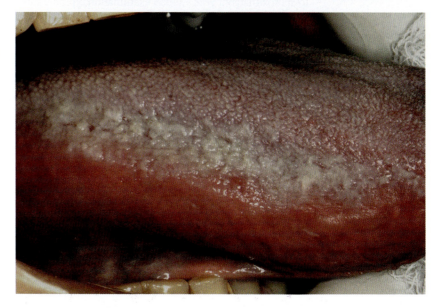

Traumatic Ulcer

Figs. **8.4 and 8.5**

A **traumatic ulcer** occurs when injury to the oral mucosa results in a complete breach of the surface epithelium. Mechanical injury is the most common cause, although chemical and thermal injuries also are possible. Mechanical trauma often results from accidental biting of the mucosa (e.g., while eating, talking, or sleeping), malocclusion, teeth with sharp cusps or incisal edges, ill-fitting prostheses, and defective restorations. Frequent sites for ulcers caused by biting trauma include the lateral border of the tongue, the lips, and the buccal mucosa. Mechanical trauma also may be caused by foreign objects (e.g., toothbrushes, sharp foodstuffs, toothpicks), surgical procedures, and dental treatment.

Clinically, the ulceration may appear erythematous, or it may be covered by a yellowish fibrinopurulent membrane. In many cases, the ulcer exhibits a white, hyperkeratotic border. Most traumatic ulcers are acute, localized lesions that resolve within 1 to 2 weeks of removal of the source of injury. However, some traumatic ulcers can exhibit a chronic course (see the next section "Traumatic Granuloma"). If an oral ulcer fails to heal within 2 to 3 weeks, biopsy should be considered to rule out malignancy.

In rare cases, oral ulceration may be caused by self-injury or self-mutilation, also known as *factitial injury*. For example, some patients may harm themselves unintentionally because of an underlying heritable condition (e.g., Lesch-Nyhan syndrome, familial dysautonomia), seizure disorder, cerebral palsy, or other organic conditions. Self-inflicted wounds also may be intentional, as in *Munchausen syndrome* (characterized by self-injury in order to seek attention, sympathy, and medical care) or other psychiatric disorders.

Traumatic Granuloma

Fig. **8.6**

Unlike conventional traumatic ulcers, the **traumatic granuloma** *(traumatic ulcerative granuloma with stromal eosinophilia, eosinophilic ulcer)* is often slow to heal. It is characterized by an exuberant inflammatory cell infiltrate that extends deeply into the connective tissue and includes eosinophils. The exact etiopathogenesis is uncertain. The lesion is presumed to be a reactive process caused by local injury, although in many cases the clinical history and examination reveal no clear source of trauma. Immunohistochemical studies suggest that a T-cell-mediated immune response plays a role.

Traumatic granulomas have been reported over a broad age range, with a slight male predominance. Most examples occur on the tongue (especially the lateral aspect), although other sites also may be involved. Pain is a variable finding. The reported duration of the lesion prior to presentation ranges from 1 week to approximately 1 year. Clinical examination typically shows a solitary ulcer with a yellowish pseudomembrane and a raised, indurated margin. An exophytic, nodular mass may be evident in some examples. The clinical presentation can mimic squamous cell carcinoma, deep fungal infections, and other chronic infections. The worrisome presentation typically prompts biopsy for microscopic diagnosis. The lesion often resolves after incisional biopsy or conservative excision. Any potential sources of oral trauma should be addressed in order to prevent recurrence. Lesions that persist or recur typically are managed by excision, although other treatments (e.g., intralesional or topical corticosteroids, cryotherapy) have been reported anecdotally in the literature.

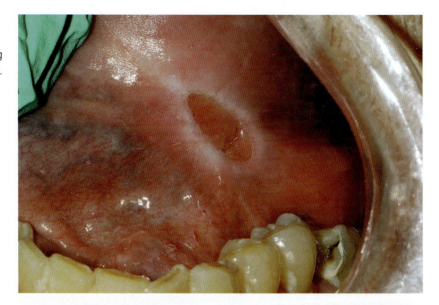

■ Figure **8.4**
Traumatic Ulcer
Trauma-induced ulcer on the ventral tongue, showing central erythema and a white, hyperkeratotic border.

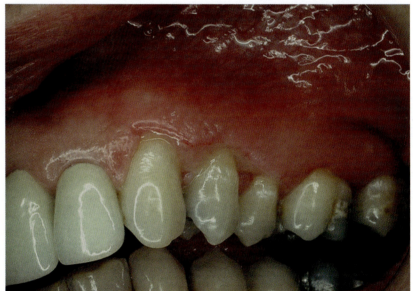

■ Figure **8.5**
Traumatic Ulcer
Ulceration of the maxillary gingiva caused by toothbrush abrasion.

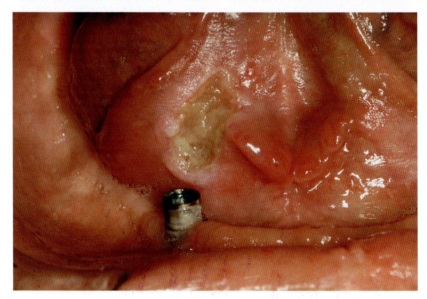

■ Figure **8.6**
Traumatic Granuloma
Chronic ulceration of the ventral tongue caused by mechanical trauma from an exposed dental implant.

Electrical Burns

Fig. **8.7**

Oral electrical burns primarily occur in young children (peak: 6 months through 5 years). Most cases result from chewing, biting, or mouthing extension cords or appliance cords. The injuries typically represent arc burns (i.e., an electrical arc flows from the voltage source to the mouth with saliva as a conducting medium), which can generate temperatures up to 3000°C. The most commonly involved sites are the lips and oral commissures, although at times the anterior regions of the tongue, gingiva, alveolar bone, and dentition also may sustain damage. Initially, the burn may be painless and appear as a charred, yellowish to gray-white zone of necrosis with surrounding erythema. Subsequently, edema develops within a few hours and may persist up to 12 days. As a brown to black eschar develops and sloughs over the next several weeks, surface ulceration may develop; during this time, there is the potential for severe bleeding. In the long-term, extensive scarring can cause limited opening, which may interfere with speaking, eating, drinking, dental care, and facial development.

Optimal treatment requires a multidisciplinary approach, including specialists in oral and maxillofacial surgery, plastic surgery, prosthodontics, and speech/swallowing therapy. In the acute period, management includes local wound care, airway maintenance, fluid and electrolyte balance, and prevention of secondary infection. After stabilization, additional considerations include fabrication of an appliance to prevent microstomia, reconstructive surgery, and functional rehabilitation. Caretakers of young children should receive education regarding electrical safety precautions.

Thermal Burns

Figs. **8.8 and 8.9**

Thermal burns in the oral cavity often result from ingestion of hot foods or liquids. Many such cases are attributed to the popularity of microwave ovens. Common culprits include microwaved pizza, potatoes, water, tea, and bottles of infant formula. Microwave electromagnetic radiation heats via a dielectric process rather than by ambient heat. This process preferentially heats substances with increased moisture content. Thus, foods with a moist interior may reach higher temperatures internally than externally, and beverages may reach temperatures greatly exceeding those of the containers in which they are heated. In addition, fats and sugars may reach temperatures far above the boiling point of water.

Common sites for oral thermal burns include the palate, posterior buccal mucosa, anterior tongue, and lips. The lesions may exhibit erythema, ulceration, and/or yellow-white epithelial necrosis. As a reflexive response, most patients spit out excessively hot foods or liquids. However, older patients with complete dentures may swallow very hot foods or liquids because of delayed heat sensation. In such cases, burn injuries also may involve the oropharynx, hypopharynx, larynx, and esophagus; resultant swelling of the upper aerodigestive tract can cause severe dyspnea and dysphagia.

Most oral thermal burns are of little consequence and resolve without treatment within 1 to 2 weeks. However, individuals who complain of pain or discomfort may be managed with nonsteroidal anti-inflammatory drugs. Patients with more extensive burns of the upper aerodigestive tract may require airway maintenance (i.e., tracheostomy, intubation), systemic steroids, and preventive antibiotic therapy.

Figure **8.7**
Electrical Burn

Young child with a severe electrical burn involving the lips and oral commissure. There are yellow-white to dark brown zones of necrosis with associated swelling and erythema.

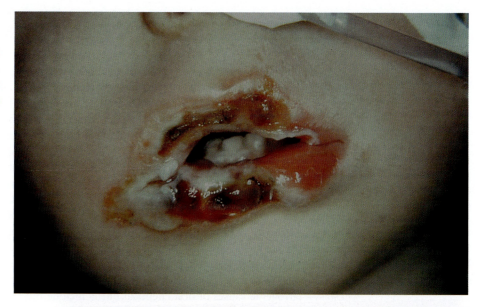

Figure **8.8**
Thermal Burn

White area of epithelial necrosis on the lower lip caused by drinking microwaved hot tea.

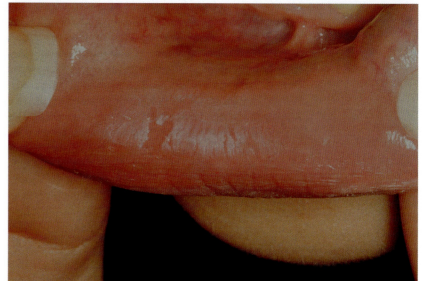

Figure **8.9**
Thermal Burn

Red and white lesion on the buccal mucosa caused by a hot mushroom.

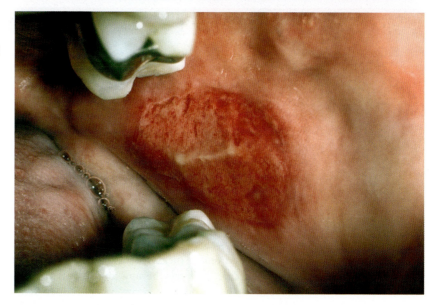

Figs. **8.10 and 8.11**

Oral burns may be caused by exposure to various types of chemical substances. For instance, some medications can cause burns when held in the mouth for an extended period. Among such agents, aspirin is particularly well known; patients may attempt to treat tooth pain by direct intraoral placement of aspirin tablets or powders. Other medications that can cause chemical burns when held in the mouth include ibuprofen, chlorpromazine, promazine, bisphosphonates, verapamil, and tetracycline hydrochloride. In other cases, patients may incur chemical injuries to the oral mucosa when using home remedies, over-the-counter products, or nontherapeutic substances for self-treatment of toothaches, gingivitis, mouth sores, or other conditions. Some examples include injudicious use of mouth wash, denture cleansers, hydrogen peroxide, carbamide peroxide (for tooth bleaching), silver nitrate, rubbing alcohol, formalin, crushed garlic, topical pain relief preparations containing phenol (and often high levels of alcohol), or Minard's liniment (a preparation of camphor, ammonia water, and medicinal turpentine). In addition, accidental or intentional ingestion of toxic substances (e.g., battery acid, household cleaning agents, pesticides) may cause oral burns plus lethal systemic effects. Furthermore, oral mucosal injury may be incurred by topical application of recreational drugs, such as cocaine or methylenedioxymethamphetamine (MDMA, Ecstasy). Iatrogenic causes of oral chemical burns include mishandling of agents used for pulp therapy (e.g., formocresol, sodium hypochlorite), dental restorative procedures (dentin bonding agents, phosphoric etching solutions, cavity varnish, calcium hydroxide), gingival retraction (e.g., trichloroacetic acid, ferric sulfate), and antisepsis or cavity sterilization (e.g., iodine, phenol, chromic acid).

Chemical burns may involve any oral mucosal surface, although the buccal and labial mucosae are injured most frequently. The severity of the burn varies, depending on the agent type, concentration, duration of exposure, and delivery method. Acidic substances tend to cause coagulation necrosis with eschar formation and limited tissue penetration, whereas alkaline substances may cause more extensive liquefaction necrosis. In mild cases, there may be painless, superficial sloughing and desquamation of the oral surface epithelium. More caustic agents can cause ulceration, white zones of epithelial necrosis, erythema, and/or edema.

Most oral chemical burns produce mild to moderate, localized tissue damage that resolves without scarring within 1 to 2 weeks. No specific treatment may be needed other than eliminating further exposure to the offending agent. Palliative measures include topical anesthetics, emollients, or protective cellulose films. More severe or extensive burns may require surgical débridement, analgesics, and antibiotics. In addition, comprehensive management of systemic adverse effects may be required for chemicals that are absorbed transorally or ingested. Preventive measures include patient education (e.g., prompt swallowing of medication, storing household chemicals out of the reach of children) and safety precautions during dental procedures (e.g., rubber dam isolation).

Chemotherapy-Induced Oral Mucositis

Fig. **8.12**

Oral mucositis represents a significant complication of cancer chemotherapy. Overall, it affects approximately 20% to 40% of patients receiving conventional chemotherapy for solid tumors and 80% of patients receiving high-dose chemotherapy before hematopoietic stem cell transplantation. Also, the risk for oral mucositis increases when chemotherapy is combined with radiation and/or targeted therapy. Examples of cytotoxic agents closely associated with oral mucositis include 5-fluorouracil, methotrexate, etoposide, irinotecan, busulfan, and melphalan.

Oral examination shows mucosal erythema, erosion, and/or ulceration. The lesions typically appear 7 to 14 days after the initiation of chemotherapy and heal within a few weeks of completion. The lesions are very painful and may interfere with the patient's ability to eat and to maintain oral hygiene. Impaired nutrition can lower resistance to secondary infection, and the ulcers may provide an entry route for life-threatening sepsis. Furthermore, severe oral mucositis may necessitate interruption or alteration of cancer therapy, which can compromise patient survival.

Suggested preventive measures for chemotherapy-induced oral mucositis include the following: pretreatment dental care, oral cryotherapy for patients receiving bolus injections of 5-fluorouracil for cancers outside of the head and neck, recombinant human keratinocyte growth factor-1 (KGF-1, palifermin) for patients receiving high-dose chemotherapy and total body irradiation before autologous stem cell transplantation for hematologic malignancy, and low-level laser therapy for patients receiving hematopoietic stem cell transplantation conditioned with high-dose chemotherapy. Mucositis management typically

Figure **8.10**
Aspirin Burn
White area of epithelial necrosis caused by aspirin placement in the lower labial vestibule.

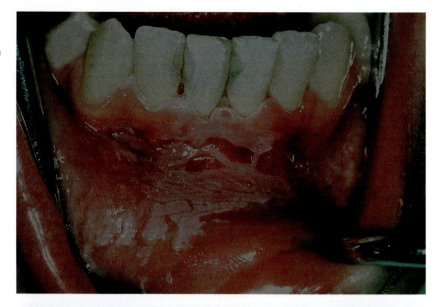

Figure **8.11**
Chemical Burn
White area of epithelial necrosis involving the buccal mucosa and vestibule. The lesion was caused by overuse of an over-the-counter topical anesthetic preparation containing phenol and alcohol.

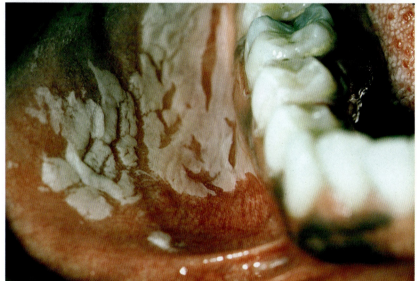

Figure **8.12**
Chemotherapy-Induced Oral Mucositis
Ulcer on the lateral tongue in a patient receiving chemotherapy.

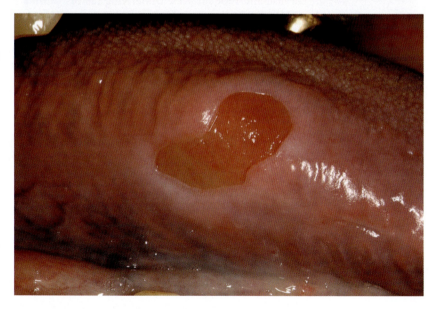

includes systemic opioids, palliative rinses (e.g., salt/soda, viscous lidocaine/diphenhydramine/bismuth subsalicylate), and oral hygiene maintenance. Various topical agents have been studied, but further research is needed.

Radiation-Induced Oral Mucositis

Fig. **8.13**

Oral mucositis affects approximately 80% of head and neck cancer patients receiving radiation therapy, and the prevalence approaches 100% among those receiving hyperfractionation or accelerated hyperfractionation regimens. Oral mucosal fields receiving weekly cumulative doses of approximately 10 Gy are at greatest risk for involvement. In the early stages, the patient exhibits oral erythema, often accompanied by a burning sensation and intolerance to spicy foods. After a cumulative radiation dose of approximately 30 Gy (usually after about 2 weeks), painful oral ulcers begin to develop. The severity of the condition typically remains at its peak for at least 2 weeks after completion of radiotherapy, and symptoms may persist up to 8 weeks after completion. The condition is similar to chemotherapy-induced oral mucositis in terms of the potential for impaired quality of life, decreased nutrition, increased hospitalization rates and treatment costs, interruption of planned cancer treatment, and increased risk for life-threatening infection. Suggested preventive measures for radiation-induced oral mucositis include the following: pretreatment dental care, benzdyamine mouthwash for those receiving ≤50 Gy without concomitant chemotherapy, low-level laser therapy for those not receiving concomitant chemotherapy, and zinc supplementation for those with oral tumors. Technological advances, such as intensity-modulated radiation therapy, may reduce the risk for severe involvement. Treatment is similar to that for chemotherapy-induced oral mucositis (see previous section).

Xerostomia-Related Caries

Fig. **8.14**

Xerostomia (dry mouth) is a common problem that can be caused by numerous factors, including drugs, radiation therapy to the head and neck, Sjögren syndrome, diabetes mellitus, human immunodeficiency virus (HIV) infection, sarcoidosis, amyloidosis, smoking, mouth breathing, and dehydration. Saliva has numerous important functions, such as food clearance, acid buffering, remineralization of enamel, and antimicrobial effects. Thus, patients with xerostomia have increased caries risk. In addition, behavioral factors may contribute to caries development. For example, patients who experience dysphagia due to dry mouth may gravitate toward soft foods high in carbohydrates, and some patients may consume sugary candies, gums, or beverages in an attempt to stimulate salivary flow and maintain moisture.

Although any tooth surface may be affected, xerostomia-related caries particularly tends to involve the cervical and root surfaces. Underlying factors causing xerostomia should be identified and, if possible, addressed. Management also may include frequent oral prophylaxis, oral hygiene reinforcement, nutritional counseling, fluoride supplementation, saliva substitutes, sugarless candies or gum, increased water intake, and sialogogues. In addition, patients may use various over-the-counter products (typically containing lactoperoxidase, lactoferrin, lysozyme, or other agents) formulated to counteract xerostomia. When performing restorative procedures, fluoride-releasing materials (e.g., glass ionomer, resin-modified glass ionomer) may be beneficial for reducing restoration failures from recurrent caries in xerostomic patients who do not routinely use topical fluoride supplements.

Osteoradionecrosis

Fig. **8.15**

Osteoradionecrosis represents another potential complication of radiation therapy to the head and neck. It is defined as exposed, nonvital, and irradiated bone that persists ≥3 months in the absence of local malignant disease. The estimated prevalence among irradiated head and neck cancer patients ranges from 5% to 15%, with greater than 70% of cases developing within the first 3 years of radiotherapy. Risk factors include radiation dose greater than 60 Gy, concomitant chemotherapy, brachytherapy, tobacco and/or alcohol use, malnutrition, poor oral hygiene, presence of teeth, and tooth extraction (especially within 21 days preceding or 2 years after radiation therapy). The risk for osteoradionecrosis is lower with intensity-modulated radiation therapy than with conventional radiotherapy.

Osteoradionecrosis affects the mandible more often than the maxilla. Pain and exposed bone are typical features but may not be evident in the early stages. Secondary infection may cause suppuration and orocutaneous sinus tract formation. Other possible findings include dysesthesia, pathologic fracture, and

Figure 8.13
Radiation-Induced Oral Mucositis

Diffuse, irregular zones of erythema with interspersed shallow ulcers involving the soft palate and uvula in a patient receiving radiation therapy to the head and neck.

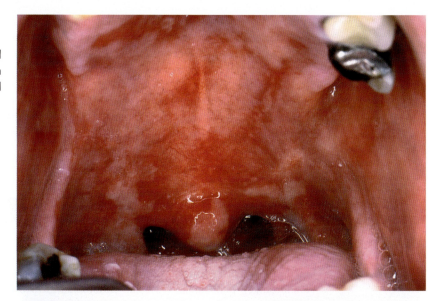

Figure 8.14
Xerostomia-Related Caries

Severe, generalized caries in a patient with xerostomia caused by radiation therapy to the head and neck.

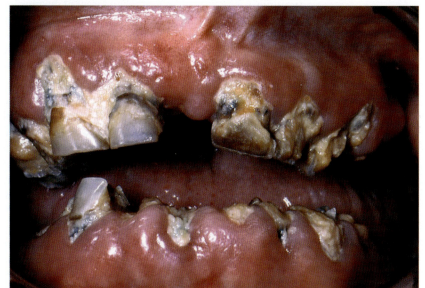

Figure 8.15
Osteoradionecrosis

Exposed, necrotic mandibular alveolar bone caused by radiation therapy for head and neck cancer. (With appreciation to Dr. Terry Day.)

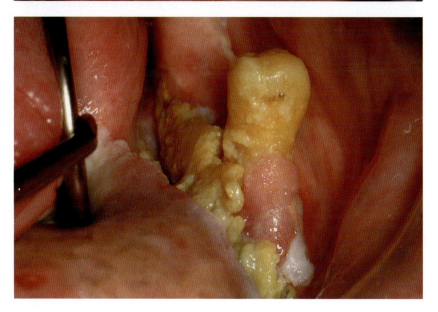

difficulty with mastication and speech. Radiographic examination shows an ill-defined, mixed radiolucency/radiopacity. Prevention entails elimination of oral infection, extraction of any unrestorable or questionable teeth, and maintenance of optimal oral hygiene. At least 3 weeks of healing are recommended between extensive dental procedures and the initiation of radiotherapy. Osteoradionecrosis often is managed by irrigation, gentle removal of exposed sequestra, systemic antibiotics for secondary infection, and oral hygiene maintenance. Severe or refractory cases may require resection and reconstruction. Adjunctive hyperbaric oxygen therapy is controversial. Some studies have shown promising results with pentoxifylline and tocopherol, ultrasound therapy, or distraction osteogenesis.

Medication-Related Osteonecrosis of the Jaws

Figs. **8.16–8.18**

Necrosis of the jawbones can occur as a complication of treatment with antiresorptive and antiangiogenic medications. Such agents include bisphosphonates (e.g., zoledronate, pamidronate, alendronate, risedronate, ibandronate), denosumab, vascular endothelial growth factor (VEGF) antagonists (e.g., bevacizumab, sunitinib, sorafenib), and mammalian target of rapamycin (mTOR) inhibitors (e.g., everolimus, sirolimus). Although the clinical applications for these agents have been expanding rapidly, these medications most commonly are used for the management of osteoporosis and cancer. According to the American Association of Oral and Maxillofacial Surgeons, the case definition for **medication-related osteonecrosis of the jaws (MRONJ)** is: (1) current or past use of antiresorptive or antiangiogenic agents, (2) exposed bone or bone that can be probed through an intraoral or extraoral fistula that has persisted greater than 8 weeks, and (3) no history of radiation therapy to the jaws or obvious metastatic disease to the jaws.

The reported prevalence of MRONJ varies across studies, and the risk increases with higher drug potency and longer duration of use. Based on a review of published studies, investigators have estimated that bisphosphonate-related osteonecrosis of the jaws occurs approximately 100 times more often among cancer patients compared to osteoporosis patients. Systemic risk factors for MRONJ include older age, diabetes, and corticosteroid use. In many cases, MRONJ develops after tooth extraction or in areas otherwise subject to trauma (e.g., traumatized tori, bone underneath an ill-fitting denture). However, some cases appear to develop spontaneously.

MRONJ exhibits a predilection for the molar and premolar regions of the jaws, and bisphosphonate-related cases exhibit a 2:1 mandible-to-maxilla ratio. Before definite bone necrosis becomes evident, the patient may have nonspecific signs and symptoms. For example, there may be a toothache or tooth mobility without associated odontogenic infection or chronic periodontal disease. Dull bone pain, maxillary sinusitis, and dysesthesia also may be present. Radiographic examination may show subtle changes in the trabecular pattern of the jawbone, regions of osteosclerosis in the alveolar or surrounding basilar bone, and thickening or obscuring of the periodontal ligament.

As the condition progresses, intraoral examination shows exposed, necrotic alveolar bone and/or an intraoral fistula that can be probed down to bone. Some patients are asymptomatic, whereas others develop pain due to secondary infection. Additional signs of infection may include suppuration and soft tissue swelling. In advanced cases, orocutaneous, oroantral, or oronasal fistula formation also is possible. Typical radiographic findings in MRONJ include ill-defined, mixed radiolucent/radiopaque areas. In advanced disease, the bone necrosis may spread to the inferior border of the mandible, the floor of the maxillary sinus, or the zygoma. At times, pathologic fracture may be evident as well.

As a preventive measure, complete dental screening with elimination of all current or potential foci of oral infection is advised prior to starting antiresorptive or antiangiogenic drug therapy. Some authorities have suggested drug holidays prior to and after surgical procedures that involve osseous injury (e.g., tooth extraction, dental implant placement, periodontal surgery); however, further studies are needed.

For patients with MRONJ, conservative treatment is recommended. If there is no evidence of infection, chlorhexidine mouth rinses and periodic clinical follow-up are advised. Patients who develop secondary infection also typically receive systemic antibiotic therapy, analgesics, and conservative débridement. More extensive surgery is reserved for advanced cases.

■ Figure 8.16
Medication-Related Osteonecrosis of the Jaws
Exposed, necrotic bone in the mandible caused by antiresorptive drug therapy.

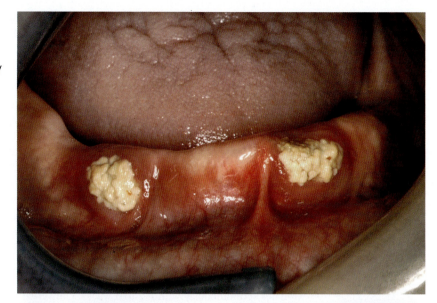

■ Figure 8.17
Medication-Related Osteonecrosis of the Jaws
Exposed, necrotic bone developing in a palatal torus as a result of antiresorptive drug therapy.

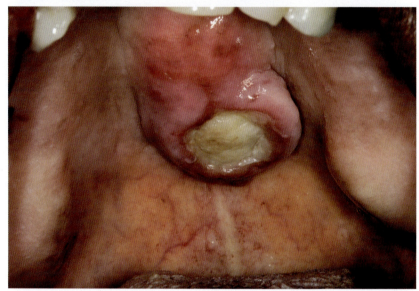

■ Figure 8.18
Medication-Related Osteonecrosis of the Jaws
Focal exposure of necrotic bone in a mandibular torus in association with denosumab administration.

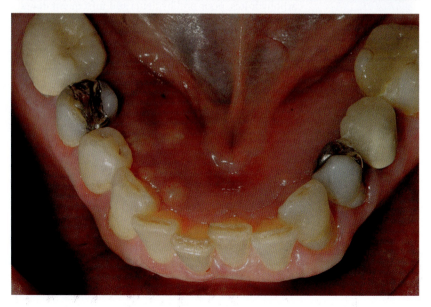

Oral Ulceration With Bone Sequestration

Fig. **8.19**

Oral ulceration with bone sequestration (*spontaneous sequestration, lingual mandibular sequestration* and *ulceration*) is an uncommon, idiopathic condition characterized by mucosal ulceration with exposure of a nonvital cortical bone fragment. Most cases occur on the lingual aspect of the posterior mandible. The condition is not related to underlying systemic disease, infection, or major trauma. However, some authors hypothesize that ulceration from minor trauma or aphthous stomatitis is the inciting event that leads to disruption of the periosteal blood supply and focal bone necrosis. There is the potential for minor alveolar trauma in patients with mandibular molars that are missing or have restorations that fail to recapitulate a normal lingual profile.

Clinical examination shows a variably painful ulcer with associated bone sequestration. Most cases involve the lingual aspect of the posterior mandible along the mylohyoid ridge. In addition, some examples involve mandibular tori or other exostoses. The ulcer may persist for a few days to several months. The sequestrum may be freely mobile or attached to the mandible. Occasionally, an occlusal radiograph exhibits a faint radiopacity overlying the lingual cortical plate.

Oral ulceration with bone sequestration is a self-limited condition. In many cases, the sequestrum exfoliates spontaneously within 2 to 4 weeks. Conservative management consists of periodic monitoring, possibly combined with an antimicrobial rinse (e.g., chlorhexidine, tetracycline) or topical steroid. Alternatively, the sequestrum may be excised. After spontaneous exfoliation or surgical removal of the nonvital bone, the ulcer typically heals promptly.

"Meth Mouth"

Fig. **8.20**

Methamphetamine (also known as *meth*, *speed*, *crank*, or *ice*) is a highly addictive central nervous system stimulant that may be smoked, snorted, injected, or taken orally in order to produce feelings of euphoria and increased energy. Recreational use of methamphetamine is a widespread problem, with recent data showing the highest levels of abuse in East Asia and Oceania. In the United States, according to the 2016 National Survey of Drug Use and Health, approximately 0.7 million individuals aged 12 years or older were current methamphetamine users. Short-term effects of the drug include insomnia, tachypnea, tachycardia, hypertension, nausea, vomiting, and hyperthermia. Debilitating long-term sequelae include psychological disturbances (e.g., paranoid psychosis, depression); structural brain damage with cognitive impairment; and cardiovascular disease.

In the oral cavity, chronic methamphetamine use can lead to rampant caries, or **"meth mouth."** This finding appears to result from drug-induced xerostomia combined with high consumption of refined carbohydrates, poor oral hygiene, and infrequent dental care. The process may begin with smooth surface and interproximal caries but eventually may progress to produce widespread coronal destruction. In addition, methamphetamine users are at increased risk for severe periodontal disease. The patient should be referred for substance abuse treatment. Dental management considerations include oral hygiene instruction, prophylaxis, nutritional counseling, and supplemental fluorides. Caution should be exercised when administering sedatives, local anesthetics with vasoconstrictors, general anesthesia, or opioids.

Opioid-Induced Palatal Perforation

Fig. **8.21**

Palatal perforation can occur as a complication of intranasal drug abuse. Although destruction of the palate and nasal septum due to intranasal cocaine abuse has been well recognized for decades, a similar pattern has been reported more recently with intranasal abuse of prescription narcotics (e.g., sustained-release oxycodone HCl [OxyContin], oxycodone/acetaminophen, hydrocodone/acetaminophen). According to the 2016 National Survey on Drug Use and Health, approximately 11.5 million individuals aged 12 years and older in the United States reported misuse of prescription pain relievers within the past year.

Patients with opioid-induced palatal perforation typically report difficulties with eating, drinking, and speech. Most exhibit perforation of the hard and/or soft palate plus the nasal septum, although isolated palatal perforation also is possible. Other findings may include pain; crusty nasal exudate, often extending into the posterior oropharynx; purulent discharge; sinonasal congestion; saddlenose deformity; and otalgia. Because many patients try to conceal their drug use, the diagnosis may not be readily apparent. Other conditions that can cause palatal perforation include lymphoma, tertiary syphilis, and granulomatosis with

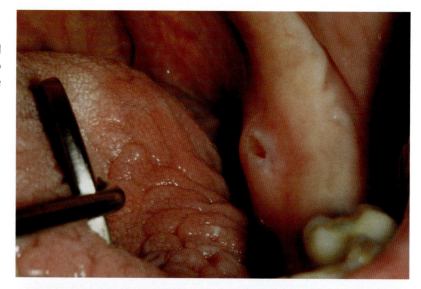

■ Figure **8.19**
Oral Ulceration With Bone Sequestration
Focal ulceration and bone sequestration on the lingual aspect of the left posterior mandible. Although no definite cause was identified, minor trauma may have been related to the absence of teeth in this area.

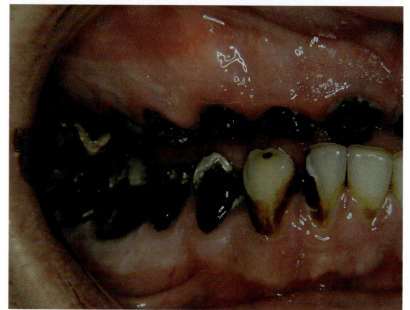

■ Figure **8.20**
"Meth Mouth"
Rampant caries in a methamphetamine abuser. (Courtesy Dr. Michael Hawks.)

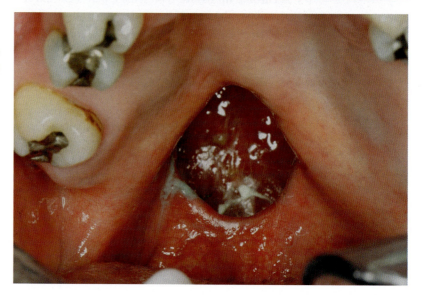

■ Figure **8.21**
Opioid-Induced Palatal Perforation
Palatal perforation in a patient who abused oxycodone by grinding up the tablets and inhaling the ground particles.

polyangiitis (Wegener granulomatosis). Evaluation may include endoscopic examination, computed tomography, incisional biopsy, cultures, PR3-ANCA (which may be elevated in patients with cocaine-induced lesions or granulomatosis with polyangiitis), serologic testing for syphilis, and toxicology screening. A palatal obturator can be fabricated, and referral for substance abuse treatment is recommended. Surgical reconstruction should not be considered until the patient demonstrates sustained drug cessation.

Exfoliative Cheilitis

Figs. 8.22 and 8.23

Exfoliative cheilitis is a condition characterized by persistent scaling and flaking of the lip vermilion. The process results from excessive keratin production and subsequent desquamation. The etiology is uncertain, although studies have noted associations with factitial/parafunctional activities (e.g., lip licking, biting, picking, sucking), stress, and psychiatric disorders (e.g., anxiety, depression, obsessive-compulsive disorder). Some case series have noted a predilection among women. Clinical examination typically shows scaling or peeling of the lip vermilion, at times accompanied by erythema, crusting, and/or bleeding. Most cases involve both lips, although involvement of only one lip also is possible. Lip dryness is a common complaint among affected patients; infrequently, there may be pain or burning as well. Many patients try to self-treat by applying lip balm, although a constantly moist environment may favor the development of superimposed candidiasis. In many examples, concurrent angular cheilitis may be evident, or secondary candidiasis may develop diffusely on the lip vermilion. Conditions that may be considered in the differential diagnosis for exfoliative cheilitis include allergic contact cheilitis and atopic cheilitis. With regard to management, the patient should be instructed to make a conscious effort to avoid lip licking or other potential sources of irritation. Some case reports have noted improvement with antifungal therapy, antibacterial agents, corticosteroids, tacrolimus ointment, pimecrolimus ointment, antidepressants, *Calendula officinalis* ointment, excimer laser therapy, or cryotherapy. In our experience, antifungal therapy in combination with the cessation of lip balm usage often induces slow resolution. However, further studies are needed to determine optimal management.

Chronic Lip Fissure

Fig. 8.24

A **chronic lip fissure** represents a persistent linear ulcer in the sagittal plane of the upper or lower lip vermilion. The condition affects approximately 0.6% of the population, and the etiology is unclear. Some authors suggest that the lesions result from physiologic weakness of tissues along embryologic planes of fusion; this theory is supported by the observation that lower lip fissures tend to occur at midline, whereas upper lip fissures often occur slightly lateral to midline. Additional proposed contributory factors include cold weather, smoking, bacterial or fungal infections, vitamin deficiency, mouth breathing, misaligned anterior teeth (possibly combined with parafunctional habits), and playing wind instruments. In addition, some investigators have noted an increased prevalence of chronic lip fissures among patients with Down syndrome, Crohn disease, or orofacial granulomatosis.

Chronic lip fissures have been reported more often in males than females. The lesion typically is not evident at birth, and most individuals present for evaluation before 45 years of age. Most cases involve one lip, although both lips occasionally may be affected. The fissure can cause pain, bleeding, and aesthetic concern. The lesion may be present continuously or intermittently, and symptoms often worsen during the winter months. Various topical treatments reported anecdotally include tacrolimus, corticosteroids, hydrocortisone and iodoquinol, aureomycin, sulfonamides, and moisturizers. However, refractory lesions may necessitate simple excision or excision with Z-plasty. Alternative treatment methods include cryotherapy and carbon dioxide laser therapy.

■ Figure **8.22**
Exfoliative Cheilitis
Generalized peeling and dryness of the lips.

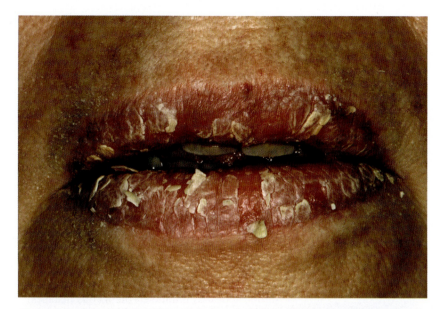

■ Figure **8.23**
Exfoliative Cheilitis
Same patient from Fig. 8.22 after treatment, which consisted of topical 1% hydrocortisone/1% iodoquinol applied to the lip vermilion plus intraoral clotrimazole troches and cessation of petrolatum-based lip balm.

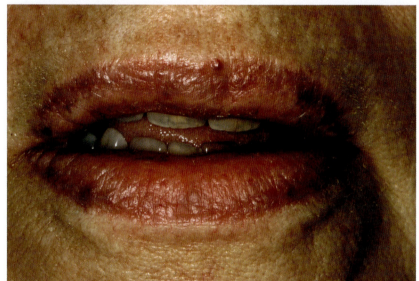

■ Figure **8.24**
Chronic Lip Fissure
Persistent, linear ulcer of the upper lip vermilion.

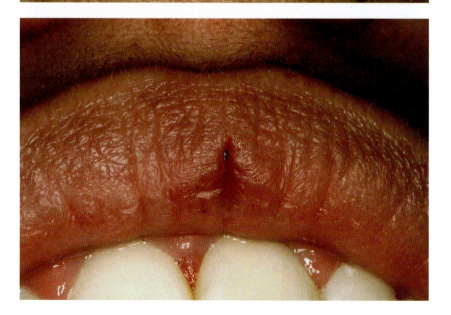

Figs. **8.25–8.27**

Hemorrhage represents the escape of blood from a ruptured blood vessel. In the oral cavity, mucosal or submucosal hemorrhage often results from trauma. Additional contributory factors may include antithrombotic drug therapy, thrombocytopenia (e.g., due to idiopathic or immune thrombocytopenic purpura, chemotherapy, leukemia), clotting disorders (e.g., hemophilia, von Willebrand disease), and vascular or perivascular connective tissue fragility (e.g., scurvy, senile purpura).

Clinically, areas of oral mucosal or submucosal hemorrhage typically appear as erythematous, purple, or blue lesions that do not blanch with pressure. In order to test for blanching, one may perform *diascopy* (application of a glass slide to apply pressure). Lesions resulting from hemorrhage will retain their color, whereas those resulting from vascular dilation will blanch. Common sites for trauma-induced hemorrhage include the buccal mucosa, lateral tongue, and labial mucosa. Sometimes significant hemorrhage may be provoked by minimal trauma in patients with an underlying blood dyscrasia or other systemic condition.

Clinical terms used to describe different patterns of hemorrhage include:

1. **petechiae** (pinpoint hemorrhagic foci measuring <3 mm; may involve the mucous membranes, skin, or serosa; appear as minute erythematous macules)
2. **purpura** (slightly larger area of hemorrhage measuring 3 mm to 1 cm; may appear as a red-purple macule or somewhat raised lesion)
3. **ecchymosis** (or "bruise") (subcutaneous or submucosal accumulation of hemorrhage measuring >1 cm; typically appears as a red-purple patch)
4. **hematoma** (accumulation of extravasated blood forming a tumor-like mass)

For example, palatal petechiae may result from various traumatic and nontraumatic causes. The lesions tend to involve the soft palate or junction of the hard and soft palate. In some cases, palatal petechiae are induced by repeated or prolonged increased intrathoracic pressure associated with coughing, vomiting, childbirth, or other activities. Petechiae induced by trauma from fellatio are discussed in the next section. In addition, palatal petechiae may be a sign of various infectious diseases, such as rubella, infectious mononucleosis, streptococcal pharyngitis, and Zika virus infection. Interestingly, a few recent reports suggest that palatal petechiae and other forms of oral hemorrhage may be caused by *Helicobacter pylori*–induced immune thrombocytopenic purpura as well.

Iatrogenic trauma also can cause mucosal or submucosal hemorrhage. For instance, during the course of dental procedures, high-speed suction tips and local anesthetic injections occasionally may cause hematomas. Also, after tooth extraction or other oral surgical procedures, some patients develop a type of hematoma commonly referred to as a *"liver clot"* (dark red, jelly-like clot that is rich in hemoglobin and typically is caused by slowly oozing venous hemorrhage). In more life-threatening cases, patients can develop upper airway obstruction due to massive hematoma formation in the floor of the mouth as a complication of surgery. Therefore, when placing dental implants, extracting teeth, removing tori, or performing osteotomies in the mandible, one should exercise caution to avoid accidental injury to the sublingual or facial arterial branches.

Clinical management depends on the cause of hemorrhage, but typically entails controlling active hemorrhage, removing sources of trauma, and/or addressing underlying systemic conditions. Liver clots usually are removed by high-speed suction or a large curette, followed by saline irrigation and the application of direct pressure. Most hemorrhagic lesions induced by minor trauma heal within 1 to 2 weeks after removal of the source of injury, although hematomas sometimes take longer to resolve.

■ Figure **8.25**
Petechiae
Numerous pinpoint spots of hemorrhage on the soft palate. (Courtesy Dr. Matt Madsen.)

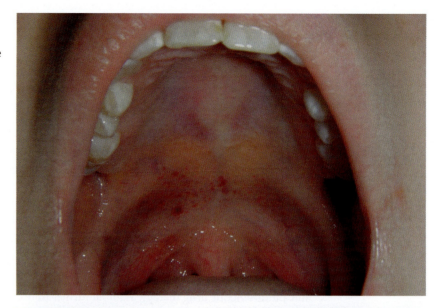

■ Figure **8.26**
Ecchymosis
Large area of hemorrhage on the left soft palate. Also present are several small hemorrhagic foci (or *petechiae*).

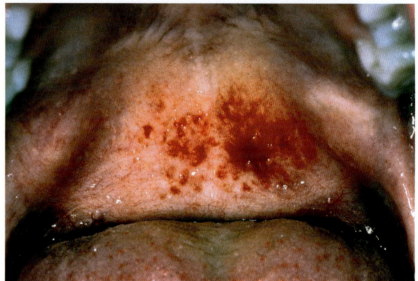

■ Figure **8.27**
Hematoma
Large, dark red "liver clot" that formed after extraction of a maxillary molar.

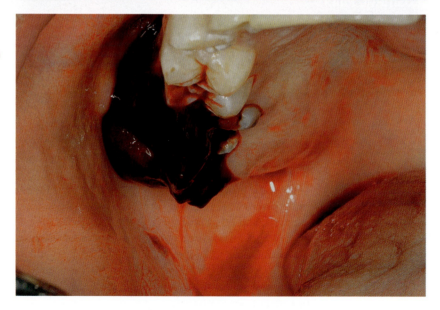

Petechiae From Fellatio

Fig. **8.28**

Negative pressure, gag reflex activation, and/or blunt force from fellatio may result in palatal *petechiae* (small, pinpoint spots of hemorrhage). In the United States, more than 80% of individuals aged 15 through 44 years report ever having oral sex with a partner of the opposite sex, and approximately 5% of males within this age range report ever having oral sex with another male. Although oral sexual activity is common, there are few cases in the scientific literature of oral lesions caused by fellatio. In addition to petechiae, other palatal lesions noted in association with fellatio include ecchymosis, nonhemorrhagic erythema (with or without candidiasis), ulcers, vesicles, and papules.

Palatal lesions from fellatio have been noted most often in women (peak in the third decade; range: 16 to 56 years). However, it is also possible to see such lesions in men or sexually abused children. The petechiae typically are asymptomatic and involve the soft palate or the hard and soft palate junction. In many cases, the hemorrhagic foci are scattered bilaterally, with or without involvement of the midline. Correlation with a clinical history of recent oral sexual activity makes the diagnosis readily apparent, although many patients are reluctant to discuss their sexual practices. The differential diagnosis for palatal petechiae also includes viral or streptococcal infection, violent coughing or vomiting, blood dyscrasias, and antithrombotic drug therapy. Without further trauma, petechiae from fellatio typically resolve within 1 to 2 weeks.

Ulceration From Cunnilingus

Fig. **8.29**

Oral trauma also may be caused by *cunnilingus* (oral stimulation of the female genitalia). The lingual frenum can develop a horizontal ulceration due to repetitive scraping against the incisal edges of the mandibular central incisors as the tongue is thrust forward. The ulceration typically heals in about a week, but recurrence is possible with repetitive injury. Smoothing the incisal edges of the mandibular incisors may reduce the risk for further ulceration. Over the long-term, this sexual practice may result in a linear band of fibrous hyperplasia on the lingual frenum.

Cosmetic Fillers

Fig. **8.30**

Cosmetic fillers have become increasingly popular over the past several decades. In the United States in 2016, more than 2.6 million cosmetic soft tissue filler procedures were performed, representing a nearly 300% increase since the beginning of the millennium. Most patients are middle-aged to older females. In order to smooth out wrinkles and creases, the fillers are injected subcutaneously into areas of the face, such as the cheeks, lips, nasolabial folds, marionette lines, and chin creases. The filler material may be nonpermanent (e.g., hyaluronic acid, collagen, poly-L-lactic acid) or permanent (e.g., silicone, polymethyl-methacrylate, hydroxyapatite). Although the procedure is minimally invasive and usually well tolerated, there is the potential for adverse reactions. During the first few hours to days following injection, possible reactions include lumps (from uneven filler distribution at the time of injection), erythema, itching, pain, swelling, bruising, recurrent herpes simplex virus infection, and localized infection. Rarely, there may be more severe acute reactions, such as anaphylaxis, local skin allergy, necrosis, scarring, myalgia, facial paralysis, and renal failure. In addition, nodules may develop weeks to months following injection as a result of foreign body reaction. Frequent sites for such nodules include the lips, labial vestibule, and anterior buccal mucosa. Occasionally, the material migrates and induces a reaction some distance from the injection site. The clinical diagnosis may not be obvious, especially if the patient does not report a history of cosmetic filler injection. Excisional biopsy is curative for small lesions. Larger lesions may be treated with intralesional or systemic corticosteroids.

■ Figure 8.28
Petechiae From Fellatio
Small spots of hemorrhage on the soft palate.

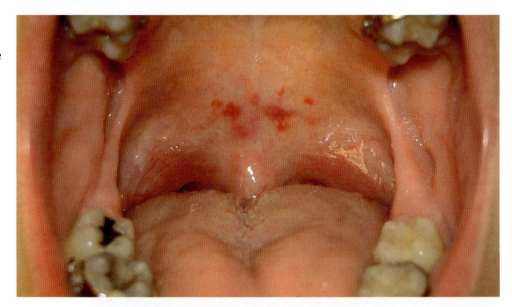

■ Figure 8.29
Ulceration From Cunnilingus
Ulceration of the lingual frenum caused by repeated trauma from the mandibular incisors as the tongue is thrust forward.

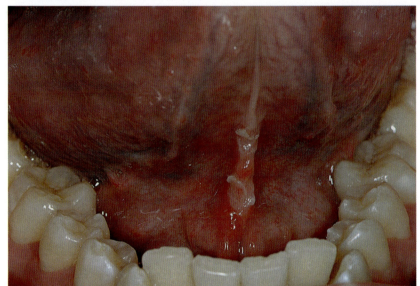

■ Figure 8.30
Cosmetic Filler
Yellowish submucosal mass in the lower labial vestibule caused by hydroxyapatite with associated foreign body reaction. (From Daley T, Damm DD, Haden JA, Kolodychak MT. Oral lesions associated with injected hydroxyapatite cosmetic filler. *Oral Surg Oral Med Oral Pathol Oral Radiol.* 2012;114:107–111.)

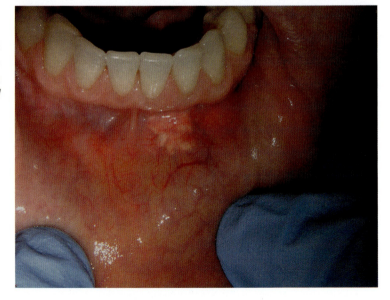

Figs. **8.31–8.33**

An **amalgam tattoo** is a pigmented oral mucosal lesion that results from implantation of dental amalgam. Amalgam represents a common source of exogenous pigmentation in the oral cavity. During the placement or removal of amalgam restorations, metallic fragments may enter the oral mucosa by various mechanisms (e.g., introduction of amalgam into mucosal abrasions or lacerations, amalgam driven by the force of high-speed air turbines, gingival contamination by dental floss passed through the contact of a recently placed filling). In addition, broken fragments of amalgam may enter the socket or periosteum during tooth extraction, and amalgam used for endodontic retrofill procedures may be left within the surgical site. The pigmentation may spread laterally for several months after implantation.

Clinically, an amalgam tattoo typically appears as a blue, gray, or black macule with well- to ill-defined borders. Although any portion of the oral mucosa may be involved, the most common sites are the gingiva, alveolar mucosa, and buccal mucosa. Unlike vascular lesions, amalgam tattoos do not blanch with diascopy; nevertheless, the absence of blanching does not completely rule out a vascular lesion. The clinical differential diagnosis may include a varix, vascular malformation, blue nevus, and melanoma. High-resolution radiographs at times may exhibit radiopaque metallic fragments. However, in many cases the fragments are too small to be detected radiographically. If a presumptive clinical diagnosis of amalgam tattoo cannot be corroborated by radiographic findings, then a biopsy with histopathologic examination should be considered. Once the diagnosis is established, no further treatment is necessary. However, amalgam tattoos involving the maxillary anterior facial gingiva or other conspicuous sites may be removed to address cosmetic concerns. Most examples are removed by conservative surgical excision, which at times is combined with grafting procedures (e.g., free gingival graft, subepithelial connective tissue graft). Laser removal also may be performed.

■ Figure 8.31
Amalgam Tattoo
Dark gray mucosal discoloration in the maxillary anterior region caused by an endodontic retrofill procedure.

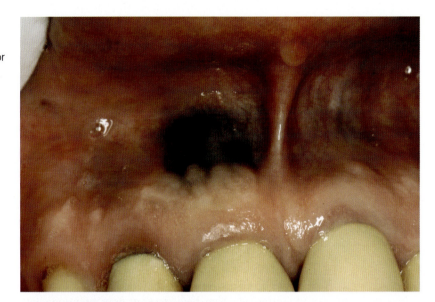

■ Figure 8.32
Amalgam Tattoo
Gray discoloration of the ventral tongue and floor of the mouth.

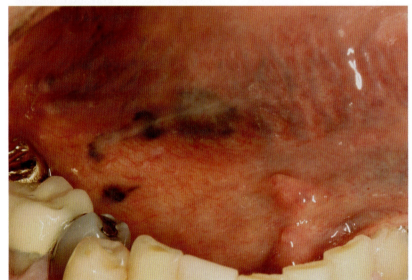

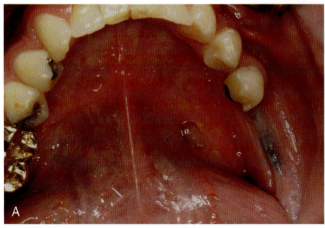

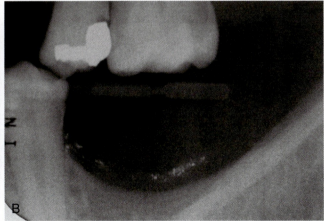

■ Figure 8.33
Amalgam Tattoo
(A) Blue-gray discoloration of the mandibular alveolar ridge. (B) Corresponding radiograph showing radiopaque metallic fragments in the area of mucosal discoloration.

Figs. 8.34 and 8.35

Intentional tattoos occasionally may be noted in the orofacial region. They can represent a cultural practice, social statement, aesthetic choice, or personal expression. In addition, tattooing may be performed by health professionals for various reasons, such as treating gingival vitiligo, color matching after surgical reconstruction, identifying landmarks for surgery or radiotherapy, hiding surgical scars, and for permanent makeup.

Permanent makeup ("cosmetic tattooing") involves dermal injection of exogenous pigments to simulate lip liner, eyeliner, or other facial cosmetics. Potential adverse reactions include swelling, burning, itching, numbness, and tenderness. Delayed-type hypersensitivity reactions may occur within days to years following tattoo application. In addition, within weeks to a year after lip tattoo placement, some patients will have developed granulomatous foreign body reactions appearing as coalescing papules or linear indurated enlargement along the vermilion border. Certain types of red pigments used for lip and other body tattoos are known to cause granulomatous, eczematous, lichenoid, or pseudolymphomatous reactions. In one reported case, a patient with no history of skin cancer or heavy sun exposure developed carcinoma of the upper lip after cosmetic lip tattoo placement.

Intraorally, blue, blue-black, or gray intentional tattoos may be evident on the maxillary facial gingiva among individuals from certain African or Middle Eastern nations. Such tattoos most often are placed in preteen and teenaged girls. This practice usually is performed for aesthetic enhancement, although at times it may be used as a homeopathic remedy for oral diseases. In addition, in the United States and other countries, some individuals have labial mucosal tattoos intended to convey personal, religious, or vulgar messages.

Patients should be advised to obtain tattoos at facilities that use sterile practices because of the risk for infection (such as hepatitis, human immunodeficiency virus [HIV], staphylococcal skin infection). Inflammatory responses to intraoral tattoos often are minor and self-limited, although surgical excision may be performed for chronic, localized, foreign body reactions. However, surgical removal of cosmetic tattoos on the lip vermilion or other aesthetic facial areas is not a viable option. For patients with persistent inflammatory reactions to permanent makeup, topical or intralesional corticosteroids may be administered, but results are variable. Laser therapy for the removal of cosmetic tattoos also has yielded inconsistent results, and this treatment carries a risk for exacerbating inflammatory reactions and causing permanent color changes. In addition, before performing magnetic resonance imaging (MRI) of the head and neck region, clinicians should be aware of the risk for ferromagnetic materials in permanent makeup to cause image artifacts and transient tingling, burning, erythema, or swelling.

Charm Needles

Fig. 8.36

A **charm needle** (or *susuk*) is a type of talisman inserted under the skin, often in the orofacial region. Such needles are used most commonly in parts of Southeast Asia. They are implanted by a *bomoh* (Malay shaman) in order to enhance the wearer's attractiveness, health, or career success. The needles consist of thin, pointed rods made of gold or other precious materials.

Charm needles usually cause no pain and are not evident clinically. However, they may be noted incidentally during radiographic examination. The needles often are implanted subcutaneously in the mandibular region, forehead, cheeks, and lips. Among cases reported in the scientific literature, the number of orofacial needles per patient ranges from 1 to greater than 80, and there may be a bilaterally symmetric distribution. It is common for the wearer to deny the charm needles' existence; according to tradition, the talismans must be kept secret to maintain their magical powers, and Muslim wearers may risk punishment by religious authorities. Clinicians should be familiar with this cultural practice in order to avoid confusion with other foreign objects (e.g., restorative pins, broken endodontic files, endodontic filling material, surgical clips) or radiographic artifact. Magnetic resonance imaging (MRI) is contraindicated for patients wearing charm needles made of ferromagnetic materials. Treatment generally is not needed. However, some patients request removal; according to legend, all charm needles must be removed before the end of life in order to avoid an excruciatingly painful death.

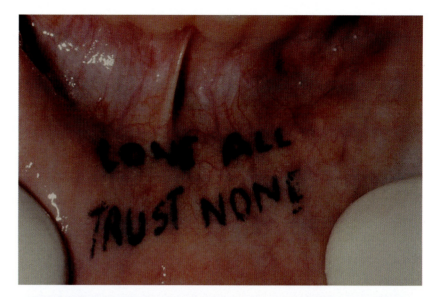

■ Figure **8.34**
Intentional Tattoo
Written message on the lower labial mucosa.

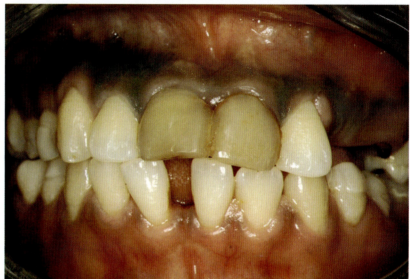

■ Figure **8.35**
Intentional Tattoo
Blue-gray tattoo of the maxillary facial gingiva in a patient from the Republic of Guinea.

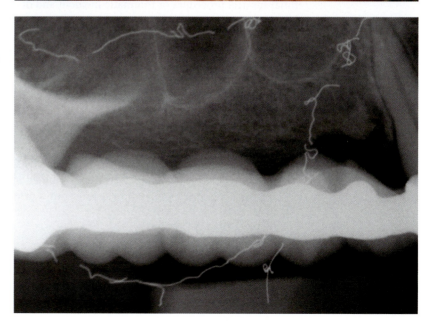

■ Figure **8.36**
Charm Needles
Radiopaque needles superimposed on the maxilla. (With appreciation to Dr. Charles Friedman.)

Antral Pseudocyst

Fig. **8.37**

An **antral pseudocyst** represents an accumulation of inflammatory serous exudate that lifts the sinus epithelial lining and periosteum away from the underlying bone to form a characteristic dome-shaped swelling. The lesion is considered a pseudocyst because it is not a pathologic cavity lined by epithelium. Many cases are caused by underlying odontogenic infection. Other proposed sources of inflammation include upper respiratory tract infection, allergy, and irritation from dry forced-air heat. Clinically, most lesions are asymptomatic, although sinus pain, headache, nasal obstruction, nasal discharge, and postnasal drip are possible. Radiographic examination typically shows a dome-shaped or spherical radiopacity involving the floor of the maxillary sinus. Infrequently, the lesion also may arise in the lateral wall or medial wall of the antrum. There is no erosion or sclerosis of the adjacent bone. The characteristic radiographic presentation usually is sufficient to form a strong presumptive diagnosis. Antral pseudocysts typically do not require treatment, other than addressing the underlying cause of inflammation. In particular, the maxillary teeth should be examined carefully, and any foci of odontogenic infection should be eliminated. If the lesion becomes unusually large, then surgical removal may be considered.

Surgical Ciliated Cyst

Figs. **8.38 and 8.39**

A **surgical ciliated cyst** (*traumatic ciliated cyst, surgical implantation cyst, respiratory implantation cyst, postoperative maxillary cyst*) is a benign cyst that typically develops as a delayed complication of sinonasal surgery, orthognathic surgery, or maxillofacial trauma. The lesion is believed to result from iatrogenic or traumatic implantation of respiratory epithelium, which subsequently may transform into a cyst. Most reported cases have developed in the posterior maxilla after a Caldwell-Luc procedure. In particular, many such reports occurred in Japanese patients who received surgical rather than medical treatment for maxillary sinusitis prior to the 1970s. In addition, some maxillary examples have arisen after midface (LeFort I, II, or III) osteotomy, antral floor augmentation, or maxillary tooth extraction with damage to the sinus floor. Infrequently, surgical ciliated cysts also may develop in the mandible, especially in the anterior region. Mandibular lesions typically arise in patients who have had surgery simultaneously involving the sinonasal region and the mandible (e.g., rhinoplasty combined with genioplasty or chin augmentation, LeFort I osteotomy combined with bilateral sagittal split osteotomy and/or genioplasty). The interval between the initial surgical procedure or traumatic incident and discovery of the lesion is variable and may be greater than 40 years.

Clinically, surgical ciliated cysts tend to cause swelling and pain or discomfort. However, some patients are asymptomatic. Lesions that become secondarily infected may exhibit purulent discharge, abscess formation, and sinus tract formation. Radiographic examination shows a unilocular or multilocular radiolucency. Cortical perforation may be evident. Surgical ciliated cysts typically are managed by simple enucleation or curettage. Marsupialization may be considered for especially large lesions. Incision and drainage should be performed when there is associated abscess formation. Suggested preventive measures include: (1) careful removal of all mucosa from harvested nasal bone or cartilage before use in autograft procedures; (2) close inspection for any aberrant tissue in a midface osteotomy site prior to fixation; (3) copious irrigation prior to closure during maxillofacial or sinonasal surgery; (4) the use of separate blades—or meticulously cleaning a single blade—when performing combined maxillary and mandibular surgical procedures; and (5) if possible, performing mandibular procedures prior to maxillary procedures in a single session.

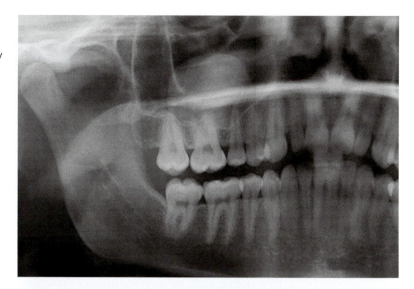

■ Figure 8.37
Antral Pseudocyst
Radiopaque, dome-shaped swelling of the right maxillary sinus floor.

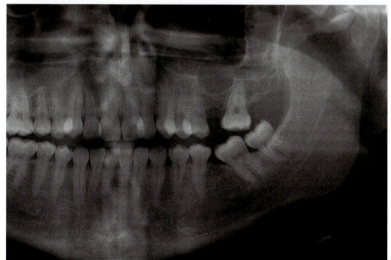

■ Figure 8.38
Surgical Ciliated Cyst
Radiolucency in the left posterior maxilla as a late complication of traumatic extraction of a maxillary molar. (Courtesy Dr. Steven Anderson.)

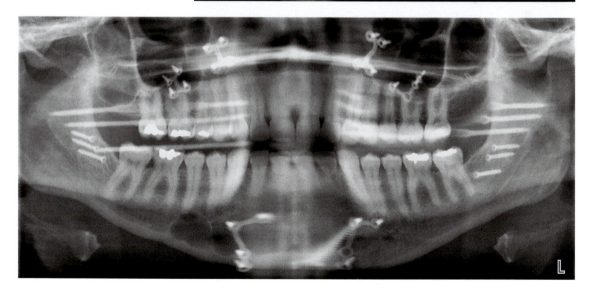

■ Figure 8.39
Surgical Ciliated Cyst
Large mandibular radiolucency noted 10 years after orthognathic surgery. (Courtesy Dr. James Lemon.)

Minocycline-Induced Pigmentation

Fig. 8.40

Minocycline is a semisynthetic tetracycline derivative often used to treat acne. Additional indications include rosacea, severe perioral dermatitis, and off-label treatment of rheumatoid arthritis. Investigational applications include minocycline granules for adjunctive treatment of periodontal disease and a triple antibiotic paste containing minocycline for regenerative endodontic therapy.

Pigmentation is a well-recognized adverse effect of minocycline and other tetracyclines. Such pigmentation may involve the bone, teeth, oral mucosa, skin, nails, sclera, conjunctiva, and thyroid. Discoloration typically occurs after prolonged minocycline use, although some cases develop after only 2 to 4 weeks of administration. Most reports of minocycline-induced pigmentation in the oral cavity involve hard tissues—especially the alveolar bone, palatal bone, and/or teeth. The stained bone typically appears blue, gray, gray-green, or black. It often shows through the overlying mucosa as blue-gray discoloration involving the entire hard palate and/or a linear band along the maxillary and mandibular facial gingiva near the mucogingival junction. Minocycline also can produce blue-gray discoloration of tooth crowns (especially in the middle third) and green-black staining of tooth roots. Unlike tetracycline, minocycline can affect fully developed teeth. Infrequently, minocycline induces pigmentation of the oral mucosa (e.g., tongue, lips, buccal mucosa, gingiva) without concurrent bone involvement.

After discontinuation of minocycline, discoloration of the oral mucosa and bone may fade or disappear over time. However, the tooth discoloration can be permanent. Some authors suggest that vitamin C may block minocycline-induced pigmentation, although further studies are needed.

Drug-Induced Pigmentation

Figs. 8.41 and 8.42

In addition to tetracylines, numerous other medications can cause pigmentation in the oral cavity. Chief examples include antimalarial drugs (e.g., chloroquine, hydrochloroquine, quinidine, quinacrine), phenothiazines, estrogens, phenolphthalein, amiodorone, chemotherapeutic agents (e.g., 5-fluoruracil, cyclophosphamide, doxorubicin, busulfan), imatinib, and certain drugs used to treat patients with human immunodeficiency virus (HIV) infection (e.g., zidovudine, clofazimine, ketoconazole). Proposed mechanisms for drug-induced pigmentation include the deposition of pigmented drug metabolites, the stimulation of increased melanin production by melanocytes, the chelation of hemosiderin to the medication, and an increased synthesis of lipofuscin or other pigments. Many systemically administered drugs can cause pigmentation of not only the oral cavity but also extraoral sites.

Antimalarial drugs are prescribed for malaria as well as various autoimmune diseases. Intraorally, they can cause diffuse blue-gray to blue-black discoloration. The discoloration typically is seen on the palate, although the tongue, gingiva, lips, and other oral sites also may be affected. In addition, similar pigmentation may be evident on the skin and nail beds. Occasionally, diffuse brown melanosis of the oral mucosa and skin may be seen as well.

More recently, mucocutaneous pigmentary changes have been reported in association with imatinib, which is a tyrosine kinase inhibitor used to treat chronic myeloid leukemia, metastatic gastrointestinal stromal tumors, and other neoplasms. Intraorally, there is typically diffuse blue-gray, blue-brown, or dark brown pigmentation of the palate. Isolated reports have described hyperpigmentation of the teeth and gingiva as well. Extraorally, imatinib may cause hypopigmentation or hyperpigmentation of the skin, hyperpigmentation of the nails, and hypopigmentation of the hair.

Drug-induced oral pigmentation is generally innocuous, although it may cause aesthetic concern. Discontinuation of the offending medication often causes gradual fading of mucosal discoloration.

■ Figure **8.40**
Minocycline-Induced Pigmentation
Linear bands of blue-gray discoloration along the maxillary and mandibular facial gingiva near the mucogingival junction due to minocycline staining of the underlying bone.

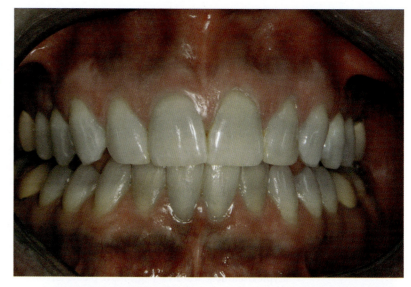

■ Figure **8.41**
Drug-Induced Pigmentation
Diffuse, blue-gray pigmentation of the palate caused by chloroquine. (Courtesy Dr. Donald R. Hoaglin.)

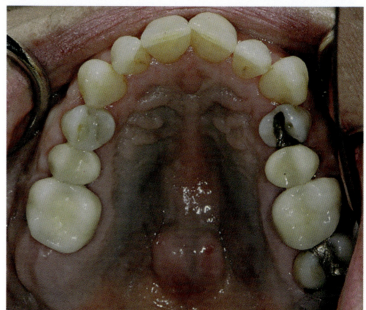

■ Figure **8.42**
Drug-Induced Pigmentation
Diffuse, dark brown pigmentation of the palate caused by imatinib. (Courtesy Dr. Walter Cólon.)

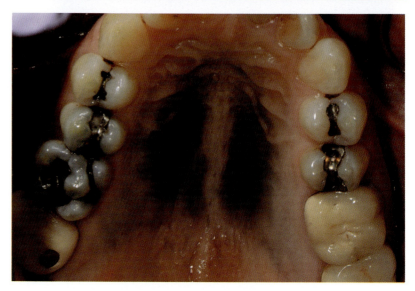

Figs. **8.43 and 8.44**

Smoker's melanosis represents oral mucosal melanin pigmentation induced by tobacco smoking. The prevalence of this condition has been estimated to be about 18% to 22% in certain European or light-skinned Asian smoking populations. There is a positive relationship between the number of cigarettes smoked per day and the frequency of individuals with oral mucosal pigmentation. The precise etiopathogenesis is uncertain, although the pigmentation is hypothesized to be a protective response to harmful substances in tobacco smoke. Toxic compounds may stimulate melanocytes to produce melanin, and melanin may bind the toxins or their resultant free radical species. Some studies have noted a predilection among females, which suggests a possible synergistic interaction between smoking and female sex hormones. Clinical examination shows brown patches or macules, often with a multifocal or diffuse distribution. Any oral mucosal surface may be affected. However, favored sites include the anterior facial gingiva in cigarette smokers, the buccal mucosa and commissures in pipe smokers, and the palatal mucosa in reverse smokers. In addition, some studies have noted increased gingival pigmentation among individuals who have been exposed to secondhand smoke. Biopsy may be considered to rule out melanoma in cases with unusual or atypical clinical features (e.g., hard palate involvement, surface elevation). Tobacco cessation typically results in gradual fading over several years.

■ Figure **8.43**
Smoker's Melanosis
Areas of brown pigmentation involving the maxillary and mandibular facial gingiva in a smoker.

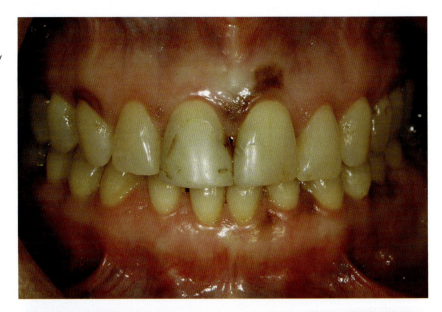

■ Figure **8.44**
Smoker's Melanosis
Brown macule on the right soft palate in a smoker.

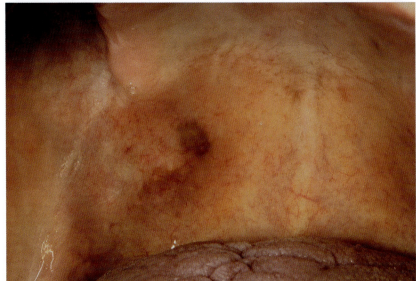

Bibliography

Linea Alba

Martínez Díaz-Canel AI, García-Pola Vallejo MJ. Epidemiological study of oral mucosa pathology in patients of the Oviedo School of Stomatology. *Med Oral*. 2002;7:4–9, 10–6.

Vieira-Andrade RG, Martins-Júnior PA, Corrêa-Faria P, et al. Oral mucosal conditions in preschool children of low socioeconomic status: prevalence and determinant factors. *Eur J Pediatr*. 2013;172:675–681.

Vieira-Andrade RG, Zuquim Guimarães Fde F, Vieira Cda S, et al. Oral mucosa alterations in a socioeconomically deprived region: prevalence and associated factors. *Braz Oral Res*. 2011;25:393–400.

Morsicatio

Kang HS, Lee HE, Ro YS, et al. Three cases of 'morsicatio labiorum'. *Ann Dermatol*. 2012;24:455–458.

Romero M, Vicente A, Bravo LA. Prevention of habitual cheek biting: a case report. *Spec Care Dentist*. 2005;25:214–216.

Woo SB, Lin D. Morsicatio mucosae oris – a chronic oral frictional keratosis, not a leukoplakia. *J Oral Maxillofac Surg*. 2009;67:140–146.

Traumatic Ulcer

Cannavale R, Itro A, Campisi G, et al. Oral self-injuries: clinical findings in a series of 19 patients. *Med Oral Patol Oral Cir Bucal*. 2015;20: e123–e129.

Limeres J, Feijoo JF, Baluja F, et al. Oral self-injury: an update. *Dent Traumatol*. 2013;29:8–14.

Traumatic Granuloma

Chatzistamou I, Doussis-Anagnostopoulou I, Georgiou G, et al. Traumatic ulcerative granuloma with stromal eosinophilia: report of a case and literature review. *J Oral Maxillofac Surg*. 2012;70:349–353.

el-Mofty SK, Swanson PE, Wick MR, et al. Eosinophilic ulcer of the oral mucosa. Report of 38 new cases with immunohistochemical observations. *Oral Surg Oral Med Oral Pathol*. 1993;75:78–722.

Fonseca FP, de Andrade BA, Coletta RD, et al. Clinicopathological and immunohistochemical analysis of 19 cases of oral eosinophilic ulcers. *Oral Surg Oral Med Oral Pathol Oral Radiol*. 2013;115:532–540.

Shen WR, Chang JY, Wu YC, et al. Oral traumatic ulcerative granuloma with stromal eosinophilia: a clinicopathological study of 34 cases. *J Formos Med Assoc*. 2015;114:881–885.

Electrical Burns

Edlich RF, Farinholt HM, Winters KL, et al. Modern concepts of treatment and prevention of electrical burns. *J Long Term Eff Med Implants*. 2005;15:511–532.

Pontini A, Reho F, Giatsidis G, et al. Multidisciplinary care in severe pediatric electrical oral burn. *Burns*. 2015;41:e41–e46.

Roberts S, Meltzer JA. An evidence-based approach to electrical injuries in children. *Pediatr Emerg Med Pract*. 2013;10:1–17.

Umstattd LA, Chang CW. Pediatric oral electrical burns: incidence of emergency department visits in the United States, 1997-2012. *Otolaryngol Head Neck Surg*. 2016;155:94–98.

Yeroshalmi F, Sidoti EJ Jr, Adamo AK, et al. Oral electrical burns in children – a model of multidisciplinary care. *J Burn Care Res*. 2011;32:e25–e30.

Thermal Burns

Cowan D, Ho B, Sykes KJ, et al. Pediatric oral burns: a ten-year review of patient characteristics, etiologies and treatment outcomes. *Int J Pediatr Otorhinolaryngol*. 2013;77:1325–1328.

Hyo Y, Fukutsuji K, Fukushima H, et al. Two cases of thermal burns of the larynx in older men. *Auris Nasus Larynx*. 2017;44:620–623.

Kafas P, Stavrianos C. Thermal burn of palate caused by microwave heated cheese-pie: A case report. *Cases J*. 2008;1:191.

Silberman M, Jeanmonod R. Aerodigestive tract burn from ingestion of microwaved food. *Case Rep Emerg Med*. 2013;2013:781809.

Wakefield Y, Pemberton MN. Oro-facial thermal injury caused by food heated in a microwave oven. *Dent Update*. 2009;36:26–27.

Chemical Burns

Dilsiz A. Self-inflicted oral soft-tissue burn due to local behavior and treatment. *J Clin Exp Dent*. 2010;2:e51–e54.

Girish MS, Latha A, Prakash C, et al. Iatrogenic injury of oral mucosa due to chemicals: a case report of formocresol injury and review. *IOSR J Dent Med Sci*. 2015;14:1–5.

Guttenberg SA. Chemical injury of the oral mucosa from verapamil. *N Engl J Med*. 1990;323:615.

Riffat F, Cheng A. Pediatric caustic ingestion: 50 consecutive cases and a review of the literature. *Dis Esophagus*. 2009;22:89–94.

Santos-Pinto L, Campos JA, Giro EM, et al. Iatrogenic chemical burns caused by chemical agents used in dental pulp therapy. *Burns*. 2004;30:614–615.

Vargo RJ, Warner BM, Potluri A, et al. Garlic burn of the oral mucosa: a case report and review of self-treatment chemical burns. *J Am Dent Assoc*. 2017;148:767–771.

Chemotherapy-Induced Oral Mucositis

De Sanctis V, Bossi P, Sanguineti G, et al. Mucositis in head and neck cancer patients treated with radiotherapy and systemic therapies: literature review and consensus statements. *Crit Rev Oncol Hematol*. 2016;100:147–166.

Elad S, Zadik Y, Yarom N. Oral complications of nonsurgical cancer therapies. *Atlas Oral Maxillofac Surg Clin North Am*. 2017;25:133–147.

Lalla RV, Bowen J, Barasch A, et al; Mucositis Guidelines Leadership Group of the Multinational Association of Supportive Care in Cancer and International Society of Oral Oncology (MASCC/ISOO). MASCC/ISOO clinical practice guidelines for the management of mucositis secondary to cancer therapy. *Cancer*. 2014;120:1453–1461.

Lalla RV, Saunders DP, Peterson DE. Chemotherapy or radiation-induced oral mucositis. *Dent Clin North Am*. 2014;58:341–349.

Riley P, Glenny AM, Worthington HV, et al. Interventions for preventing oral mucositis in patients with cancer receiving treatment: oral cryotherapy. *Cochrane Database Syst Rev*. 2015;(12):CD011552.

Radiation-Induced Oral Mucositis

De Sanctis V, Bossi P, Sanguineti G, et al. Mucositis in head and neck cancer patients treated with radiotherapy and systemic therapies: literature review and consensus statements. *Crit Rev Oncol Hematol*. 2016;100:147–166.

Elad S, Zadik Y, Yarom N. Oral complications of nonsurgical cancer therapies. *Atlas Oral Maxillofac Surg Clin North Am*. 2017;25: 133–147.

Lalla RV, Bowen J, Barasch A, et al; Mucositis Guidelines Leadership Group of the Multinational Association of Supportive Care in Cancer and International Society of Oral Oncology (MASCC/ISOO). MASCC/ISOO clinical practice guidelines for the management of mucositis secondary to cancer therapy. *Cancer*. 2014;120:1453–1461.

Lalla RV, Saunders DP, Peterson DE. Chemotherapy or radiation-induced oral mucositis. *Dent Clin North Am*. 2014;58:341–349.

Maria OM, Eliopoulos N, Muanza T. Radiation-induced oral mucositis. *Front Oncol*. 2017;7:89.

Moslemi D, Nokhandani AM, Otaghsaraei MT, et al. Management of chemo/radiation-induced oral mucositis in patients with head and neck cancer: a review of the current literature. *Radiother Oncol*. 2016;120:13–20.

Xerostomia-Related Caries

Guggenheimer J, Moore PA. Xerostomia: etiology, recognition and treatment. *J Am Dent Assoc*. 2003;134:61–69, 118–119.

Gupta N, Pal M, Rawat S, et al. Radiation-induced dental caries, prevention and treatment - a systematic review. *Natl J Maxillofac Surg*. 2015;6:160–166.

Haveman CW, Summitt JB, Burgess JO, et al. Three restorative materials and topical fluoride gel used in xerostomic patients: a clinical comparison. *J Am Dent Assoc*. 2003;134:177–184.

Plemons JM, Al-Hashimi I, Marek CL. American Dental Association Council on Scientific Affairs: Managing xerostomia and salivary gland hypofunction: executive summary of a report from the American Dental Association Council on Scientific Affairs. *J Am Dent Assoc*. 2014;145:867–873.

Osteoradionecrosis

Buglione M, Cavagnini R, Di Rosario F, et al. Oral toxicity management in head and neck cancer patients treated with chemotherapy and radiation: dental pathologies and osteoradionecrosis (part 1) literature review and consensus statement. 2016;97:131–142.

Costa DA, Costa TP, Netto EC, et al. New perspectives on the conservative management of osteoradionecrosis of the mandible: a literature review. *Head Neck.* 2016;38:1708–1716.

Nadella KR, Kodali RM, Guttikonda LK, et al. Osteoradionecrosis of the jaws: clinico-therapeutic management: a literature review and update. *J Maxillofac Oral Surg.* 2015;14:891–901.

Owosho AA, Estilo CL, Huryn JM, et al. Pentoxifylline and tocopherol in the management of cancer patients with medication-related osteonecrosis of the jaw: an observational retrospective study of initial case series. *Oral Surg Oral Med Oral Pathol Oral Radiol.* 2016;122:455–459.

Owosho AA, Tsai CJ, Lee RS, et al. The prevalence and risk factors associated with osteoradionecrosis of the jaw in oral and oropharyngeal cancer patients treated with intensity-modulated radiation therapy (IMRT): the Memorial Sloan Kettering Cancer Center experience. *Oral Oncol.* 2017;64:44–51.

Medication-Related Osteonecrosis of the Jaws

American College of Prosthodontists. *Medication-Related Osteonecrosis of the Jaw.* Chicago, IL: American College of Prosthodontists; 2016. Available at: https://www.prosthodontics.org/assets/1/7/Medication-Related_Osteonecrosis_of_the_Jaw.pdf. Accessed November 1, 2017.

Kim KM, Rhee Y, Kwon YD, et al. Medication related osteonecrosis of the jaw: 2015 position statement of the Korean Society for Bone and Mineral Research and the Korean Association of Oral and Maxillofacial Surgeons. *J Bone Metab.* 2015;22:151–165.

Otto S, Kwon TG, Saaf AT. Chapter 4 Definition, Clinical Features and Staging of Medication-related Osteonecrosis of the Jaws. In: Otto S, ed. *Medication-related Osteonecrosis of the Jaws. Bisphosphonates, Denosumab, and New Agents.* Berlin: Springer-Verlag; 2015:43–54.

Ruggiero SL, Dodson TB, Fantasia J, et al. American Association of Oral and Maxillofacial Surgeons: American Association of Oral and Maxillofacial Surgeons position paper on medication-related osteonecrosis of the jaw – 2014 update. *J Oral Maxillofac Surg.* 2014;72:1938–1956.

Oral Ulceration With Bone Sequestration

Farah CS, Savage NW. Oral ulceration with bone sequestration. *Aust Dent J.* 2003;48:61–64.

Khan AA, Morrison A, Hanley DA, et al. International Task Force on Osteonecrosis of the Jaw: Diagnosis and management of osteonecrosis of the jaw: a systematic review and international consensus. *J Bone Miner Res.* 2015;30:3–23.

Palla B, Burian E, Klecker JR, et al. Systematic review of oral ulceration with bone sequestration. *J Craniomaxillofac Surg.* 2016;44:257–264.

"Meth Mouth"

Chomchai C, Chomchai S. Global patterns of methamphetamine use. *Curr Opin Psychiatry.* 2015;28:269–274.

Clague J, Belin TR, Shetty V. Mechanisms underlying methamphetamine-related dental disease. *J Am Dent Assoc.* 2017;148:377–386.

Hamamoto DT, Rhodus NL. Methamphetamine abuse and dentistry. *Oral Dis.* 2009;15:27–37.

Shetty V, Harrell L, Murphy DA, et al. Dental disease patterns in methamphetamine users: findings in a large urban sample. *J Am Dent Assoc.* 2015;146:875–885.

Substance Abuse and Mental Health Services Administration: Key Substance Use and Mental Health Indicators in the United States: Results from the 2016 National Survey on Drug Use and Health, HHS Publication No. SMA 17-5044, NSDUH Series H-52, Rockville, MD, 2017, Center for Behavioral Health Statistics and Quality, Substance Abuse and Mental Health Services Administration. Available at: https://www.samhsa.gov/data/. Accessed October 27, 2017.

Opioid-Induced Palatal Perforation

Center for Behavioral Health Statistics and Quality. *2016 National Survey on Drug Use and Health: Detailed Tables.* Rockville, MD: Substance Abuse and Mental Health Services Administration; 2017. Available at: https://www.samhsa.gov/data/sites/default/files/NSDUH-DetTabs-2016/NSDUH-DetTabs-2016.pdf. Accessed October 27, 2017.

Greene D. Total necrosis of the intranasal structures and soft palate as a result of nasal inhalation of crushed OxyContin. *Ear Nose Throat J.* 2005;84:512, 514, 516.

Hardison SA, Marcum KK, Lintzenich CR. Severe necrosis of the palate and nasal septum resulting from intranasal abuse of acetaminophen. *Ear Nose Throat J.* 2015;94:E40–E42.

Jewers WM, Rawal YB, Allen CM, et al. Palatal perforation associated with intranasal prescription narcotic abuse. *Oral Surg Oral Med Oral Pathol Oral Radiol Endod.* 2005;99:594–597.

Vosler PS, Ferguson BJ, Contreras JI, et al. Clinical and pathologic characteristics of intranasal abuse of combined opioid-acetaminophen medications. *Int Forum Allergy Rhinol.* 2014;4:839–844.

Exfoliative Cheilitis

Almazrooa SA, Woo SB, Mawardi H, et al. Characterization and management of exfoliative cheilitis: a single-center experience. *Oral Surg Oral Med Oral Pathol Oral Radiol.* 2013;116:e485–e489.

Bhatia BK, Bahr BA, Murase JE. Excimer laser therapy and narrowband ultraviolet B therapy for exfoliative cheilitis. *Int J Womens Dermatol.* 2015;1:95–98.

Reade PC, Sim R. Exfoliative cheilitis–a factitious disorder? *Int J Oral Maxillofac Surg.* 1986;15:313–317.

Roveroni-Favaretto LH, Lodi KB, Almeida JD. Topical *Calendula officinalis* L. successfully treated exfoliative cheilitis: a case report. *Cases J.* 2009;2:9077.

Chronic Lip Fissure

Axéll T, Skoglund A. Chronic lip fissures. Prevalence, pathology and treatment. *Int J Oral Surg.* 1981;10:354–358.

Combes J, Mellor TK. Treatment of chronic lip fissures with carbon dioxide laser. *Br J Oral Maxillofac Surg.* 2009;47:102–105.

Kluemper GT, White DK, Slevin JT. Chronic fissural cheilitis: a manifestation of anterior crowding. *Am J Orthod Dentofacial Orthop.* 2001;119:71–75.

Rosenquist BE. Median lip fissure. *J Craniofac Surg.* 1995;6:390–391.

Mucosal or Submucosal Hemorrhage

Del Castillo-Pardo de Vera JL, López-Arcas Calleja JM, Burgueño-García M. Hematoma of the floor of the mouth and airway obstruction during mandibular dental implant placement: a case report. *Oral Maxillofac Surg.* 2008;12:223–226.

Derrington SM, Cellura AP, McDermott LE, et al. Mucocutaneous findings and course in an adult with zika virus Infection. *JAMA Dermatol.* 2016;152:691–693.

Druckman RF, Fowler EB, Breault LG. Post-surgical hemorrhage: formation of a "liver clot" secondary to periodontal plastic surgery. *J Contemp Dent Pract.* 2001;2:62–71.

Jomen W, Sato T, Maesawa C. Improvement in platelet count after 3rd-line and 4th-line eradication therapy for *Helicobacter pylori* in patients with immune thrombocytopenia. *Rinsho Ketsueki.* 2017;58:126–131.

Law C, Alam P, Borumandi F. Floor-of-mouth hematoma following dental implant placement: literature review and case presentation. *J Oral Maxillofac Surg.* 2017;75:2340–2346.

Mergoni G, Sarraj A, Merigo E, et al. Oral submucosal hemorrhage as first clinical manifestation of *H. Pylori*-associated idiopathic thrombocytopenic purpura. *Ann Stomatol (Roma).* 2013;4(suppl 2):31.

Mitchell RN. Hemorrhage. In: Kumar V, Abbas AK, Fausto N, et al, eds. *Robbins and Cotran Pathologic Basis of Disease.* 8th ed. Philadelphia: Saunders Elsevier; 2010:114–115.

Nibhanipudi KV. A study to determine if addition of palatal petechiae to Centor criteria adds more significance to clinical diagnosis of acute strep pharyngitis in children. *Glob Pediatr Health.* 2016;3:2333794X16657943.

Petechiae From Fellatio

Cohen PR, Miller VM. Fellatio-associated petechiae of the palate: report of purpuric palatal lesions developing after oral sex. *Dermatol Online J.* 2013;19:18963.

Damm DD, White DK, Brinker CM. Variations of palatal erythema secondary to fellatio. *Oral Surg Oral Med Oral Pathol.* 1981;52:417–421.

National Center for Health Statistics. *Key Statistics from the National Survey of Family Growth.* Hyattsville, MD: National Center for Health Statistics; 2011-2015. Available at: https://www.cdc.gov/nchs/nsfg/key_statistics/s.htm#sexualfemales. Accessed October 10, 2017.

Oliveira SC, Slot DE, Van der Weijden GA. What is the cause of palate lesions? A case report. *Int J Dent Hyg.* 2013;11:306–309.

Ulceration From Cunnilingus

Leider AS. Intraoral ulcers of questionable origin. *J Am Dent Assoc.* 1976;92:1177–1178.

Mader CL. Lingual frenum ulcer resulting from orogenital sex. *J Am Dent Assoc.* 1981;103:888–890.

Cosmetic Fillers

American Society of Plastic Surgeons National Clearinghouse of Plastic Surgery Procedural Statistics: 2016 Plastic Surgery Statistics Report, Arlington, IL, 2016. American Society of Plastic Surgeons. Available at: https://www.plasticsurgery.org/documents/News/Statistics/2016/plastic-surgery-statistics-full-report-2016.pdf. Accessed October 28, 2017.

Daley T, Damm DD, Haden JA, et al. Oral lesions associated with injected hydroxyapatite cosmetic filler. *Oral Surg Oral Med Oral Pathol Oral Radiol.* 2012;114:107–111.

Eversole R, Tran K, Hansen D, et al. Lip augmentation dermal filler reactions, histopathologic features. *Head Neck Pathol.* 2013;7:241–249.

Lombardi T, Samson J, Plantier F, et al. Orofacial granulomas after injection of cosmetic fillers. Histopathologic and clinical study of 11 cases. *J Oral Pathol Med.* 2004;33:115–120.

Sanchis-Bielsa JM, Bagán JV, Poveda R, et al. Foreign body granulomatous reactions to cosmetic fillers: a clinical study of 15 cases. *Oral Surg Oral Med Oral Pathol Oral Radiol Endod.* 2009;108:237–241.

Amalgam Tattoo

Buchner A. Amalgam tattoo (amalgam pigmentation) of the oral mucosa: clinical manifestations, diagnosis and treatment. *Refuat Hapeh Vehashinayim* (1993). 2004;21:25–28, 92.

Buchner A, Hansen LS. Amalgam pigmentation (amalgam tattoo) of the oral mucosa. A clinicopathologic study of 268 cases. *Oral Surg Oral Med Oral Pathol.* 1980;49:139–147.

Meleti M, Vescovi P, Mooi WJ, et al. Pigmented lesions of the oral mucosa and perioral tissues: a flow-chart for the diagnosis and some recommendations for the management. *Oral Surg Oral Med Oral Pathol Oral Radiol Endod.* 2008;105:606–616.

Owens BM, Johnson WW, Schuman NJ. Oral amalgam pigmentations (tattoos): a retrospective study. *Quintessence Int.* 1992;23:805–810.

Thumbigere-Math V, Johnson DK. Treatment of amalgam tattoo with a subepithelial connective tissue graft and acellular dermal matrix. *J Int Acad Periodontol.* 2014;16:50–54.

Yilmaz HG, Bayindir H, Kusacki-Seker B, et al. Treatment of amalgam tattoo with an Er,Cr:YSGG laser. *J Investig Clin Dent.* 2010;1:50–54.

Intentional Tattoos

Batstone MD, Fox CM, Dingley ME, et al. Cosmetic tattooing of free flaps following head and neck reconstruction. *Craniomaxillofac Trauma Reconstr.* 2013;6:61–64.

Duke D, Urioste SS, Dover JS, et al. A reaction to a red lip cosmetic tattoo. *J Am Acad Dermatol.* 1998;39:488–490.

Garcovich S, Carbone T, Avitabile S, et al. Lichenoid red tattoo reaction: histological and immunological perspectives. *Eur J Dermatol.* 2012;22:93–96.

Ortiz A, Yamauchi PS. Rapidly growing squamous cell carcinoma from permanent makeup tattoo. *J Am Acad Dermatol.* 2009;60:1073–1074.

Shin JB, Seo SH, Kim BK, et al. Cutaneous T cell pseudolymphoma at the site of a semipermanent lip-liner tattoo. *Dermatology.* 2009;218:75–78.

Telang LA. Body art: intraoral tattoos. *Br Dent J.* 2015;218:212–213.

Tirelli G, Cova MA, Zanconati F, et al. Charcoal suspension tattoo: new tool for the localization of malignant laterocervical lymph nodes. *Eur Arch Otorhinolaryngol.* 2016;273:3973–3978.

Tope WD, Shellock FG. Magnetic resonance imaging and permanent cosmetics (tattoos): survey of complications and adverse events. *J Magn Reson Imaging.* 2002;15:180–184.

Wenzel SM, Welzel J, Hafner C, et al. Permanent make-up colorants may cause severe skin reactions. *Contact Dermatitis.* 2010;63:223–227.

Charm Needles

Jurkiewicz MT, Lim CCT, Mohan S. Clandestine charisma of the charm needles: a radiologist's challenge. *Emerg Radiol.* 2017;24:427–430.

Nor MM, Yushar M, Razali M, et al. Incidental radiological findings of susuk in the orofacial region. *Dentomaxillofac Radiol.* 2006;35:473–474.

Sharif MO, Horner K, Chadwick S, et al. Susuk charms? A case report. *Br Dent J.* 2013;215:13–15.

Tandjung YR, Hong CP, Nambiar P, et al. Uncommon radiological findings: a case report. *Int Dent J.* 2007;57:173–176.

Antral Pseudocyst

Carter LC, Calamel A, Haller A, et al. Seasonal variation in maxillary antral pseudocysts in a general clinic population. *Dentomaxillofac Radiol.* 1998;27:22–24.

Gardner DG. Pseudocysts and retention cysts of the maxillary sinus. *Oral Surg Oral Med Oral Pathol.* 1984;58:561–567.

Meer S, Altini M. Cysts and pseudocysts of the maxillary antrum revisited. *SADJ.* 2006;61:10–13.

Parks ET. Cone beam computed tomography for the nasal cavity and paranasal sinuses. *Dent Clin North Am.* 2014;58:627–651.

Sette-Dias AC, Naves MD, Mesquita RA, et al. Differential diagnosis of antral pseudocyst. A case report. *Stomatologija.* 2013;15:92–94.

Sultan M, Haberland CM, Skrip L, et al. Prevalence of antral pseudocysts in the pediatric population. *Pediatr Dent.* 2015;37:541–544.

Surgical Ciliated Cyst

Bourgeois SL Jr, Nelson BL. Surgical ciliated cyst of the mandible secondary to simultaneous Le Fort I osteotomy and genioplasty: report of case and review of the literature. *Oral Surg Oral Med Oral Pathol Oral Radiol Endod.* 2005;100:36–39.

Kaneshiro S, Nakajima T, Yoshikawa Y, et al. The postoperative maxillary cyst: report of 71 cases. *J Oral Surg.* 1981;39:191–198.

Leung YY, Wong WY, Cheung LK. Surgical ciliated cysts may mimic radicular cysts or residual cysts of maxilla: report of 3 cases. *J Oral Maxillofac Surg.* 2012;70:e264–e269.

Li CC, Feinerman DM, MacCarthy KD, et al. Rare mandibular surgical ciliated cysts: report of two new cases. *J Oral Maxillofac Surg.* 2014;72:1736–1743.

Ragsdale BD, Laurent JL, Janette AJ, et al. Respiratory implantation cyst of the mandible following orthognathic surgery. *J Oral Maxillofac Pathol.* 2009;13:30–34.

Yoshikawa Y, Nakajima T, Kaneshiro S, et al. Effective treatment of the postoperative maxillary cyst by marsupialization. *J Oral Maxillofac Surg.* 1982;40:487–491.

Minocycline Staining

Filitis DC, Graber EM. Minocycline-induced hyperpigmentation involving the oral mucosa after short-term minocycline use. *Cutis.* 2013;92:46–48.

Kahler B, Rossi-Fedele G. A review of tooth discoloration after regenerative endodontic therapy. *J Endod.* 2016;42:563–569.

LaPorta VN, Nikitakis NG, et al. Minocycline-associated intra-oral soft-tissue pigmentation: clinicopathologic correlations and review. *J Clin Periodontol.* 2005;32:119–122.

Sánchez AR, Rogers RS 3rd, Sheridan PJ. Tetracycline and other tetracycline-derivative staining of the teeth and oral cavity. *Int J Dermatol.* 2004;43:709–715.

Treister NS, Magalnick D, Woo SB. Oral mucosal pigmentation secondary to minocycline therapy: report of two cases and a review of the literature. *Oral Surg Oral Med Oral Pathol Oral Radiol Endod.* 2004;97:718–725.

Drug-Induced Pigmentation

Agrawal P, Singh O, Nigam AK, et al. Imatinib-induced dental hyperpigmentation in chronic myeloid leukemia in an adult female. *Indian J Pharmacol.* 2015;47:685–686.

de Andrade BA, Fonseca FP, Pires FR, et al. Hard palate hyperpigmentation secondary to chronic chloroquine therapy: report of five cases. *J Cutan Pathol.* 2013;40:833–838.

de Melo Filho MR, da Silva CA, da Rocha Dourado M, et al. Palate hyperpigmentation caused by prolonged use of the anti-malarial chloroquine. *Head Neck Pathol.* 2012;6:48–50.

Kleinegger CL, Hammond HL, Finkelstein MWL. Oral mucosal hyperpigmentation secondary to antimalarial drug therapy. *Oral Surg Oral Med Oral Pathol Oral Radiol Endod.* 2000;90:189–194.

Lerman MA, Karimbux N, Guze KA, et al. Pigmentation of the hard palate. *Oral Surg Oral Med Oral Pathol Oral Radiol Endod.* 2009;107:8–12.

Li CC, Malik SM, Blaeser BF, et al. Mucosal pigmentation caused by imatinib: report of three cases. *Head Neck Pathol.* 2012;6:290–295.

Mattsson U, Halbritter S, Mörner Serikoff E, et al. Oral pigmentation in the hard palate associated with imatinib mesylate therapy: a report of three cases. *Oral Surg Oral Med Oral Pathol Oral Radiol Endod.* 2011;111:e12–e16.

Singh N, Bakhshi S. Imatinib-induced dental hyperpigmentation in childhood chronic myeloid leukemia. *J Pediatr Hematol Oncol.* 2007;29:208–209.

Smoker's Melanosis

Axéll T, Hedin CA. Epidemiologic study of excessive oral melanin pigmentation with special reference to the influence of tobacco habits. *Scand J Dent Res.* 1982;90:434–442.

Hanioka T, Tanaka K, Ojima M, et al. Association of melanin pigmentation in the gingiva of children with parents who smoke. *Pediatrics.* 2005;116:e186–e190.

Hedin CA, Axéll T. Oral melanin pigmentation in 467 Thai and Malaysian people with special emphasis on smoker's melanosis. *J Oral Pathol Med.* 1991;20:8–12.

Hedin CA, Pindborg JJ, Axéll T. Disappearance of smoker's melanosis after reducing smoking. *J Oral Pathol Med.* 1993;22:228–230.

Sridharan S, Ganiger K, Satyanarayana A, et al. Effect of environmental tobacco smoke from smoker parents on gingival pigmentation in children and young adults: a cross-sectional study. *J Periodontol.* 2011;82: 956–962.

9

Allergies and Immunologic Diseases

Recurrent Aphthous Stomatitis

Recurrent aphthous stomatitis represents one of the most common intraoral pathoses with a reported prevalence of approximately 20%. The lesions appear to be an immune-mediated reaction in which the mucosal destruction is caused by cytotoxic T-lymphocytes (CD8+). A wide variety of triggers have been described that can be categorized into one of three groups: antigenic sensitivity, thinned mucosa, or immune dysregulation. In contrast to intraoral recurrent herpes simplex viral infection, the lesions occur almost exclusively on mucosa not bound to bone. Common therapies for mild cases include topical anesthetics, coating or occlusive agents, topical cauterizing agents, laser cauterization, antiseptics (e.g., chlorhexidine gluconate), antibiotic solutions (e.g., tetracycline or minocycline), and topical corticosteroid rinses and gels. Treatments for severe disease include systemic corticosteroids, colchicine, dapsone, thalidomide, pentoxifylline, monoclonal antibodies directly against tumor necrosis factor, and many others. Three clinical variants are seen: minor, major, and herpetiform.

Minor Aphthous Stomatitis

Figs. **9.1 and 9.2**

Minor aphthous stomatitis is by far the most common variant, representing the pattern reported in more than 80% of affected patients. The lesion often begins as a tender red macule that evolves into a highly painful yellowish ulcer surrounded by an erythematous border. The ulcerations vary from 3 to 10 mm in diameter and typically heal within 7 to 14 days. Although diffuse disease may be seen, most patients present with one to five lesions per episode. Minor aphthae can occur at any age but are seen more often in children and young adults. The frequency of recurrence is highly variable.

Major Aphthous Stomatitis

Fig. **9.3**

Major aphthous stomatitis *(Sutton disease, periadenitis mucosa necrotica recurrens [PMNR])* is far less common than the minor variant and is seen in 10% to 15% of affected patients. The lesions vary from 1 to 3 cm in diameter, take from 2 to 6 weeks to resolve, and tend to heal with scarring. The attacks tend to arise after puberty and often continue for decades unless an associated trigger can be eliminated. Compared to minor aphthae, major aphthae are more resistant to therapy and often require more potent topical or systemic therapy.

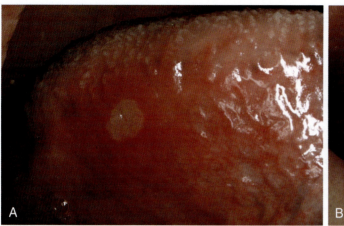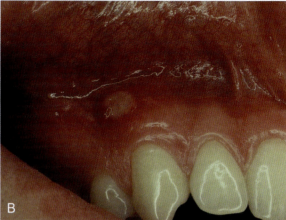

■ Figure **9.1**
Minor Aphthous Stomatitis
(A) Focal yellow zone of ulceration with surrounding erythema of the lateral border of the tongue on the right side. (B) Focal zone of ulceration noted in the movable mucosa of the anterior maxillary vestibule on the right side.

■ Figure **9.2**
Minor Aphthous Stomatitis
Multiple ulcerations of the dorsal surface of the tongue.

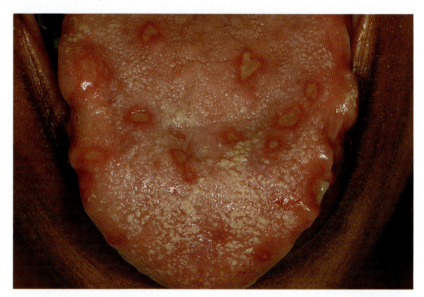

■ Figure **9.3**
Major Aphthous Stomatitis
Large mucosal ulceration of the soft palate on the right side.

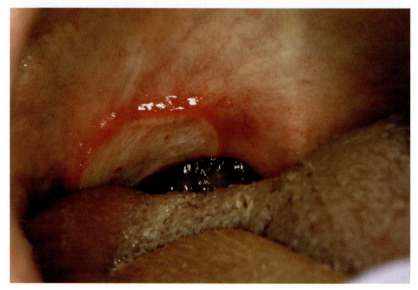

Fig. **9.4**

Herpetiform aphthous stomatitis is the least common variant of aphthous stomatitis, representing the pattern noted in 5% to 10% of affected patients. The name is not meant to imply an association with a herpes simplex virus. This nomenclature was chosen because the pattern of mucosal ulceration resembles that seen in herpes simplex. However, these two disorders can be separated easily by anatomic distribution. Aphthae tend to spare intraoral mucosa bound to bone. In contrast, primary herpes simplex virus infection consistently demonstrates diffuse and highly symptomatic gingival involvement, whereas recurrent intraoral herpes simplex infection tends to affect the attached gingiva or hard palate. Individual herpetiform aphthae are small with a diameter of 1 to 3 mm. In contrast to the other variants, the number of ulcers per recurrence tends to be high, often approaching as many as 100. The lesions usually heal within 7 to 10 days, but recurrences often are spaced closely. The ulcerations tend to present as mild disease that is responsive to topical corticosteroid therapy. A liquid oral suspension usually is preferable to a gel because of the widespread distribution of the lesions.

Behçet Syndrome

Figs. **9.5 and 9.6**

In 1937 a Turkish dermatologist, Hulusi Behçet, described a syndrome characterized by recurrent oral ulcerations, genital ulcerations, and uveitis. With time, it has become clear that **Behçet syndrome** is a more widespread disease with potential cutaneous, articular, vascular, cardiac, pulmonary, gastrointestinal, and neurologic involvement. Although the cause is unknown, it has been theorized that the disorder represents an abnormal immune response triggered by a cross-reaction of one or more infectious agents with the host tissues of a genetically predisposed individual. HLA B51 has been associated strongly with the disease. Although the syndrome is seen worldwide, the prevalence is highest along the old *silk route,* extending from Japan to the Middle Eastern and Mediterranean nations, with the highest frequency seen in Behçet's Turkish homeland.

The oral ulcers appear similar to minor, major, or herpetiform aphthae and exhibit a predilection for the soft palate and oropharynx. The genital ulcers frequently involve the labia majora and the scrotum. The most common skin alterations are erythema nodosum–like or papulopustular lesions. Two sets of diagnostic criteria are popular. The first requires recurrent oral ulcers plus two of the following: (1) recurrent genital ulcers, (2) ocular involvement, (3) skin lesions, or (4) a positive pathergy test (abnormal skin response to a sterile needle prick). Another uses a point system, with a total of 4 points required for the definitive diagnosis. Oral, genital, and ocular lesions receive 2 points each, whereas skin lesions, vascular involvement, neurologic manifestations, and a positive pathergy test each receive 1 point.

■ Figure **9.4**
Herpetiform Aphthous Stomatitis
Numerous small ulcerations and clusters of coalesced ulcerations noted on the maxillary labial mucosa.

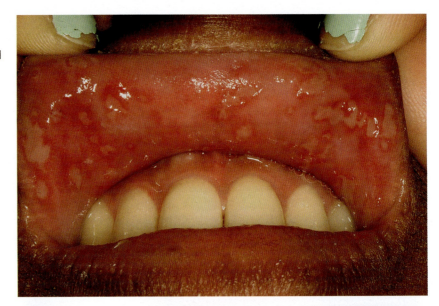

■ Figure **9.5**
Behçet Syndrome
Large, deep ulceration of the left buccal mucosa.

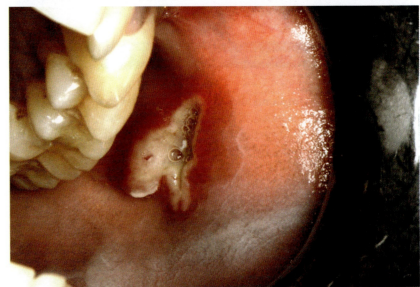

■ Figure **9.6**
Behçet Syndrome
Ulceration of the scrotum.

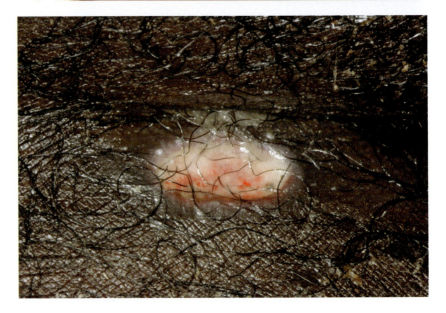

Transient Lingual Papillitis

Figs. **9.7 and 9.8**

Transient lingual papillitis refers to an acute and temporary enlargement of one or more fungiform papillae. Although the causation is unknown, the process has been associated with chronic irritation, thermal injury, heavy tobacco or alcohol use, spicy or acidic foods, allergies, gastrointestinal disorders, cyclic hormonal changes, lack of sleep, and stress.

The process may be localized to one or several papillae in an isolated area or generalized with numerous altered papillae involving a significant portion of the tongue. The altered papillae appear erythematous, white, or yellow and may or may not be painful. In most patients, the papillae are painful and exhibit inflammatory hyperplasia. Examples of the generalized pattern spreading to other family members have been reported. In contrast to the more common symptomatic variants, there is a generalized papulokeratotic variant in which the altered papillae are painless and appear whitish because of overlying hyperparakeratosis.

The symptomatic variants of transient lingual papillitis usually resolve within 4 days. Some patients have admitted to removing the lesions with fingernail clippers. In addition to elimination of any predisposing factors, recommended therapies include local anesthetics, coating agents, antiseptic mouth rinses, and topical corticosteroids.

Allergic Contact Stomatitis to Toothpaste

Fig. **9.9**

Intraoral allergic contact stomatitis (*stomatitis venenata*) arises from a wide variety of antigens. When secondary to an ingredient in toothpaste, the most common presentation is cheilitis with or without eczema of the perioral skin. Affected lips feel dry and often demonstrate mild erythema, cracks, or mild fissuring. Less frequently, erythema, swelling, focal ulceration, or areas of erosion may occur on the gingiva, tongue, or other mucosal surfaces. On occasion, the buccal mucosa and vestibules may demonstrate an asymptomatic sloughing of the superficial layers of the epithelium.

Reactions to toothpaste occur in both genders but demonstrate a female predominance. The duration of use prior to recognition of the mucosal changes can vary from less than 2 weeks to as much as several years. In most affected patients, the alterations clear with replacement of the offending toothpaste with plain baking soda or a toothpaste that is free of flavorings, preservatives, and sodium lauryl sulfate.

■ Figure **9.7**
Transient Lingual Papillitis
Enlarged, yellowish, and painful fungiform papillae of the anterior dorsal surface of the tongue on the right side.

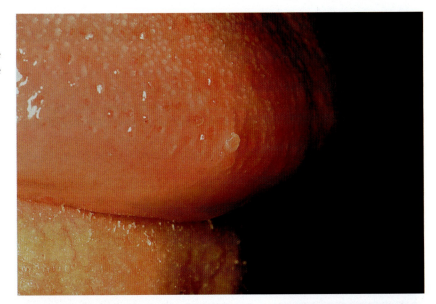

■ Figure **9.8**
Transient Lingual Papillitis
Numerous enlarged and painful fungiform papillae of the dorsal surface of the tongue on the right side. (Courtesy Dr. Courtney Shelbourne.)

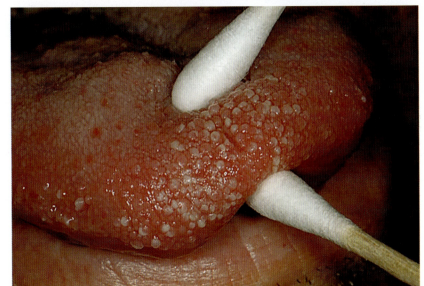

■ Figure **9.9**
Allergic Contact Stomatitis to Toothpaste
White, stringy, and removable strips of sloughed epithelium noted in the mandibular vestibule on the left side.

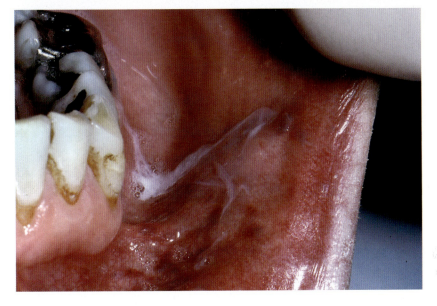

Fig. **9.10**

Oral lichenoid reactions refer to mucosal lesions that resemble lichen planus clinically and microscopically, but they can be associated with a specific etiological factor. Frequently mentioned causes include other systemic diseases, drug reactions, food allergies, and mucosal contact with dental restorations. A wide variety of dental materials may result in lichenoid contact reactions, but amalgams are implicated in the vast majority of the cases. Cutaneous patch testing to the metals within amalgam has proven to be inconsistently positive, possibly because some examples are secondary to the local irritant effect of mercury rather than a systemic allergy.

Although lichen planus and some other lichenoid reactions often are migratory, symmetrical, and bilateral, lichenoid reactions to amalgam typically are nonmigratory and localized to the site of contact. The altered mucosa may be present as a red or white patch, with or without striae and erosion. Although many affected patients report rapid improvement following removal of the offending amalgam, some lesions slowly resolve over several months.

Figs. **9.11 and 9.12**

Sarcoidosis is a systemic disease characterized by noncaseating granulomatous inflammation. The disorder is idiopathic; however, evidence suggests the process represents an abnormal immune response to infectious or environmental agents in genetically predisposed individuals.

Although any anatomic site may be affected, the lungs, lymph nodes, skin, and eyes are involved most frequently. Oral lesions are uncommon, but when present, they can lead to the initial diagnosis. Any mucosal site may be affected, presenting as a brownish–red, purplish, or normal-colored macule, papule, or submucosal mass. Intraosseous lesions also may be seen and present as ill-defined radiolucencies that may be associated with loosening of teeth.

Since spontaneous resolution is noted in a majority of patients with sarcoidosis, systemic therapy is reserved for severe or progressive disease. Corticosteroids are first-line therapy, followed by other immunosuppressive medications or antimalarials. When localized, oral mucosal lesions often are surgically excised, whereas osseous lesions receive thorough curettage.

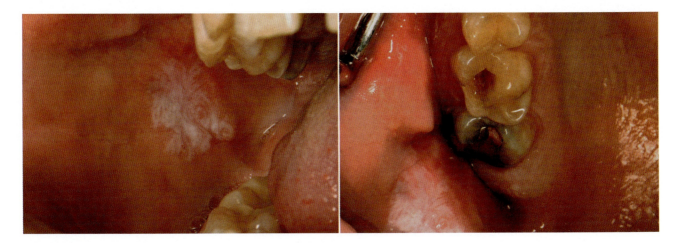

■ Figure **9.10**
Lichenoid Reaction to Amalgam
Irregular white plaque of the right buccal mucosa in contact with a large amalgam restoration present in the maxillary right second molar.

■ Figure **9.11**
Sarcoidosis
Brownish–red macules of the soft palate.

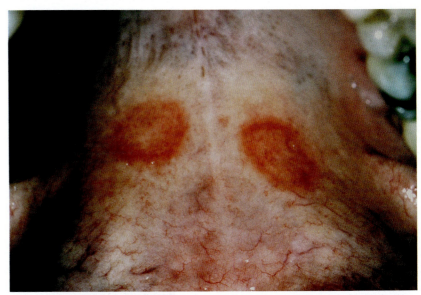

■ Figure **9.12**
Sarcoidosis
Ill-defined radiolucency associated with the maxillary right first molar. (Courtesy Dr. Chad Matthews.)

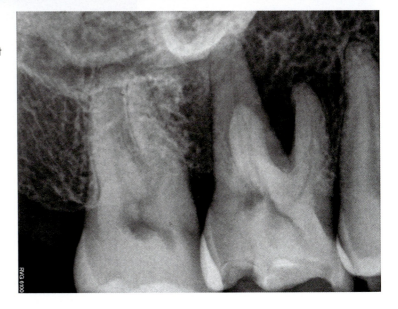

Figs. **9.13–9.16**

Orofacial granulomatosis refers to orofacial swellings created by granulomatous inflammation in the absence of a previously diagnosed local or systemic disease. The disorder should not be considered a final diagnosis, but a potential sign of an underlying and not yet discovered process. After the pathologist has searched for foreign material and stained for mycobacterial and deep fungal organisms, the clinician must evaluate the patient for pathoses known to be associated with granulomatous inflammation, such as local foci of infection, food allergies, berylliosis, Crohn disease, sarcoidosis, granulomatosis with polyangiitis (Wegener granulomatosis), and chronic granulomatous disease.

Although orofacial granulomatosis may arise at any age, young adults are affected most frequently. In young children, the condition often is associated with Crohn disease, although the onset of bowel symptoms may be delayed for years. When orofacial granulomatosis is seen in association with Crohn disease, the gastrointestinal manifestations often are pan-enteric and more severe than those noted in patients without oral involvement.

The most common clinical presentation is painless enlargement of the lips. Isolated lip involvement has been termed *cheilitis granulomatosa* or *Miescher cheilitis*. When enlarged lips are seen in combination with facial paralysis and fissured tongue, the triad has been termed *Melkersson-Rosenthal syndrome*. Orofacial granulomatosis also may be associated with gingival hyperplasia, cobblestone buccal mucosa, and vestibular linear hyperplastic folds, often with associated ulceration.

Primary therapy should be directed at discovering and appropriately managing any underlying associated disorder. If thorough local and systemic evaluations fail to identify an underlying causation, intralesional triamcinolone injections or systemic corticosteroids may be administered.

■ Figure **9.13**
Orofacial Granulomatosis
Chronically enlarged lower lip.

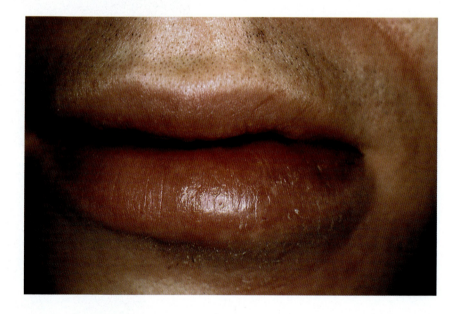

Figure 9.14
Orofacial Granulomatosis
Hyperplastic folds of tissue involving the upper and lower vestibular mucosa and gingiva. (Courtesy Dr. Steven Anderson.)

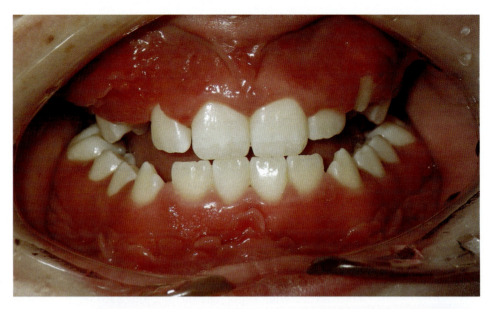

Figure 9.15
Orofacial Granulomatosis
Prominent diffuse enlargement of the lower lip.

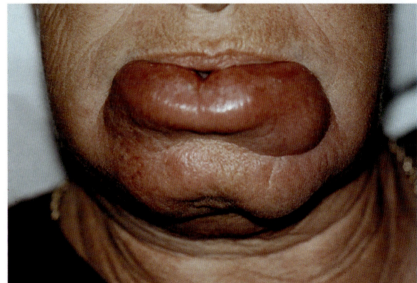

Figure 9.16
Orofacial Granulomatosis
The same patient depicted in Fig. 9.15 after treatment with intralesional triamcinolone.

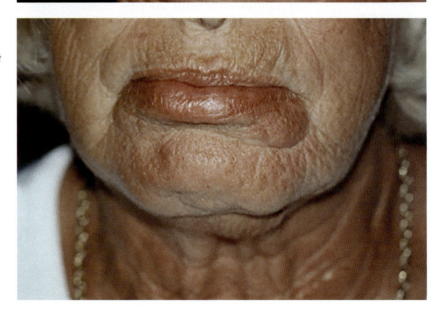

Figs. 9.17 and 9.18

Granulomatosis with polyangiitis *(Wegener granulomatosis)* is a systemic, necrotizing, and granulomatous vasculitis affecting the small- and medium-sized blood vessels. Two major patterns are seen: (1) a classical form affecting the kidneys plus the upper and lower respiratory tracts and (2) a localized form limited to the upper and/or lower respiratory tract. Approximately 85% of affected patients will demonstrate anti-neutrophil cytoplasmic antibodies directed against proteinase 3 (PR3-ANCA, previously termed *C-ANCA*), with a higher frequency noted in patients with generalized disease.

Oral lesions are uncommon, but they may precede other manifestations and lead to early diagnosis. Patterns of oral involvement include clinically nonspecific ulcerations, labial mucosal nodules, palatal perforation, and "strawberry gingivitis." Strawberry gingivitis is a clinically distinctive pattern of hyperplasia that demonstrates a finely papular surface created by numerous short, bulbous, hemorrhagic, and friable projections.

The disease is serious, with 90% of untreated patients with renal involvement dying within 2 years of diagnosis. Therefore, early diagnosis and treatment are critical. Treatment depends on disease severity and often consists of systemic corticosteroids combined with cyclophosphamide, methotrexate, rituximab, or other agents. With appropriate therapy, prolonged remission is achieved in up to 75% of patients, but recurrences are common without maintenance therapy.

Angioedema

Fig. 9.19

Angioedema refers to an acute onset of diffuse edematous swelling, which most commonly affects the subcutaneous and submucosal soft tissues. The most common cause is an allergic reaction that triggers mast cell degranulation with histamine release. Other triggers unrelated to histamine release include side effects of angiotensin-converting enzyme inhibitors, the use of tissue plasminogen activator, hereditary alterations in the complement pathway, lymphoproliferative diseases, and acquired autoimmunity against C1-inhibitor (first stage of the complement cascade).

Angioedema presents with rapid onset of soft, nontender tissue swellings. In the head and neck region, the face, lips, tongue, floor of mouth, pharynx, and larynx may be affected. The process is potentially life threatening because of the possibility of airway compromise. Treatment depends on the underlying cause, and known triggers should be avoided. The classic therapy for cases associated with allergies is antihistamines and corticosteroids, which are often combined with epinephrine. Patients with hereditary or acquired C1-inhibitor deficiency often respond to C1-inhibitor concentrate and bradykinin antagonists such as icatibant.

■ Figure **9.17**
Granulomatosis With Polyangiitis
Hyperplastic and hemorrhagic gingiva noted on the facial mandibular surface on the left side. A necrotic area of ulceration also is present on the facial gingiva of the right maxillary premolars. (Courtesy Dr. James Wilson.)

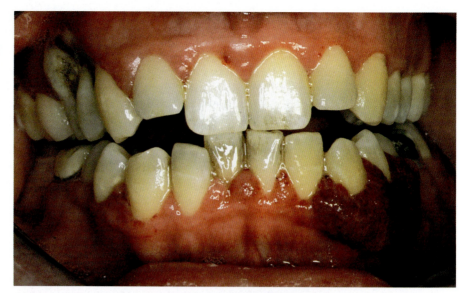

■ Figure **9.18**
Granulomatosis With Polyangiitis
Edentulous patient with diffuse, bumpy, and hemorrhagic hyperplasia of the maxillary alveolar mucosa and palate. (Courtesy Dr. Woodrow Merritt.)

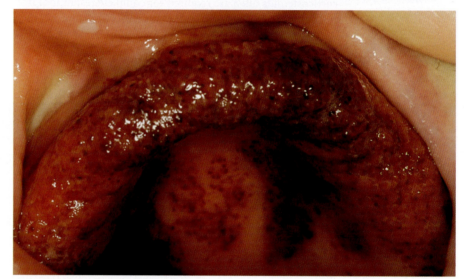

■ Figure **9.19**
Angioedema
Diffuse enlargement of the lower lip. This swelling came up rapidly during dental therapy in a patient taking an angiotensin-converting enzyme inhibitor. The swelling did not respond to antihistamine and epinephrine.

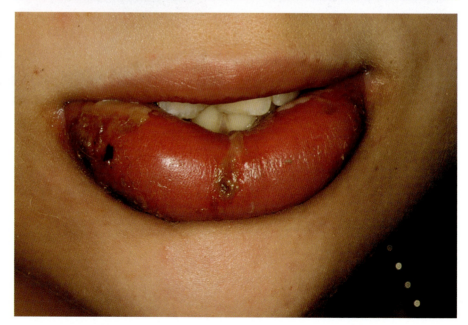

Figs. **9.20–9.23**

Secondary to an aging and well-medicated population, **drug reactions** are not rare. The use of two medications by a patient is correlated with a 6% risk of an adverse drug reaction. If the number of drugs increases to five, the risk increases to 50%, whereas taking eight or more medications is associated with an almost 100% chance of an adverse reaction. Alteration of the oral mucosa secondary to a medication is termed *stomatitis medicamentosa*. The patterns of mucosal damage vary almost as much as the number of medications that result in the alterations. Drug reactions may mimic aphthous ulcerations, lichen planus, pemphigoid, pemphigus, lupus erythematosus, and many other less common patterns of mucosal disease.

When investigating the possibility of a drug reaction, many clinicians will review lists of offending medications, but this can be an inefficient approach. Due to the rapidly expanding number of new medications, most lists are out of date before they are published. The best approach is to obtain the list of medications utilized by the affected patient and investigate each drug with a powerful drug reference program that includes not only the common reactions, but also a thorough review of the entire medical literature related to each suspect medication.

Chronic mucosal drug reactions may resolve following cessation of the offending medication, but topical corticosteroids often are required for complete resolution. If the medication cannot be stopped for health reasons, control often is very difficult, even with appropriate corticosteroid therapy.

■ Figure **9.20**
Chronic Mucosal Drug Reaction
Diffuse white striae of the dorsal surface of the tongue, which ultimately proved to be a lichenoid reaction to allopurinol.

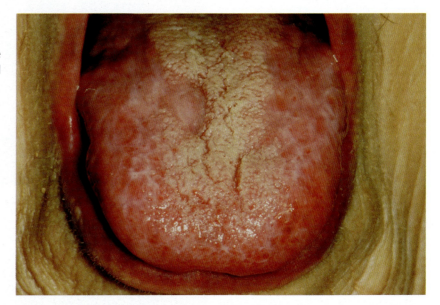

■ Figure **9.21**
Chronic Mucosal Drug Reaction
Large zone of erosion with surrounding atrophy and reticular striae of the right buccal mucosa, which was ultimately proven to be a lichenoid drug reaction to metformin. (Courtesy Dr. Matthew Marshall.)

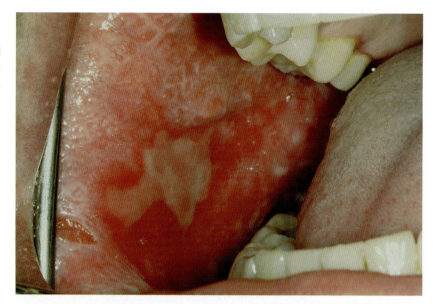

■ Figure **9.22**
Chronic Mucosal Drug Reaction
Striae of the vermilion border of the lower lip and erythematous atrophy of the mandibular facial gingiva, which was ultimately proven to be a lichenoid reaction to a statin medication.

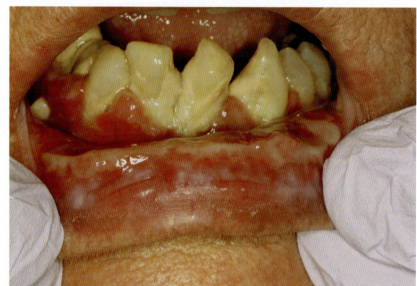

■ Figure **9.23**
Chronic Mucosal Drug Reaction
The same patient depicted in Fig. 9.22 after discontinuation of the offending medication.

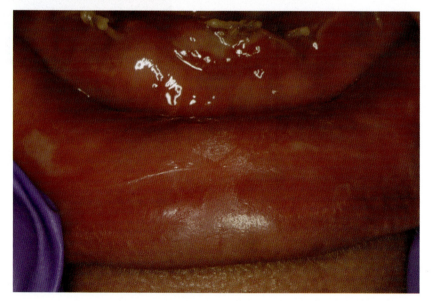

Figs. **9.24–9.27**

Cinnamic aldehyde has been ranked as the 20th most common allergen by the North American Contact Dermatitis Group. This artificial form of cinnamon is a flavoring agent in foods, candy, chewing gum, lip balm, mouthwash, toothpaste, and dental floss. Reactions to the natural spice are rare but known to occur.

The features of intraoral cinnamon reactions vary widely due to the diverse methods of delivery. The altered mucosa may be erythematous, white, thickened, vesicular, ulcerative, or sloughing. Burning or mucosal swelling sometimes may occur. When isolated to a localized area, the mucositis often is related to agents such as candy or gum. When the mucosal alterations are more widespread, often a toothpaste or mouthwash is involved.

One classic pattern associated with use of cinnamon gum presents on the buccal mucosa in a linear pattern that coincides with the occlusal plane. The adjacent lateral border of the tongue frequently may be similarly affected. Often, the clinical alterations resemble morsicatio, but associated burning is an important clue to the appropriate diagnosis.

Appropriate therapy is obvious: discontinuation of the cinnamon product and avoidance of other items that may contain the allergen. Complete resolution often is rapid but may be delayed for as long as 3 weeks. Rarely, severe examples require a short course of topical corticosteroids.

■ Figure **9.24**
Contact Stomatitis to Cinnamic Aldehyde
Linear white lesion with surrounding erythema in a patient with a chief complaint of mucosal burning. The patient chewed two packs of cinnamon gum every day, and the mucosal alterations cleared after cessation of the habit.

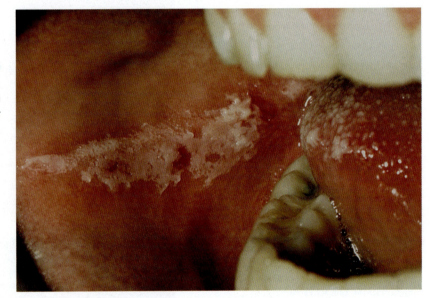

■ Figure **9.25**
Contact Stomatitis to Cinnamic Aldehyde

The same patient depicted in Fig. 9.24 with a white alteration of the right lateral border of the tongue that was associated with mucosal burning.

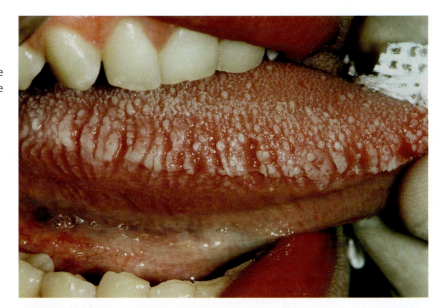

■ Figure **9.26**
Contact Stomatitis to Cinnamic Aldehyde

A burning linear white patch with surrounding mucosal erythema on the left buccal mucosa.

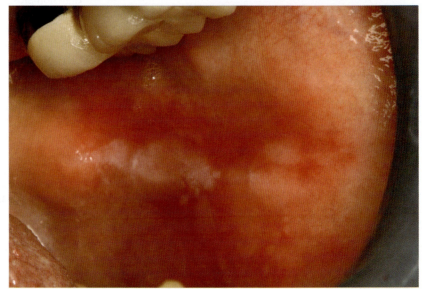

■ Figure **9.27**
Contact Stomatitis to Cinnamic Aldehyde

The same patient as in Fig. 9.26 showing resolution of the lesion after cessation of chewing cinnamon gum.

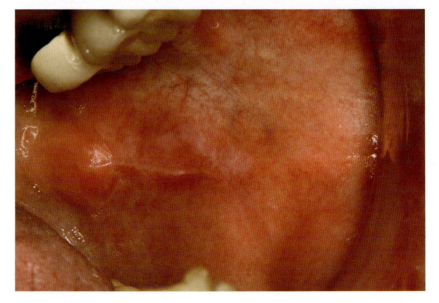

Bibliography

Aphthous Ulcerations

Ranganath SP, Pai A. Is optimal management of recurrent aphthous stomatitis possible? A reality check. *J Clin Diagn Res.* 2016;10:ZE8–ZE13.

Scully C, Porter S. Oral mucosal disease: recurrent aphthous stomatitis. *Br J Oral Maxillofac Surg.* 2008;46:198–206.

Ship JA. Recurrent aphthous stomatitis: an update. *Oral Surg Oral Med Oral Pathol Oral Radiol Endod.* 1996;81:141–147.

Tarakji B, Gazal G, Al-Maweri SA, et al. Guidelines for the diagnosis and treatment of recurrent aphthous stomatitis for dental practitioners. *J Int Oral Health.* 2015;7:74–80.

Vincent SD, Lilly GE. Clinical, historic, and therapeutic features of aphthous stomatitis: literature review and open clinical trial employing steroids. *Oral Surg Oral Med Oral Pathol.* 1992;74:79–86.

Behçet Syndrome

Alpsoy E. Behçet disease: a comprehensive review with a focus on epidemiology, etiology and clinical features, and management of mucocutaneous disease. *J Dermatol.* 2016;43:620–632.

Helm TN, Camisa C, Allen C, et al. Clinical features of Behçet's disease: report of four cases. *Oral Surg Oral Med Oral Pathol.* 1991;72:30–34.

Nair JR, Moots RJ. Behçet's disease. *Clin Med.* 2017;17:71–77.

Yazici Y, Yurdakul S, Yasici H. Behçet's syndrome. *Curr Rheumatol Rep.* 2010;12:429–435.

Transient Lingual Papillitis

Brannon RB, Flaitz CM. Transient lingual papillitis: a papulokeratotic variant. *Oral Surg Oral Med Oral Pathol Oral Radiol Endod.* 2003;96:187–191.

Kalogirou E-M, Tosios KI, Nititakis NG, et al. Transient lingual papillitis: a retrospective study of 11 cases and review of the literature. *J Clin Exp Dent.* 2017;9:e157–e162.

Kornerup IM, Senye M, Peters E. Transient lingual papillitis. *Quintessence.* 2016;47:871–875.

Whitaker SB, Krupa JJ, Singh BB. Transient lingual papillitis. *Oral Surg Oral Med Oral Pathol Oral Radiol Endod.* 1996;82:441–445.

Allergic Contact Stomatitis to Toothpaste

Berton F, Stacchi C, Bussani R, et al. Toothpaste-induced oral mucosal desquamation. *Dermatitis.* 2017;28:162–163.

de Groot A. Contact allergy to (ingredients of) toothpaste. *Dermatitis.* 2017;28:95–114.

Macdonald JB, Tobin CA, Burkemper NM, et al. Oral leukoedema with mucosal desquamation caused by toothpaste containing sodium lauryl sulfate. *Cutis.* 2016;97:e4–e5.

Oral Lichenoid Reactions to Amalgam

Finne K, Göransson K, Winckler L. Oral lichen planus and contact allergy to mercury. *Int J Oral Surg.* 1982;11:236–239.

Henriksson E, Mattsson U, Håkansson J. Healing of lichenoid reactions following removal or amalgam. A clinical follow-up. *J Clin Periodontol.* 1995;22:287–294.

Luiz AC, Hirota SK, Dal Vechio A, et al. Diagnosing oral lichenoid contact reaction: clinical judgment versus skin-patch test. *Minerva Stomatol.* 2012;61:311–317.

Sharma R, Handa S, De D, et al. Role of dental restoration materials in oral mucosal lichenoid lesions. *Indian J Dermatol Venereol Leprol.* 2015;81:478–484.

Suter VGA, Warnakulasuriya S. The role of patch testing in the management of oral lichenoid lesions. *J Oral Pathol Med.* 2016;45:48–57.

Thornhill MH, Pemberton MN, Simmons RK, et al. Amalgam-contact hypersensitivity lesions and oral lichen planus. *Oral Surg Oral Med Oral Pathol Oral Radiol Endod.* 2003;95:291–299.

Oral Sarcoidosis

Bouaziz A, Le Scanff J, Chapelon-Abric C, et al. Oral involvement in sarcoidosis: report of 12 cases. *Q J Med.* 2012;105:755–767.

Kasamatsu A, Kanazawa H, Watanabe T, et al. Oral sarcoidosis: report of a case and review of the literature. *J Oral Maxillofac Surg.* 2007;65:1256–1259.

Poate TWJ, Sharma R, Moutasim KA, et al. Orofacial presentations of sarcoidosis – a case series and review of the literature. *Br Dent J.* 2008;205:437–442.

Suresh L, Radfar L. Oral sarcoidosis: a review of the literature. *Oral Dis.* 2005;11:138–145.

Orofacial Granulomatosis

Fedele S, Fung PPL, Bamashmous N, et al. Long-term effectiveness of intralesional triamcinolone acetonide therapy in orofacial granulomatosis: an observational cohort study. *Brit J Dermatol.* 2014;170:794–801.

Gale G, Sigurdsson GV, Östman S, et al. Does Crohn's disease with concomitant orofacial granulomatosis represent a distinctive disease subtype? *Inflamm Bowel Dis.* 2016;22:1071–1077.

Grave B, McCullough M, Wiesenfeld D. Orofacial granulomatosis – a 20-year review. *Oral Dis.* 2009;15:46–51.

Miest R, Bruce A, Rogers RS. Orofacial granulomatosis. *Clin Dermatol.* 2016;34:505–513.

Tilakaratne WM, Freysdottir J, Fortune F. Orofacial granulomatosis: review on aetiology and pathogenesis. *J Oral Pathol Med.* 2008;37:191–195.

Wiesenfeld D, Ferguson M, Mitchell D, et al. Oro-facial granulomatosis – a clinical and pathologic analysis. *Q J Med.* 1985;54:101–113.

Granulomatosis With Polyangiitis

Allen CM, Camisa C, Salewski C, et al. Wegener's granulomatosis: report of three cases with oral lesions. *J Oral Maxillofac Surg.* 1991;49:294–298.

Knight JM, Hayduk MJ, Summerlin D-J. "Strawberry" gingival hyperplasia: a pathognomonic mucocutaneous finding in Wegener's granulomatosis. *Arch Dermatol.* 2000;136:171–173.

Stewart C, Cohen D, Bhattacharyya I, et al. Oral manifestations of Wegener's granulomatosis: a report of three cases and a literature review. *J Am Dent Assoc.* 2007;138:338–348.

Weed LW Jr, Coffey SA. Wegener's granulomatosis. *Oral Maxillofac Surg Clin North Am.* 2008;20:643–649.

Angioedema

Bas M, Greve J, Stelter K, et al. A randomized trial of icatibant in ACE-inhibitor-induced angioedema. *N Engl J Med.* 2015;372:418–425.

Greaves M, Lawlor F. Angioedema: manifestations and management. *J Am Acad Dermatol.* 1991;25:155–165.

Megerian CA, Arnold JE, Berer M. Angioedema: 5 years' experience, with a review of the disorder's presentation and treatment. *Laryngoscope.* 1992;102:256–260.

Pahs L, Droege C, Kneale H, et al. A novel approach to the treatment of orolingual angioedema after tissue plasminogen activator administration. *Ann Emerg Med.* 2016;68:345–348.

Rees SR, Gibson J. Angioedema and swellings of the orofacial region. *Oral Dis.* 1997;3:39–42.

Chronic Mucosal Drug Reactions

Femiano F, Lanza A, Buonaiuto C, et al. Oral manifestations of adverse drug reactions: guidelines. *J Eur Acad Dermatol Venereol.* 2008;22:681–691.

Parks ET. Disorders affecting the oral cavity. Lesions associated with drug reactions. *Dermatol Clin.* 1996;14:327–337.

Seymour RA, Rudralingham M. Oral and dental adverse drug reactions. *Periodontol.* 2008;46:9–26.

Wright JM. Oral manifestations of drug reactions. *Dent Clin North Am.* 1984;28:529–543.

Contact Stomatitis to Cinnamic Aldehyde

Allen CM, Blozis GG. Oral mucosal reactions to cinnamon-flavored chewing gum. *J Am Dent Assoc.* 1988;116:664–667.

Drake TE, Maibach HI. Allergic contact dermatitis and stomatitis caused by a cinnamic aldehyde-flavored toothpaste. *Arch Dermatol.* 1976;112:202–203.

Endo H, Rees TD. Clinical features of cinnamon-induced contact stomatitis. *Compend Contin Educ Dent.* 2006;27:403–409.

Isaac-Renton M, Li MK, Parsons LM. Cinnamon spice and everything not nice: many features of intraoral allergy to cinnamic aldehyde. *Dermatitis.* 2015;26:116–121.

Miller RL, Gould AR, Bernstein ML. Cinnamon-induced stomatitis venenataL clinical and characteristic histopathologic features. *Oral Surg Oral Med Oral Pathol.* 1992;73:708–716.

10

Epithelial Pathology

Squamous Papilloma

Figs. **10.1** and **10.2**

The **squamous papilloma** represents a benign squamous epithelial proliferation induced by human papillomavirus (HPV). Most examples harbor HPV types 6 and 11 (which are nononcogenic or "low-risk" types) and exhibit low infectivity. Squamous papillomas are relatively common and comprise approximately 3% of biopsy specimens submitted to oral and maxillofacial pathology laboratories. They can develop at any age, with a peak in the fourth and fifth decades. Frequently involved subsites include the palate/uvula, tongue, and lips. The patient is usually asymptomatic. Clinical examination shows a papule or nodule with numerous pointed ("warty"), blunted ("cauliflower-like"), or filiform ("threadlike") surface projections. The base may be pedunculated or sessile. Depending on the amount of surface keratinization, the lesion may appear white, red, or normal in color. Most papillomas reach a maximum diameter of about 0.5 cm, although some examples become larger. The clinical differential diagnosis may include verruca vulgaris, verruciform xanthoma, and condyloma acuminatum. Treatment consists of conservative excision, and recurrence is uncommon.

Verruca Vulgaris (Common Wart)

Fig. **10.3**

Verruca vulgaris is another type of benign squamous epithelial proliferation induced by human papillomavirus (HPV) (especially HPV types 2 and 4). Verrucae are contagious and can be spread via person-to-person contact, autoinoculation, or contaminated surfaces/objects. Most cases arise on the skin, with a predilection for the hands, but oral lesions also are possible. Oral examples resulting from autoinoculation tend to involve the lip vermilion, labial mucosa, or anterior tongue. Verrucae most often develop in young patients, with a peak during adolescence. Clinical examination shows a papule or nodule with pointed projections or a rough, pebbly surface. Most lesions measure <1 cm in diameter, and they may be solitary or multiple. Cutaneous lesions can appear pink, yellow, gray-brown, or white, whereas oral examples are typically white. Up to two-thirds of cutaneous cases in children resolve spontaneously within 2 years; thus, clinical observation is a viable management option. However, active treatment often is rendered because the lesions can be unsightly or irritating. First-line therapy for cutaneous verrucae consists of topical salicylic acid or cryotherapy. Treatment options for recurrent or recalcitrant cases include topical 5-fluorouracil, intralesional bleomycin, photodynamic therapy, and immunotherapy (e.g., intralesional *Candida* or mumps antigen, topical squaric acid, or dinitrochlorobenzene). Oral verrucae usually are removed by conservative excision; alternative treatments include laser therapy, cryotherapy, and electrosurgery.

■ Figure **10.1**
Papilloma
White papule with short surface projections on the soft palate.

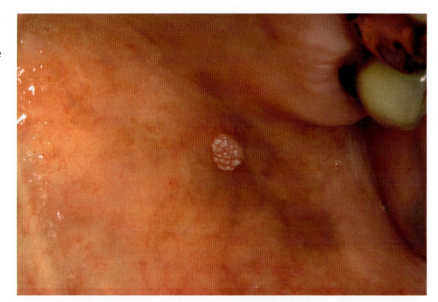

■ Figure **10.2**
Papilloma
White lesion with elongated, thread-like surface projections on the left posterior ventrolateral tongue.

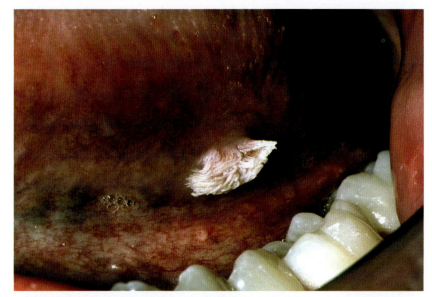

■ Figure **10.3**
Verruca Vulgaris
White papule with pointed surface projections on the anterior dorsal tongue.

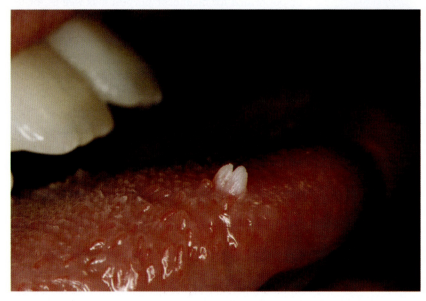

Condyloma Acuminatum

Fig. 10.4

Condyloma acuminatum is a human papillomavirus (HPV)–induced squamous epithelial proliferation mainly involving the anogenital region, although oral lesions are also possible. Most cases are caused by HPV types 6 and 11; however, coinfection with other HPV types (including oncogenic or "high-risk" types 16 and 18) is frequent. Condyloma acuminatum is a common sexually transmitted disease, with an estimated global annual incidence of 160 to 289 cases per 100,000 population. The condition exhibits a predilection for teenagers and young adults. The presence of condyloma acuminatum in a child may indicate sexual abuse. In addition, perinatal transmission of condylomata is possible.

In the oral cavity, condylomata tend to arise on the labial mucosa, lingual frenum, and soft palate. The lesions typically appear as pink, sessile masses with blunted or pointed surface projections. There is often a cluster of several lesions, although some examples are solitary. The average size (about 1 to 1.5 cm) is somewhat larger than that for the squamous papilloma.

Oral condylomata typically are treated by conservative excision. Alternative treatments include cryotherapy and laser ablation; however, there is concern regarding the potential for lasers to produce an infectious plume. External genital lesions often are managed by patient-applied topical agents (e.g., imiquimod, podophyllotoxin, sinatecatechins). In the United States, routine HPV vaccination is recommended for girls and boys 11 to 12 years old. Currently, a 9-valent vaccine is being distributed that protects against HPV types associated with condyloma acuminatum as well as cervical, anal, and oropharyngeal cancers.

Multifocal Epithelial Hyperplasia (Heck Disease, Focal Epithelial Hyperplasia)

Fig. 10.5

Multifocal epithelial hyperplasia is a squamous epithelial proliferation mainly caused by human papillomavirus (HPV) types 13 and 32. Potential contributory factors include genetic predisposition, crowded living conditions, poor hygiene, malnutrition, and human immunodeficiency virus infection. Among reported cases, there is a predilection for Inuits and Native Americans; however, the condition has been described in various other populations and ethnic groups as well.

Multifocal epithelial hyperplasia most commonly arises in children and adolescents, but adults also can be affected. The lesions can involve any oral site, with many patients exhibiting bilateral involvement of the labial mucosa, dorsolateral tongue, and/or buccal mucosa. Clinical examination shows multiple painless papules, nodules, or plaques with pebbly to flat-topped surfaces. The lesions may appear pink or white. At times, individual lesions coalesce to produce a cobblestone pattern or fissured appearance. Spontaneous regression may occur within months to several years. However, conservative excision may be performed for diagnostic purposes, as well as for lesions that cause aesthetic concerns or are subject to recurrent trauma. Alternative treatment methods include cryotherapy, laser therapy, electrocoagulation, systemic interferon-alpha, and topical interferon-beta. Recurrence is possible.

Sinonasal Papillomas

Fig. 10.6

Sinonasal papillomas are uncommon, benign proliferations of the *Schneiderian membrane* (epithelium lining the paranasal sinuses and much of the nasal cavity). There are three types: (1) *inverted* (nearly two-thirds of cases), (2) *fungiform (exophytic)* (about one-third of cases), and (3) *cylindrical cell (oncocytic Schneiderian)* (about 5% of cases). The etiopathogenesis is uncertain. However, human papillomavirus (HPV) has been detected in approximately two-thirds of fungiform papillomas and in a smaller proportion of the other types. Other proposed contributory factors (e.g., chronic sinusitis, tobacco smoke, occupational exposures) remain unproven.

Sinonasal papillomas usually arise in adults. The fungiform and inverted types exhibit a male predilection, whereas the cylindrical cell type has an approximately even gender distribution. Fungiform papillomas occur almost exclusively on the nasal septum. In contrast, inverted and cylindrical cell papillomas exhibit a predilection for the lateral nasal wall, maxillary sinus, and ethmoid sinus. Some patients are asymptomatic, whereas others experience epistaxis, unilateral nasal obstruction, rhinorrhea, and/or headache. In particular, inverted papillomas exhibit significant growth potential; they can cause pressure erosion of the underlying bone and, at times, extend into adjacent structures. Thorough microscopic examination is warranted to rule out transformation into carcinoma.

■ Figure **10.4**
Condyloma Acuminatum
Hard palate exhibiting a nodule with a rough, warty surface. A second smaller lesion also is present on the other side of the midline.

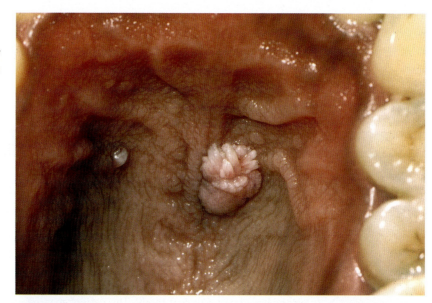

■ Figure **10.5**
Multifocal Epithelial Hyperplasia
Multiple, flat-topped papules and nodules on the lower labial mucosa.

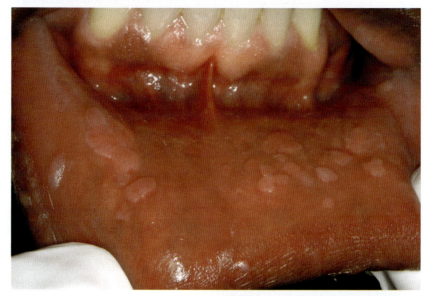

■ Figure **10.6**
Carcinoma Arising in an Inverted Papilloma
This inverted sinonasal papilloma transformed into squamous cell carcinoma. Magnetic resonance imaging showed a large tumor that arose from the right sinonasal region and invaded the adjacent soft tissue, orbital rim, and palate. (Courtesy Dr. Carla Penner.)

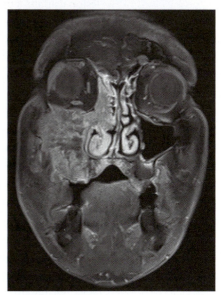

Sinonasal papillomas are treated by complete surgical removal via an external or endoscopic approach. Lateral rhinotomy and medial maxillectomy often are required for inverted and cylindrical cell papillomas. Recurrence is possible. In addition, malignant transformation may occur in about 2% to 27% of inverted papillomas and 4% to 17% of cylindrical cell papillomas.

Molluscum Contagiosum

Fig. **10.7**

Molluscum contagiosum is an epithelial condition caused by the molluscum contagiosum virus (MCV), a member of the Poxviridae family. It affects about 5% to 7.5% of the world population. MCV is transmitted via skin-to-skin contact, contaminated fomites (e.g., shared clothing or towels), autoinoculation, or sexual contact. Warm, humid environments (e.g., swimming pools, saunas) may favor disease spread. Risk factors include atopic dermatitis and human immunodeficiency virus infection.

Molluscum contagiosum exhibits a predilection for children and adolescents. In children, the condition often involves the skin of the trunk, extremities, and face. In adults, the genitalia tend to be affected. Oral lesions have been reported rarely. The patient may be asymptomatic or may experience tenderness and itching. Clinical examination typically shows a cluster of pink-white, waxy papules, each measuring 2 to 4 mm in diameter. The papules exhibit central depressions from which one can express creamy, white-gray material. There are usually <20 lesions; however, eruptions of >100 lesions are possible, especially in immunocompromised patients. Atopic patients are prone to developing adjacent eczema.

Molluscum contagiosum typically resolves spontaneously within 6 to 18 months. Thus, some clinicians advocate watchful waiting. However, active treatment may be considered to prevent disease spread, provide symptomatic relief, address cosmetic concerns, or eliminate severe/persistent disease. Treatment options include curettage, cryotherapy, and topical agents (e.g., salicylic acid, potassium hydroxide, benzoyl peroxide). For immunocompromised individuals with refractory lesions, topical cidofivir may be considered.

Verruciform Xanthoma

Figs. **10.8 and 10.9**

The **verruciform xanthoma** is an uncommon, benign condition characterized by papillary epithelial hyperplasia and subepithelial accumulation of lipid-laden histiocytes (*xanthoma cells* or "*foam cells*"). The lesion exhibits a predilection for the oral mucosa, although skin and genital lesions also are possible. The etiology is unknown. Some investigators propose that verruciform xanthomas represent an unusual reaction or immune response to local epithelial disturbances; this hypothesis is supported by reported examples that have developed in association with other pathologic conditions (e.g., lichen planus, discoid lupus erythematosus, epithelial dysplasia, squamous cell carcinoma, pemphigus vulgaris, warty dyskeratoma, graft-versus-host disease). The lesion is not caused by human papillomavirus (HPV), diabetes, or hyperlipidemia. However, there is a single reported case of multiple verruciform xanthomas arising in the upper aerodigestive tract of a child with an undefined systemic lipid storage disorder.

Oral verruciform xanthomas have been reported over a broad age range, with a peak in the fifth through seventh decades and no marked gender predilection. Lesions most often arise on the gingiva, alveolar ridge, and hard palate. In addition, the buccal mucosa, tongue, and other subsites may be involved. Clinical examination typically shows a painless, well-delineated plaque or nodule with a warty, papillary, or granular surface. However, some examples appear as smooth, flat-topped nodules. The lesions can be white, yellow, red, or pink and usually measure <2 cm in diameter. Most patients exhibit solitary lesions, although multifocal involvement has been reported infrequently. The clinical differential diagnosis may include squamous papilloma, verruca vulgaris, condyloma acuminatum, and early squamous cell carcinoma.

Verruciform xanthomas typically are treated by conservative excision, and recurrence is rare. The removed lesion should be submitted for microscopic diagnosis. Although the condition is benign and does not undergo malignant transformation, some reported cases have developed in association with carcinoma *in situ* or squamous cell carcinoma.

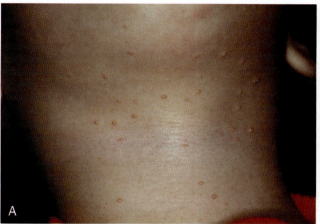
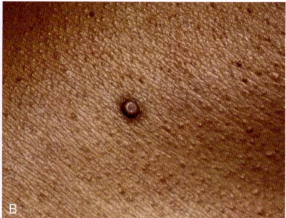

■ Figure **10.7**
Molluscum Contagiosum
(A) Child with multiple pink papules on the skin of the neck. (B) Pink, waxy papule with a central depression.

■ Figure **10.8**
Verruciform Xanthoma
Raised, pink-white lesion with a rough surface on the lingual marginal gingiva.

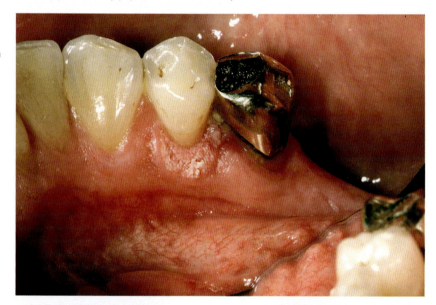

■ Figure **10.9**
Verruciform Xanthoma
Yellow-red nodule with a rough, papillary surface on the posterior maxillary alveolar ridge.

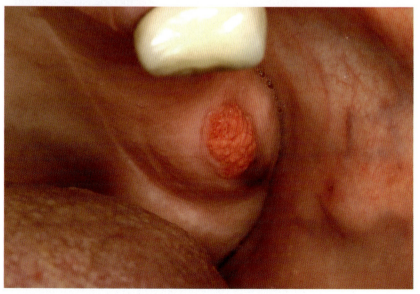

Seborrheic Keratosis

Fig. **10.10**

Seborrheic keratosis is a very common, benign skin lesion. It has been noted in 80% to 100% of individuals >50 years old. Although the etiopathogenesis is uncertain, some investigators have noted an association with chronic sun exposure and a possible genetic predisposition.

Seborrheic keratosis exhibits a predilection for white adults. Typically, the onset of lesions occurs around the fourth decade, and the lesions increase in number with age. Initially, seborrheic keratoses appear as small, tan to brown macules. Subsequently, they gradually enlarge to form well-demarcated plaques with fissured, pitted, verrucous, or smooth surfaces. The plaques characteristically appear "stuck onto" the skin and usually measure <2 cm in diameter. Most examples are asymptomatic, although persistent mechanical irritation (e.g., from clothing) can cause inflammation, bleeding, and pruritus. In rare cases, sudden onset of numerous pruritic seborrheic keratoses develops in patients with an underlying internal malignancy. This phenomenon is known as the *Leser-Trélat sign*.

A strong presumptive diagnosis of seborrheic keratosis often can be made based on the clinical findings, although biopsy and microscopic diagnosis should be considered for lesions exhibiting atypical clinical features. In addition, cosmetic concerns and persistent mechanical irritation are indications for removal. Common treatment methods include curettage, shave excision, and cryotherapy. However, cryotherapy does not allow for histopathologic evaluation and should be reserved for unequivocal cases as determined by a qualified professional.

Dermatosis Papulosa Nigra

Fig. **10.11**

Dermatosis papulosa nigra represents a variant of seborrheic keratosis (see previous section). This condition is especially common among blacks, although it also can be found in Asians, Hispanics, and other ethnic groups. The etiopathogenesis is not well understood. However, there appears to be a strong genetic predisposition, with >50% of patients reporting a family history of such lesions.

Dermatosis papulosa nigra exhibits a female predilection, with an approximate female-to-male ratio of 2:1. In contrast to conventional seborrheic keratosis, which typically begins to appear during the fourth decade of life, this variant usually develops during adolescence. Subsequently, the number of lesions increases with age. Patients typically exhibit multiple asymptomatic, dark brown to black papules on the skin of the face, neck, upper back, and chest. Facial lesions tend to involve the malar regions and temples.

Dermatosis papulosa nigra is a benign condition with no malignant potential. Therefore, treatment is not necessary, although some patients request removal for cosmetic reasons. Treatment options include scissors excision, curettage, laser therapy, electrodessication, cryotherapy, and microdermabrasion. However, one should exercise caution when treating the lesions, because there is a risk for inducing hypertrophic scar formation, hyperpigmentation, or hypopigmentation in dark-skinned individuals.

Sebaceous Hyperplasia

Fig. **10.12**

Sebaceous hyperplasia is a localized, benign proliferation of sebaceous glands, with a predilection for the facial skin (especially involving the nose, cheeks, and forehead). The etiology is uncertain. An increased prevalence has been noted among transplant patients taking cyclosporine. In addition, sebaceous hyperplasia may arise in association with *Muir-Torre syndrome* (a rare, autosomal-dominant disorder characterized by visceral malignancies, sebaceous adenomas and carcinomas, and keratoacanthomas).

Sebaceous hyperplasia typically develops in adults >40 years old, and the prevalence increases with age. The lesion usually is asymptomatic and grows slowly. Clinical examination shows a soft, yellow-white to normal-colored papule, often with central umbilication (corresponding to the sebaceous duct ostium). The clinical appearance can mimic basal cell carcinoma. However, the ability to express sebum from the central depression aids in distinguishing sebaceous hyperplasia from basal cell carcinoma. If the diagnosis is uncertain, then excisional biopsy should be considered. Otherwise, treatment generally is reserved for patients with cosmetic concerns. Alternative treatment options include cryosurgery, photodynamic therapy, laser therapy, electrodessication, and isotretinoin.

In addition, intraoral sebaceous hyperplasia has been reported rarely. It tends to occur on the buccal mucosa or retromolar pad of adults (mean age, 36 years). Clinically, the lesion presents as a soft, yellow-white

■ Figure **10.10**
Seborrheic Keratosis
Skin showing a brown, well-demarcated plaque with a rough surface.

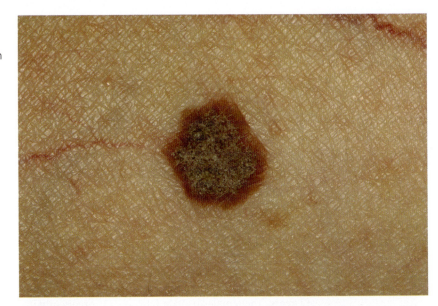

■ Figure **10.11**
Dermatosis Papulosa Nigra
Multiple dark brown papules on the facial skin.

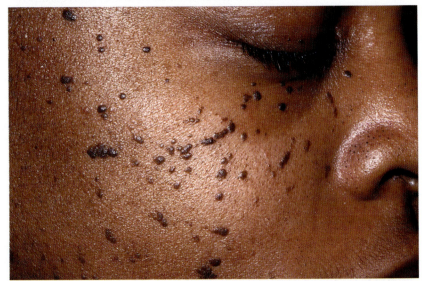

■ Figure **10.12**
Sebaceous Hyperplasia
Skin of the left cheek showing a papule with central umbilication.

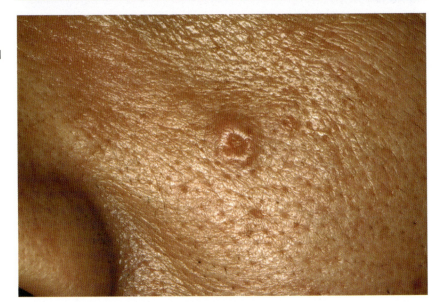

papule or "cauliflower-like" nodule. Compared to Fordyce granules, the lesions of intraoral sebaceous hyperplasia tend to be somewhat larger and are usually solitary rather than multifocal. Simple excision is appropriate treatment.

Oral Melanotic Macule (Oral Focal Melanosis)

Figs. **10.13 and 10.14**

The **oral melanotic macule** appears as a flat, brown area of mucosal discoloration and represents the most common oral lesion of melanocytic origin. In one study, melanotic macules comprised 86% of all solitary oral melanocytic lesions submitted to an oral pathology laboratory over a 19-year period. The etiopathogenesis is unclear. Intraoral lesions are not associated with sun exposure, and it is disputed whether examples arising on the lip vermilion exhibit such an association. The condition apparently results from melanocytic hyperactivity; characteristic microscopic findings include increased melanin deposition in the basal layer of the surface epithelium and melanin incontinence in the superficial connective tissue.

Oral melanotic macules occur over a broad age range, with a mean age at diagnosis of approximately 47 years. The female-to-male ratio is 2 : 1. Frequently involved subsites include the lower lip, gingiva, and buccal mucosa. Clinical examination typically shows a solitary, brown to brown-black macule with well-demarcated borders. The lesion tends to reach its maximum size (mean, 7 mm) relatively rapidly and then remains constant thereafter. The clinical differential diagnosis may include a melanocytic nevus, amalgam tattoo, oral melanoacanthoma, and early melanoma.

In terms of clinical management, biopsy and histopathologic examination typically should be considered for unexplained, persistent, and solitary pigmented oral lesions—especially those involving the hard palate and maxillary gingiva (which are high-risk sites for melanoma). In addition, patients may request removal of melanotic macules involving aesthetic areas. In order to obtain tissue suitable for microscopic evaluation, conventional surgical excision is preferred over electrocautery, laser ablation, or other destructive methods. After removal, melanotic macules typically do not recur. There is only a single reported case of an apparent oral melanotic macule that transformed into a melanoma.

Laugier-Hunziker Syndrome

Fig. **10.15**

Laugier-Hunziker syndrome represents a rare, acquired mucocutaneous pigmentary disorder of unknown etiology. Fewer than 200 cases have been reported in the literature. The condition has been described most often in Europe, with a predilection for white females. It occurs over a broad age range, with a mean age at diagnosis of approximately 49 years and a peak in the fifth through seventh decades. Oral examination shows multiple brown, black, or gray macules, often involving the lips, hard palate, tongue, gingiva, and buccal mucosa. The lesions typically exhibit a smooth surface and may be lenticular, oval, or irregular in shape. The macules tend to be small (<5 mm in diameter) and discrete, but occasionally they may coalesce to form large, confluent areas of pigmentation. In addition, approximately 60% of patients exhibit nail pigmentation, appearing as longitudinal streaks (*longitudinal melanonychia*) or homogeneous discoloration of the radial or ulnar half. Occasionally, pigmented lesions may be noted in other sites, such as the skin (especially on the palms and soles), anogenital region, conjunctiva, and oropharynx. The clinical differential diagnosis may include Peutz-Jeghers syndrome, Addison disease, McCune-Albright syndrome, drug-induced pigmentation, and physiologic (racial) pigmentation. Treatment is not necessary but may be considered for aesthetic reasons. Treatment methods include laser ablation and cryotherapy. Recurrence is possible but may be minimized by avoiding exposure to sunlight. The condition is not associated with an increased risk for malignancy.

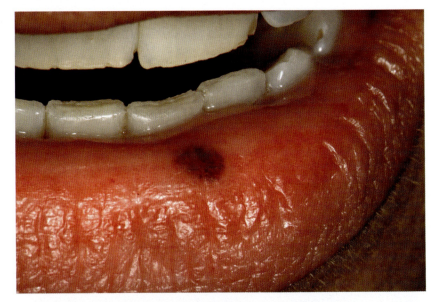

■ Figure 10.13
Oral Melanotic Macule
A well-demarcated, brown macule on the lower lip.

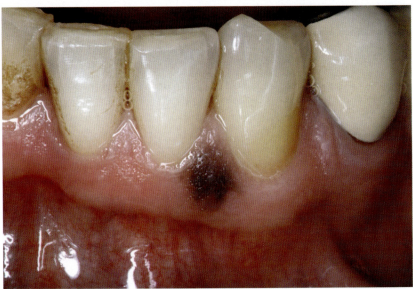

■ Figure 10.14
Oral Melanotic Macule
Brown macule on the anterior mandibular gingiva.

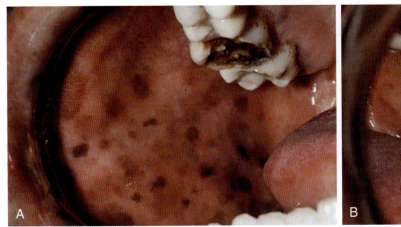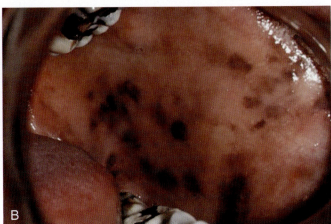

■ Figure 10.15
Laugier–Hunziker Syndrome
Multiple brown macules on the (A) right and (B) left buccal mucosa.

Oral Melanoacanthoma (Melanoacanthosis)

Fig. **10.16**

Oral melanoacanthoma is an uncommon, benign pigmented lesion, characterized by numerous dendritic melanocytes dispersed throughout the surface epithelium. Although the etiopathogenesis is uncertain, it appears to represent a reactive process. Oral melanoacanthoma exhibits a predilection for black females, with a mean age at diagnosis of 35 years. The buccal mucosa is the most common location, although any area of the oral mucosa can be affected. The clinical presentation can be alarming. There is typically a rapidly enlarging and ill-defined area of dark brown to black pigmentation, with a flat to slightly raised surface. Within just a few weeks, the lesion may reach a size of several centimeters. The patient usually experiences no symptoms, although pain, burning, and pruritus have been reported in some cases. Most lesions are solitary, but multifocal involvement is possible. The concerning clinical presentation often prompts incisional biopsy in order to rule out melanoma. Once the diagnosis has been established, no further treatment is necessary. Many cases exhibit spontaneous regression after incisional biopsy and/or removal of potential sources of local irritation.

Ephelides (Freckles)

Fig. **10.17**

Ephelides (singular, *ephelis*) are small, brown macules commonly found on the skin. The lesions result from increased melanin deposition in the basilar region of the epidermis, with no increase in the number of melanocytes. The development of ephelides appears to be determined primarily by genetic factors. In addition, sun exposure seems to play a contributory role; the lesions usually are most pronounced in the summer and fade in the winter. Ephelides tend to occur on the face, neck, arms, and shoulders of fair-skinned, blue-eyed, and red- or blond-haired individuals. Typically, ephelides appear during the first decade of life, and they may increase in size, number, and color intensity during adolescence. Subsequently, they usually become less prominent in adulthood. Clinical examination shows multiple small (approximately 1 to 2 mm in diameter), well-defined, and uniformly light brown macules. The number of lesions may vary from <10 to several hundred. Ephelides are benign and do not require treatment. However, in order to address cosmetic concerns, they may be treated by cryotherapy, hydroquinone, chemical peels, or laser therapy. Sunscreens may prevent the development of new lesions and the darkening of existing ones.

Actinic Lentigines (Solar Lentigines, Age Spots)

Fig. **10.18**

Actinic lentigines are brown macules that commonly arise on sun-exposed areas of the skin in middle-aged to elderly adults. The number of lesions increases with age, and they are considered a hallmark of photodamaged skin. Individuals with ephelides (see previous section) in childhood and adolescence tend to develop actinic lentigines later in life. In addition, actinic lentigines exhibit a predilection for whites and Asians. Commonly involved sites include the face, dorsa of the hands, forearms, shoulders, and upper back. The lesions typically present as asymptomatic, uniformly pigmented, and light to dark brown macules with well-demarcated but irregular borders. The lesions may range from a few millimeters to >1 cm in diameter. The pigmented nature of actinic lentigines results from a local proliferation of basal melanocytes within the epidermis. Treatment is not necessary but may be desired for cosmetic reasons. Treatment options include cryotherapy, laser therapy, and topical agents (e.g., hydroquinone, tretinoin, tazarotene). In addition, biopsy and microscopic diagnosis should be considered for apparent actinic lentigines with atypical clinical features (e.g., rapid growth, change in appearance, pain, ulceration, bleeding, itching). Although actinic lentigo is a benign lesion, it is a clinical marker of photodamage and may indicate an increased risk for skin cancer. Therefore, clinical monitoring is warranted.

■ Figure **10.16**
Oral Melanoacanthoma
Dark brown patch on the right buccal mucosa.

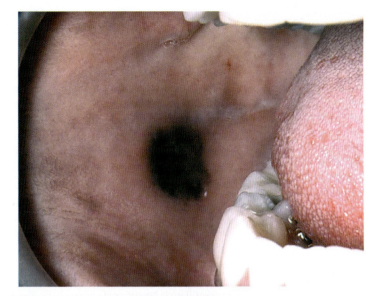

■ Figure **10.17**
Ephelides
Multiple light brown macules on the facial skin.

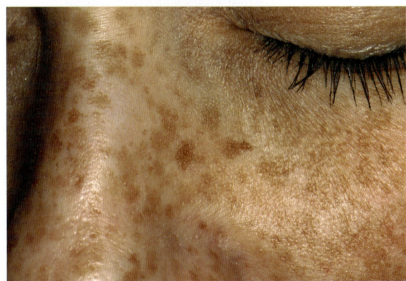

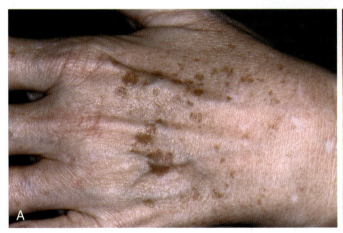

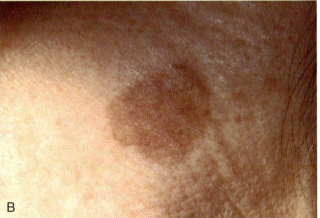

■ Figure **10.18**
Actinic Lentigines
(A) Brown macules on the skin of the dorsal hand in an older adult. (B) Flat, light brown, and well-demarcated lesion on the skin of the forehead in an older adult.

Figs. **10.19 and 10.20**

A **melanocytic nevus** represents a benign proliferation of nevus cells that are derived from the neural crest. Melanocytic nevi most often occur on the skin, although occasionally they may involve the oral mucosa. There are numerous types of melanocytic nevi. The remainder of this section will focus on the most common type, referred to as the *acquired melanocytic nevus* (or "common mole").

Acquired melanocytic nevi usually appear on the skin during adolescence or early adulthood. The natural history includes initiation, growth, stabilization, and involution. Accordingly, the lesions become less prevalent with advancing age. Cutaneous nevi tend to be more numerous in whites compared to Asians or blacks. The average white adult exhibits approximately 10 to 40 cutaneous melanocytic nevi, with most lesions distributed above the waist. In addition, females often have a few more nevi than males. Clinically, a nevus may appear as a macule, smooth-surfaced papule, or papillary nodule. Most examples measure <6 mm, and the lesions may appear brown, black, or normal in color. In some cases, hairs may protrude from the lesion surface. Microscopically, acquired melanocytic nevi may be classified into the following developmental stages: (1) *junctional* (nevus cells confined to the junction of the epithelium and connective tissue), (2) *compound* (nevus cells in both the junctional zone and underlying connective tissue), and (3) *intradermal* or *intramucosal* (nevus cells confined to the connective tissue). Although cutaneous acquired melanocytic nevi typically do not require treatment, conservative excision may be considered in some cases (e.g., for cosmetic reasons, lesions subject to chronic irritation from clothing, lesions exhibiting a change in size or color). Recurrence is rare, and the risk for malignant transformation of an individual acquired melanocytic nevus is low. However, patients with a large number (>100) of cutaneous nevi are at increased risk for developing melanoma and should be monitored periodically.

Oral melanocytic nevi are relatively rare, with approximately two-thirds occurring in females. The average age at diagnosis is about 35 years. Intramucosal nevi (the intraoral counterpart of intradermal nevi) are seen most commonly, comprising approximately 64% of oral melanocytic nevi. Oral intramucosal nevi are found most frequently on the buccal mucosa, hard palate, gingiva, and lip vermilion. Most oral melanocytic nevi appear brown or black, although about 20% of cases do not exhibit clinically evident pigmentation. The clinical differential diagnosis for a pigmented nevus in the oral cavity may include a melanotic macule, amalgam tattoo, oral melanoacanthoma, and early melanoma. Typically, biopsy of a persistent, unexplained pigmented lesion of the oral mucosa should be considered in order to rule out malignancy. Nonpigmented lesions may mimic a papilloma or fibroma, and typically they are removed by simple excision.

Fig. **10.21**

The **blue nevus** is a melanocytic nevus variant in which the lesional cells are found deep within the connective tissue. Its characteristic blue hue is attributed to the *Tyndall effect* (the scattering of light as it passes through a colloidal suspension). Light is reflected by the deeply located melanin particles and passes through the overlying tissue; the cells within the overlying tissue act as a suspension, absorbing long wavelengths of light but allowing the shorter-wavelength blue light to pass. Most blue nevi occur on the skin, especially in the head and neck region, sacral region, and dorsal aspects of the distal extremities. In addition, oral lesions are possible; approximately one-third of all intraoral melanocytic nevi are blue nevi. There are two major histopathologic subtypes: *common blue nevus* and *cellular blue nevus*. The common blue nevus represents the second most common type of oral melanocytic nevus, whereas cellular blue nevi are exceedingly rare in the oral cavity.

Among oral cases of blue nevi, there is a marked predilection for the palate. Females are affected more often than males, and the mean age at diagnosis is approximately 38 to 43 years. Clinical examination typically shows a blue to blue-black macule or nodule. Most lesions measure <1 cm, although some examples (especially cellular blue nevi) can become larger. The clinical differential diagnosis may include an amalgam tattoo, varix, or early melanoma. In general, biopsy of unexplained pigmented lesions of the oral mucosa should be considered in order to rule out malignancy. Oral blue nevi typically are treated by conservative excision, and there is a low risk for recurrence. However, periodic clinical follow-up is prudent after removal of cellular blue nevi because of rare reports of malignant transformation.

■ Figure **10.19**
Melanocytic Nevus
Light brown, slightly raised lesion with protruding hairs on the skin adjacent to the upper lip vermilion.

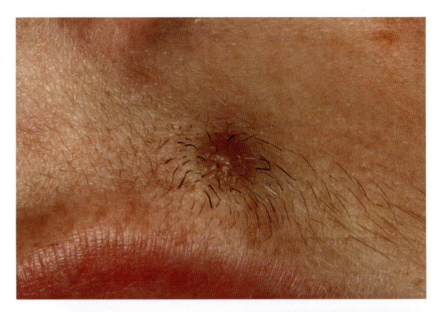

■ Figure **10.20**
Melanocytic Nevus
Dark brown macule on the soft palate. (Courtesy Dr. Molly Rosebush.)

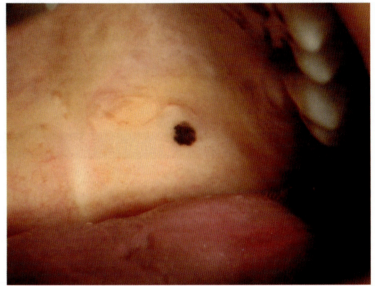

■ Figure **10.21**
Blue Nevus
Blue macule on the palate.

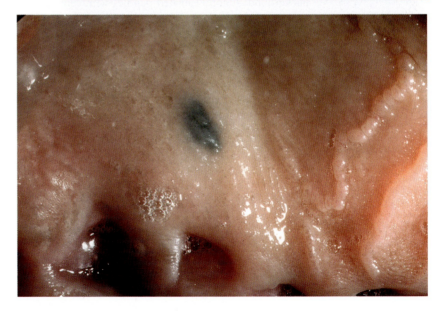

Figs. **10.22 and 10.23**

Alveolar ridge keratosis is a benign, hyperkeratotic patch or plaque that commonly develops on the retromolar pad or edentulous alveolar ridge. It is believed to represent a response to chronic, frictional trauma (i.e., from opposing teeth, prostheses, or foodstuffs during mastication). The condition has been likened to a cutaneous callus or lichen simplex chronicus. Because it presents as a white lesion that cannot be wiped away, alveolar ridge keratosis often is included in studies of oral leukoplakia. However, it appears to represent a distinct, benign clinicopathologic entity rather than an oral, potentially malignant disorder.

Clinically, alveolar ridge keratosis usually is noted in adults, with a mean age of approximately 50 to 55 years and a male predilection. About 50% to 60% of cases involve the retromolar pads, sometimes bilaterally. Other lesions arise on edentulous areas of the mandibular or maxillary alveolar ridge. Clinical examination typically shows a white patch or plaque with a rough, warty, wrinkled, or corrugated surface. In addition, some examples may appear as white papules. A strong presumptive clinical diagnosis often can be made in cases with a classic presentation. However, biopsy may be considered to rule out epithelial dysplasia or carcinoma in cases with the following findings: (1) patient history of tobacco and/or alcohol use; (2) concurrent or prior oral leukoplakia involving areas other than the retromolar pad or edentulous alveolar ridge; or (3) atypical clinical features (e.g., erythema, ulceration, markedly verrucous or papillary surface, lesion borders extending beyond the retromolar pad or edentulous ridge). Microscopic findings characteristic of alveolar ridge keratosis include hyperorthokeratosis, a pebbly surface architecture, wedge-shaped hypergranulosis, acanthosis (epithelial thickening) with tapered rete ridges, no dysplastic changes, and absent or scant inflammation. Once the diagnosis has been established, no further treatment is needed other than periodic clinical observation.

Fig. **10.24**

Nicotine stomatitis is an alteration of the palatal mucosa associated with tobacco smoking. The condition arises much more frequently in pipe and cigar smokers compared to cigarette smokers. It appears to develop in response to heat rather than chemicals in the tobacco smoke. In addition, electronic cigarette use and the consumption of very hot beverages (such as tea or maté) may be contributory factors.

Clinically, nicotine stomatitis most often occurs in middle-aged to older adult males. The palatal mucosa becomes diffusely hyperkeratotic, producing a leathery and white or gray change. Within this hyperkeratotic background, slightly elevated papules with central erythematous punctae form; these papules represent inflamed minor salivary glands and their associated ductal orifices. In severe cases, the palatal mucosa becomes diffusely thickened and fissured, imparting a "dried mud" appearance.

Nicotine stomatitis itself is not a premalignant condition, although tobacco use does confer an increased risk for oral leukoplakia (see the following section) and cancer. Therefore, tobacco counseling, thorough examination, and periodic clinical follow-up are advised. Nicotine stomatitis typically regresses after tobacco cessation. However, if any portion of the lesion persists longer than 1 month after discontinuation, then biopsy and microscopic evaluation should be considered.

■ Figure **10.22**
Alveolar Ridge Keratosis
White, rough plaque on an edentulous area of the mandibular alveolar ridge.

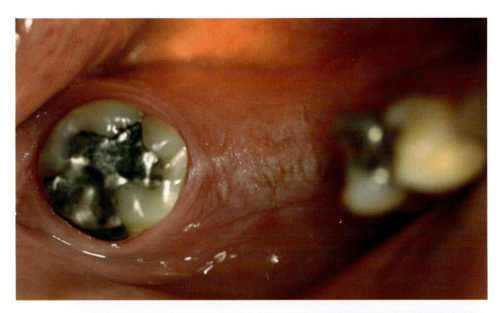

■ Figure **10.23**
Alveolar Ridge Keratosis
White, rough plaque on the left mandibular alveolar ridge in an edentulous patient.

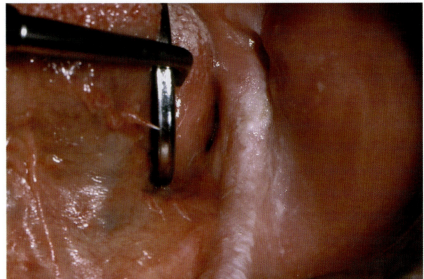

■ Figure **10.24**
Nicotine Stomatitis
Extensive leathery, white change of the palatal mucosa, with slightly elevated papules and erythematous punctae. (Courtesy Dr. Manuel LaRosa.)

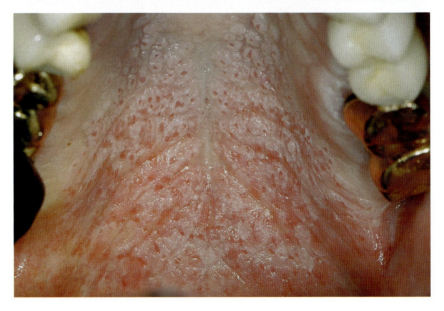

Traditionally, oral **leukoplakia** has been defined as a white patch or plaque that cannot be characterized clinically or pathologically as another other disease. This definition requires the exclusion of other conditions that can cause white oral mucosal changes (e.g., candidiasis, morsicatio, frictional keratosis, lichen planus, tobacco pouch keratosis, nicotine stomatitis, oral hairy leukoplakia). The estimated worldwide prevalence of oral leukoplakia is 2%. Tobacco use is a major risk factor, with leukoplakia occurring up to six times more often among smokers than nonsmokers. Additional risk factors include alcohol consumption and areca nut product use. The significance of oral leukoplakia is that it carries an increased risk of becoming or already harboring invasive carcinoma; thus, it is considered an *oral potentially malignant disorder*. According to a recent systematic review of the literature, the mean malignant transformation rate is approximately 3.5% (range, 0.13% to 34%), although this rate likely is dependent on what clinical lesions are classified as leukoplakia. If a stricter definition of leukoplakia is applied (excluding such lesions as alveolar ridge keratosis tobacco pouch keratosis, and morsicatio), then a higher transformation rate will be seen.

Clinically, oral leukoplakia exhibits a predilection for middle-aged to older men. As many as 8% of males >70 years old are affected. Frequently involved subsites include the lip vermilion, buccal mucosa, and gingiva. Among lesions with dysplasia or carcinoma, the most commonly involved locations are the tongue, lip vermilion, and floor of the mouth. Most patients are asymptomatic. The inability to wipe away the lesion aids in distinguishing oral leukoplakia from pseudomembranous candidiasis. Over time, individual lesions may exhibit regression, progression, or no significant change. Initially, the lesion may appear as a *thin leukoplakia* (flat to slightly elevated, white to gray plaque with a translucent, fissured, or wrinkled surface). Subsequently, the lesion may become a *thick (or homogeneous) leukoplakia*, appearing as a leathery, opaque, white plaque with deepened fissures. In addition, some examples may develop a granular, warty, or nodular surface. If the lesion appears white and red, it may be termed *speckled leukoplakia* or *erythro-leukoplakia*. Clinical features that are worrisome for high-grade dysplasia or invasive carcinoma include an erythematous component and verrucous, granular, or nodular surface change. However, even subtle or seemingly innocuous leukoplakias may exhibit dysplasia or carcinoma. Therefore, biopsy should be considered for any unexplained oral white lesion.

Microscopically, oral leukoplakias are characterized by hyperkeratosis, acanthosis (epithelial thickening), and/or hyperplasia (elongated epithelial rete). In addition, about 16% to 39% of cases exhibit epithelial dysplasia, and 3% may show unsuspected squamous cell carcinoma. In particular, leukoplakias of the lateral tongue and floor of the mouth have a greater risk for harboring dysplasia or carcinoma compared to those in other oral subsites.

Treatment of oral leukoplakia is guided by the clinical findings and microscopic diagnosis. General management considerations include risk factor control, surgical/medical interventions, and clinical surveillance. However, there is a paucity of evidence from well-designed clinical trials, and further studies are needed. Habit cessation should be encouraged for patients who use tobacco, consume alcohol heavily, or chew areca nut products. These habits are established etiologic factors for oral, potentially malignant disorders and oral squamous cell carcinoma. Also, some tobacco-related leukoplakias may resolve after smoking cessation. For leukoplakias with no or mild dysplasia, careful clinical follow-up typically is provided. For cases exhibiting moderate to severe dysplasia or carcinoma *in situ*, surgical excision usually is performed. Alternative treatments include laser ablation, photodynamic therapy, and cryotherapy; however, unlike surgical excision, destructive treatments do not allow for histopathologic examination. In addition, various topical or systemic agents (e.g., vitamin A, beta carotene, lycopene) have been studied; although such agents may improve the clinical appearance of lesions, relapse is common.

Notably, there is currently no strong evidence that conventional or alternative treatments for oral leukoplakia can reduce the risk for progression to malignancy. Patients with oral leukoplakia and other oral potentially malignant disorders can exhibit *field cancerization* (diffuse or multifocal fields of altered epithelial cells caused by exposure to carcinogens). Thus, the risk for cancer development may persist despite treatments aimed at eradicating clinically evident lesions. Considering that the risk for malignant transformation can persist despite previous treatment for oral leukoplakia, lifelong clinical surveillance is recommended.

■ Figure **10.25**
Leukoplakia
Ill-defined, white plaque on the lateral and ventral tongue. A biopsy showed hyperkeratosis with severe epithelial dysplasia.

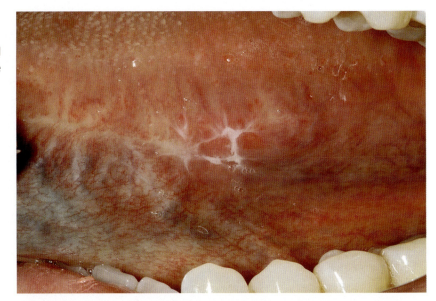

■ Figure **10.26**
Leukoplakia
Extensive white plaque on the lateral and ventral tongue. A biopsy showed hyperkeratosis with mild epithelial dysplasia, and the lesion subsequently transformed into squamous cell carcinoma.

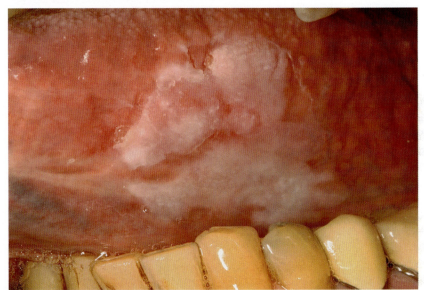

■ Figure **10.27**
Leukoplakia
White plaque in the sublingual caruncle region. A biopsy showed hyperkeratosis with moderate epithelial dysplasia.

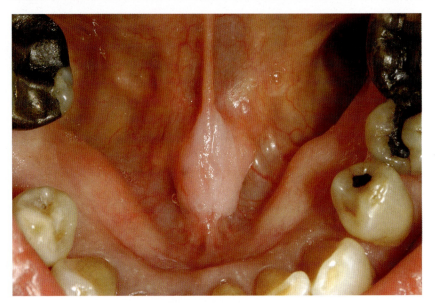

■ Figure **10.28**
Leukoplakia
White, thick plaque with a corrugated surface on the floor of the mouth. A biopsy showed hyperkeratosis with moderate epithelial dysplasia.

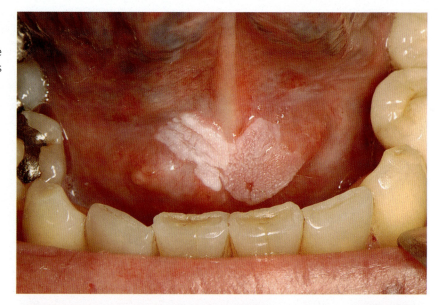

■ Figure **10.29**
Leukoplakia
White plaque with a rough, wrinkled surface on the palate and retromolar trigone. (Because there is focal erythema, the lesion also could be termed *erythroleukoplakia*.)

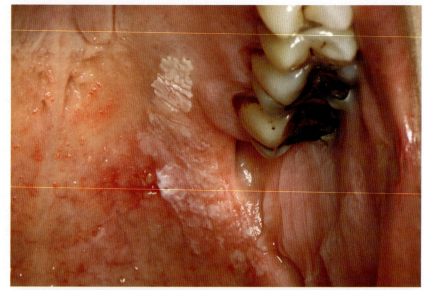

■ Figure **10.30**
Leukoplakia
Soft palate exhibiting an extensive white plaque with irregular borders.

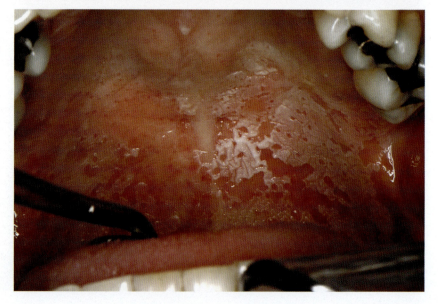

Figure **10.31**
Leukoplakia
White plaque with a rough surface on the right buccal mucosa. A biopsy showed hyperkeratosis with moderate epithelial dysplasia.

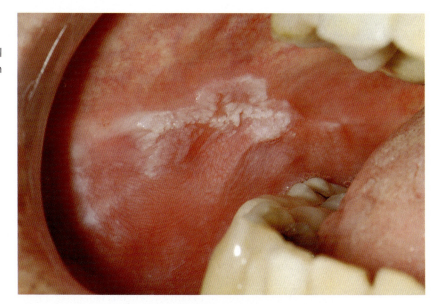

Figure **10.32**
Leukoplakia
Large white plaque on the right buccal mucosa. The lesion exhibits thick and thin areas. A biopsy showed hyperkeratosis with moderate epithelial dysplasia. (Courtesy Dr. Manuel LaRosa.)

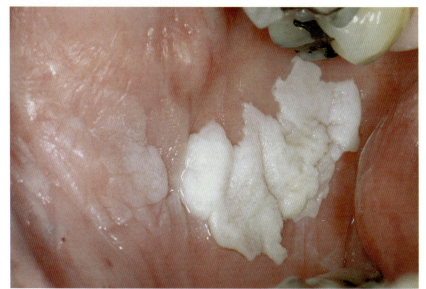

Figure **10.33**
Speckled Leukoplakia
White and red plaque with a granular surface.

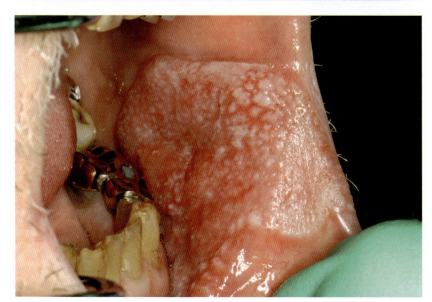

Figs. **10.34–10.37**

Proliferative verrucous leukoplakia represents a rare and potentially very aggressive form of oral leukoplakia. The etiopathogenesis is uncertain. No definite causative role has been established for tobacco, alcohol, human papillomavirus (HPV), or Epstein-Barr virus. The diagnosis can be challenging and typically is made in retrospect after a patient develops multiple lesions over the course of many years with eventual progression to squamous cell carcinoma.

Proliferative verrucous leukoplakia exhibits a predilection for women (female-to-male ratio, 2.7 : 1 to 4 : 1), with a mean age at diagnosis of 67 years. Frequently involved sites include the gingiva, alveolar mucosa, buccal mucosa, and tongue. Initially, the patient may exhibit a solitary, homogenous white lesion that mimics conventional oral leukoplakia. Occasionally, an erythematous component also may be evident. However, over time the patient develops additional and/or more extensive lesions, often with bilateral involvement. Early lesions tend to be relatively flat, whereas later lesions tend to exhibit rough, granular, or warty surfaces. Typically, after many years, there is progression to verrucous carcinoma or conventional squamous cell carcinoma. Clinical signs that are worrisome for malignancy include erythema, a warty or papillary surface, ulceration, pain, and paresthesia.

Diagnosis of proliferative verrucous leukoplakia requires clinicopathologic correlation. Depending on lesion stage, the microscopic findings may include hyperkeratosis (with no to varying degrees of dysplasia), verrucous hyperplasia, verrucous carcinoma, or conventional squamous cell carcinoma. Although diagnostic criteria vary across studies, some authors have proposed the following: (1) leukoplakia with verrucous or wart-like areas involving >2 oral subsites; (2) when adding all involved sites, minimum size >3 cm; (3) well-documented period of disease evolution >5 years, with lesion spread/enlargement and >1 recurrence in a previously treated area; and (4) at least one biopsy. The index of suspicion is especially high among older women with no identifiable risk factors for oral cancer.

Unfortunately, there is currently no cure for proliferative verrucous leukoplakia. Various approaches (e.g., conventional surgery, laser ablation, photodynamic therapy, topical bleomycin, systemic chemotherapy, radiation, antiviral therapy) have been reported in the literature. However, even with treatment, recurrence rates range from 87% to 100%, and malignant transformation rates are >70%. Thus, clinical management focuses on close, lifelong clinical surveillance with selective biopsies to provide the best chance of early oral cancer detection. Biopsies should be considered for new lesions or lesions with significant changes in appearance, size, and/or symptoms. Overall disease-related mortality is approximately 30% to 50%.

■ Figure **10.34**
Proliferative Verrucous Leukoplakia
White, linear plaque involving the facial marginal gingiva in the anterior mandibular region.

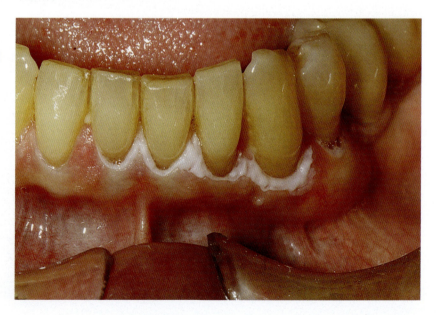

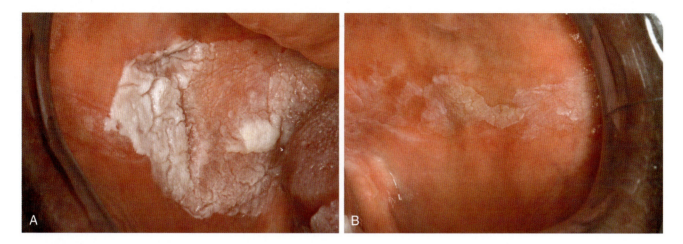

■ Figure **10.35**
Proliferative Verrucous Leukoplakia
This patient had extensive white plaques on the (A) right and (B) left buccal mucosa.

■ Figure **10.36**
Proliferative Verrucous Leukoplakia
Same patient depicted in Fig. 10.35. Ventral tongue exhibiting a large, white plaque with a rough, warty surface.

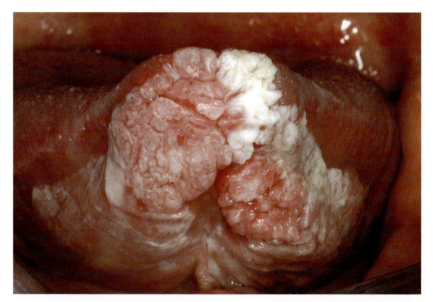

■ Figure **10.37**
Proliferative Verrucous Leukoplakia
Diffuse, thick, white plaque involving the facial mandibular gingiva and adjacent vestibule.

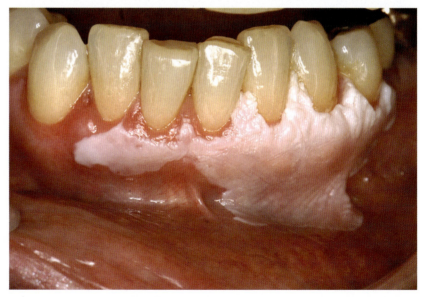

Figs. **10.38–10.40**

Erythroplakia is defined as a red patch or plaque that cannot be characterized clinically or pathologically as any other condition. It is analogous to leukoplakia (see previous section) and represents an *oral potentially malignant disorder*. Notably, most true oral erythroplakias demonstrate dysplasia or carcinoma at initial presentation. According to various large-scale epidemiologic surveys in the United States and Asia, the prevalence of oral erythroplakia ranges from 0.02% to 0.83%. Major risk factors include tobacco and alcohol use.

Oral erythroplakia predominantly is noted among middle-aged to elderly adults, with no significant gender predilection. Frequently involved sites include the soft palate, floor of the mouth, and buccal mucosa. Many patients are asymptomatic, although pain or burning is possible. Clinical examination typically shows a well-demarcated, erythematous patch or plaque with a soft to velvety texture. In some cases, a combination of erythematous and white features may be evident (termed *erythroleukoplakia*).

Red lesions of the oral mucosa should be viewed with suspicion, especially when occurring in high-risk sites for oral cancer (such as the ventrolateral tongue and floor of the mouth). Biopsy typically is warranted for erythematous lesions that have no identifiable cause or do not resolve within 2 weeks of removal of potential sources of irritation. Microscopic examination aids in ruling out other erythematous conditions (e.g., candidiasis, nonspecific mucositis, vascular lesions) and assessing for epithelial dysplasia or carcinoma. For erythroleukoplakias, biopsy sampling should include the red component, which exhibits a greater risk for harboring significant dysplasia or carcinoma compared to the white component.

Clinical management of erythroplakia is guided by the microscopic diagnosis. Surgical excision typically is performed for lesions exhibiting moderate dysplasia, severe dysplasia, or carcinoma *in situ*. Laser ablation or other destructive methods also may be considered, although surgical excision is preferable in order to allow for histopathologic examination. Management of invasive squamous cell carcinoma is discussed separately. After treatment, the patient should receive long-term clinical follow-up, because of the risk for recurrence or additional lesions.

■ Figure **10.38**
Erythroplakia

Right posterior buccal mucosa showing an erythematous lesion with ulceration. A biopsy showed carcinoma *in situ*.

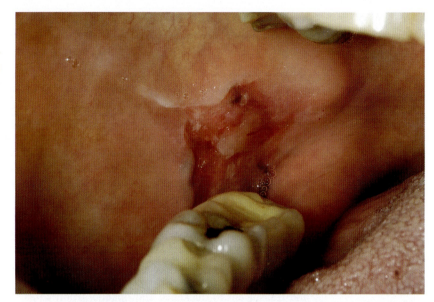

■ Figure **10.39**
Erythroplakia

Mostly erythematous plaque on the soft and hard palate.

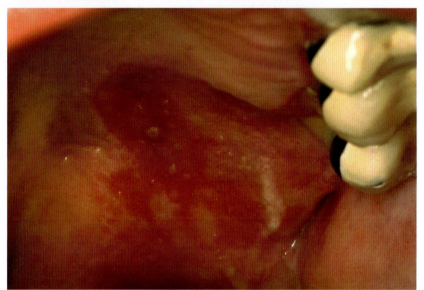

■ Figure **10.40**
Erythroleukoplakia

Red and white plaque involving the left posterior ventrolateral tongue. A biopsy showed squamous cell carcinoma. (Courtesy Dr. Bradley Gregory.)

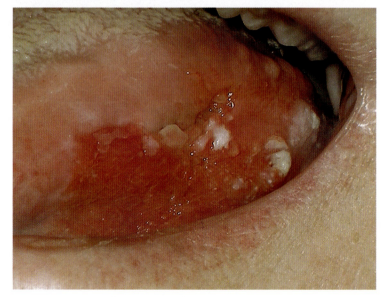

Figs. **10.41–10.43**

Tobacco pouch keratosis is an oral mucosal alteration that develops in areas of chronic smokeless tobacco placement. In the United States, according to the 2016 National Survey on Drug Use and Health, approximately 3.3% of people (or 8.8 million individuals) 12 years and older use smokeless tobacco. The highest prevalence rates are seen in the Midwestern and Southern regions. In addition, recent studies suggest that, although cigarette smoking rates have been declining in the United States, smokeless tobacco use has remained relatively constant. Major types of smokeless tobacco include moist snuff, dry snuff, and chewing tobacco. In Western cultures, tobacco pouch keratosis has been noted in 60% of snuff users and 15% of chewing tobacco users. The lesion often arises in young adult men and men >65 years old; however, in some subpopulations there is a predilection for older women.

Clinically, tobacco pouch keratosis affects areas (such as the buccal vestibular mucosa or lower labial mucosa) that come into direct contact with smokeless tobacco. The altered mucosa typically is flaccid, with wrinkles or fissures likened to the appearance of rippled sand on a beach after an ebbing tide. Depending on the degree of hyperkeratosis and acanthosis, the lesion may appear white, gray, or normal in color. Sometimes an erythematous component also is evident. The altered mucosa may range from thin and translucent to thickened and opaque. Upon palpation, the lesion may feel soft, velvety, or leathery. Similar mucosal alterations may be induced by chronic placement of bulky materials (e.g., hard candy, sunflower seeds, beef jerky).

Tobacco pouch keratosis is associated with a low risk for developing high-grade dysplasia or carcinoma, and a strong presumptive clinical diagnosis often can be made based on the clinical findings. However, biopsy and histopathologic examination should be considered for lesions with severe or atypical mucosal alterations (e.g., ulceration, intense whiteness, granular or verrucous surface, nodularity, induration, bleeding).

Although smokeless tobacco use is associated with a lower risk for cancer than cigarette smoking, cessation of all tobacco habits should be encouraged. Tobacco pouch keratosis typically will resolve several weeks after cessation of smokeless tobacco use. If any portion of the lesion persists longer than 6 weeks without smokeless tobacco contact, then biopsy is indicated to rule out significant dysplasia or squamous cell carcinoma. Oral cancers related to smokeless tobacco typically develop after several decades of use, with dry snuff tending to be more carcinogenic than moist snuff and chewing tobacco.

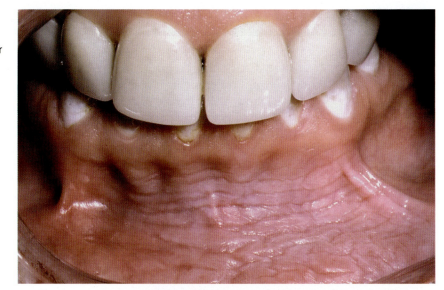

■ Figure **10.41**
Tobacco Pouch Keratosis
Gray-white, fissured lesion involving the anterior mandibular vestibule and lower labial mucosa.

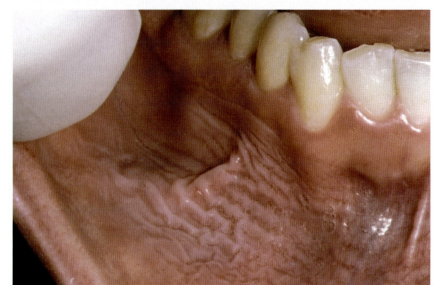

■ Figure **10.42**
Tobacco Pouch Keratosis
Gray-white, fissured lesion involving the right mandibular buccal vestibule.

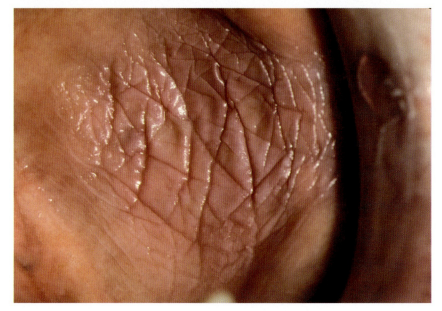

■ Figure **10.43**
Mint Candy Pouch
The left buccal mucosa appears wrinkled and flaccid because of chronic placement of mint candy.

Figs. **10.44–10.46**

Oral submucous fibrosis is a chronic, precancerous, and often debilitating condition characterized by slowly progressive fibrosis of the oral cavity and oropharynx. It is noted mainly in the Indian subcontinent, South/Southeast Asia, Taiwan, and southern China. The condition is caused primarily by areca nut chewing—an addictive habit practiced by 10% to 20% of the world's population. Depending on regional customs, this nut from the *Areca catechu* palm tree may be chewed alone or in combination with other substances, in order to relieve stress and produce a feeling of euphoria. In India, areca nut traditionally is incorporated into a betel quid (i.e., betel leaf wrapped around a mixture of areca nut, slaked lime, possibly tobacco, and sometimes condiments). In addition, the use of commercially freeze-dried areca nut products (such as gutkha) has become increasingly popular; such products contain especially high concentrations of areca nut and may cause more rapid development of oral submucous fibrosis compared to conventional betel quid. A genetic predisposition also may play a role in disease development.

Individuals with oral submucous fibrosis are often young adult betel quid users. Initially, the patient may complain of a burning sensation or intolerance to spicy foods. Oral examination during early disease stages may reveal vesicles, petechiae, xerostomia, and melanosis. With progression of the condition, fibrosis results in mucosal pallor, rigidity, and trismus. Swallowing and speaking can become very difficult. In advanced cases, submucosal fibrous bands may be evident upon palpation of the buccal mucosa, labial mucosa, and soft palate. Additional possible findings include a shrunken uvula, depapillated tongue, ulceration, and erythema. Sometimes mucosal alterations can extend into the upper esophagus.

Clinical management of oral submucous fibrosis can be challenging, and further studies are needed. Patients should be advised to discontinue areca nut use; however, once trismus has developed, habit cessation does not induce regression of the condition. Mild cases can be treated with intralesional corticosteroids. Severe cases may require surgical intervention and physiotherapy, although relapse is common. Alternative treatments include interferon gamma, proteolytic enzymes, pentoxyfilline, antioxidants, vitamins, and minerals. Close clinical follow-up is essential because of the risk for development of oral squamous cell carcinoma. Estimated malignant transformation rates for oral submucous fibrosis range from 2% to 8%.

■ Figure **10.44**
Oral Submucous Fibrosis
Gutkha user with limited mouth opening and pale palatal mucosa.

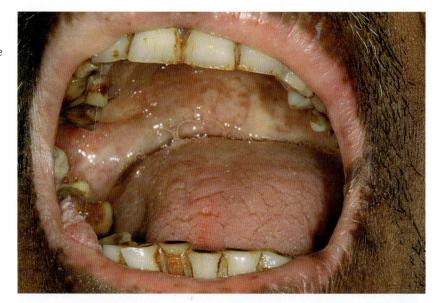

■ Figure **10.45**
Oral Submucous Fibrosis
Same patient depicted in Fig. 10.44. Pallor of the left buccal mucosa.

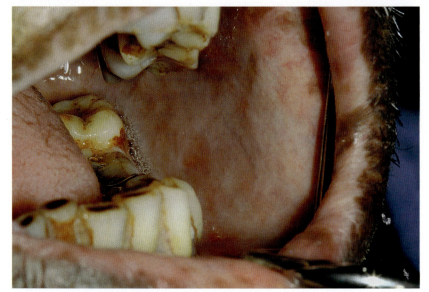

■ Figure **10.46**
Squamous Cell Carcinoma in a Patient With Oral Submucous Fibrosis
Same patient depicted in Figs. 10.44 and 10.45. Extensive mass involving the right buccal mucosa and right lower labial mucosa.

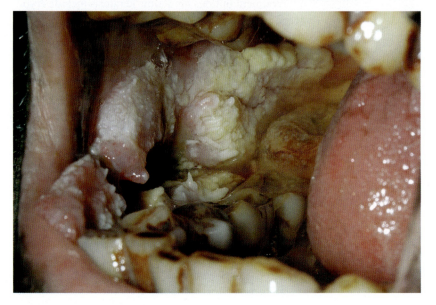

Actinic Cheilosis (Actinic Cheilitis)

Fig. **10.47**

Actinic cheilosis is a common, premalignant lesion of the lower lip vermilion caused by chronic ultraviolet light exposure. Similar lesions on the skin are called *actinic keratoses* (see next section). Major risk factors for actinic cheilosis include increased age, male gender, outdoor occupational/leisure activities, proximity to the equator, and light-complexioned skin. In addition, patients with certain genetic disorders (e.g., xeroderma pigmentosum, albinism) are at increased risk for developing actinic cheilosis and skin cancer. Cofactors that may increase the likelihood of actinic cheilosis transforming into squamous cell carcinoma include tobacco use and immunosuppression.

Actinic cheilosis exhibits a predilection for men >40 years old. Early lesions often appear as ill-defined, pale areas on the lower lip vermilion. Fissures and dryness also may be evident, and the transition between the vermilion and adjacent skin often becomes blurred. With progression, the lesion can develop into a rough, crusted, white and/or red plaque. Persistent ulceration, nodularity, and bleeding may indicate either actinic cheilosis with severe dysplasia or transformation into squamous cell carcinoma.

Clinical management of actinic cheilosis includes patient education (e.g., sun avoidance, wide-brimmed hat and sunscreen when outdoors). For lesions with severe dysplasia, vermilionectomy can be performed. Conventional surgery allows for microscopic examination to rule out carcinoma. For lesions with mild to moderate dysplasia, alternative treatments include topical agents (e.g., 5-fluorouracil, imiquimod), laser ablation, electrosurgery, cryotherapy, and photodynamic therapy. After treatment, long-term clinical follow-up is recommended.

Actinic Keratosis

Fig. **10.48**

Actinic keratosis is a common, premalignant skin lesion caused by chronic ultraviolet light exposure. Risk factors for actinic keratosis are similar to those for actinic cheilosis (see previous section); such factors include increased age, male gender, outdoor occupational/leisure activities, proximity to the equator, light-complexioned skin, and certain rare genetic disorders (e.g., xeroderma pigmentosum, albinism).

Actinic keratosis seldom occurs in individuals younger than 40 years. The condition typically involves the skin of sun-exposed areas (e.g., face, balding scalp, ears, neck, dorsa of the hands, forearms). There is often a cluster of lesions, although solitary lesions are possible. Many patients are asymptomatic, whereas others experience tenderness, pruritus, or burning. Clinical examination shows irregular macules or plaques with rough, scaly surfaces. Sometimes an actinic keratosis can be difficult to visualize, although its "sandpaper-like" texture is readily evident upon palpation. The lesions may range from a few millimeters to several centimeters in diameter, and they may be white, red, brown, or normal in color.

Treatment options for actinic keratosis include cryotherapy, curettage, surgical excision, topical agents (e.g., 5-fluorouracil, imiquimod), chemical peels, laser ablation, and photodynamic therapy. In addition, patients should be counseled to avoid sun exposure, apply sunscreens, and wear protective clothing. Although the risk of an individual lesion undergoing malignant transformation is low, the risk for squamous cell carcinoma developing in patients with multiple actinic keratoses is high (6% to 10% over a 10-year period). Therefore, treatment and long-term follow-up are advised.

Keratoacanthoma

Fig. **10.49**

Keratoacanthoma is a controversial epithelial proliferation. Some authorities consider it to represent a well-differentiated variant of squamous cell carcinoma, whereas others regard it as a benign neoplasm or borderline malignancy. Most examples occur on the skin, where they apparently originate from the follicular isthmus and infundibulum. Intraoral lesions are extremely rare. Ultraviolet light exposure is the major risk factor for keratoacanthoma. Other possible factors include radiation therapy, immunosuppression, trauma, and certain medications (e.g., *BRAF* inhibitors). Most lesions are solitary, although multiple keratoacanthomas can develop, either sporadically or in association with certain heritable conditions (e.g., Ferguson-Smith syndrome, Muir-Torre syndrome, xeroderma pigmentosum).

Solitary keratoacanthomas typically develop on the sun-exposed skin of older, light-complexioned adults. Approximately 8% of cases involve the outer edge of the lip vermilion border. Males are affected more often than females. Initially, the lesion exhibits rapid growth, reaching a maximum size of 1 to 2 cm within about 6 weeks. A fully developed lesion usually appears as a dome-shaped nodule with a central

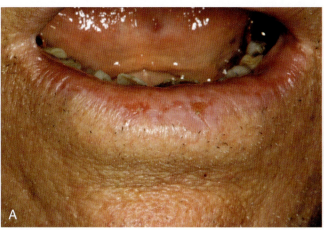
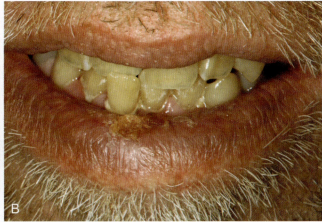

■ Figure **10.47**
Actinic Cheilosis
(A) Lower lip exhibiting pallor with focal erythema and crusting. (B) Crusted lesion on the lower lip.

■ Figure **10.48**
Actinic Keratosis
Erythematous, slightly raised lesion on the skin of the forehead.

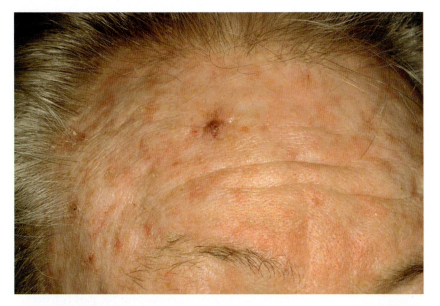

■ Figure **10.49**
Keratoacanthoma
Skin of the nose exhibiting a pink-red nodule with a central keratin plug.

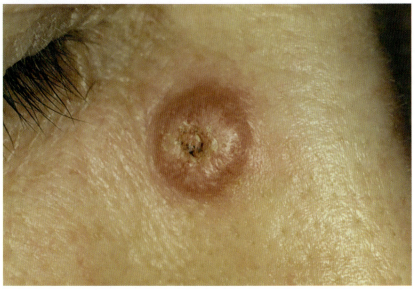

keratin plug. Subsequently, there is a period of stabilization, followed by spontaneous regression. Involution usually occurs within 6 to 12 months of lesion onset and often results in a depressed scar.

Keratoacanthomas typically are treated by surgical excision. Alternative treatments include intralesional chemotherapy, topical imiquimod, topical 5-fluorouracil, and systemic retinoids. The recurrence rate is approximately 1% to 8%. There are unusual reports of malignant transformation, although such cases may represent difficulties in microscopic distinction between keratoacanthoma and squamous cell carcinoma.

Oral and Oropharyngeal Squamous Cell Carcinoma

Figs. **10.50–10.67**

Squamous cell carcinoma is a malignancy of squamous epithelial cells and accounts for approximately 90% of oral and oropharyngeal cancers. According to data collected by the International Agency for Research on Cancer, worldwide in 2012 there were >529,000 new cases of lip/oral cavity/pharyngeal cancer and >292,000 deaths from these tumors. The incidence varies by region, with the highest rates noted in South-Central, Eastern, and Southeast Asia. In the United States, the American Cancer Society estimates that in 2018 there will be >51,000 newly diagnosed cases of oral cavity/pharyngeal cancer and >10,000 deaths from these tumors. Risk factors for oral cavity and oropharyngeal squamous cell carcinoma include tobacco use, heavy alcohol consumption, and betel quid chewing. With regard to tobacco use, one meta-analysis reported a relative risk of 6.76 for oropharyngeal squamous cell carcinoma and 3.43 for oral squamous cell carcinoma among current tobacco smokers compared with nonsmokers. Also, a synergistic effect has been noted when cigarette smoking is combined with alcohol consumption, and an especially high oral cancer risk (approximate pooled odds ratio, 40) has been noted among individuals who smoke, drink alcohol, and chew betel quid. Additional important etiologic factors include ultraviolet radiation exposure for lip vermilion cancers and high-risk human papillomavirus (HPV) infection (most frequently HPV type 16) for oropharyngeal tumors. Although the HPV-attributable fraction of oropharyngeal squamous cell carcinoma varies by geographic region and study method, it has been estimated to be 40% globally and >60% in the United States. In contrast, a much smaller proportion (<7%) of oral squamous cell carcinomas has been attributed to HPV. Other potential contributory factors for oral and pharyngeal cancer include poor diet, vitamin/mineral deficiencies, immunosuppression, environmental pollutants, occupational exposures, and certain heritable conditions (e.g., Fanconi anemia, dyskeratosis congenita, Bloom syndrome).

Epidemiologic trends for oral and oropharyngeal cancers are influenced by trends in underlying causative factors. Over the past several decades, the incidence of oropharyngeal cancer has been rising dramatically in many developed nations as a result of an increase in HPV-related tumors. In contrast, trends in the incidence of oral cavity cancer largely coincide with tobacco use trends. For example, in the United States, declining oral cancer incidence over the past two decades mirrors declining smoking rates.

The risk for oral cancer is greater among males than females and generally increases with age. Approximately 90% of oral/pharyngeal cancers are diagnosed in patients older than 40 years, and >50% of cases occur in patients older than 65 years. However, among oropharyngeal squamous cell carcinomas, HPV-related tumors tend to occur in somewhat younger patients compared to non–HPV-related tumors (mean age difference, approximately 5 to 10 years). In addition, in the United States and other Western countries, an increased frequency of oral tongue cancer has been noted among adults <40 years—especially young adult females with no history of smoking or alcohol use.

The clinical presentation of intraoral squamous cell carcinoma varies. In the Western world, frequently involved subsites include the tongue (especially the lateral and ventrolateral aspects) and floor of the mouth. In contrast, in areas of the world where betel quid use is prevalent, the most frequently involved subsites are the tongue and buccal mucosa. During early stages of disease, many patients are asymptomatic. However, with disease progression, the patient may develop pain, paresthesia, and cervical lymphadenopathy. Upon examination, the lesion can appear white, red, and/or normal in color, and any of the following clinical patterns may be evident: *leukoplakia* (white plaque), *erythroplakia* (red plaque), *erythroleukoplakia* (red and white plaque), *exophytic growth* (fungating, papillary, or verruciform mass, often with induration and surface ulceration), and *endophytic growth* (central ulceration with a raised, "rolled" border). Endophytic lesions can mimic a traumatic granuloma or deep fungal infection. Upon radiographic examination, lesions that have invaded the underlying bone may exhibit significant resorption, often with a "moth-eaten," ill-defined, or ragged appearance.

Squamous cell carcinomas of the lip vermilion tend to develop in fair-skinned individuals with a history of chronic sun exposure. The lower lip is affected much more often than the upper lip. Clinical examination often shows a crusted, indurated lesion with associated ulceration. Lip vermilion tumors tend to grow relatively slowly, and regional metastasis (typically to the submental region) is usually a late event. In some cases, perineural invasion may result in extension of the tumor into the mandible via the mental foramen.

Oropharyngeal squamous cell carcinomas may involve the tonsillar region, base of tongue, soft palate, and/or posterior pharyngeal wall. Among HPV-related cases, the tonsillar region and base of tongue are favored subsites. Clinical signs and symptoms of oropharyngeal cancer may include persistent sore throat, dysphagia, odynophagia, and cervical lymphadenopathy. In particular, HPV-related oropharyngeal squamous cell carcinomas exhibit a propensity for regional metastasis, even though the primary tumor may be small or undetectable. In some cases, the patient initially presents for evaluation of an enlarged cervical lymph node, which may be treated at first with antibiotics. However, if the lesion does not resolve within 2 weeks, then referral for fine-needle aspiration and further evaluation should be considered.

In general, the clinical management of oral and oropharyngeal squamous cell carcinoma is guided by tumor stage. Lip vermilion cancers often are diagnosed at an early stage and treated by wedge resection. Resectable intraoral tumors typically are treated by surgery, which may be combined with radiation therapy, chemotherapy, and/or targeted agents. Oropharyngeal squamous cell carcinomas detected at an early stage may be managed by either surgery or definitive radiation therapy; however, more advanced tumors typically require various combinations of surgery, radiation therapy, chemotherapy, and/or targeted agents. Among oropharyngeal squamous cell carcinomas, HPV-positive lesions tend to exhibit better responses to chemotherapy and/or radiation therapy and more favorable patient outcomes compared to HPV-negative lesions; accordingly, clinical trials evaluating less intensive treatment regimens for HPV-related oropharyngeal squamous cell carcinoma are an active area of investigation.

In the United States, the overall 5-year relative survival rate for patients with oral and pharyngeal cancers is approximately 67%. Because most lip vermilion tumors are diagnosed at an early stage, the overall 5-year relative survival rate for lip tumors is excellent (approximately 88%). In contrast, intraoral and oropharyngeal cancers tend to be diagnosed at later stages, with lower 5-year relative survival rates (61% for floor-of-mouth lesions, 69% for tongue lesions, and 73% for oropharyngeal lesions).

■ Figure **10.50**
Oral Squamous Cell Carcinoma
Ulcerated, crusted nodule on the lower lip vermilion.

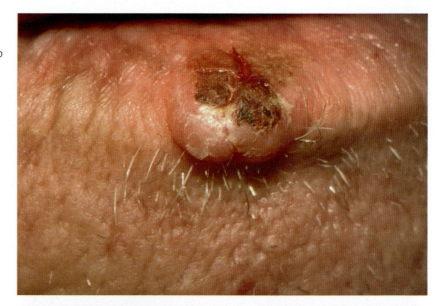

■ Figure **10.51**
Oral Squamous Cell Carcinoma
Crusted, white lesions on the lower lip vermilion. The patient was receiving immunosuppressive therapy for bone marrow transplantation.

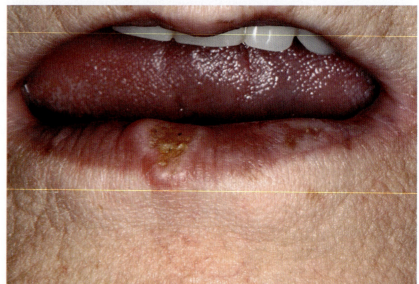

■ Figure **10.52**
Oral Squamous Cell Carcinoma
After 6 weeks, the lower lip lesions depicted in Fig. 10.51 exhibited enlargement and ulceration.

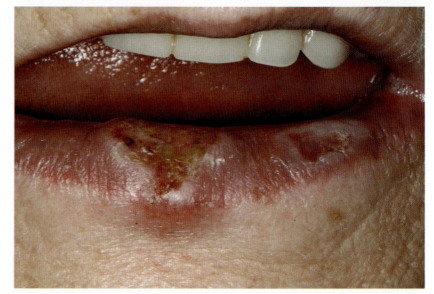

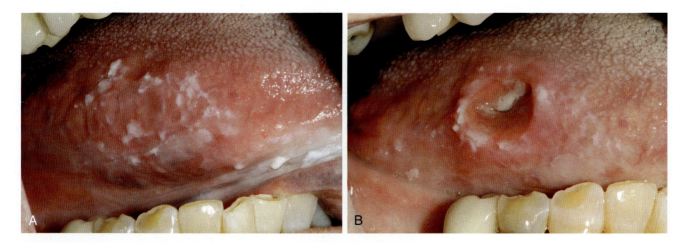

■ Figure **10.53**
Oral Squamous Cell Carcinoma Developing in Leukoplakia
(A) Ill-defined, extensive white plaque on the right lateral and ventral tongue. A biopsy showed hyperkeratosis with moderate epithelial dysplasia. Because of the patient's poor overall health, further surgical management was deferred, and the patient was placed on regular periodic recall. (B) After 1 year, the lesion transformed into squamous cell carcinoma. The tumor exhibited an ulcerated, endophytic crater.

■ Figure **10.54**
Oral Squamous Cell Carcinoma
Erythematous mass on the right ventrolateral tongue in a 20-year-old male. A suture from the biopsy can be seen. (With appreciation to Dr. Terry Day.)

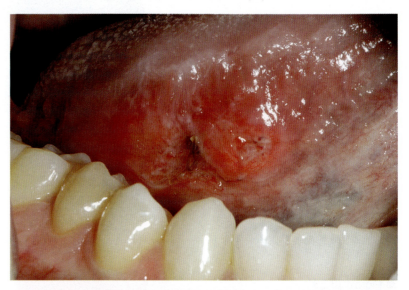

■ Figure **10.55**
Oral Squamous Cell Carcinoma
Extensive, ill-defined leukoplakia on the left ventrolateral tongue with focal erythema.

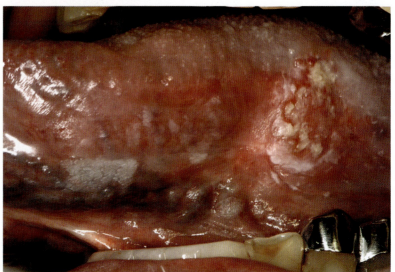

■ Figure **10.56**
Oral Squamous Cell Carcinoma
Right ventrolateral tongue showing an erythematous mass with focal ulceration.

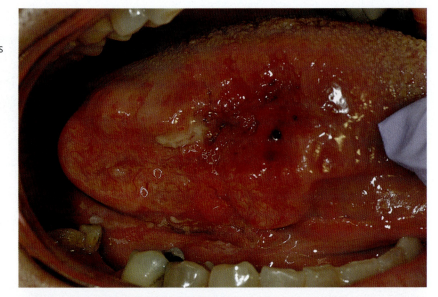

■ Figure **10.57**
Oral Squamous Cell Carcinoma
Extensive mass involving much of the tongue.

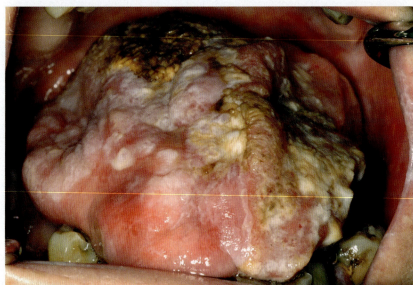

■ Figure **10.58**
Human Papillomavirus–Related Oropharyngeal Squamous Cell Carcinoma
Ulcerated, erythematous lesion involving the right tonsillar region.

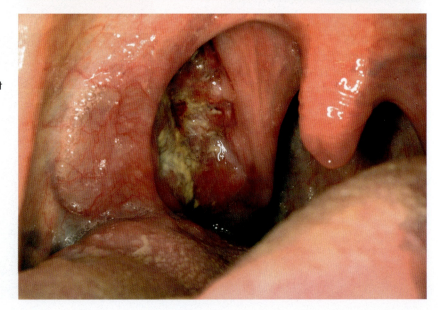

■ Figure **10.59**
Oral Squamous Cell Carcinoma
Floor of the mouth exhibiting ulceration and erythema.

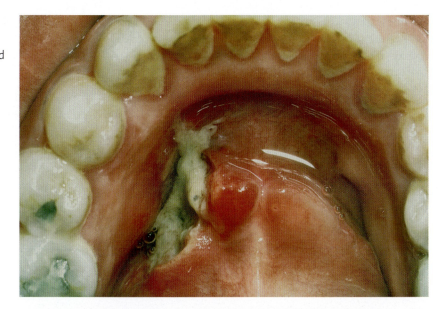

■ Figure **10.60**
Oral Squamous Cell Carcinoma
White mass with a rough, irregular surface on the lower alveolar ridge and floor of the mouth.

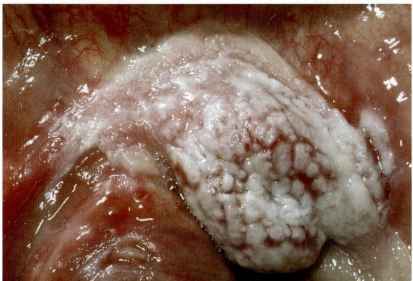

■ Figure **10.61**
Oral Squamous Cell Carcinoma
Extensive mass involving the right buccal mucosa, mandibular vestibule, and mandibular ridge. The patient was a long-time user of chewing tobacco. (With appreciation to Dr. Terry Day.)

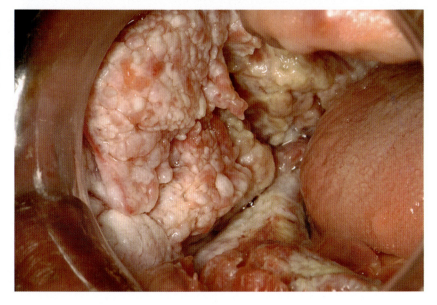

■ Figure **10.62**
Oral Squamous Cell Carcinoma
Anterior maxillary facial gingiva showing a white and red mass with an irregular surface. (With appreciation to Dr. Terry Day.)

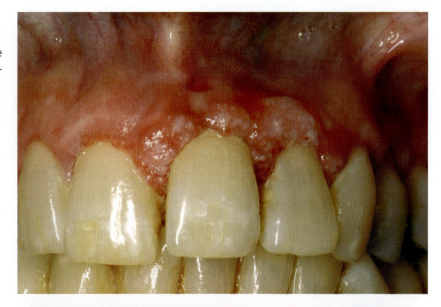

■ Figure **10.63**
Oral Squamous Cell Carcinoma
Palatal aspect of the same lesion depicted in Fig. 10.62. (With appreciation to Dr. Terry Day.)

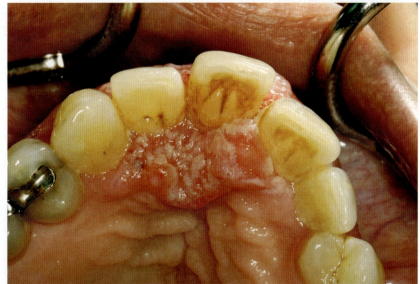

■ Figure **10.64**
Oral Squamous Cell Carcinoma
Erythematous, ulcerated mass involving the mandibular alveolar ridge and vestibule.

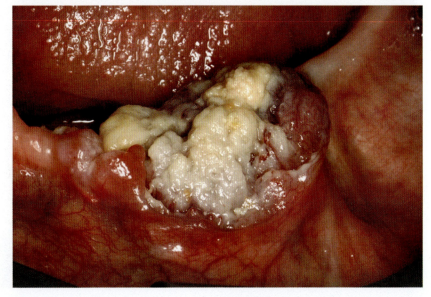

■ Figure **10.65**
Oral Squamous Cell Carcinoma
Erythematous mass involving the floor of the mouth and mandibular alveolar ridge.

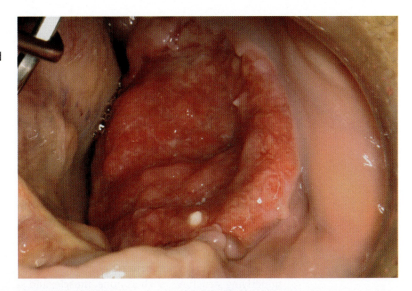

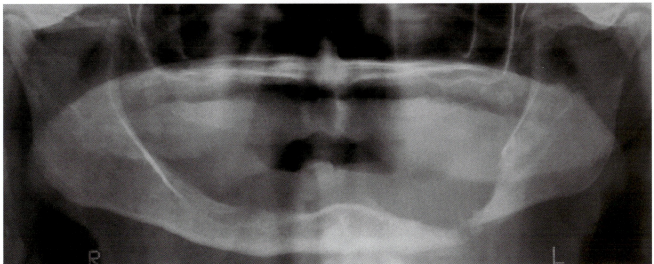

■ Figure **10.66**
Oral Squamous Cell Carcinoma
Panoramic radiograph of the same patient depicted in Fig. 10.65. The tumor invaded the mandible, resulting in pathologic fracture.

■ Figure **10.67**
Oropharyngeal Squamous Cell Carcinoma
Right cervical lymph node enlargement caused by metastatic carcinoma from the base of the tongue. (With appreciation to Dr. Terry Day.)

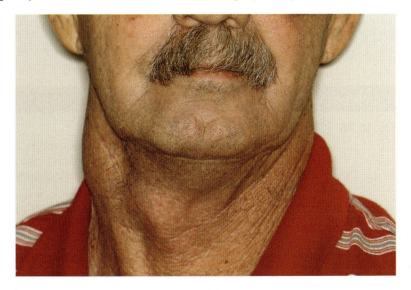

Verrucous Carcinoma

Fig. **10.68**

Verrucous carcinoma is a low-grade variant of squamous cell carcinoma and comprises approximately 2% to 12% of all oral carcinomas. This tumor variant most commonly arises in the oral cavity but also can occur in other sites (e.g., larynx, oropharynx, sinonasal region, anogenital region). It is characterized by a warty clinical appearance, tendency for slow growth, and locally aggressive behavior. Although the exact etiopathogenesis is unclear, studies have demonstrated associations with tobacco (both inhaled and smokeless), alcohol, and/or betel quid use. Human papillomavirus (HPV) has been found in a minority of head and neck verrucous carcinomas, but current evidence does not support HPV-driven tumorigenesis.

In the oral cavity, verrucous carcinoma most often develops in older males. Frequently involved subsites include the mandibular vestibule, buccal mucosa, gingiva, and tongue. Clinical examination typically shows a plaque-like or exophytic mass with a warty, papillary, or pebbly surface. Most examples are white, although some tumors may appear pink or erythematous. The tumor tends to grow slowly and may be present for several years before the diagnosis is established. When left untreated, the lesion can destroy underlying structures, such as bone, muscle, and salivary glands.

Oral verrucous carcinoma usually is treated by surgical excision. Metastasis is rare, and the 5-year survival rate is >80% for patients with localized disease. However, it is possible for conventional squamous cell carcinoma to arise within a verrucous carcinoma; for such "hybrid tumors," more aggressive therapy typically is indicated.

Spindle Cell Carcinoma (Sarcomatoid Carcinoma, Carcinosarcoma)

Fig. **10.69**

Spindle cell carcinoma represents a rare variant of squamous cell carcinoma, characterized by spindled tumor cells that simulate a sarcoma but are epithelial in nature. The tumor can arise anywhere within the upper aerodigestive tract, with a predilection for the larynx and oral cavity. Risk factors for spindle cell carcinoma of the upper aerodigestive tract include tobacco use, alcohol consumption, and previous radiotherapy.

Spindle cell carcinoma exhibits a predilection for older adult males, with a peak in the fifth and sixth decades. Within the oral cavity, frequently involved sites include the tongue, gingiva/alveolar mucosa, buccal mucosa, floor of the mouth, and lip. The patient may complain of swelling, pain, paresthesia, persistent ulceration, or bleeding. Clinical examination often shows an exophytic, polypoid mass with a smooth, ulcerated surface. Based on its clinical appearance, sometimes the tumor may be mistaken for a fibroma or other benign lesion. Microscopic examination exhibits a proliferation of invasive spindle cells, typically accompanied by a squamous epithelial component (consisting of dysplastic surface epithelium, carcinoma *in situ*, or conventional invasive squamous cell carcinoma).

Oral spindle cell carcinomas usually are treated by surgical resection, alone or combined with radiotherapy. Spindle cell carcinoma generally exhibits a worse prognosis than conventional squamous cell carcinoma. Although reported survival rates vary, one recent study based on epidemiologic data from the United States reported 5-year disease-specific survival of 39% for spindle cell carcinoma of the oral cavity.

Carcinoma of the Maxillary Sinus

Fig. **10.70**

Only about 3% to 5% of head and neck cancers arise from the sinonasal tract. Among paranasal sinus cancers, the majority (70% to 80%) develop in the antrum. In this location, the most common malignant tumor type is squamous cell carcinoma. In addition, various other carcinomas can occur in the maxillary sinus, such as salivary gland-type adenocarcinomas, sinonasal adenocarcinomas, and sinonasal undifferentiated carcinoma. The etiology of paranasal sinus carcinomas is not well understood and varies by tumor type. Contributory factors may include occupational exposures (e.g., to wood and leather dust), cigarette smoking, preexisting sinonasal papilloma, and high-risk human papillomavirus (HPV) infection.

Squamous cell carcinomas of the maxillary sinus exhibit a predilection for older adult males. In many cases, the patient remains asymptomatic until the tumor has reached a considerable size and has begun to invade adjacent structures. At initial presentation, sinonasal obstruction is a common complaint. Other clinical findings may include swelling, tooth mobility, pain, paresthesia, proptosis, diplopia, and trismus. Radiographic examination may show a cloudy sinus with destruction of the surrounding bone. Most

■ Figure **10.68**
Verrucous Carcinoma
Large, exophytic, warty mass on the buccal and labial mucosa.

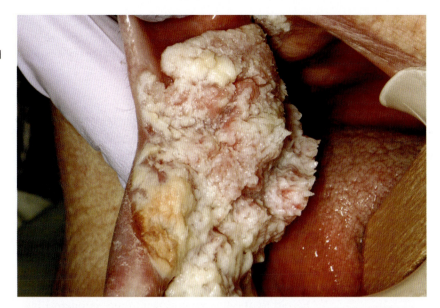

■ Figure **10.69**
Spindle Cell Carcinoma
Lingual mandibular gingiva showing a polypoid, nodular mass with a smooth surface. (Courtesy Dr. Michael Kolodychak.)

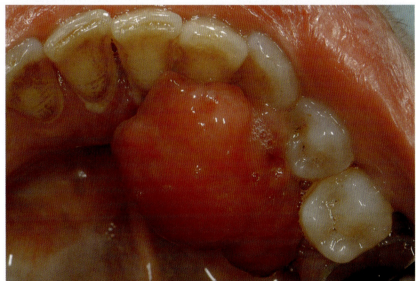

■ Figure **10.70**
Carcinoma of the Maxillary Sinus
This patient had a squamous cell carcinoma that arose in the maxillary sinus and produced this bulging, ulcerated mass of the maxillary alveolar ridge.

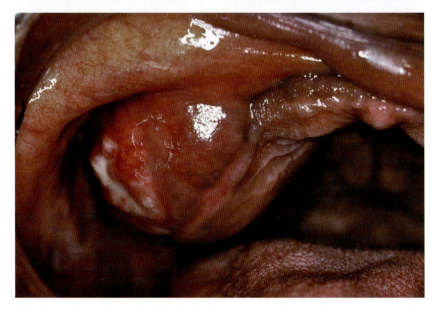

patients have advanced (stage III or IV) disease at diagnosis. Treatment depends on tumor stage but typically consists of surgical resection with postoperative radiotherapy. The overall 5-year survival rate for patients with squamous cell carcinoma of the paranasal sinuses is approximately 30%.

Basal Cell Carcinoma

Figs. **10.71–10.73**

Basal cell carcinoma is a locally invasive, epithelial malignancy that arises from the basal cell layer of the skin and its appendages. It represents the most common form of skin cancer, as well as the most common type of cancer overall. The most important etiologic factor for basal cell carcinoma is ultraviolet light exposure—especially intermittent, intense sun exposure during childhood and adolescence. An increased risk for basal cell carcinoma has been associated with fair skin, severe sunburns and freckling during childhood, a tendency to burn rather than tan, proximity to the equator, tanning bed use, psoralen and ultraviolet A (PUVA) therapy, and certain photosensitizing medications. Additional risk factors include ionizing radiation exposure, immunosuppression, arsenic ingestion, and various genodermatoses (e.g., nevoid basal cell carcinoma syndrome, xeroderma pigmentosum, albinism, and Bazex–Dupré–Christol syndrome). The underlying molecular pathogenesis involves mutations in genes related to the sonic hedgehog signaling pathway and the *TP53* tumor suppressor gene.

Clinically, basal cell carcinoma predominantly arises in sun-exposed areas of the skin, with about 80% of cases occurring in the head and neck region. The lesion tends to develop in older individuals, although it can occur over a broad age range. Men are affected more often than women. There are several clinico-pathologic variants. The *nodular (noduloulcerative) variant* is most common and accounts for about 50% to 79% of basal cell carcinomas. It presents as a slowly enlarging papule or nodule with central ulceration ("rodent ulcer") and raised, rolled borders. Crusting, periodic bleeding, associated telangiectasias, and a pearly opalescent appearance are frequent findings. Commonly involved sites include the cheeks, nasolabial folds, and forehead. Sometimes a noduloulcerative tumor can become colonized by melanocytes and exhibit spotty areas of brown to black pigmentation; such lesions have been termed the *pigmented variant*. The *superficial variant* comprises about 15% of cases and typically appears as a well-circumscribed, scaly, erythematous-pink macule or patch. This variant is unusual in that it favors the trunk and extremities. Multifocal involvement is possible, and the lesions may mimic an inflammatory condition (such as eczema or psoriasis). The *morpheaform (sclerosing) variant* appears as an ill-defined, indurated, and ivory-colored plaque or depression, at times accompanied by telangiectasias, small crusts, or erosions. Because it may mimic a scar, delay in diagnosis is common.

Oral examples of basal cell carcinoma have been reported but are extremely rare. The diagnosis of basal cell carcinoma in the oral cavity is controversial. Some reported cases may represent misdiagnosed salivary or odontogenic neoplasms.

Cutaneous basal cell carcinomas with a low risk for recurrence usually are treated by surgical excision or electrodessication and curettage. Alternative treatment methods for superficial tumors with low risk for recurrence include topical agents (e.g., 5-fluorouracil, imiquimod), cryosurgery, and photodynamic therapy. Lesions with a high risk for recurrence often are managed by Mohs micrographic surgery (a procedure that entails staged resection under local anesthesia and frozen section evaluation of surgical margins). Features associated with increased recurrence among cutaneous basal cell carcinomas of the head and neck include the following: lesions >6 mm in diameter and occurring in the "H-zone" of the face (nose, ear, temple, and periorbital areas), lesions >1 cm and occurring in head and neck sites outside of the "H-zone," ill-defined clinical borders, aggressive growth pattern (e.g., morpheaform), perineural invasion, immunosuppression, site of prior radiotherapy, and recurrent lesions. Basal cell carcinomas exhibit an extremely low rate of metastasis (0.028% to 0.55%). Death potentially may result from direct extension into adjacent vital structures; however, mortality rarely is seen today because of early detection and improved treatment. Periodic clinical evaluation is important for patients with a history of basal cell carcinoma because they are at risk for developing additional primary nonmelanoma skin cancers.

■ Figure **10.71**
Basal Cell Carcinoma
Noduloulcerative lesion on the skin of the forehead. Note the central ulceration and raised, rolled borders with telangiectasias.

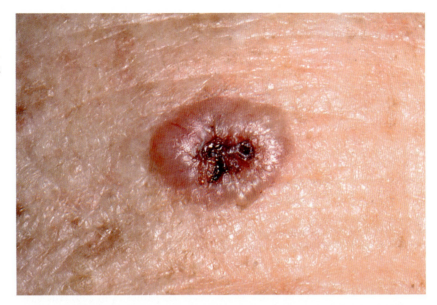

■ Figure **10.72**
Basal Cell Carcinoma
Noduloulcerative lesion with pigmentation.

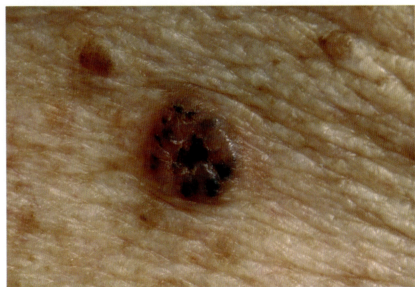

■ Figure **10.73**
Basal Cell Carcinoma
Ulcerated lesion that arose from the skin behind the right ear.

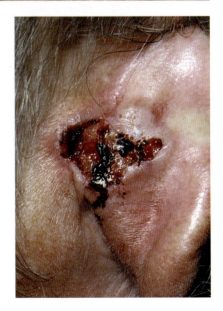

Figs. **10.74–10.76**

Melanoma represents a malignant neoplasm of melanocytic origin. It predominantly arises on the skin, although mucosal lesions rarely occur. This neoplasm represents the third most common skin cancer, and its incidence has been increasing in many parts of the world over the past several decades. In the United States, epidemiologic data for 2005 through 2014 shows increasing annual incidence among older individuals but stable or decreasing annual incidence among those younger than 50 years. Although melanoma is not nearly as common as basal cell carcinoma and squamous cell carcinoma of the skin, it is responsible for the vast majority of deaths due to skin cancer. In the United States, the American Cancer Society estimates that in 2018 that there will be >91,000 newly diagnosed cases of melanoma and >9000 melanoma-related deaths.

Cutaneous melanoma primarily is caused by ultraviolet radiation exposure. Risk factors include a history of sunburns, psoralen and ultraviolet A (PUVA) treatment, tanning bed use, a personal or family history of melanoma, a large number (>100) of melanocytic nevi, and a history of dysplastic or atypical nevi. Cutaneous melanoma most often arises in fair-complexioned, white adults. In the United States, the lifetime risk of developing melanoma is estimated to be 2.5% for whites (1 in 40), 0.1% for blacks (1 in 1000), and 0.5% for Hispanics (1 in 200). The lesion occurs over a broad age range, with most cases diagnosed in individuals >50 years old. The most common primary sites are the back for men and the lower extremities for women. Clinical examination often shows an asymmetric macule or nodule with irregular borders and color variegation. Many lesions appear brown or black, although some examples can appear gray, erythematous, or flesh-colored. Advanced tumors may exhibit ulceration and bleeding. Clinical features that may aid in distinguishing melanoma from a benign melanocytic nevus include the "ABCDE" criteria (*A*symmetry, *B*order irregularity, *C*olor variegation, *D*iameter >6 mm, *E*volution in size/shape/color or a "mole" that looks different from the rest). These criteria are designed to help the layperson or primary care practitioner detect pigmented lesions that warrant further evaluation by a dermatologist. Major clinicopathologic subtypes of cutaneous melanoma include *superficial spreading, nodular, lentigo maligna*, and *acral lentiginous*. These subtypes differ in their propensity for radial (i.e., horizontally spreading) versus vertical (i.e., deeply invasive) growth. Clinical management of cutaneous melanoma is guided by tumor staging. Wide excision is the mainstay of therapy. Sentinel lymph node biopsy, lymph node dissection, adjuvant immunotherapy, targeted agents, and radiation therapy also may be considered. Five-year survival rates for patients with cutaneous melanomas that are thin and confined to the skin are >90%, whereas patients with regional or distant metastasis exhibit 5-year survival rates of approximately 40% to 78% and 15% to 20%, respectively.

Primary oral mucosal melanoma accounts for <1% of all melanomas, and its etiology is uncertain. The lesion can occur over a broad age range, with a mean age of approximately 68 years. Most authors report either a slight male predilection or an even gender distribution, and patients of any race can be affected. The most commonly involved subsites are the hard palate and maxillary gingiva. Clinical examination often shows a flat or nodular lesion with brown to black pigmentation and ill-defined, irregular borders. In addition, some examples may appear gray, blue, erythematous, white, or pink. Color variegation often is noted within an individual lesion. Hemorrhage and ulceration also are possible, especially in more advanced tumors. Occasionally, there is multifocal involvement due to satellite tumor formation. In many cases, cervical lymph node metastasis is evident at initial presentation. Clinical management of oral mucosal melanoma depends on tumor stage. The mainstay of treatment is wide resection. Lymph node dissection, postoperative radiotherapy, and systemic therapy (e.g., interferon, interleukin, c-kit inhibitors) also may be considered. The overall prognosis is poor, with a mean survival of approximately 28 months.

■ Figure **10.74**
Melanoma
Pigmented skin lesion exhibiting asymmetry, border irregularity, color variegation, and diameter >6 mm.

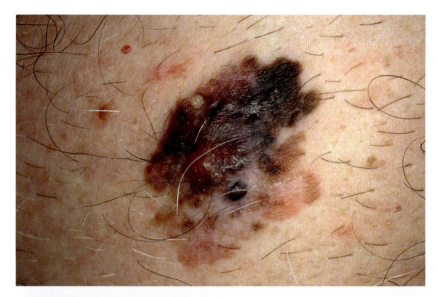

■ Figure **10.75**
Melanoma
Ill-defined, splotchy, gray-brown pigmentation of the palate.

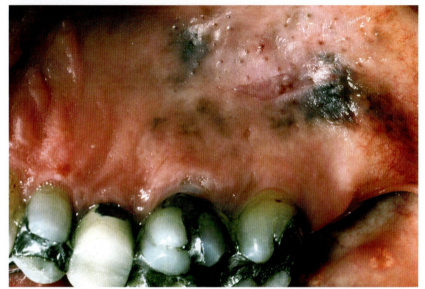

■ Figure **10.76**
Melanoma
Maxillary gingiva showing an extensive pigmented mass with an exophytic, nodular component. (Courtesy Dr. Neetha Santosh.)

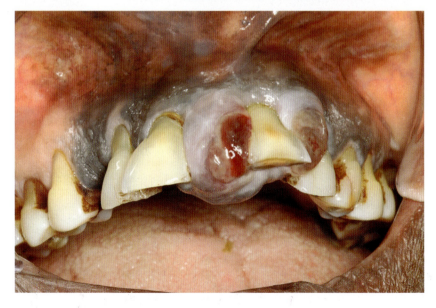

Bibliography

Squamous Papilloma

Abbey LM, Page DG, Sawyer DR. The clinical and histopathologic features of a series of 464 oral squamous cell papillomas. *Oral Surg Oral Med Oral Pathol*. 1980;49:419–428.

Carneiro TE, Marinho SA, Verli FD, et al. Oral squamous papilloma: clinical, histologic and immunohistochemical analyses. *J Oral Sci*. 2009;51:367–372.

Jones AV, Franklin CD. An analysis of oral and maxillofacial pathology found in adults over a 30-year period. *J Oral Pathol Med*. 2006;35:392–401.

Jones AV, Franklin CD. An analysis of oral and maxillofacial pathology found in children over a 30-year period. *Int J Paediatr Dent*. 2006;16:19–30.

Verruca Vulgaris

Green TL, Eversole LR, Leider AS. Oral and labial verruca vulgaris: clinical, histologic, and immunohistochemical evaluation. *Oral Surg Oral Med Oral Pathol*. 1986;62:410–416.

Kwok CS, Gibbs S, Bennett C, et al. Topical treatments for cutaneous warts. *Cochrane Database Syst Rev*. 2012;(9):CD001781.

Lynch MD, Cliffe J, Morris-Jones R. Management of cutaneous viral warts. *BMJ*. 2014;348:g3339.

Mulhem E, Pinelis S. Treatment of nongenital cutaneous warts. *Am Fam Physician*. 2011;84:288–293.

Condyloma Acuminatum

Grillo-Ardila CF, Angel-Müller E, Salazar-Díaz LC, et al. Imiquimod for anogenital warts in non-immunocompromised adults. *Cochrane Database Syst Rev*. 2014;(11):CD010389.

Kui LL, Xiu HZ, Ning LY. Condyloma acuminatum and human papilloma virus infection in the oral mucosa of children. *Pediatr Dent*. 2003;25:149–153.

Meites E, Kempe A, Markowitz LE. Use of a 2-dose schedule for human papillomavirus vaccination — updated recommendations of the Advisory Committee on Immunization Practices. *MMWR Morb Mortal Wkly Rep*. 2016;65:1405–1408.

Park IU, Introcaso C, Dunne EF. Human papillomavirus and genital warts: a review of the evidence for the 2015 Centers for Disease Control and Prevention sexually transmitted diseases treatment guidelines. *Clin Infect Dis*. 2015;61(suppl 8):S849–S855.

Multifocal Epithelial Hyperplasia

Feller L, Khammissa RA, Wood NH, et al. Focal epithelial hyperplasia (Heck disease) related to highly active antiretroviral therapy in an HIV-seropositive child. A report of a case, and a review of the literature. *SADJ*. 2010;65:172–175.

Khanal S, Cole ET, Joh J, et al. Human papillomavirus detection in histologic samples of multifocal epithelial hyperplasia: a novel demographic presentation. *Oral Surg Oral Med Oral Pathol Oral Radiol*. 2015;120:733–743.

Ledesma-Montes C, Vega-Memije E, Garcés-Ortíz M, et al. Multifocal epithelial hyperplasia. Report of nine cases. *Med Oral Patol Oral Cir Bucal*. 2005;10:394–401.

Said AK, Leao JC, Fedele S, et al. Focal epithelial hyperplasia – an update. *J Oral Pathol Med*. 2013;42:435–442.

Yasar S, Mansur AT, Serdar ZA, et al. Treatment of focal epithelial hyperplasia with topical imiquimod: report of three cases. *Pediatr Dermatol*. 2009;26:465–468.

Sinonasal Papillomas

Barnes L. Schneiderian papillomas and nonsalivary glandular neoplasms of the head and neck. *Mod Pathol*. 2002;15:279–297.

Barnes L, Tse LLY, Hunt JL. Schneiderian papillomas. In: El-Naggar AK, Chan JK, Grandis JR, et al, eds. *WHO Classification of Head and Neck Tumours*. 4th ed. Lyon: IARC; 2017:28–32.

Bullock MJ. Low-grade epithelial proliferations of the sinonasal tract. *Head Neck Pathol*. 2016;10:47–59.

Kaufman MR, Brandwein MS, Lawson W. Sinonasal papillomas: clinicopathologic review of 40 patients with inverted and oncocytic schneiderian papillomas. *Laryngoscope*. 2002;112:1372–1377.

Leoncini G, Zanetti L. The papillomas of the sinonasal tract. A comprehensive review. *Pathologica*. 2017;109:31–34.

Vorasubin N, Vira D, Suh JD, et al. Schneiderian papillomas: comparative review of exophytic, oncocytic, and inverted types. *Am J Rhinol Allergy*. 2013;27:287–292.

Molluscum Contagiosum

de Carvalho CH, de Andrade AL, de Oliveira DH, et al. Intraoral molluscum contagiosum in a young immunocompetent patient. *Oral Surg Oral Med Oral Pathol Oral Radiol*. 2012;114:e57–e60.

Leung AKC, Barankin B, Hon KLE. Molluscum contagiosum: an update. *Recent Pat Inflamm Allergy Drug Discov*. 2017;11:22–31.

Nguyen HP, Franz E, Stiegel KR, et al. Treatment of molluscum contagiosum in adult, pediatric, and immunodeficient populations. *J Cutan Med Surg*. 2014;18:299–306.

Olsen JR, Gallacher J, Finlay AY, et al. Time to resolution and effect on quality of life of molluscum contagiosum in children in the UK: a prospective community cohort study. *Lancet Infect Dis*. 2015;15:190–195.

van der Wouden JC, van der Sande R, Kruithof EJ, et al. Interventions for cutaneous molluscum contagiosum. *Cochrane Database Syst Rev*. 2017;(5):CD004767.

Verruciform Xanthoma

de Andrade BA, Agostini M, Pires FR, et al. Oral verruciform xanthoma: a clinicopathologic and immunohistochemical study of 20 cases. *J Cutan Pathol*. 2015;42:489–495.

Philipsen HP, Reichart PA, Takata T, et al. Verruciform xanthoma—biological profile of 282 oral lesions based on a literature survey with nine new cases from Japan. *Oral Oncol*. 2003;39:325–336.

Yu CH, Tsai TC, Wang JT, et al. Oral verruciform xanthoma: a clinicopathologic study of 15 cases. *J Formos Med Assoc*. 2007;106:141–147.

Seborrheic Keratosis

Hafner C, Vogt T. Seborrheic keratosis. *J Dtsch Dermatol Ges*. 2008;6:664–677.

Jackson JM, Alexis A, Berman B, et al. Current understanding of seborrheic keratosis: prevalence, etiology, clinical presentation, diagnosis, and management. *J Drugs Dermatol*. 2015;14:1119–1125.

Noiles K, Vender R. Are all seborrheic keratoses benign? Review of the typical lesion and its variants. *J Cutan Med Surg*. 2008;12:203–210.

Dermatosis Papulosa Nigra

Hafner C, Vogt T. Seborrheic keratosis. *J Dtsch Dermatol Ges*. 2008;6:664–677.

Kundu RV, Patterson S. Dermatologic conditions in skin of color: part II. Disorders occurring predominantly in skin of color. *Am Fam Physician*. 2013;87:859–865.

Metin SA, Lee BW, Lambert WC, et al. Dermatosis papulosa nigra: a clinically and histopathologically distinct entity. *Clin Dermatol*. 2017;35:491–496.

Sebaceous Hyperplasia

Azevedo RS, Almeida OP, Netto JN, et al. Comparative clinicopathological study of intraoral sebaceous hyperplasia and sebaceous adenoma. *Oral Surg Oral Med Oral Pathol Oral Radiol Endod*. 2009;107:100–104.

Daley TD. Intraoral sebaceous hyperplasia. Diagnostic criteria. *Oral Surg Oral Med Oral Pathol S*. 1993;75:343–347.

Eisen DB, Michael DJ. Sebaceous lesions and their associated syndromes: part I. *J Am Acad Dermatol*. 2009;61:549–560.

Oral Melanotic Macule

Buchner A, Merrell PW, Carpenter WM. Relative frequency of solitary melanocytic lesions of the oral mucosa. *J Oral Pathol Med*. 2004;33:550–557.

Kahn MA, Weathers DR, Hoffman JG. Transformation of a benign oral pigmentation to primary oral melanoma. *Oral Surg Oral Med Oral Pathol Oral Radiol Endod.* 2005;100:454–459.

Kaugars GE, Heise AP, Riley WT, et al. Oral melanotic macules. A review of 353 cases. *Oral Surg Oral Med Oral Pathol.* 1993;76:59–61.

Shen ZY, Liu W, Bao ZX, et al. Oral melanotic macule and primary oral malignant melanoma: epidemiology, location involved, and clinical implications. *Oral Surg Oral Med Oral Pathol Oral Radiol Endod.* 2011;112:e21–e25.

Laugier-Hunziker Syndrome

Nayak RS, Kotrashetti VS, Hosmani JV. Laugier-Hunziker syndrome. *J Oral Maxillofac Pathol.* 2012;16:245–250.

Nikitakis NG, Koumaki D. Laugier-Hunziker syndrome: case report and review of the literature. *Oral Surg Oral Med Oral Pathol Oral Radiol.* 2013;116:e52–e58.

Wang WM, Wang X, Duan N, et al. Laugier-Hunziker syndrome: a report of three cases and literature review. *Int J Oral Sci.* 2012;4:226–230.

Wei Z, Li GY, Ruan HH, et al. Laugier-Hunziker syndrome: a case report. *J Stomatol Oral Maxillofac Surg.* 2017;doi:10.1016/j.jormas.2017.12.003. [Epub ahead of print].

Oral Melanoacanthoma

Cantudo-Sanagustín E, Gutiérrez-Corrales A, Vigo-Martínez M, et al. Pathogenesis and clinicohistopathological characteristics of melanoacanthoma: a systematic review. *J Clin Exp Dent.* 2016;8:e327–e336.

das Chagas E, Silva de Carvalho LF, Farina VH, et al. Immunohistochemical features of multifocal melanoacanthoma in the hard palate: a case report. *BMC Res Notes.* 2013;6:30.

Fornatora ML, Reich RF, Haber S, et al. Oral melanoacanthoma: a report of 10 cases, review of the literature, and immunohistochemical analysis for HMB-45 reactivity. *Am J Dermatopathol.* 2003;25:12–15.

Yarom N, Hirshberg A, Buchner A. Solitary and multifocal oral melanoacanthoma. *Int J Dermatol.* 2007;46:1232–1236.

Ephelides

Hernando B, Ibañez MV, Deserio-Cuesta JA, et al. Genetic determinants of freckle occurrence in the Spanish population: towards ephelides prediction from human DNA samples. *Forensic Sci Int Genet.* 2017;33:38–47.

Plensdorf S, Martinez J. Common pigmentation disorders. *Am Fam Physician.* 2009;79:109–116.

Actinic Lentigines

Byrom L, Barksdale S, Weedon D, et al. Unstable solar lentigo: a defined separate entity. *Australas J Dermatol.* 2016;57:229–234.

Ortonne JP, Pandya AG, Lui H, et al. Treatment of solar lentigines. *J Am Acad Dermatol.* 2006;54(5 suppl 2):S262–S271.

Plensdorf S, Martinez J. Common pigmentation disorders. *Am Fam Physician.* 2009;79:109–116.

Melanocytic Nevus

Buchner A, Hansen LS. Pigmented nevi of the oral mucosa: a clinicopathologic study of 36 new cases and review of 155 cases from the literature. Part I: a clinicopathologic study of 36 new cases. *Oral Surg Oral Med Oral Pathol.* 1987;63:566–572.

Buchner A, Hansen LS. Pigmented nevi of the oral mucosa: a clinicopathologic study of 36 new cases and review of 155 cases from the literature. Part II: analysis of 191 cases. *Oral Surg Oral Med Oral Pathol.* 1987;63:676–682.

Buchner A, Leider AS, Merrell PW, et al. Melanocytic nevi of the oral mucosa: a clinicopathologic study of 130 cases from northern California. *J Oral Pathol Med.* 1990;19:197–201.

Buchner A, Merrell PW, Carpenter WM. Relative frequency of solitary melanocytic lesions of the oral mucosa. *J Oral Pathol Med.* 2004;33:550–557.

Ferreira L, Jham B, Assi R, et al. Oral melanocytic nevi: a clinicopathologic study of 100 cases. *Oral Surg Oral Med Oral Pathol Oral Radiol.* 2015;120:358–367.

Meleti M, Vescovi P, Mooi WJ, et al. Pigmented lesions of the oral mucosa and perioral tissues: a flow-chart for the diagnosis and some recommendations for the management. *Oral Surg Oral Med Oral Pathol Oral Radiol Endod.* 2008;105:606–616.

Blue Nevus

Ojha J, Akers JL, Akers JO, et al. Intraoral cellular blue nevus: report of a unique histopathologic entity and review of the literature. *Cutis.* 2007;80:189–192.

Ferreira L, Jham B, Assi R, et al. Oral melanocytic nevi: a clinicopathologic study of 100 cases. *Oral Surg Oral Med Oral Pathol Oral Radiol.* 2015;120:358–367.

Phadke PA, Zembowicz A. Blue nevi and related tumors. *Clin Lab Med.* 2011;31:345–458.

Shumway BS, Rawal YB, Allen CM, et al. Oral atypical cellular blue nevus: an infiltrative melanocytic proliferation. *Head Neck Pathol.* 2013;7:171–177.

Alveolar Ridge Keratosis

Bellato L, Martinelli-Kläy CP, Martinelli CR, et al. Alveolar ridge keratosis—a retrospective clinicopathological study. *Head Face Med.* 2013;9:12.

Chi AC, Lambert PR 3rd, Pan Y, et al. Is alveolar ridge keratosis a true leukoplakia?: A clinicopathologic comparison of 2,153 lesions. *J Am Dent Assoc.* 2007;138:641–651.

Natarajan E, Woo SB. Benign alveolar ridge keratosis (oral lichen simplex chronicus): a distinct clinicopathologic entity. *J Am Acad Dermatol.* 2008;58:151–157.

Nicotine Stomatitis

Bardellini E, Amadori F, Conti G, et al. Oral mucosal lesions in electronic cigarettes consumers versus former smokers. *Acta Odontol Scand.* 2017;1–3. [Epub ahead of print].

dos Santos RB, Katz J. Nicotinic stomatitis: positive correlation with heat in maté tea drinks and smoking. *Quintessence Int.* 2009;40:537–540.

Rossie KM, Guggenheimer J. Thermally induced 'nicotine' stomatitis. A case report. *Oral Surg Oral Med Oral Pathol.* 1990;70:597–599.

Taybos G. Oral changes associated with tobacco use. *Am J Med Sci.* 2003;326:179–182.

Leukoplakia

Chi AC, Day TA, Neville BW. Oral cavity and oropharyngeal squamous cell carcinoma–an update. *CA Cancer J Clin.* 2015;65:401–421.

Lingen MW, Abt E, Agrawal N, et al. Evidence-based clinical practice guideline for the evaluation of potentially malignant disorders in the oral cavity: a report of the American Dental Association. *J Am Dent Assoc.* 2017;148:712–727.

Lodi G, Franchini R, Warnakulasuriya S, et al. Interventions for treating oral leukoplakia to prevent oral cancer. *Cochrane Database Syst Rev.* 2016;(7):CD001829.

Nadeau C, Kerr AR. Evaluation and management of oral potentially malignant disorders. *Dent Clin North Am.* 2018;62:1–27.

Warnakulasuriya S, Ariyawardana A. Malignant transformation of oral leukoplakia: a systematic review of observational studies. *J Oral Pathol Med.* 2016;45:155–166.

Proliferative Verrucous Leukoplakia

Akrish S, Ben-Izhak O, Sabo E, et al. Oral squamous cell carcinoma associated with proliferative verrucous leukoplakia compared with conventional squamous cell carcinoma–a clinical, histologic and immunohistochemical study. *Oral Surg Oral Med Oral Pathol Oral Radiol.* 2015;119:318–325.

Capella DL, Gonçalves JM, Abrantes AAA, et al. Proliferative verrucous leukoplakia: diagnosis, management and current advances. *Braz J Otorhinolaryngol.* 2017;83:585–593.

Carrard VC, Brouns ER, van der Waal I. Proliferative verrucous leukoplakia; a critical appraisal of the diagnostic criteria. *Med Oral Patol Oral Cir Bucal.* 2013;18:e411–e413.

Gillenwater AM, Vigneswaran N, Fatani H, et al. Proliferative verrucous leukoplakia (PVL): a review of an elusive pathologic entity! *Adv Anat Pathol.* 2013;20:416–423.

Munde A, Karle R. Proliferative verrucous leukoplakia: an update. *J Cancer Res Ther.* 2016;12:469–473.

Erythroplakia

Nadeau C, Kerr AR. Evaluation and management of oral potentially malignant disorders. *Dent Clin North Am.* 2018;62:1–27.

Reichart PA, Philipsen HP. Oral erythroplakia–a review. *Oral Oncol.* 2005;41:551–561.

Shafer WG, Waldron CA. Erythroplakia of the oral cavity. *Cancer.* 1975;36:1021–1028.

Tobacco Pouch Keratosis

Chang JT, Levy DT, Meza R. Examining the transitions between cigarette and smokeless tobacco product use in the United States using the 2002-2003 and 2010-2011 longitudinal cohorts. *Nicotine Tob Res.* 2017;doi:10.1093/ntr/ntx251. [Epub ahead of print].

Greer RO Jr. Oral manifestations of smokeless tobacco use. *Otolaryngol Clin North Am.* 2011;44:31–56.

Substance Abuse and Mental Health Services Administration. *Results from the 2016 National Survey on Drug Use and Health: Detailed Tables.* Rockville, MD: Substance Abuse and Mental Health Services Administration; 2017. Available at: https://www.samhsa.gov/data/sites/default/files/NSDUH-DetTabs-2016/NSDUH-DetTabs-2016.htm#tab2-28A. Accessed January 4, 2018.

Taybos G. Oral changes associated with tobacco use. *Am J Med Sci.* 2003;326:179–182.

Oral Submucous Fibrosis

Angadi PV, Rekha KP. Oral submucous fibrosis: a clinicopathologic review of 205 cases in Indians. *Oral Maxillofac Surg.* 2011;15:15–19.

Arakeri G, Brennan PA. Oral submucous fibrosis: an overview of the aetiology, pathogenesis, classification, and principles of management. *Br J Oral Maxillofac Surg.* 2013;51:587–593.

Ray JG, Ranganathan K, Chattopadhyay A. Malignant transformation of oral submucous fibrosis: overview of histopathological aspects. *Oral Surg Oral Med Oral Pathol Oral Radiol.* 2016;122:200–209.

Tilakaratne WM, Ekanayaka RP, Warnakulasuriya S. Oral submucous fibrosis: a historical perspective and a review on etiology and pathogenesis. *Oral Surg Oral Med Oral Pathol Oral Radiol.* 2016;122:178–191.

Warnakulasuriya S, Kerr AR. Oral submucous fibrosis: a review of the current management and possible directions for novel therapies. *Oral Surg Oral Med Oral Pathol Oral Radiol.* 2016;122:232–241.

Actinic Cheilosis

Cavalcante AS, Anbinder AL, Carvalho YR. Actinic cheilitis: clinical and histological features. *J Oral Maxillofac Surg.* 2008;66:498–503.

Jadotte YT, Schwartz RA. Solar cheilosis: an ominous precursor: part I. Diagnostic insights. *J Am Acad Dermatol.* 2012;66:173–184.

Jadotte YT, Schwartz RA. Solar cheilosis: an ominous precursor: part II. Therapeutic perspectives. *J Am Acad Dermatol.* 2012;66:187–198.

Lopes ML, Silva Júnior FL, Lima KC, et al. Clinicopathological profile and management of 161 cases of actinic cheilitis. *An Bras Dermatol.* 2015;90:505–512.

Actinic Keratosis

Goldberg LH, Mamelak AJ. Review of actinic keratosis. Part I: etiology, epidemiology and clinical presentation. *J Drugs Dermatol.* 2010;9:1125–1132.

Rigel DS, Stein Gold LF. The importance of early diagnosis and treatment of actinic keratosis. *J Am Acad Dermatol.* 2013;68(1 suppl 1):S20–S27.

Rosen T, Lebwohl MG. Prevalence and awareness of actinic keratosis: barriers and opportunities. *J Am Acad Dermatol.* 2013;68(1 suppl 1):S2–S9.

Keratoacanthoma

Gleich T, Chiticariu E, Huber M, Hohl D. Keratoacanthoma: a distinct entity? *Exp Dermatol.* 2016;25:85–91.

Ko CJ. Keratoacanthoma: facts and controversies. *Clin Dermatol.* 2010;28:254–261.

Kwiek B, Schwartz RA. Keratoacanthoma (KA): an update and review. *J Am Acad Dermatol.* 2016;74:1220–1233.

Oral and Oropharyngeal Squamous Cell Carcinoma

Chaturvedi AK, Anderson WF, Lortet-Tieulent J, et al. Worldwide trends in incidence rates for oral cavity and oropharyngeal cancers. *J Clin Oncol.* 2013;31:4550–4559.

Chi AC, Day TA, Neville BW. Oral cavity and oropharyngeal squamous cell carcinoma–an update. *CA Cancer J Clin.* 2015;65:401–421.

Guha N, Warnakulasuriya S, Vlaanderen J, et al. Betel quid chewing and the risk of oral and oropharyngeal cancers: a meta-analysis with implications for cancer control. *Int J Cancer.* 2014;135:1433–1443.

Lingen MW, Xiao W, Schmitt A, et al. Low etiologic fraction for high-risk human papillomavirus in oral cavity squamous cell carcinomas. *Oral Oncol.* 2013;49:1–8.

Ndiaye C, Mena M, Alemany L, et al. HPV DNA, E6/E7 mRNA, and p16INK4a detection in head and neck cancers: a systematic review and meta-analysis. *Lancet Oncol.* 2014;15:1319–1331.

Rhodus NL, Kerr AR, Patel K. Oral cancer: leukoplakia, premalignancy, and squamous cell carcinoma. *Dent Clin North Am.* 2014;58:315–340.

Shield KD, Ferlay J, Jemal A, et al. The global incidence of lip, oral cavity, and pharyngeal cancers by subite in. *CA Cancer J Clin.* 2012;67:51–64, 2017.

Siegel RL, Miller KD, Jemal A. Cancer statistics, 2018. *CA Cancer J Clin.* 2018;68:7–30.

Surveillance Research Program, National Cancer Institute. Fast Stats: an interactive tool for access to SEER cancer statistics. Available at: https://seer.cancer.gov/faststats. Accessed February 5, 2018.

Taberna M, Mena M, Pavón MA, et al. Human papillomavirus-related oropharyngeal cancer. *Ann Oncol.* 2017;28:2386–2398.

Vigneswaran N, Williams MD. Epidemiologic trends in head and neck cancer and aids in diagnosis. *Oral Maxillofac Surg Clin North Am.* 2014;26:123–141.

Warnakulasuriya S. Global epidemiology of oral and oropharyngeal cancer. *Oral Oncol.* 2009;45:309–316.

Verrucous Carcinoma

Ackerman LV. Verrucous carcinoma of the oral cavity. *Surgery.* 1948;23:670–678.

Alonso JE, Kuan EC, Arshi A, et al. A population-based analysis of verrucous carcinoma of the oral cavity. *Laryngoscope.* 2018;128:393–397.

Koch BB, Trask DK, Hoffman HT, et al. Commission on Cancer, American College of Surgeons, American Cancer Society: National survey of head and neck verrucous carcinoma: patterns of presentation, care, and outcome. *Cancer.* 2001;92:110–120.

Patel KR, Chernock RD, Zhang TR, et al. Verrucous carcinomas of the head and neck, including those with associated squamous cell carcinoma, lack transcriptionally active high-risk human papillomavirus. *Hum Pathol.* 2013;44:2385–2392.

Peng Q, Wang Y, Quan H, et al. Oral verrucous carcinoma: from multifactorial etiology to diverse treatment regimens (review). *Int J Oncol.* 2016;49:59–73.

Spindle Cell Carcinoma

Bice TC, Tran V, Merkley MA, et al. Disease-specific survival with spindle cell carcinoma of the head and neck. *Otolaryngol Head Neck Surg.* 2015;153:973–980.

Ellis GL, Corio RL. Spindle cell carcinoma of the oral cavity. A clinicopathologic assessment of fifty-nine cases. *Oral Surg Oral Med Oral Pathol.* 1980;50:523–533.

Gerry D, Fritsch VA, Lentsch EJ. Spindle cell carcinoma of the upper aerodigestive tract: an analysis of 341 cases with comparison to conventional squamous cell carcinoma. *Ann Otol Rhinol Laryngol.* 2014;123:576–583.

Lewis JS Jr. Spindle cell lesions–neoplastic or non-neoplastic?: spindle cell carcinoma and other atypical spindle cell lesions of the head and neck. *Head Neck Pathol.* 2008;2:103–110.

Viswanathan S, Rahman K, Pallavi S, et al. Sarcomatoid (spindle cell) carcinoma of the head and neck mucosal region: a clinicopathologic review of 103 cases from a tertiary referral cancer centre. *Head Neck Pathol.* 2010;4:265–275.

Carcinoma of the Maxillary Sinus

Ansa B, Goodman M, Ward K, et al. Paranasal sinus squamous cell carcinoma incidence and survival based on Surveillance, Epidemiology, and End Results data, 1973 to 2009. *Cancer.* 2013;119:2602–2610.

Bossi P, Farina D, Gatta G, et al. Paranasal sinus cancer. *Crit Rev Oncol Hematol.* 2016;98:45–61.

Lewis JS Jr. Sinonasal squamous cell carcinoma: a review with emphasis on emerging histologic subtypes and the role of human papillomavirus. *Head Neck Pathol.* 2016;10:60–67.

Youlden DR, Cramb SM, Peters S, et al. International comparisons of the incidence and mortality of sinonasal cancer. *Cancer Epidemiol.* 2013;37:770–779.

Basal Cell Carcinoma

Bichakjian CK, Olencki T, Aasi SZ, et al. Basal cell skin cancer, version 1.2016, NCCN Clinical Practice Guidelines in Oncology. *J Natl Compr Canc Netw.* 2016;14:574–597.

Gandhi SA, Kampp J. Skin cancer epidemiology, detection, and management. *Med Clin North Am.* 2015;99:1323–1335.

Marzuka AG, Book SE. Basal cell carcinoma: pathogenesis, epidemiology, clinical features, diagnosis, histopathology, and management. *Yale J Biol Med.* 2015;88:167–179.

Shumway BS, Kalmar JR, Allen CM, et al. Basal cell carcinoma of the buccal mucosa in a patient with nevoid basal cell carcinoma syndrome. *Int J Surg Pathol.* 2011;19:348–354.

Melanoma

Aguas SC, Quarracino MC, Lence AN, et al. Primary melanoma of the oral cavity: ten cases and review of 177 cases from literature. *Med Oral Patol Oral Cir Bucal.* 2009;14:E265–E271.

American Academy of Dermatology Ad Hoc Task Force for the ABCDEs of Melanoma, Tsao H, Olazagasti JM, et al. Early detection of melanoma: reviewing the ABCDEs. *J Am Acad Dermatol.* 2015;72:717–723.

Haigentz M Jr, Strojan P, Pellitteri PK, et al. Update on primary head and neck mucosal melanoma. *Head Neck.* 2016;38:147–155.

Mohan M, Sukhadia VY, Pai D, et al. Oral malignant melanoma: systematic review of literature and report of two cases. *Oral Surg Oral Med Oral Pathol Oral Radiol.* 2013;116:e247–e254.

National Comprehensive Care Network. NCCN Clinical Practice Guidelines in Oncology (NCCN Guidelines): Head and Neck Cancers Version 2.2017, Fort Washington, PA, 2017, National Comprehensive Cancer Network. Available at: https://www.nccn.org/professionals/physician_gls/pdf/head-and-neck.pdf. Accessed January 24, 2018.

National Comprehensive Care Network. NCCN Clinical Practice Guidelines in Oncology (NCCN Guidelines): Melanoma Version 2.2018, Fort Washington, PA, 2018, National Comprehensive Cancer Network. Available at: https://www.nccn.org/professionals/physician_gls/PDF/melanoma.pdf. Accessed January 24, 2018.

Siegel RL, Miller KD, Jemal A. Cancer statistics, 2018. *CA Cancer J Clin.* 2018;68:7–30.

Williams MD. Update from the 4th edition of the *World Health Organization Classification of Head and Neck Tumours*: mucosal melanomas. *Head Neck Pathol.* 2017;11:110–117.

Mucocele (Mucus Extravasation Phenomenon)

Figs. **11.1–11.4**

The **mucocele** is a common lesion of the oral mucosa in which rupture of an excretory salivary gland duct results in an accumulation of spilled mucin beneath the mucosal surface. The lesion often arises secondary to trauma, although spontaneous examples also can occur.

Mucoceles are seen most frequently in children and young adults. They show a strong predilection for the lower labial mucosa, which accounts for 67% to 82% of all cases. The second most common site is the floor of the mouth, followed by the ventral tongue (from the glands of Blandin-Nuhn) and buccal mucosa. Surprisingly, the upper labial mucosa is an extremely rare site for mucoceles despite the presence of numerous minor salivary glands. Mucoceles in the floor of the mouth usually arise from the sublingual gland and are often known as *ranulas*. These lesions are discussed in more detail later in this chapter.

A mucocele presents as a soft nodular swelling that can vary from 1 to 2 mm to several centimeters in size. The lesion often has a bluish translucent color due to the accumulation of spilled mucin. However, some examples may appear pink, especially if the spilled mucin is located deeper in the tissue. The patient may report that the lesion fluctuates in size, periodically undergoing rupture and drainage.

The *superficial mucocele* is a clinical variant that tends to occur most often on the soft palate, retromolar area, and posterior buccal mucosa. These small lesions arise from rupture of a salivary duct just as it merges with the mucosal surface. They appear as small, tense, vesicle-like papules, measuring 1 to 4 mm in diameter, which may appear at mealtimes. Usually the lesion bursts and heals within a few days, although periodic recurrences may develop at the same site. On the buccal mucosa, superficial mucoceles may occur secondary to lichen planus or other inflammatory disorders.

Some mucoceles are transitory lesions that resolve on their own within a few days. Persistent mucoceles usually are treated by surgical excision, which should include removal of the underlying feeding glands. It is important to submit the excised tissue for microscopic examination to confirm the diagnosis and to rule out a salivary gland neoplasm. In most cases the prognosis is excellent, although the lesion sometimes recurs if the feeding gland is not removed.

■ **Figure 11.1**
Mucocele
Small, bluish, translucent nodule on the lower labial mucosa.

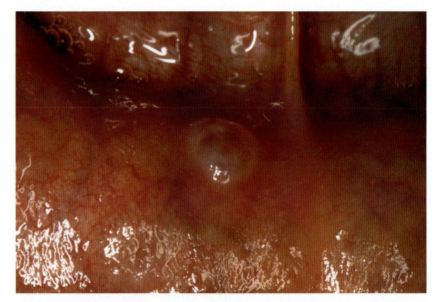

■ Figure 11.2
Mucocele
Bluish swelling on the lower labial mucosa.

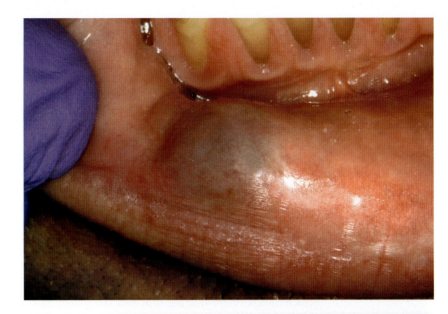

■ Figure 11.3
Mucocele
Nodular mass on the anterior ventral tongue.

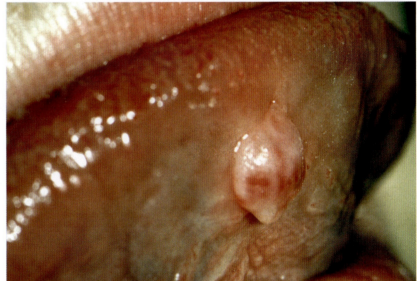

■ Figure 11.4
Superficial Mucocele
Translucent vesicle-like papule on the lateral soft palate.

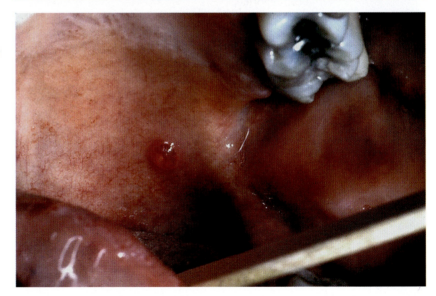

Ranula

The **ranula** is a variant of the mucocele that occurs in the floor of the mouth. Mucin spillage arises from rupture of one of the multiple ducts of the sublingual gland that empty into the oral floor on each side. The term *ranula* is derived from the Latin word *rana* ("frog"), because the lesion resembles the swollen belly of a frog. Because the spillage arises from one of the larger major salivary glands, ranulas usually are larger than mucoceles of minor gland origin.

Ranulas occur most often in children and young adults. The lesion usually appears as a soft, compressible, bluish swelling in the floor of the mouth lateral to the midline. Some patients report periodic rupture and recurrence of the lesion. Larger examples may fill the floor of the mouth on the affected side and elevate the tongue. In some cases the spilled mucin dissects through the mylohyoid muscle, resulting in a swelling in the anterior neck known as a *plunging ranula*. In this situation the diagnosis of ranula may not be suspected, especially if no associated intraoral swelling is present.

Several different treatments have been used for ranulas. The most common approach involves surgical removal of the associated sublingual gland, which is usually successful even without removal of the actual mucin spillage and its inflamed lining. Other surgeons may elect to marsupialize (or exteriorize) the lesion, which involves removing the roof over the spilled mucin and allowing the site to granulate in. However, this approach has a higher recurrence rate, especially for large ranulas. Other clinicians have advocated sclerotherapy, such as injection of OK-432 or ethanol into the lesion.

Salivary Duct Cyst

Fig. **11.7**

In contrast to the mucocele, the **salivary duct cyst** is a true cystic lesion lined by epithelium. Such cysts may be developmental in origin, or they may occur secondary to ductal obstruction that increases intraluminal pressure.

Salivary duct cysts can arise from either the major or minor salivary glands. Major gland cysts are most common in the parotid gland and present as slowly enlarging painless swellings. Minor gland examples occur most often in the floor of the mouth, buccal mucosa, and lips. They are usually seen in middle-aged and older adults, with a median age of 56 years. In the floor of the mouth, a salivary duct cyst often appears as a translucent, amber swelling immediately adjacent to the submandibular duct. In other locations, the swelling may exhibit a bluish color that often is mistaken for a mucocele. Multifocal examples rarely have been reported.

Salivary duct cysts of the minor glands are treated by conservative surgical excision. In the major glands, treatment may involve partial or total removal of the associated gland. Recurrence is rare.

■ Figure **11.5**
Plunging Ranula
(A) Soft swelling in the midline region of the neck just below the chin. (B) Coronal computed tomography image of the patient showing a central radiolucent cyst-like cavity containing mucinous fluid. Note the narrow tract extending down through the mylohyoid muscle from the oral cavity *(arrow)*. (Courtesy Dr. Steven Anderson.)

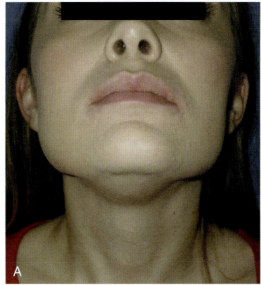
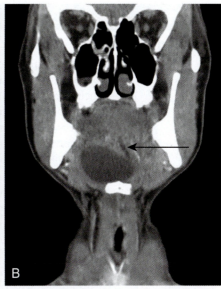

■ Figure **11.6**
Ranula
Child with a soft blue swelling in the left floor of the mouth.

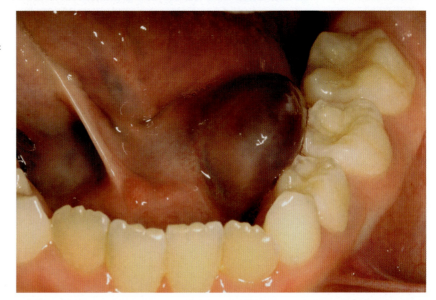

■ Figure **11.7**
Salivary Duct Cyst
Amber-colored nodule immediately adjacent to the submandibular duct.

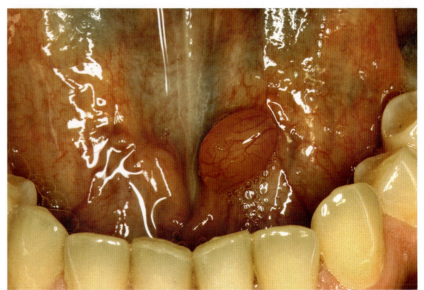

Figs. **11.8–11.11**

The formation of calcifications within the salivary ductal system is known as **sialolithiasis**. These calcifications are thought to arise from the deposition of calcium salts around a nidus of debris, such as inspissated mucin, epithelial cells, bacteria, or foreign matter. Decreased salivary flow or stasis of secretions is thought to contribute to the formation of sialoliths. However, the tendency to form salivary stones does not appear to be related to systemic disturbances in calcium and phosphate metabolism. Although some studies have suggested that sialolithiasis occurs more often in patients who also have cholelithiasis or nephrolithiasis, other studies have found no such relationship.

Sialoliths develop most often in the ductal system of the submandibular gland, which accounts for 72% to 95% of cases. When compared with the parotid gland, the higher frequency of stone formation in the submandibular gland is thought to be due to several factors: (1) saliva from the submandibular gland is more mucoid and viscous than parotid saliva; (2) the submandibular duct has a longer, tortuous, upward path that can contribute to saliva stasis; and (3) saliva from the submandibular gland has a higher pH and contains more calcium than parotid saliva.

Major gland sialoliths usually present with pain and swelling of the affected gland, which is exacerbated at mealtimes, when salivary flow is stimulated. If the stone is located near the terminal portion of the excretory duct, then a hard mass may be palpable. Radiographic examination usually will reveal a circumscribed radiopaque mass in the duct or the gland itself. On panoramic films, the calcification may appear superimposed on the mandible, so that it can be mistaken for an intrabony lesion. An occlusal radiograph can be helpful to confirm the presence of a sialolith in the terminal portion of the submandibular duct. However, not all sialoliths can be visualized radiographically, probably related to the degree of calcification.

Sialoliths of the minor salivary glands are less common, occurring most often in the upper lip (47%), buccal mucosa (35%), and lower lip (10%). Such a lesion may be palpable as a tiny firm bump that can be associated with local tenderness.

Small sialoliths of the major glands can sometimes be treated by gentle massage or by the use of sialagogues to stimulate salivary flow and encourage passage of the stone. Larger lesions will require surgical removal, sialendoscopic retrieval, or a combination of sialendoscopy and surgical excision. In some instances, extracorporeal shock wave lithotripsy can be used to facilitate removal of a stone. If the associated gland has sustained significant inflammatory damage, the gland also may have to be removed. Minor gland sialoliths are treated by simple excision of the stone along with the associated gland.

■ Figure **11.8**
Sialolithiasis
Radiopacity in the submandibular gland region, which is superimposed on the mandible.

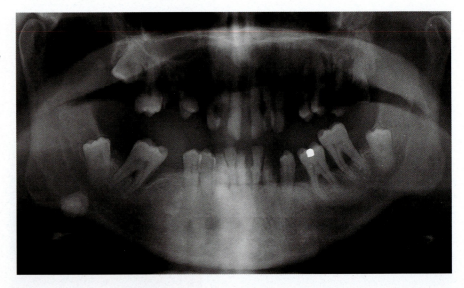

■ Figure **11.9**
Sialolithiasis
Small, hard, yellowish mass located near the orifice of the submandibular duct.

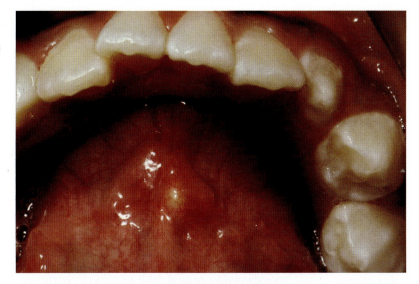

■ Figure **11.10**
Sialolithiasis
Radiograph of the patient seen in Fig. 11.9, showing a small radiopacity *(arrow)* in the floor of the mouth.

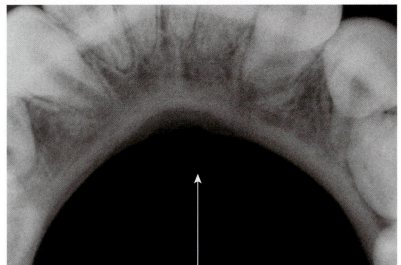

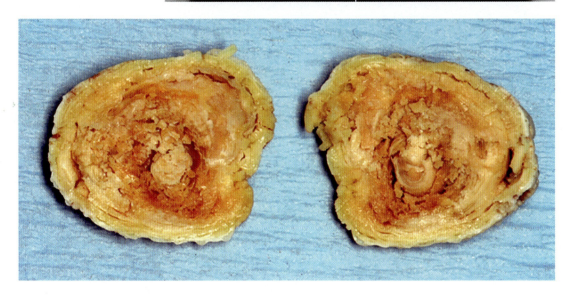

■ Figure **11.11**
Sialolithiasis
Gross specimen of a decalcified sialolith showing the laminated internal structure.

Sialadenitis, or inflammation of the salivary glands, can occur in a variety of situations. Acute sialadenitis can result from both bacterial infections (e.g., retrograde spread of bacteria secondary to decreased salivary flow) and viral infections (e.g., mumps, cytomegalovirus). Chronic sialadenitis can develop secondary to ductal obstruction (e.g., sialolithiasis) or in certain immune-related disorders, such as Sjögren syndrome and sarcoidosis.

Bacterial sialadenitis most commonly affects the parotid gland and presents as a painful swelling of the cheek that may be associated with trismus and low-grade fever. When the gland is massaged, a purulent exudate may be expressed from the parotid duct. Such infections sometimes develop after a surgical procedure and are therefore known as "surgical mumps." Because fluid intake is suppressed prior to surgery and atropine is given during surgery, patients have decreased salivary flow and are more susceptible to a retrograde bacterial infection.

Juvenile recurrent parotitis is the most common inflammatory salivary disorder of children in the United States. The cause is uncertain. It is characterized by recurring episodes of unilateral or bilateral, nonsuppurative parotid swelling typically occurring between the ages of 2 and 6 years. The condition is usually self-limiting and improves after puberty.

Acute bacterial sialadenitis should be treated with appropriate antibiotic therapy. Viral mumps is managed with supportive care; although routine vaccinations have greatly reduced the incidence of mumps, no specific antiviral agent is available for the treatment of such infections. Juvenile recurrent parotitis can often be managed successfully by sialendoscopy with saline irrigation, which has been shown to reduce the number of recurring episodes.

Cheilitis Glandularis

Fig. **11.13**

Cheilitis glandularis is a rare inflammatory disorder of the minor salivary glands. The cause is uncertain, although actinic damage is thought to be the most significant etiologic factor in most cases. The condition occurs most often in middle-aged and older men.

Most cases of cheilitis glandularis have been reported on the lower lip vermilion, although rare examples also have been described on the upper lip and palate. Inflammation and hypertrophy of the glandular tissue results in swelling and eversion of the lower lip, with dilation of the orifices of the minor salivary gland ducts. When the lip is squeezed, mucopurulent secretions can be expressed from these ductal openings.

Some cases of cheilitis glandularis have been associated with the subsequent development of squamous cell carcinoma on the lower lip. However, these examples may simply reflect the fact that both conditions are related to chronic sun damage to the lip vermilion. Problematic cases of cheilitis glandularis can be treated successfully by vermilionectomy (lip shave).

Sialadenosis

Fig. **11.14**

Sialadenosis is a noninflammatory, hypertrophic process characterized by enlargement of the salivary glands secondary to an underlying systemic disorder. The most commonly related conditions include diabetes mellitus, bulimia, alcoholism, and general malnutrition. It is thought that these disorders may cause dysregulation of the autonomic neural innervation of salivary acinar cells, which leads to the accumulation of secretory granules and resultant enlargement.

Sialadenosis typically presents with gradual enlargement of the parotid glands, which may or may not be painful. In most cases this enlargement is bilateral, although unilateral cases also can occur. The submandibular glands also may be affected in some patients. However, involvement of the minor salivary glands is extremely rare. Although glandular enlargement is present, patients may complain of diminished salivary flow.

Management of patients with sialadenosis centers around control of the underlying disorder. Mild examples may not require any treatment. If the degree of enlargement creates a cosmetic concern, then partial parotidectomy could be performed. Pilocarpine has been used to reduce the salivary enlargement in patients with bulimia.

■ Figure 11.12
Sialadenitis
Purulent exudate milked from the parotid duct in a patient with a bacterial infection of the parotid gland.

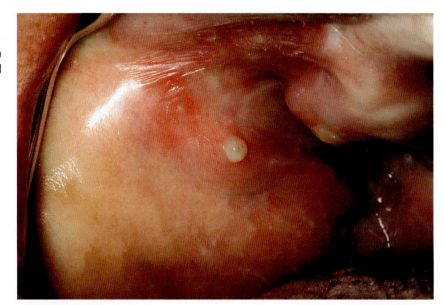

■ Figure 11.13
Cheilitis Glandularis
Mucoid secretions have been expressed from the openings of multiple minor salivary gland ducts on the lower lip.

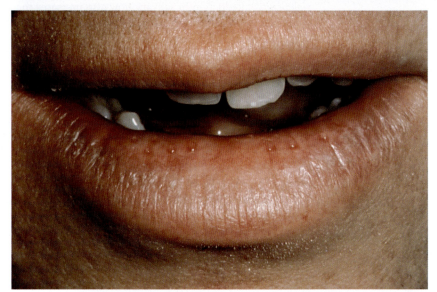

■ Figure 11.14
Sialadenosis
Painless bilateral enlargement of the parotid glands in a patient with alcoholism.

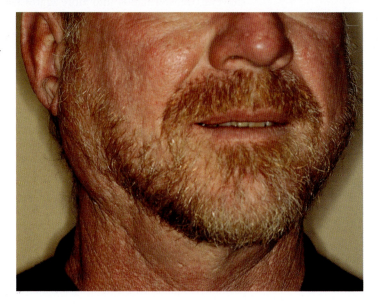

Figs. 11.15 and 11.16

Sjögren syndrome is an autoimmune disorder that primarily affects exocrine glands. Lymphocytic infiltration of the salivary and lacrimal glands leads to diminished secretions, evidenced clinically by xerostomia and xerophthalmia. This combination of symptoms sometimes is known as the *sicca syndrome* (*sicca*, meaning dry). Like many autoimmune diseases, Sjögren syndrome is seen most frequently in middle-aged adults and shows a strong female predilection (9:1 female-to-male ratio). Two subtypes are recognized. *Primary* Sjögren syndrome shows only the sicca syndrome without any other autoimmune disorder. The term *secondary* Sjögren syndrome is used when the disease develops in a patient who also has another autoimmune disease. Approximately 15% of patients with rheumatoid arthritis and 30% of patients with systemic lupus erythematosus also suffer from Sjögren syndrome.

Dryness of the mouth may contribute to difficulty in swallowing, atrophy of tongue papillae, altered taste, and difficulty wearing a denture. Patients are more susceptible to candidiasis, which may be manifested by a denture-sore mouth and angular cheilitis. Because of the loss of salivary cleansing action, affected individuals are prone to develop dental caries, especially cervical decay. Up to half of affected patients will develop firm enlargement of the major salivary glands secondary to a lymphocytic infiltration that destroys the acinar units. This pattern of inflammation microscopically is known as a *benign lymphoepithelial lesion (myoepithelial sialadenitis)*. Reduction in salivary flow also increases the risk for a retrograde bacterial sialadenitis.

Ocular dryness *(keratoconjunctivitis sicca)* affects the epithelial surface of the eye, producing a scratchy, gritty sensation and blurred vision. In addition, dryness of the skin, nasal mucosa, and vaginal mucosa can occur. Other potential features include fatigue, depression, lymphadenopathy, Raynaud phenomenon, vasculitis, and peripheral neuropathy.

Patients with Sjögren syndrome have elevated serum immunoglobulin levels (especially IgG) and erythrocyte sedimentation rates. A variety of autoantibodies may be produced, including antinuclear antibodies (ANA) and rheumatoid factor. Two particular nuclear autoantibodies, known as anti-SS-A (anti-Ro) and anti-SS-B (anti-La), are often identified. In many centers, biopsy of minor salivary glands from the lower lip is used to support the diagnosis by demonstrating multiple foci of lymphocytic inflammation within the glandular tissue. Sialography may show punctate sialectasia with lack of arborizing ducts—a pattern likened to a "fruit-laden branchless tree."

Symptoms of xerostomia and xerophthalmia can be managed by the use of artificial saliva and tears. Sugarless candy, gum, and sialagogue medications (pilocarpine and cevimeline) can also be used to stimulate salivary secretions. Periodic fluoride applications may be warranted to help prevent xerostomia-related caries.

Patients with Sjögren syndrome are at increased risk for the development of lymphoma, which is estimated to occur in 5% to 15% of cases. These tumors are primarily low-grade non-Hodgkin lymphomas known as *extranodal marginal zone B-cell lymphomas of mucosa-associated lymphoid tissue (MALT lymphomas)*. However, transformation into more aggressive high-grade lymphomas can occur.

Necrotizing Sialometaplasia

Fig. 11.17

Necrotizing sialometaplasia is a destructive inflammatory process caused by an infarction within salivary gland tissue. The etiology is uncertain, although a variety of possible predisposing factors have been suggested, including local trauma. Necrotizing sialometaplasia occurs most often in the minor salivary glands of the posterior palate, which accounts for more than 75% of cases. The condition also sometimes develops at other minor salivary gland sites. Involvement of major salivary gland tissue is distinctly rare, usually being reported in the parotid gland.

Two-thirds of palatal cases are unilateral, with the remainder being bilateral or midline in location. An initial swelling may be noted, which is followed in 2 to 3 weeks by necrosis and sloughing of the surface mucosal tissue. In some instances, the patient may actually describe a piece of the palate falling out. At this point, a crater-like ulceration will be noted, which may have a raised, rolled border. This ulcer can range in size from less than 1 cm to larger than 5 cm in diameter.

Because of its rapid evolution and ulcerated appearance, necrotizing sialometaplasia often is worrisome clinically for malignancy. In addition, because the residual salivary ducts of the infarcted glands undergo prominent squamous metaplasia, the microscopic appearance easily can be mistaken for a carcinoma if the pathologist is not aware of this histopathologic pattern.

The prognosis for necrotizing sialometaplasia is excellent. In most cases, an incisional biopsy is performed initially to confirm the diagnosis. After biopsy, the lesion should heal on its own accord over a period of 4 to 6 weeks.

■ Figure **11.15**
Sjögren Syndrome
Bilateral enlargement of the parotid and submandibular glands, representing benign lymphoepithelial lesions.

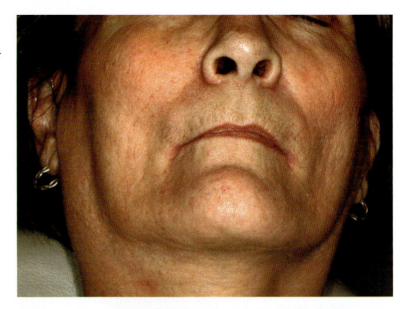

■ Figure **11.16**
Sjögren Syndrome
Parotid sialogram showing atrophy and punctate sialectasia ("fruit-laden branchless tree").

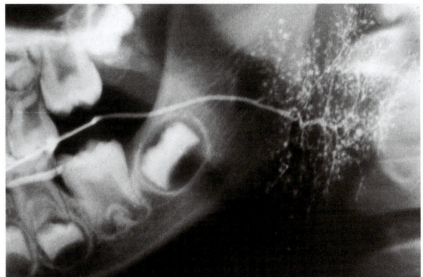

■ Figure **11.17**
Necrotizing Sialometaplasia
Ulcerated lesion with a raised rolled border at the junction of the hard and soft palate. (With appreciation to Dr. Martin Steed.)

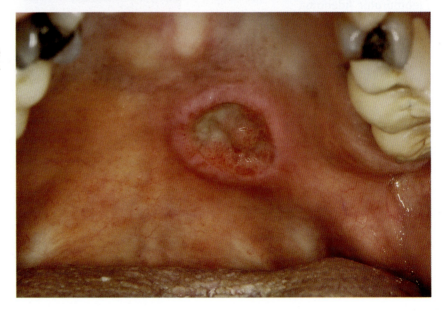

Figs. **11.18–11.21**

The most common tumor of salivary gland origin is the **pleomorphic adenoma**, also known as a **benign mixed tumor**. This lesion comprises 50% to 77% of parotid tumors, 53% to 72% of submandibular tumors, and 33% to 41% of minor salivary gland tumors. The tumor occurs over a wide age range, with a peak prevalence between the ages of 30 and 60 years. Approximately 60% of cases occur in females.

The pleomorphic adenoma typically is a slowly growing neoplasm that presents as a firm, painless mass. Parotid tumors occur much more often in the superficial lobe of the gland, producing a swelling of the cheek in front of or below the ear. Although the tumor shows slow enlargement, pleomorphic adenomas have an almost unlimited growth potential, with the ability to grow to a tremendous size if neglected by the patient. About 10% of parotid cases involve the deep lobe of the gland beneath the facial nerve, sometimes presenting as a mass of the lateral soft palate or pharyngeal wall. The most common minor gland location is the posterior lateral hard and soft palate, which accounts for over half of intraoral cases. The upper lip is the second most common minor gland site (19% to 27% of cases), followed by the buccal mucosa (13% to 17% of cases).

Treatment for the pleomorphic adenoma is complete surgical excision. Although the tumor is circumscribed, the surrounding capsule is often incomplete or may show infiltration by tumor cells. Therefore, conservative resection or enucleation of a parotid tumor may result in seeding of tumor into the surgical bed with a high risk for multiple recurrences. Because of this, tumors of the superficial lobe usually are treated by superficial parotidectomy with preservation of the facial nerve. Tumors in the deep lobe may require total removal of the gland while also attempting to preserve the nerve. Pleomorphic adenomas of the submandibular gland are best treated by total removal of the gland with the tumor. Tumors of the hard palate are managed by total excision extending down to the periosteum.

Overall, the prognosis of pleomorphic adenomas is excellent, with a cure rate of more than 95% after adequate surgery. The risk for recurrence appears to be much lower for tumors arising in the minor salivary glands. One rare (albeit significant) complication is malignant transformation, resulting in a *carcinoma ex pleomorphic adenoma*. One recent review reported malignant transformation in 0.15% of a large series of pleomorphic adenomas. The risk for malignant change appears to increase with the duration of the tumor.

■ Figure **11.18**
Pleomorphic Adenoma
Firm nodular mass of the left parotid gland just below the ear at the angle of the mandible. (With appreciation to Dr. Terry Day.)

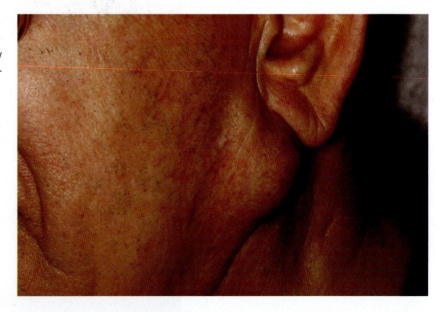

Figure **11.19**
Pleomorphic Adenoma
Nodular mass of the left posterior hard palate, immediately adjacent to a central palatal torus. *Arrows* point to edges of the oval midline torus; the tumor is located lateral and posterior to this central bony growth. (Courtesy Dr. Peter Franco.)

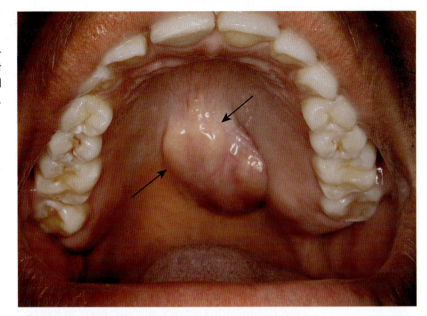

Figure **11.20**
Pleomorphic Adenoma
Large mass of the hard palate.

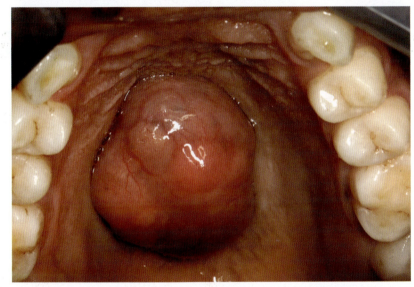

Figure **11.21**
Pleomorphic Adenoma
Nodular mass on the upper labial mucosa. (With appreciation to Dr. Ashleigh Briody.)

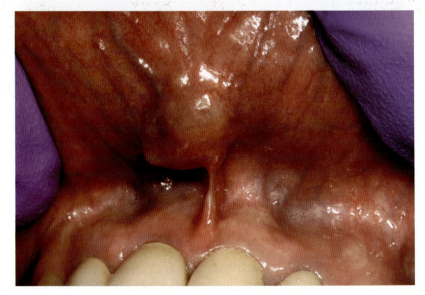

Warthin Tumor (Papillary Cystadenoma Lymphomatosum)

Fig. **11.22**

The **Warthin tumor** is the second most common neoplasm in the parotid gland, accounting for 5% to 22% of parotid tumors. In contrast, it comprises only 0.6% to 1.3% of submandibular gland tumors and is distinctly rare in the minor salivary glands. The tumor shows a strong relationship to smoking, as evidenced by an eight times greater risk in smokers versus nonsmokers. Earlier studies showed the tumor to be 10 times more common in men than in women; however, this male/female ratio has become less pronounced in recent decades, probably because the prevalence of smoking in men and women has become more equalized. Based on its unusual clinical and microscopic features, some authors have suggested that the Warthin tumor may not represent a true neoplasm but instead be a reactive process.

Warthin tumors usually develop in older adults, with a peak prevalence in the sixth and seventh decades of life. The lesion presents as a slowly growing, painless mass. More than 98% of parotid Warthin tumors develop in the superficial lobe of the gland, especially in the tail of the parotid. In addition, from 5% to 17% of affected patients will develop bilateral or multicentric tumors.

Warthin tumors are benign growths that are usually treated by surgical resection. However, if a reliable preliminary diagnosis can be made with diagnostic imaging or by fine-needle aspiration biopsy, some clinicians will recommend clinical follow-up rather than surgery. A 2% to 6% recurrence rate has been reported following surgery, although many of these cases may represent multicentric tumors rather than true recurrences.

Canalicular Adenoma

Fig. **11.23**

The **canalicular adenoma** is an uncommon benign salivary gland neoplasm that develops almost exclusively in the oral minor salivary glands. The tumor shows a strong predilection for the upper lip, which accounts for approximately 70% of reported cases. The next most common site is the buccal mucosa, followed by the palatal glands. Only rare examples have been documented in the parotid gland. The lesion usually occurs in older adults, with a mean age of approximately 66 years. The tumor is more common in women (the female-to-male ratio is 1.7:1).

The canalicular adenoma typically presents as a slow-growing, painless mass ranging from several millimeters to 2 cm in diameter. Sometimes the tumor will exhibit a bluish color, which might be mistaken clinically for a mucocele. However, it should be recalled that mucoceles in the upper lip are exceedingly rare. One interesting finding is that 13% of canalicular adenomas occur as multifocal tumors.

Treatment for the canalicular adenoma consists of conservative local excision. The lesion rarely recurs and the prognosis is excellent.

Acinic Cell Carcinoma

Fig. **11.24**

The **acinic cell carcinoma** is a malignant salivary gland neoplasm that shows serous acinar differentiation with zymogen granules. Based on its serous cell composition, it should not be surprising that the parotid gland is the most common site for this tumor. Acinic cell carcinoma comprises approximately 3% of all parotid tumors and 15% of parotid malignancies. Less frequently, examples have been reported in the submandibular gland and the minor salivary glands, sometimes being described microscopically as poor in zymogen granules. However, with the recent recognition of (mammary analogue) secretory carcinoma of salivary origin, most cases of acinic cell carcinoma reported at these other sites likely would be reclassified today as secretory carcinomas.

Acinic cell carcinoma occurs over a wide age range, with a median age of 52 years. The tumor is seen more often in females than in males (the female-to-male ratio is approximately 1.5:1). The lesion usually is reported as a slowly enlarging, painless mass that often is present for months or years prior to diagnosis.

Acinic cell carcinomas of the superficial lobe of the parotid gland usually are treated by superficial parotidectomy, whereas deep lobe tumors often require total removal of the gland. Elective neck dissection usually is not warranted, although it may be considered for locally aggressive tumors or tumors with high-grade microscopic features. The role of radiation therapy remains controversial. The overall prognosis is good, with 5-year survival rates of more than 90%. However, approximately 8% to 10% of patients will die from their disease, most often secondary to distant metastases.

■ Figure **11.22**
Warthin Tumor
Large mass arising in the tail of the parotid gland.

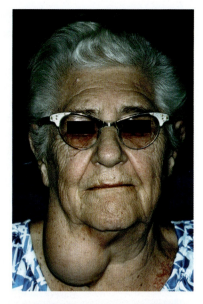

■ Figure **11.23**
Canalicular Adenoma
Nodular mass arising in the upper labial mucosa. (Courtesy Dr. John Wright.)

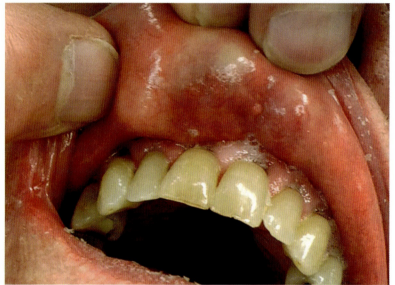

■ Figure **11.24**
Acinic Cell Carcinoma
Large mass arising in the superficial lobe of the parotid gland. (Courtesy Dr. Román Carlos.)

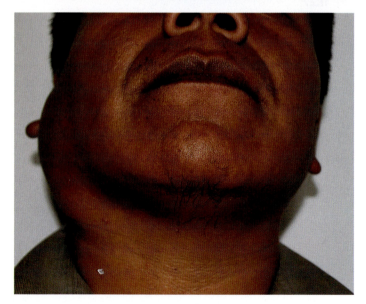

Mucoepidermoid Carcinoma

Figs. **11.25 and 11.26**

The most common malignancy of salivary gland origin is the **mucoepidermoid carcinoma**—a neoplasm that includes a mixture of mucin-producing cells and squamous (epidermoid) cells. This tumor comprises 4% to 10% of major gland tumors and 13% to 23% of minor gland tumors. Mucoepidermoid carcinomas occur predominantly in adults, but they develop over a wide age range. The tumor is rare in children, although it represents the most common salivary malignancy in this age group.

In the major salivary glands, mucoepidermoid carcinomas are most common in the parotid. The lesion often appears as a slowly enlarging painless swelling, although aggressive, high-grade tumors may be associated with pain or facial nerve paralysis. The most common site for minor gland tumors is the posterior lateral palate, where the lesion also typically presents as a slow-growing, painless mass. Because the tumor often contains cystic spaces filled with mucin, the lesion may exhibit a bluish discoloration of the mucosa that can be mistaken for a mucocele or vascular tumor. Although salivary neoplasms are uncommon in the lower lip, retromolar pad, tongue, and floor of the mouth, mucoepidermoid carcinoma represents the most common salivary tumor in each of these subsites.

Microscopic grading of mucoepidermoid carcinoma is important in determining treatment and prognosis. Based on the tumor growth pattern and the relative numbers of mucous cells versus epidermoid cells, tumors are usually placed into one of three categories: low-grade, intermediate-grade, and high-grade. The prognosis for low-grade and intermediate-grade tumors usually is good, with 5-year survival rates as high as 92% to 98%. However, survival for high-grade tumors is significantly lower, ranging from 38% to 67%.

Treatment for mucoepidermoid carcinoma depends not only on the tumor grade but also on the size, location, and clinical stage of the tumor. Early-stage tumors in the superficial lobe of the parotid gland may be treated by superficial parotidectomy with preservation of the facial nerve. However, more advanced tumors may require sacrifice of the nerve. Neck dissection is indicated for patients with evidence of regional metastatic disease. Adjunctive radiation therapy may also be used for aggressive, high-grade tumors. Surgical management of mucoepidermoid carcinoma of the submandibular gland consists of total removal of the gland. Most mucoepidermoid carcinomas of the minor glands are lower-grade tumors that can be treated by assured surgical excision including a margin of surrounding normal tissue. Palatal tumors that involve the underlying maxilla may require resection of the involved bone to ensure clean margins.

Intraosseous Mucoepidermoid Carcinoma

Fig. **11.27**

Approximately 2% to 3% of mucoepidermoid carcinomas will arise primarily within the jaws. The most likely source for these rare tumors is thought to be odontogenic epithelium, especially because odontogenic cysts often include mucus-producing cells. In addition, the **intraosseous mucoepidermoid carcinoma** sometimes arises in association with an impacted tooth. However, it is possible that some examples could arise from salivary tissue entrapped within bone or, in the case of maxillary tumors, from sinonasal glands.

Intraosseous mucoepidermoid carcinomas occur more frequently in the mandible than in the maxilla, with the most common site being the molar/ramus region. The tumor occurs over a wide age range, with an average age at diagnosis of 48 years. The lesion often presents as a painless cortical swelling, although some examples are discovered as incidental findings during routine radiographic examination. Less commonly, the tumor is associated with pain or paresthesia. Radiographically, the lesion usually appears as a well-circumscribed unilocular or multilocular radiolucency that is likely to be mistaken for an odontogenic cyst or tumor.

Most intraosseous mucoepidermoid carcinomas are low-grade and intermediate-grade tumors; only 10% to 15% of examples are classified as high-grade lesions. Treatment consists primarily of radical surgical resection, which is associated with a much better prognosis than more conservative therapy such as enucleation or curettage. Adjunctive radiation therapy also may be used. The overall prognosis is relatively good; approximately 10% of patients die from the tumor, usually as a result of local recurrence.

■ Figure **11.25**
Mucoepidermoid Carcinoma
Tiny blue papule of the lateral soft palate. This early tumor might be mistaken for a small mucocele. (Courtesy Dr. David Schmidt.)

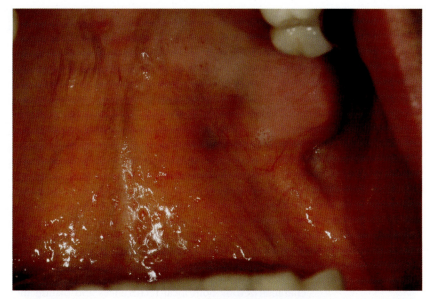

■ Figure **11.26**
Mucoepidermoid Carcinoma
Nodular mass on the left posterior lateral hard palate.

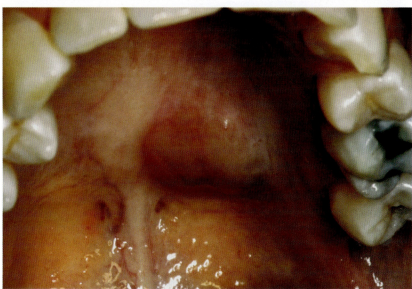

■ Figure **11.27**
Intraosseous Mucoepidermoid Carcinoma
Loculated radiolucency of the right posterior mandible in the second and third molar region.

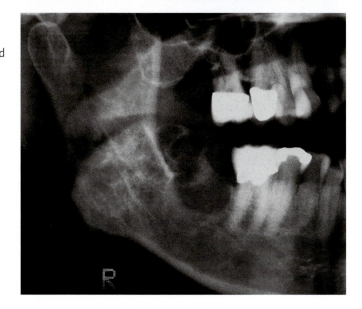

Figs. **11.28–11.31**

Adenoid cystic carcinoma is an uncommon but well-recognized salivary gland malignancy. This tumor develops most often in the various minor salivary glands, which account for 40% to 45% of cases. Most of the remaining cases are divided between the parotid and submandibular glands. On a relative percentage basis, adenoid cystic carcinoma comprises only 2% of all parotid neoplasms; in contrast, it represents the most common malignancy of the submandibular gland, accounting for 11% to 17% of all tumors in this gland. The most common minor gland site is the posterior lateral palate, where it comprises 8% to 15% of salivary tumors. Adenoid cystic carcinoma develops most frequently in middle-aged adults and is rare in children. The tumor occurs more frequently in females than in males (the female-to-male ratio is 1.4:1).

Adenoid cystic carcinoma usually presents as a slowly enlarging mass. Because of its tendency to invade nerves, patients frequently complain of increasingly intense pain. With lesions in the parotid gland, facial nerve paralysis can develop. Palatal tumors may be covered by intact mucosa, although secondary ulceration can occur. Adenoid cystic carcinomas arising on the hard palate or in the maxillary sinus can cause significant adjacent bone destruction.

Despite its slow growth, adenoid cystic carcinoma tends to pursue a relentless and unpredictable course characterized by both local recurrences and distant metastases. Treatment consists primarily of radical surgical resection in an attempt to achieve clear margins, although tumor often demonstrates deceptive infiltrative invasion into adjacent tissues, especially along nerve bundles. Because regional lymph node metastasis is uncommon (3% to 16% of cases), neck dissection is usually not required. Adjuvant radiation therapy is often utilized to improve local disease control.

Adenoid cystic carcinoma shows a propensity for distant blood-borne metastasis, especially to the lungs, bone, and brain. Although 5-year survival rates may range as high as 68% to 82%, such figures are deceptive because of the tendency of this tumor for late recurrence and delayed metastases. The 10-year survival rate drops to 52% to 69%, and it continues to decline to as low as 28% to 35% by 20 years.

■ Figure **11.28**
Adenoid Cystic Carcinoma
Firm mass in the left parotid gland. (With appreciation to Dr. Terry Day.)

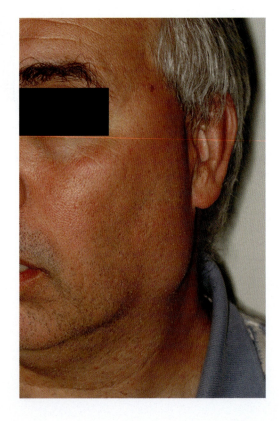

■ Figure **11.29**
Adenoid Cystic Carcinoma
Small nodular swelling of the left posterior lateral hard palate.

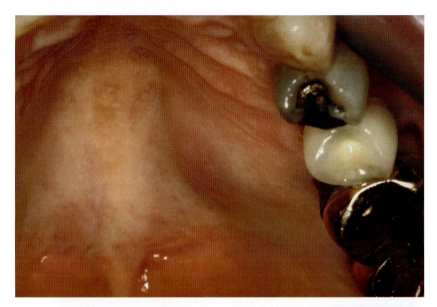

■ Figure **11.30**
Adenoid Cystic Carcinoma
Large ulcerated mass of the palate.

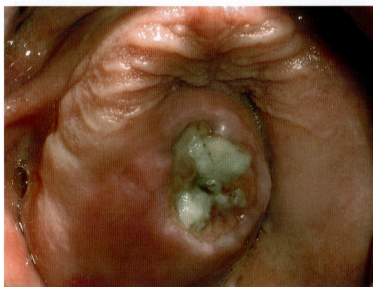

■ Figure **11.31**
Adenoid Cystic Carcinoma
Axial computed tomography scan of a patient with a large adenoid cystic carcinoma of the palate. The tumor has invaded the nasal cavity and both maxillary sinuses. (Courtesy Dr. Kevin Riker.)

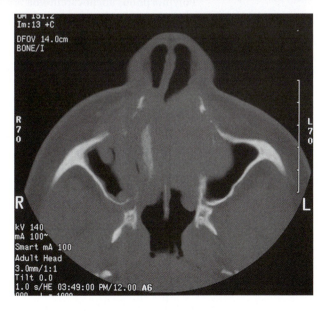

Carcinoma ex pleomorphic adenoma is a high-grade salivary gland carcinoma in which malignant transformation occurs in a previously benign pleomorphic adenoma. This tumor most often develops in the parotid gland, where it represents 2% to 3% of all parotid neoplasms. It is less common in the submandibular gland and in the minor salivary glands. Minor gland examples are seen most frequently on the palate.

Several features support the concept that this lesion represents malignant degeneration within a previously benign tumor. Carcinoma ex pleomorphic adenoma usually occurs in middle-aged and older adults, and the mean age is about 15 years older than for benign pleomorphic adenoma. Sometimes the patient will report a history of a slowly enlarging mass for a number of years, which then exhibits rapid growth with pain or ulceration. Finally, when the tumor is examined microscopically, residual features typical of benign pleomorphic adenoma often are found within the lesion.

Treatment and prognosis for carcinoma ex pleomorphic adenoma depend on both the degree of invasion and the histopathologic subtype of the malignant component. Early "noninvasive" tumors that have not violated the capsule of the original pleomorphic adenoma have an excellent prognosis, with almost 100% survival. Such malignant change often is discovered incidentally upon microscopic examination of a lesion thought to represent a pleomorphic adenoma. If only minimal extracapsular invasion is present (≤1.5 mm), the prognosis also is excellent, with a 5-year survival rate of 98%. In contrast, tumors showing wider invasion have a much more guarded prognosis. For these patients, the 5-year survival rates range from 25% to 65%, and these rates drop to 10% to 35% at 15 years. However, the prognosis for widely invasive carcinoma ex pleomorphic adenoma also depends on the specific histopathologic subtype of the malignancy. For example, if the malignant component is a low-grade tumor, such as polymorphous (low-grade) adenocarcinoma, the 5-year survival can be as high as nearly 90%.

Noninvasive and minimally invasive tumors may be treated in a manner similar to benign pleomorphic adenomas (e.g., lobectomy for tumors in the superficial lobe of the parotid gland). However, widely invasive tumors require more aggressive resection, often in conjunction with regional lymph node dissection and adjunctive radiation therapy.

Polymorphous (Low-Grade) Adenocarcinoma

Fig. **11.34**

Polymorphous adenocarcinoma is a salivary gland malignancy that arises almost exclusively in the minor salivary glands. Only rare examples have been described in the major glands, sometimes representing the malignant component of a carcinoma ex pleomorphic adenoma. Prior to the 2017 release of the fourth edition of the *World Health Organization Classification for Head and Neck Tumours*, this lesion was known as *polymorphous low-grade adenocarcinoma*. However, because occasional examples may act in a more aggressive fashion, the "low-grade" designation was dropped.

Polymorphous adenocarcinoma represents one of the more common minor salivary malignancies, comprising 5% to 11% of minor gland tumors. The lesion is most common in middle-aged and older adults, with a mean age of 61 years. Two-thirds of all cases occur in females. The most common location is the hard or soft palate, which accounts for 57% to 73% of cases. The upper lip and buccal mucosa are the next most common sites. The lesion usually appears as a slowly enlarging nonulcerated mass. Palatal tumors sometimes may exhibit a slightly rough and papillary appearance of the overlying mucosa, which can be a clinical clue to the diagnosis. Despite the frequent presence of perineural invasion microscopically, pain is not a common clinical finding.

Most patients are diagnosed with only localized tumor and have an excellent prognosis. Regional lymph node metastases have been described in 9% to 17% of patients, and distant metastasis is rare. Treatment usually consists of wide surgical excision, which may require resection of the underlying bone if bony invasion is present. Recurrence has been reported in 9% to 29% of patients, although most examples can still be controlled with reexcision. The 5-year and 10-year disease-specific survival rates are 98.6% and 96.4%, respectively.

■ Figure 11.32
Carcinoma ex Pleomorphic Adenoma

Massive tumor of the right parotid gland. The patient related a 10-year history of a slowly enlarging mass that demonstrated sudden rapid growth over the preceding 3 months. (Courtesy Dr. Román Carlos.)

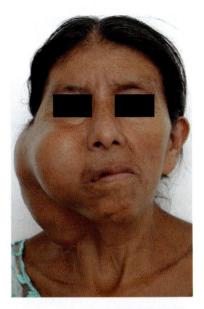

■ Figure 11.33
Carcinoma ex Pleomorphic Adenoma

Large ulcerated mass involving almost the entire hard palate.

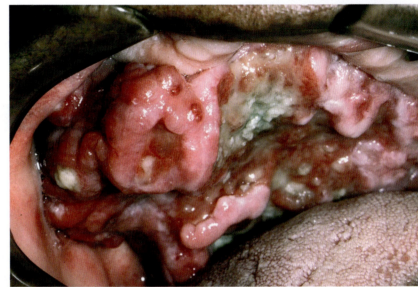

■ Figure 11.34
Polymorphous (Low-Grade) Adenocarcinoma

Nodular mass of the left posterior hard and soft palate. (With appreciation to Dr. Terry Day.)

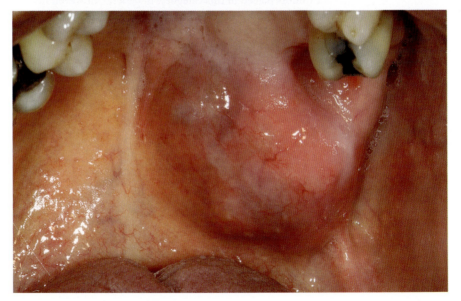

(Mammary Analogue) Secretory Carcinoma

Fig. **11.35**

Secretory carcinoma is a recently recognized salivary gland malignancy that was first described in 2010. It was originally termed *mammary analogue secretory carcinoma (MASC)* because of its similarity to secretory carcinoma of the breast, including the presence of a chromosomal translocation that results in the formation of an *ETV6-NTRK3* gene fusion. However, in an effort to standardize terminology at different organ sites, the fourth edition of the *World Health Organization Classification for Head and Neck Tumours* (2017) recommends the simpler term *secretory carcinoma*. Previously, most examples of this tumor had been categorized as either acinic cell carcinoma or simply as salivary adenocarcinoma.

Secretory carcinoma usually occurs in adults; the mean age at diagnosis is 47 years. The tumor develops most often in the parotid gland (58% of cases), followed by the minor salivary glands (31%) and the submandibular gland (9%). The most common minor gland sites are the lips, soft palate, and buccal mucosa. The lesion usually presents as a slowly enlarging painless mass, although some examples may produce some discomfort.

Because of its recent recognition, data on treatment and prognosis for secretory carcinoma are somewhat limited. Current evidence suggests that most examples of this tumor are low-grade malignancies that have a favorable prognosis. However, some cases have shown local tumor recurrence and metastasis, including occasional deaths. In addition, examples microscopically showing tumor dedifferentiation have acted in a more aggressive fashion. Most cases can be treated successfully by local surgical resection, with adjuvant radiation therapy reserved for examples showing more aggressive clinical or microscopic features.

Salivary Adenocarcinoma, Not Otherwise Specified

Fig. **11.36**

Despite the variety of salivary gland malignancies that have been recognized, pathologists still encounter tumors that defy current classification schemes. Such tumors typically are categorized as **salivary adenocarcinoma, not otherwise specified (NOS)**. Similar to salivary neoplasms in general, such malignancies are described most often in the parotid gland, followed by the minor glands and the submandibular gland.

Because salivary adenocarcinoma NOS represents a "dumping ground" for a variety of unclassifiable tumors, it is impossible to describe typical clinical features for these lesions. In most instances, the clinical presentation (e.g., growth rate; presence of pain, neural deficits, or overlying ulceration) for any particular tumor likely would depend on its inherent biologic potential. Likewise, it can be difficult to predict behavior for tumors placed in this category. In general, however, neoplasms with a poorly differentiated microscopic pattern would be expected to act in a more aggressive fashion than better differentiated tumors. Most tumors would be treated by surgical resection, possibly supplemented with adjuvant radiation therapy, especially for more aggressive lesions.

■ Figure **11.35**
(Mammary Analogue) Secretory Carcinoma

Bluish mass on the lower labial mucosa, which could be mistaken for a mucocele.

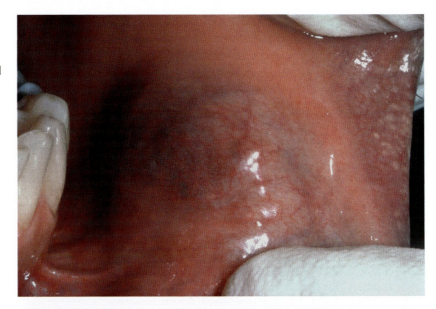

■ Figure **11.36**
Salivary Adenocarcinoma, NOS

Mass on the right posterior lateral hard palate. (The central ulcer represents the biopsy site.)

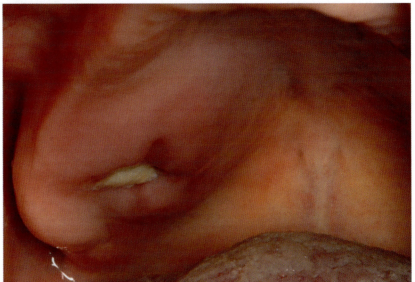

Bibliography

Mucocele

Bezerra TM, Monteiro BV, Henriques AC, et al. Epidemiological survey of mucus extravasation phenomenon at an oral pathology referral center during a 43 year period. *Braz J Otorhinolaryngol.* 2016;82:536–542.

Chi AC, Lambert PR 3rd, Richardson MS, et al. Oral mucoceles: a clinicopathologic review of 1,824 cases, including unusual variants. *J Oral Maxillofac Surg.* 2011;69:1086–1093.

Jinbu Y, Kusama M, Itoh H, et al. Mucocele of the glands of Blandin-Nuhn: clinical and histopathologic analysis of 26 cases. *Oral Surg Oral Med Oral Pathol Oral Radiol Endod.* 2003;95:467–470.

Ranula

Harrison JD. Modern management and pathophysiology of ranula: literature review. *Head Neck.* 2010;32:1310–1320.

Kono M, Satomi T, Abukawa H, et al. Evaluation of OK-432 injection therapy as possible primary treatment of intraoral ranula. *J Oral Maxillofac Surg.* 2017;75:336–342.

Lyly A, Castrén E, Aronniemi J, et al. Plunging ranula – patient characteristics, treatment, and comparison between different populations. *Acta Otolaryngol.* 2017;137:1271–1274.

Yang Y, Hong K. Surgical results of the intraoral approach for plunging ranula. *Acta Otolaryngol.* 2014;134:201–205.

Salivary Duct Cyst

Eversole LR. Oral sialocysts. *Arch Otolaryngol.* 1987;113:51–56.

Stojanov IJ, Malik UA, Woo SB. Intraoral salivary duct cyst: clinical and histopathologic features of 177 cases. *Head Neck Pathol.* 2017;11(4): 469–476. doi:10.1007/s12105-017-0810-5. [Epub 2017 Mar 27].

Takeda Y, Yamamoto H. Salivary duct cyst: its frequency in a certain Japanese population group (Tohoku districts), with special reference to adenomatous proliferation of the epithelial lining. *J Oral Sci.* 2001;43:9–13.

Sialolithiasis

Kopeć T, Wierzbicka M, Kałużny J, et al. Sialadenoscopy and sialendoscopically-assisted operations in the treatment of lithiasis of the submandibular and parotid glands: our experience of 239 cases. *Br J Oral Maxillofac Surg.* 2017;54:767–771.

Kraaij S, Karagozoglu KH, Forouzanfar T, et al. Salivary stones: symptoms, aetiology, biochemical composition and treatment. *Br Dent J.* 2014;217:E23.

Kraaij S, Karagozoglu KH, Kenter YA, et al. Systemic diseases and the risk of developing salivary stones: a case control study. *Oral Surg Oral Med Oral Pathol Oral Radiol.* 2015;119:539–543.

Sigismund PE, Zenk J, Koch M, et al. Nearly 3,000 salivary stones: some clinical and epidemiologic aspects. *Laryngoscope.* 2015;125:1879–1882.

Sialadenitis

Francis CL, Larsen CG. Pediatric sialadenitis. *Otolaryngol Clin N Am.* 2014;47:763–778.

Hernandez S, Busso C, Walvekar RR. Parotitis and sialendoscopy of the parotid gland. *Otolaryngol Clin N Am.* 2016;49:381–393.

Ramakrishna J, Strychowsky J, Gupta M, et al. Sialendoscopy for the management of juvenile recurrent parotitis: a systematic review and meta-analysis. *Laryngoscope.* 2015;125:1472–1479.

Cheilitis Glandularis

Lourenço SV, Kos E, Nunes TB, et al. In vivo reflectance confocal microscopy evaluation of cheilitis glandularis: a report of 5 cases. *Am J Dermatopathol.* 2015;37:197–202.

Nico MMS, Nakano de Melo J, Lourenço SV. Cheilitis glandularis: a clinicopathological study in 22 patients. *J Am Acad Dermatol.* 2010;62:233–238.

Reiter S, Vered M, Yarom N, et al. Cheilitis glandularis: clinico-histopathological diagnostic criteria. *Oral Dis.* 2011;17:335–339.

Sialadenosis

Guggenheimer J, Close JM, Eghtesad B. Sialadenosis in patients with advanced liver disease. *Head Neck Pathol.* 2009;3:100–105.

Ihrler S, Rath C, Zengel P, et al. Pathogenesis of sialadenosis: possible role of functionally deficient myoepithelial cells. *Oral Surg Oral Med Oral Pathol Oral Radiol Endod.* 2010;110:218–223.

Mignogna MD, Fedele S, Lo Russo L. Anorexia/bulimia-related sialadenosis of palatal minor salivary glands. *J Oral Pathol Med.* 2004;33:441–442.

Sjögren Syndrome

Aljanobi H, Sabharwal A, Krishnakumar B, et al. Is it Sjögren's syndrome or burning mouth syndrome? Distinct pathoses with similar oral symptoms. *Oral Surg Oral Med Oral Pathol Oral Radiol.* 2017;123:482–495.

Bolstad AI, Skarstein K. Epidemiology of Sjögren's syndrome – from an oral perspective. *Curr Oral Health Rep.* 2016;3:328–336.

Patel R, Shahane A. The epidemiology of Sjögren's syndrome. *Clin Epidemiol.* 2014;6:247–255.

Shiboski CH, Shiboski SC, Seror R, et al. 2016 American College of Rheumatology/European League Against Rheumatism classification criteria for primary Sjögren's syndrome: a consensus and data-driven methodology involving three international patient cohorts. *Arthritis Rheumatol.* 2017;69:35–45.

Necrotizing Sialometaplasia

Brannon RB, Fowler CB, Hartman KS. Necrotizing sialometaplasia: a clinicopathologic study of sixty-nine cases and review of the literature. *Oral Surg Oral Med Oral Pathol.* 1991;72:317–325.

Carlson DL. Necrotizing sialometaplasia: a practical approach to the diagnosis. *Arch Pathol Lab Med.* 2009;133:692–698.

Kaplan I, Alterman M, Kleinman S, et al. The clinical, histologic, and treatment spectrum in necrotizing sialometaplasia. *Oral Surg Oral Med Oral Pathol Oral Radiol.* 2012;114:577–585.

Pleomorphic Adenoma

Friedrich RE, Li L, Knop J, et al. Pleomorphic adenoma of the salivary glands: analysis of 94 patients. *Anticancer Res.* 2005;25:1703–1705.

Mendenhall WM, Mendenhall CM, Werning JW, et al. Salivary gland pleomorphic adenoma. *Am J Clin Oncol.* 2008;31:95–99.

Valstar MH, de Ridder M, van den Broek EC, et al. Salivary gland pleomorphic adenoma in the Netherlands: a nationwide observational study of primary tumor incidence, malignant transformation, recurrence, and risk factors for recurrence. *Oral Oncol.* 2017;66:93–99.

Wu Y-C, Wang Y-P, Cheng S-J, et al. Clinicopathological study of 74 palatal pleomorphic adenomas. *J Formos Med Assoc.* 2016;115:25–30.

Warthin Tumor

Espinoza S, Felter A, Malinvaud D, et al. Warthin's tumor of parotid gland: surgery or follow-up? Diagnostic value of a decisional algorithm with functional MRI. *Diagn Interv Imaging.* 2016;97:37–43.

Klussmann JP, Wittekindt C, Preuss SF, et al. High risk for bilateral Warthin tumor in heavy smokers—review of 185 cases. *Acta Otolaryngol.* 2006;126:1213–1217.

Sagiv D, Witt RL, Glikson E, et al. Warthin tumor within the superficial lobe of the parotid gland: a suggested criterion for diagnosis. *Eur Arch Otorhinolaryngol.* 2017;274:1993–1996.

Thangarajah T, Reddy VM, Castellanos-Arango F, et al. Current controversies in the management of Warthin tumour. *Postgrad Med J.* 2009;85:3–8.

Canalicular Adenoma

Peraza AJ, Wright J, Gómez R. Canalicular adenoma: a systematic review. *J Craniomaxillofac Surg.* 2017;45:1754–1758.

Thompson LD, Bauer JL, Chiosea S, et al. Canalicular adenoma: a clinicopathologic and immunohistochemical analysis of 67 cases with a review of the literature. *Head Neck Pathol.* 2015;9:181–195.

Yoon AJ, Beller DE, Woo VL, et al. Bilateral canalicular adenomas of the upper lip. *Oral Surg Oral Med Oral Pathol Oral Radiol Endod.* 2006;102:341–343.

Acinic Cell Carcinoma

Biron VL, Lentsch EJ, Gerry DR, et al. Factors influencing survival in acinic cell carcinoma: a retrospective survival analysis of 2061 patients. *Head Neck.* 2015;37:870–877.

Ellis GL, Corio RL. Acinic cell adenocarcinoma: a clinicopathologic analysis of 294 cases. *Cancer*. 1983;52:542–549.

Neskey DM, Klein JD, Hicks S, et al. Prognostic factors associated with decreased survival in patients with acinic cell carcinoma. *JAMA Otolaryngol Head Neck Surg*. 2013;139:1195–1202.

Vander Poorten V, Triantafyllou A, Thompson LD, et al. Salivary acinic cell carcinoma: reappraisal and update. *Eur Arch Otorhinolaryngol*. 2016;273:3511–3531.

Mucoepidermoid Carcinoma

Coca-Pelaz A, Rodrigo JP, Triantafyllou A, et al. Salivary mucoepidermoid carcinoma revisited. *Eur Arch Otorhinolaryngol*. 2015;272:799–819.

Goode RK, Auclair PL, Ellis GL. Mucoepidermoid carcinoma of the major salivary glands: clinical and histopathologic analysis of 234 cases with evaluation of grading criteria. *Cancer*. 1998;82:1217–1224.

Liu S, Ow A, Ruan M, et al. Prognostic factors in primary salivary gland mucoepidermoid carcinoma: an analysis of 376 cases in an Eastern Chinese population. *Int J Oral Maxillofac Surg*. 2014;43:667–673.

McHugh CH, Roberts DB, El-Naggar AK, et al. Prognostic factors in mucoepidermoid carcinoma of the salivary glands. *Cancer*. 2012;118:3928–3936.

Intraosseous Mucoepidermoid Carcinoma

Bell D, Lewis C, El-Naggar AK, et al. Primary intraosseous mucoepidermoid carcinoma of the jaw: reappraisal of the MD Anderson Cancer Center experience. *Head Neck*. 2016;38:E1312–E1317.

Chan KC, Pharoah M, Lee L, et al. Intraosseous mucoepidermoid carcinoma: a review of the diagnostic imaging features of four jaw cases. *Dentomaxillofac Radiol*. 2013;42:20110162.

Merna C, Kita A, Wester J, et al. Intraosseous mucoepidermoid carcinoma: outcome review. *Laryngoscope*. 2018;doi:10.1002/lary.26832.

Zhou CX, Chen XM, Li TJ. Central mucoepidermoid carcinoma: a clinicopathologic and immunohistochemical study of 39 Chinese patients. *Am J Surg Pathol*. 2012;36:18–26.

Adenoid Cystic Carcinoma

Coca-Pelaz A, Rodrigo JP, Bradley PJ, et al. Adenoid cystic carcinoma of the head and neck – an update. *Oral Oncol*. 2015;51:652–661.

Ellington CL, Goodman M, Kono SA, et al. Adenoid cystic carcinoma of the head and neck: incidence and survival trends based on the 1973-2007 Surveillance, Epidemiology, and End Results data. *Cancer*. 2012;118:4444–4451.

Lloyd S, Yu JB, Wilson LD, et al. Determinants and patterns of survival in adenoid cystic carcinoma of the head and neck, including an analysis of adjuvant radiation therapy. *Am J Clin Oncol*. 2011;34:76–81.

Suárez C, Barnes L, Silver CE, et al. Cervical lymph node metastasis in adenoid cystic carcinoma of the oral cavity and oropharynx: a collective international review. *Auris Nasus Larynx*. 2016;43:477–484.

van Weert S, Bloemena E, van der Waal I, et al. Adenoid cystic carcinoma of the head and neck: a single-center analysis of 105 consecutive cases over a 30-year period. *Oral Oncol*. 2013;49:824–829.

Carcinoma ex Pleomorphic Adenoma

Antony J, Gopalan V, Smith RA, et al. Carcinoma ex pleomorphic adenoma: a comprehensive review of clinical, pathological and molecular data. *Head Neck Pathol*. 2012;6:1–9.

Chen MM, Roman SA, Sosa JA, et al. Predictors of survival in carcinoma ex pleomorphic adenoma. *Head Neck*. 2014;36:1324–1328.

Hu YH, Zhang CY, Xiz RH, et al. Prognostic factors of carcinoma ex pleomorphic adenoma of the salivary glands, with emphasis on the widely invasive carcinoma: a clinicopathologic analysis of 361 cases in a Chinese population. *Oral Surg Oral Med Oral Pathol Oral Radiol*. 2016;122:598–608.

Polymorphous (Low-Grade) Adenocarcinoma

Chi AC, Neville BW. Surface papillary epithelial hyperplasia (rough mucosa) is a helpful clue for identification of polymorphous low-grade adenocarcinoma. *Head Neck Pathol*. 2015;9:244–252.

Elhakim MT, Breinholt H, Godballe C, et al. Polymorphous low-grade adenocarcinoma: a Danish national study. *Oral Oncol*. 2016;55:6–10.

Patel TD, Vazquez A, Marchiano E, et al. Polymorphous low-grade adenocarcinoma of the head and neck: a population-based study of 460 cases. *Laryngoscope*. 2015;125:1644–1649.

Seethala RR, Johnson JT, Barnes EL, et al. Polymorphous low-grade adenocarcinoma: the University of Pittsburgh experience. *Arch Otolaryngol Head Neck Surg*. 2010;136:385–392.

Fonseca I, Assaad A, Katabi N, et al. Polymorphous adenocarcinoma. In: El-Naggar AK, Chan JK, Grandis JR, et al, eds. *WHO Classification of Head and Neck Tumours*. 4th ed. Lyon: IARC; 2017:167.

(Mammary Analogue) Secretory Carcinoma

Baghai F, Yazdani F, Etebarian A, et al. Clinicopathologic and molecular characterization of mammary analogue secretory carcinoma of salivary gland origin. *Pathol Res Pract*. 2017;213:1112–1118.

Bishop JA, Yonescu R, Batista D, et al. Most nonparotid "acinic cell carcinomas" represent mammary analog secretory carcinomas. *Am J Surg Pathol*. 2013;37:1053–1057.

Majewska H, Skálová A, Stodulski D, et al. Mammary analogue secretory carcinoma of salivary glands: a new entity associated with ETV6 gene rearrangement. *Virchows Arch*. 2015;466:245–254.

Skálová A, Vanecek T, Sima R, et al. Mammary analogue secretory carcinoma of salivary glands, containing the ETV6-NTRK3 fusion gene: a hitherto undescribed salivary gland tumor entity. *Am J Surg Pathol*. 2010;34:599–608.

Skálová A, Bell D, Bishop JA, et al. Secretory carcinoma. In: El-Naggar AK, Chan JK, Grandis JR, et al, eds. *WHO Classification of Head and Neck Tumours*. 4th ed. Lyon: IARC; 2017:177.

Salivary Adenocarcinoma, Not Otherwise Specified (NOS)

Li J, Wang BY, Nelson M, et al. Salivary adenocarcinoma, not otherwise specified: a collection of orphans. *Arch Pathol Lab Med*. 2004;128:1385–1394.

Matsuba HM, Mauney M, Simpson JR, et al. Adenocarcinomas of major and minor salivary gland origin: a histopathologic review of treatment failure patterns. *Laryngoscope*. 1988;98:784–788.

Spiro RH, Huvos AG, Strong EW. Adenocarcinoma of salivary origin: clinicopathologic study of 204 patients. *Am J Surg*. 1982;144:423–431.

12

Soft Tissue Tumors

Fibroma (Irritation Fibroma; Traumatic Fibroma)

Figs. 12.1–12.5

The **fibroma** is the most common tumor-like soft tissue growth in the oral cavity. The lesion is not considered to be a true neoplasm but rather a reactive overgrowth of fibrous connective tissue that develops in response to local irritation or trauma. It is most common along the bite line of the buccal mucosa, presumably secondary to biting trauma. Other common locations include the labial mucosa, gingiva, and lateral border of the tongue. The lesion typically appears as a soft to firm nodular growth that is similar in color to the adjacent mucosa. However, fibromas that are subject to ongoing irritation may exhibit secondary ulceration or a white, hyperkeratotic surface. In patients of color, the presence of overlying mucosal pigmentation may result in a gray to brown color.

Fibromas can develop at any age but are diagnosed most frequently in middle-aged adults. They can vary in size from tiny lesions only a couple of millimeters in diameter to larger masses that can measure several centimeters in diameter. On occasion patients may develop more than one lesion. Treatment consists of conservative surgical excision and recurrence is rare. However, the tissue should be submitted for microscopic examination to confirm the diagnosis and to rule out other tumors that may have a similar clinical appearance.

■ **Figure 12.1**
Fibroma
Smooth-surfaced pink nodule on the anterior buccal mucosa.

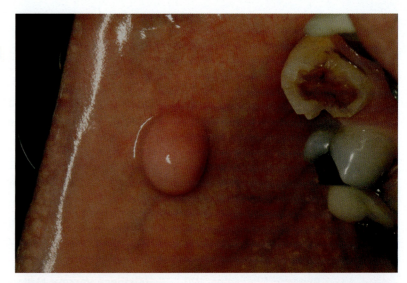

■ **Figure 12.2**
Fibroma
Large nodule on the buccal mucosa.

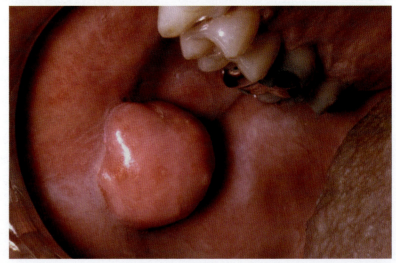

■ Figure **12.3**
Fibroma
Nodular mass on the maxillary buccal gingiva.

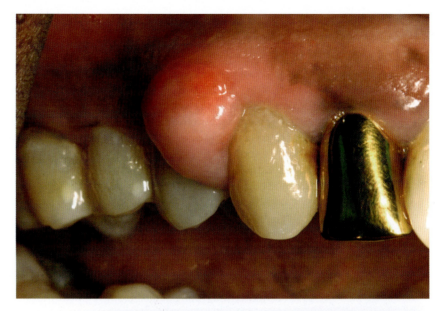

■ Figure **12.4**
Fibroma
Pink nodule on the ventrolateral border of the tongue.

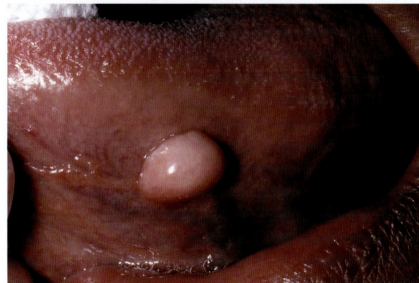

■ Figure **12.5**
Fibroma
Small nodule on the lower labial mucosa.

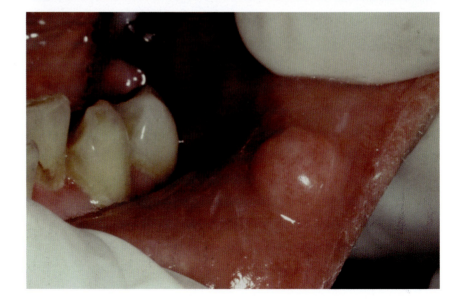

Giant Cell Fibroma

Figs. 12.6 and 12.7

The **giant cell fibroma** is another oral tumor-like growth that is composed of fibrous connective tissue. It exhibits distinctive clinical and microscopic features that warrant its separation from the more common "irritation" fibroma (discussed previously). Its name is derived from the presence of large stellate, multinucleated fibroblasts on histopathologic examination. Unlike the irritation fibroma, the giant cell fibroma does not appear to be caused by trauma. The lesion represents approximately 2% to 5% of oral fibrous growths submitted for biopsy.

In contrast to the irritation fibroma, the giant cell fibroma occurs most frequently on the gingiva rather than the buccal mucosa. The hard palate and tongue are also common locations. Most examples appear as small sessile or pedunculated growths that are less than 1 cm in diameter. Many examples demonstrate a rough, bosselated surface that can be mistaken for a papilloma. The lesion may be pink or of a whitish hue. Treatment usually consists of conservative surgical excision, and recurrence is rare.

Interestingly, the developmental *retrocuspid papilla* shows microscopic features that are similar to those of the giant cell fibroma. Retrocuspid papillae are frequently bilateral lesions that occur as small, pink papules on the lingual gingiva of the lower cuspids. Such lesions are common, being reported in 25% to 99% of children and young adults. However, their prevalence drops to 6% to 19% in older patients, which suggests that they are an anatomic variation that disappears with age. Such lesions should be recognized clinically, but they do not require excision.

Oral Focal Mucinosis

Fig. 12.8

Oral focal mucinosis is an uncommon oral soft tissue growth composed of markedly loose connective tissue. Because this tissue is relatively acellular and contains abundant ground substance, it has a myxomatous (mucinous) appearance microscopically. It is believed to represent the oral counterpart of cutaneous focal mucinosis or cutaneous myxoid cyst. The cause is unknown.

Oral focal mucinosis occurs most often in young adults and shows a 2:1 female-to-male predilection. The most common location is the gingiva, which accounts for two-thirds to three-quarters of all cases. The lesion appears as a sessile or pedunculated, painless nodule that can measure from several millimeters to 2 cm in diameter. Because the color is typically similar to the adjacent mucosa, the lesion often mimics an ordinary fibroma. Treatment consists of excisional biopsy, and the lesion should not recur.

■ Figure **12.6**
Giant Cell Fibroma
Pebbly white lesion on the mandibular lingual gingiva. Such a lesion easily can be mistaken for a papilloma. (Courtesy Dr. Collin Bryant.)

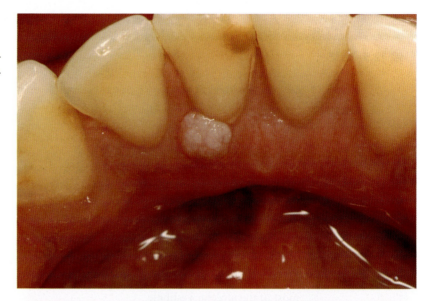

■ Figure **12.7**
Giant Cell Fibroma
Pedunculated nodule of the midline posterior hard palate.

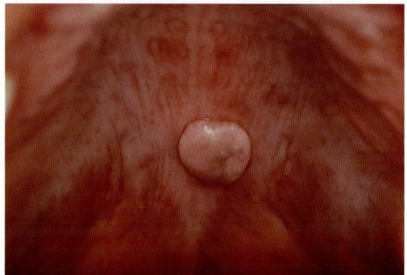

■ Figure **12.8**
Oral Focal Mucinosis
Nodular mass of the incisive papilla area, which mimics a fibroma.

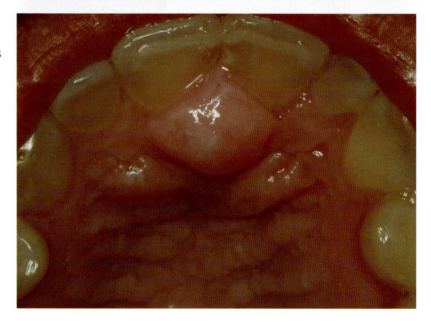

Figs. **12.9–12.12**

The word *epulis* is a generic term that refers to a growth on the gingiva or alveolar mucosa. However, the best-known usage of this term is in **epulis fissuratum**, which is a reactive overgrowth of fibrous connective tissue in response to an ill-fitting denture.

The epulis fissuratum appears as a single fold or multiple folds of hyperplastic tissue in the alveolar vestibule adjacent to a denture flange. When multiple folds are present, they have fissure-like grooves to accommodate the denture—hence the term *epulis fissuratum*. Logically such lesions occur most frequently in middle-aged and older adults because this segment of the population is most likely to become edentulous and to wear a denture. There is a significant predilection for women, who account for two-thirds to three-fourths of reported cases.

Epulis fissuratum can develop in either arch, and lesions are seen more frequently along the anterior portion of the alveolar ridge than in the posterior region. On occasion, such lesions can develop in the floor of the mouth in association with the lingual flange of a lower denture. The redundant tissue is typically pink and firm, although ulceration is often noted at the depth of the fissures. The size of an epulis fissuratum can vary from small, early growths less than 1 cm in length to large, multilobulated masses that involve most of the alveolar vestibule.

Treatment for the epulis fissuratum consists of surgical excision with microscopic examination of the excised tissue. The poorly fitting denture should be remade or relined to prevent recurrence of the tissue overgrowth.

■ Figure **12.9**
Epulis Fissuratum
Hyperplastic folds of tissue in the anterior mandibular vestibule.

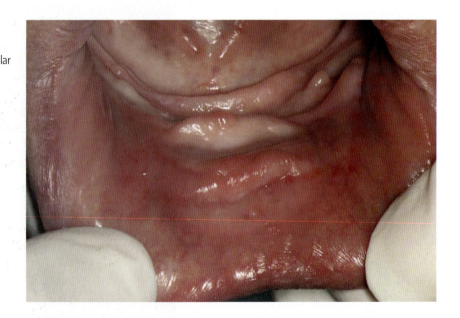

Figure 12.10
Epulis Fissuratum
Multiple redundant folds of hyperplastic tissue in the anterior mandibular vestibule. (With appreciation to Dr. Pete Kobes.)

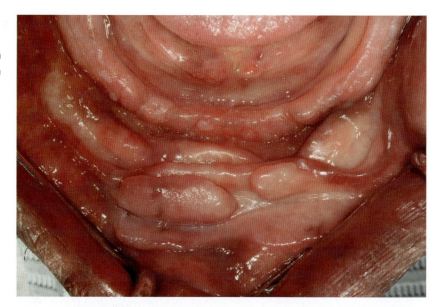

Figure 12.11
Epulis Fissuratum
Same patient as seen in Fig. 12.10, showing the denture fitting in place between the tissue folds. (With appreciation to Dr. Pete Kobes.)

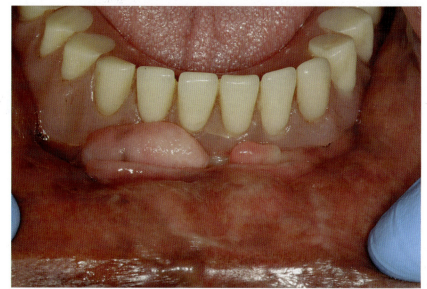

Figure 12.12
Epulis Fissuratum
Hyperplastic tissue in the anterior floor of the mouth.

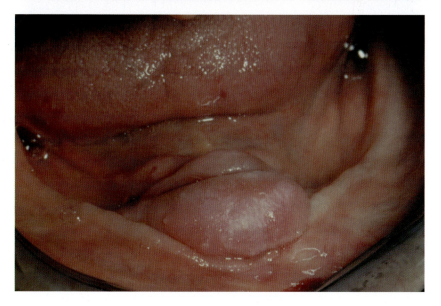

Inflammatory Papillary Hyperplasia

Fig. **12.13**

Inflammatory papillary hyperplasia is a pebbly overgrowth of the oral mucosa, which usually occurs beneath a denture. It may be related to an ill-fitting denture, poor denture hygiene, or a denture that is worn 24 hours a day. *Candida* can be found in up to 20% of cases, although it is uncertain whether these organisms play a role in pathogenesis or are simply secondary pathogens. On occasion the condition also may develop in dentate patients who have high-arched palates or who are mouth breathers.

Inflammatory papillary hyperplasia usually develops on the hard palate, although some examples may occur on the alveolar ridge or on the surface of an epulis fissuratum. The condition typically presents as an asymptomatic red, pebbly hyperplasia of the mucosal surface. Early examples may be localized to the palatal vault, whereas advanced cases may involve virtually the entire hard palate.

Treatment depends on the severity of the condition. Mild examples may be managed by removal of the denture, which can reduce inflammation and allow the mucosa to return to a more normal appearance. Cases related to *Candida* may show some improvement after appropriate antifungal therapy. More advanced cases may require surgical removal prior to fabrication of a new denture. When the tissue is examined microscopically, the epithelium sometimes demonstrates prominent, irregular hyperplasia of the rete ridges (*pseudoepitheliomatous hyperplasia*), which potentially could be mistaken for squamous cell carcinoma. Clinical correlation and good communication between the clinician and pathologist are important to avoid this possibility.

Leaflike Denture Fibroma

Figs. **12.14 and 12.15**

Like the epulis fissuratum and inflammatory papillary hyperplasia, the **leaflike denture fibroma** is another reactive tissue overgrowth related to a poorly fitting denture. Also known as a fibroepithelial polyp, the lesion develops as a pedunculated growth on the hard palate beneath a complete maxillary denture. The lesion appears as a flattened, pink mucosal mass attached to the palate by a narrow stalk. When the denture is in place, this mass is compressed against the roof of the mouth. However, when the denture is removed, the growth can be lifted away from an underlying cupped-out mucosal depression. Often the periphery of the mass will exhibit a serrated edge that makes it resemble a tree leaf. Sometimes adjacent inflammatory papillary hyperplasia also may be present. Treatment consists of excisional biopsy followed by relining the existing denture or fabrication of a new prosthesis.

Figure **12.13**
Inflammatory Papillary Hyperplasia
Red, pebbly mucosal change in the palatal vault. (Courtesy Dr. Rhet Tucker.)

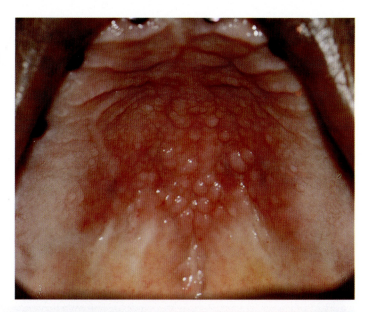

Figure **12.14**
Leaflike Denture Fibroma
Flat soft tissue mass pressed against the palatal mucosa beneath a denture.

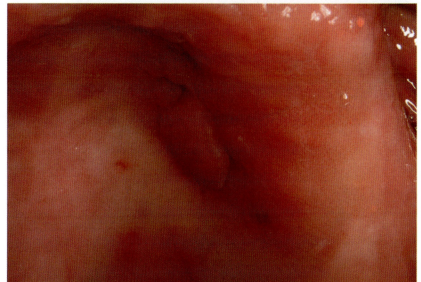

Figure **12.15**
Leaflike Denture Fibroma
Same patient as seen in Fig. 12.14, showing the pedunculated nature of the lesion.

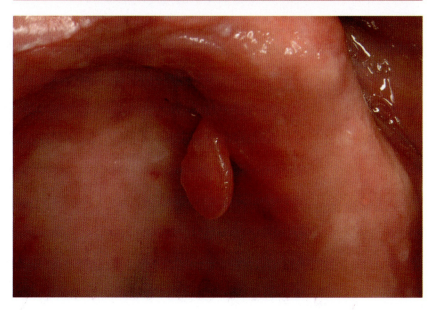

Solitary Fibrous Tumor

Fig. **12.16**

The **solitary fibrous tumor** is a rare soft tissue neoplasm that exhibits fibroblastic or myofibroblastic differentiation. Originally described in 1931 as a pleural tumor, it now has been described in a variety of other sites, including the oral cavity. Tumors previously categorized under the name *hemangiopericytoma* are thought to represent cellular variants of solitary fibrous tumor.

The solitary fibrous tumor occurs most often in middle-aged adults and does not show a gender predilection. Oral examples develop most frequently on the buccal mucosa, although cases also have been reported at a number of other sites including the lip, tongue, alveolar mucosa, and floor of mouth. The lesion appears as a firm, painless nodular mass that is indistinguishable clinically from a variety of other soft tissue neoplasms. The tumor usually is well circumscribed and separates easily from the surrounding tissues at the time of surgery.

Treatment for the solitary fibrous tumor usually consists of local surgical excision, although wider resection may be required if microscopic features of malignancy are identified. Most oral examples behave in a benign fashion, although up to 10% of extrapleural tumors at other sites have demonstrated malignant behavior.

Myofibroma

Fig. **12.17**

The **myofibroma** is a tumor composed of myofibroblasts, which are cells showing fibroblastic and smooth muscle features. Although such tumors are rare, the head and neck region is one of the most common locations. Myofibromas can occur at any age, but lesions develop most frequently in the first and second decades of life (the mean age is 23.1 years). Most examples occur as single tumors, although some patients develop multicentric lesions *(myofibromatosis)*. The most common site for oral lesions is within the mandible, followed by the alveolar/gingival mucosa, buccal mucosa, and tongue.

An oral myofibroma typically presents as a firm, painless mass that is difficult to distinguish from a variety of other soft tissue growths. Soft tissue examples are usually pink to red, and ulceration sometimes will occur secondary to trauma. Intrabony lesions may appear as either unilocular or poorly defined radiolucent defects. Multicentric myofibromatosis usually is diagnosed in neonates and infants, who may develop from several to over a hundred of such tumors throughout the body.

Solitary myofibromas should be treated by conservative surgical excision. Only a small percentage of tumors recur, which usually can be managed by reexcision. Multifocal examples also rarely recur, and sometimes such lesions can undergo spontaneous regression. However, neonatal myofibromatosis involving the viscera or vital organs sometimes acts aggressively and can result in death within the first few days of life.

Aggressive Fibromatosis

Fig. **12.18**

The term *fibromatosis* has been used for a variety of fibrous tissue growths in different anatomic locations. For example, one well-recognized benign fibrous overgrowth limited to the gingival tissues is known by the term *gingival fibromatosis*, although this condition is not considered neoplastic. However, more cellular and infiltrative fibrous soft tissue tumors can occur; these are termed **aggressive fibromatosis**, or sometimes **juvenile fibromatosis**, because they are seen most frequently in children and young adults. These locally aggressive lesions have a biologic behavior considered to be intermediate between common benign fibrous growths and fibrosarcoma. A similar intrabony counterpart is known as a *desmoplastic fibroma*.

Aggressive fibromatosis in the head and neck region usually appears as a firm painless mass that can grow to considerable size, with resultant facial deformity. The most common site is the paramandibular soft tissue region, which may be associated radiographically with irregular underlying bone erosion. In some instances, the mass develops gradually, although other examples show more rapid growth. Treatment consists of surgical resection, which often requires a generous margin of adjacent normal tissue. Recurrence has been reported in approximately 30% of head and neck cases, but metastasis does not occur. Adjuvant chemotherapy or radiation therapy sometimes may be employed for recurrent or incompletely resected tumors.

■ Figure **12.16**
Solitary Fibrous Tumor
Nodular mass on the lower labial mucosa. (Courtesy Dr. Tom McDonald.)

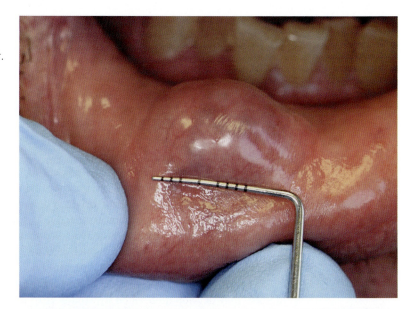

■ Figure **12.17**
Myofibroma
Ulcerated mass arising on the maxillary buccal gingiva. (Courtesy Dr. Patrick Coleman.)

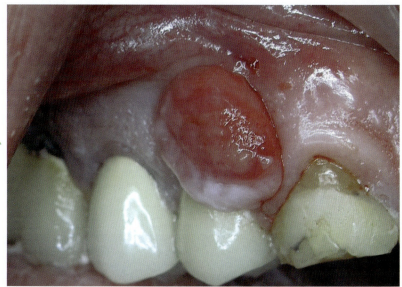

■ Figure **12.18**
Aggressive Fibromatosis
Panoramic radiograph showing bony destruction of the right posterior body and ramus of the mandible. (Courtesy Dr. Khaled Abughazaleh.)

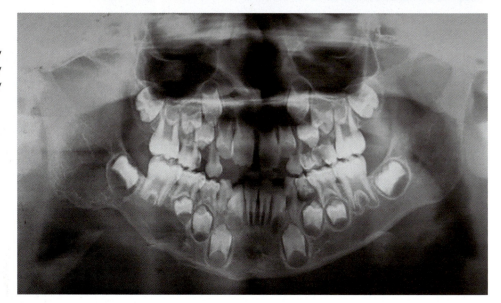

Figs. **12.19–12.22**

The **pyogenic granuloma** is a common tumor-like overgrowth of granulation tissue thought to represent a reactive lesion to local irritation rather than a true neoplasm. However, because many examples microscopically demonstrate a lobular arrangement of capillary blood vessels, the term *lobular capillary hemangioma* also sometimes is used. The name "pyogenic granuloma" is actually inaccurate and misleading. Such lesions are not pyogenic (pus-producing), nor are they composed of true granulomatous inflammation microscopically.

Oral pyogenic granulomas usually present as ulcerated masses that initially may demonstrate rapid growth. Lesions are typically painless, but they often will bleed easily because of their prominent vascularity. Early pyogenic granulomas appear bright red, although later lesions may become pink as blood vessels gradually are replaced by fibrous connective tissue. The size can vary from small growths only a few millimeters in diameter to large exophytic, pedunculated masses several centimeters in diameter. The most common location is the gingiva, which accounts for approximately 75% to 85% of oral cases. Other examples may occur on the tongue, lips, and buccal mucosa.

Pyogenic granulomas can occur at any age, but they are seen most frequently in children and young adults. They develop more often in women than in men, which often is attributed to the effect of female hormones. It is well known that the prevalence is higher in women during pregnancy—so much so that such lesions have been called *pregnancy tumors* or *granuloma gravidarum*. Following pregnancy, these lesions may shrink and undergo fibrous maturation to resemble a fibroma.

Pyogenic granulomas usually are treated by complete surgical excision. For examples associated with pregnancy, removal sometimes is deferred until after childbirth unless the lesion is causing significant functional or cosmetic problems. For pyogenic granulomas of the gingiva, the excision should extend down to the periosteum, and the adjacent teeth should be scaled to remove any underlying source of irritation, such as dental calculus. The reported recurrence rate ranges from 3% to 15%, with a higher risk of recurrence for lesions removed during pregnancy. It is important to submit the excised tissue for microscopic examination because both primary and metastatic malignancies can mimic pyogenic granulomas.

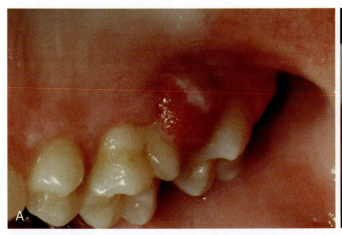 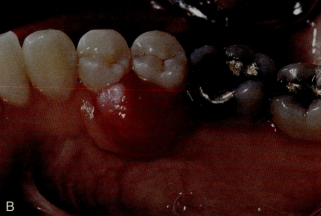

■ Figure **12.19**
Pyogenic Granuloma
(A) Red, ulcerated mass on the palatal gingiva. (B) Ulcerated mass on the mandibular lingual gingiva.

■ Figure **12.20**
Pyogenic Granuloma
Large pink mass arising on the mandibular buccal gingiva.

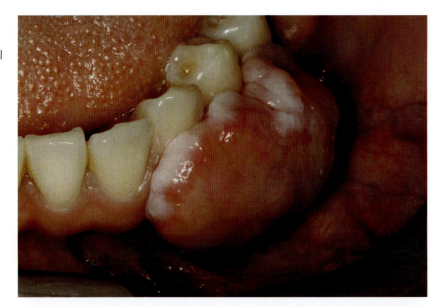

■ Figure **12.21**
Pyogenic Granuloma
Ulcerated red mass on the anterior dorsal tongue.

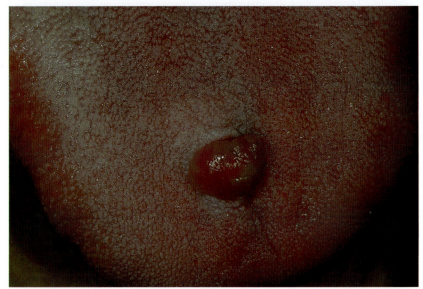

■ Figure **12.22**
Pyogenic Granuloma
Large pedunculated, ulcerated mass on the anterior dorsal tongue.

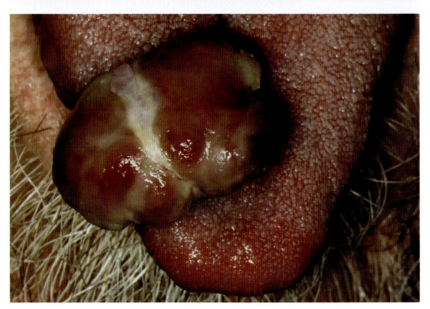

Epulis Granulomatosa

Fig. **12.23**

The term **epulis granulomatosa** is used for overgrowths of hyperplastic granulation tissue that develop in extraction sockets. Such lesions resemble pyogenic granulomas and often arise secondary to the presence of small bony sequestra within the granulation tissue of the healing extraction site. Clinically, the epulis granulomatosa presents as an ulcerated, nodular growth of pinkish red tissue that emanates from a recent extraction socket. Treatment consists of surgical excision of the mass and curettage of the socket to remove any remaining bone spicules. Microscopic examination of the excised tissue is important to rule out the possibility of unsuspected malignancy, including both primary and metastatic tumors of the oral cavity.

Peripheral Ossifying Fibroma

Figs. **12.24 and 12.25**

The **peripheral ossifying fibroma** is a common, tumor-like growth of the gingiva characterized by a core of fibrous connective tissue exhibiting the formation of variable amounts of mineralized product. The lesion is considered to be reactive rather than neoplastic, and the mineralized product probably arises from either periosteal or periodontal ligament cells. Many examples produce obvious woven or lamellar bone, but other cases show formation of cementum-like material or dystrophic calcifications. It is possible that some lesions develop initially as pyogenic granulomas that subsequently demonstrate fibrous maturation and mineralization. Despite the similarity in names, this lesion is unrelated to the central ossifying fibroma of bone.

Peripheral ossifying fibromas occur most frequently in teenagers and young adults, with a peak prevalence during the second decade of life. They show a nearly 2:1 female-to-male ratio. Lesions are slightly more common in the maxillary arch, and over half of cases develop in the incisor/canine region. An early peripheral ossifying fibroma appears as a red ulcerated mass that often mimics a pyogenic granuloma of the gingiva. The growth typically appears to arise from the interdental papilla, and it can be sessile or pedunculated. As the lesion matures, it may undergo fibrous maturation with reepithelialization of the ulcerated surface, assuming an appearance more suggestive of an irritation fibroma. Most peripheral ossifying fibromas are less than 2 cm in diameter, although rare examples measure as large as 6 to 9 cm. The adjacent teeth are usually unaffected, although occasional examples have been associated with tooth loosening or migration.

Treatment for the peripheral ossifying fibroma consists of surgical removal, which should include microscopic examination of the excised tissue. The potential for recurrence ranges from 8% to as high as 30%. To minimize the risk of recurrence, the excision should extend down to periosteum and the adjacent teeth should be scaled thoroughly to remove any potential source of irritation.

Figure **12.23**
Epulis Granulomatosa
Hyperplastic granulation tissue that developed at the site of recent tooth extractions.

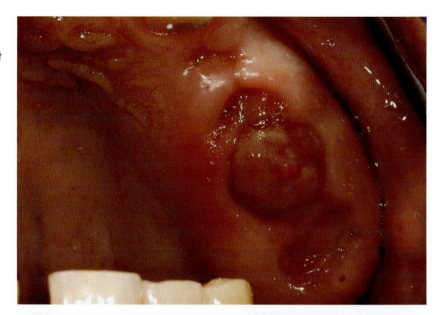

Figure **12.24**
Peripheral Ossifying Fibroma
Red, ulcerated mass on the maxillary buccal gingiva.

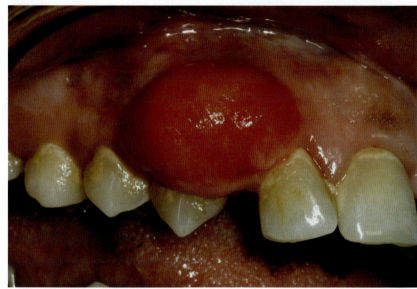

Figure **12.25**
Peripheral Ossifying Fibroma
Pinkish red nodule on the anterior maxillary gingiva.

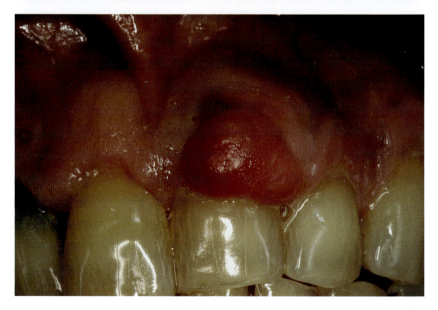

Peripheral Giant Cell Granuloma

Fig. 12.26

The **peripheral giant cell granuloma** is a relatively common tumor-like growth that develops on the gingiva or alveolar ridge. It is microscopically similar to the central giant cell granuloma of bone, being characterized by a proliferation of multinucleated giant cells that resemble osteoclasts. Peripheral giant cell granulomas occur over a wide age range, with a mean age ranging from 31 to 46 years. There is no significant gender predilection. The lesion occurs slightly more often on the mandibular than on the maxillary gingiva.

The peripheral giant cell granuloma presents as a red to blue-purple mass that may or may not be ulcerated. The lesion often has been present for many months before the diagnosis is made. Most lesions measure less than 2 cm in diameter, but larger examples occasionally occur. The clinical appearance frequently mimics a pyogenic granuloma; however, peripheral giant cell granulomas often exhibit a more blue to purple hue rather than the bright red color typical of a pyogenic granuloma. On occasion, cupping resorption of the underlying alveolar bone may be noted.

Treatment for the peripheral giant cell granuloma consists of complete surgical excision, which should extend down to the underlying bone. The adjacent teeth should be scaled to remove any source of irritation that might contribute to recurrence of the lesion, which has been estimated to develop in 10% to 18% of cases. On rare occasions, peripheral giant cell lesions have been reported in patients with hyperparathyroidism. However, "brown tumors" of hyperparathyroidism are more likely to occur within bone and mimic a central giant cell granuloma.

Lipoma

Figs. 12.27 and 12.28

The most common true neoplasm of mesenchymal origin is the **lipoma**—a benign tumor of fat. Such tumors often develop on the trunk and proximal extremities, although they occur less frequently in the oral and maxillofacial regions. Lipomas are more common in obese patients, although their metabolism is not related to normal body fat; if a patient with a lipoma loses weight, the tumor will not reduce in size even though body fat is lost.

Lipomas develop most often in middle-aged and older adults. The tumor presents as a slowly growing soft, nodular mass that may be sessile or pedunculated. The most common oral locations are the buccal mucosa and buccal vestibule, which account for almost half of all cases. However, it is speculated that occasional reported buccal examples actually may represent herniation of the buccal fat pad through the buccinator muscle, which results in a mass that resembles a tumor. Less common intraoral sites include the tongue, floor of mouth, and lips. The lipoma frequently will demonstrate a yellowish hue, although deeper tumors may appear pink. Treatment consists of local surgical excision, and recurrence is rare.

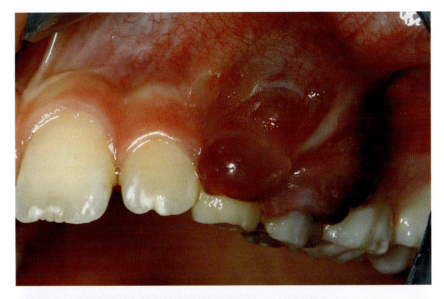

■ Figure 12.26
Peripheral Giant Cell Granuloma
Blue-purple mass on the maxillary buccal gingiva.

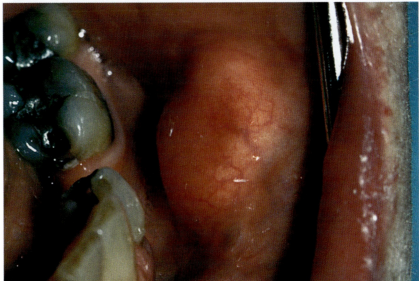

■ Figure 12.27
Lipoma
Yellowish submucosal mass in the buccal mucosa.

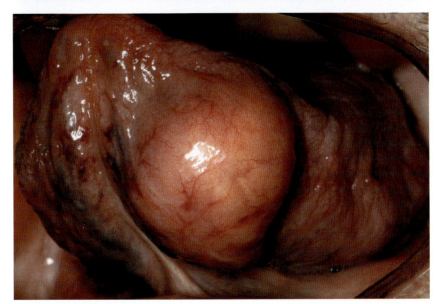

■ Figure 12.28
Lipoma
Large yellowish pink mass of the anterior tongue.

Schwannoma (Neurilemoma)

Figs. **12.29–12.31**

The **schwannoma** is a benign neural tumor derived from Schwann cells—the cells responsible for producing the myelin sheath around nerve axons. Although these tumors are uncommon, from one-quarter to nearly one-half of all cases occur in the head and neck region. Schwannomas may occur as isolated neoplasms, but they also can develop as part of two hereditary syndromes: *neurofibromatosis type II* and *schwannomatosis*.

Schwannomas are diagnosed most often in young and middle-aged adults. An isolated schwannoma frequently arises as a slow-growing, rubbery, firm, encapsulated mass along a nerve trunk. The tumor is usually asymptomatic, although some cases are associated with tenderness or pain. Schwannomas can occur anywhere in the oral cavity, but the most common location is the tongue. Rare intrabony examples also may develop, usually presenting as unilocular or multilocular radiolucencies.

Neurofibromatosis type II is an autosomal dominant condition caused by mutation of a tumor suppressor gene (known as *NF2*) on chromosome 22, which is responsible for production of the protein *merlin*. Individuals with this disorder develop bilateral schwannomas ("acoustic neuromas") of the auditory-vestibular nerve (cranial nerve VIII), which result in deafness, tinnitus, and dizziness. Patients also may develop additional schwannomas of peripheral nerves as well as meningiomas and gliomas in the central nervous system. Schwannomatosis is related to mutation of a different gene on chromosome 22 known as *SMARCB1*. Patients with this condition develop multiple noncutaneous schwannomas but without tumors of the auditory-vestibular nerve. Interestingly, the tumors in this condition usually cause chronic pain.

Treatment for a solitary peripheral schwannoma consists of local surgical excision, and recurrence is rare. Surgical management for acoustic neuromas associated with neurofibromatosis type II, because of their location, is much more difficult, often resulting in deafness and possible facial nerve damage. Stereotactic radiosurgery is an alternative approach that sometimes is used for older or frail patients with such tumors.

■ **Figure 12.29**
Schwannoma
Parapharyngeal tumor resulting in bulging asymmetry of the patient's left soft palate.

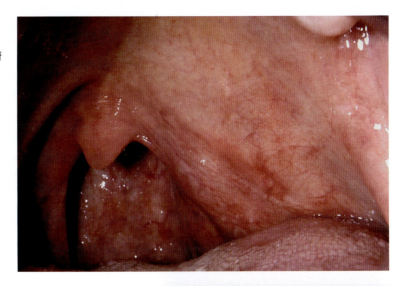

■ **Figure 12.30**
Schwannoma
Computed tomography scan showing a tumor in the left parapharyngeal space *(arrow)*. (With appreciation to Dr. Terry Day.)

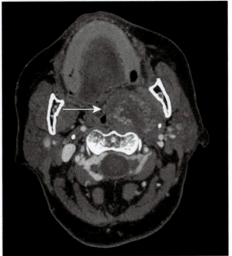

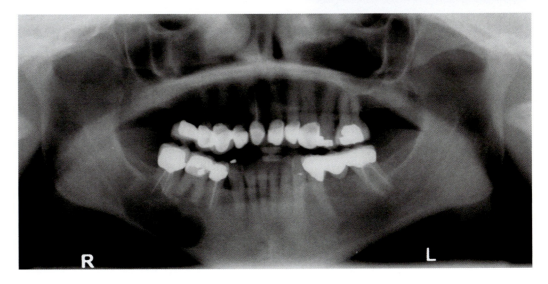

■ **Figure 12.31**
Schwannoma
Large unilocular radiolucency of the right mandible apical to the molar teeth, representing a schwannoma that arose from the mandibular nerve. (Courtesy Dr. Brent Mortenson.)

Traumatic Neuroma (Amputation Neuroma)

Fig. 12.32

The **traumatic neuroma** is a tumor-like proliferation of neural tissue that develops after a nerve has been severed or otherwise damaged. When a nerve is damaged, the nerve bundle distal to the site of trauma typically undergoes degeneration. As the proximal end of the nerve tries to grow along the old nerve pathway and reestablish innervation, it may encounter scar tissue that blocks its path. Growth of the nerve in the area of the scar then produces a mass at the site.

A traumatic neuroma of the oral mucosa presents as a smooth-surfaced nodular mass. Frequently, the patient will complain of altered nerve sensation or pain, which can be spontaneous or may be triggered by manipulation of the lesion. However, not all traumatic neuromas are painful. The most common oral site is the mental foramen area, presumably secondary to either tooth extraction or subsequent trauma from wearing a denture. Patients may report numbness along the distribution of the nerve distal to the site of damage. Other common oral locations include the tongue and lower lip. Intraosseous examples also can occur; such a lesion may be noted as a radiolucent defect on routine oral radiographs.

Treatment for the traumatic neuroma consists of surgical excision, which should include a small portion of the proximal nerve bundle. Most such lesions do not recur, although some examples may return or be associated with persistent pain at the site.

Palisaded Encapsulated Neuroma (Solitary Circumscribed Neuroma)

Fig. 12.33

The **palisaded encapsulated neuroma** is an uncommon nerve tumor that has a predilection for the head and neck region. Because most examples are not truly encapsulated and may show only focal palisading of the lesional cells, some authors prefer the term *solitary circumscribed neuroma*. This lesion may not represent a true neoplasm, and it has been speculated that trauma may play a role in its etiology.

The palisaded encapsulated neuroma develops most often on the face, especially on the nose and cheeks. Oral examples most frequently occur on the hard palate, gingiva, and labial mucosa. The lesion typically presents as a smooth, dome-shaped, painless nodule that is usually less than 1 cm in diameter. Treatment consists of conservative local excision, and the lesion rarely recurs.

Neurofibroma

Fig. 12.34

The **neurofibroma** is a benign neoplasm that is composed of a mixed population of Schwann cells, perineural fibroblasts, and axons. It is the most common peripheral nerve tumor. The lesion is diagnosed most frequently on the skin, but intraoral neurofibromas also occur.

A neurofibroma presents as a soft, painless, nodular mass that grows slowly. Size can vary from small lesions that are only a few millimeters in diameter to large, diffuse masses several centimeters in size. Solitary tumors are diagnosed most frequently in young adults. If a patient has multiple tumors, the possibility of neurofibromatosis type I must be strongly considered (see next topic). Intrabony neurofibromas also have been reported; these can appear as either unilocular or multilocular radiolucencies.

The possibility of neurofibromatosis should be ruled out in any patient with a neurofibroma. Treatment for solitary tumors consists of surgical excision, and recurrence is uncommon. Malignant transformation of an isolated neurofibroma is rare, although a significant risk for the development of a peripheral malignant nerve sheath tumor does exist for patients with neurofibromatosis.

■ Figure **12.32**
Traumatic Neuroma
Small pink nodule on the upper lip.

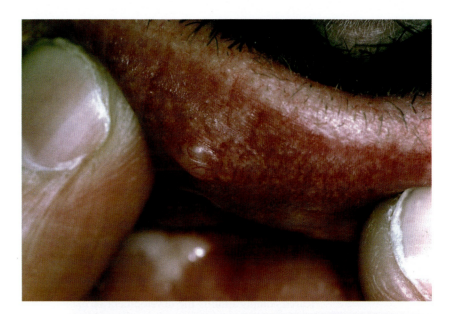

■ Figure **12.33**
Palisaded Encapsulated Neuroma
Nodular mass of the anterior hard palate in the incisive papilla area.

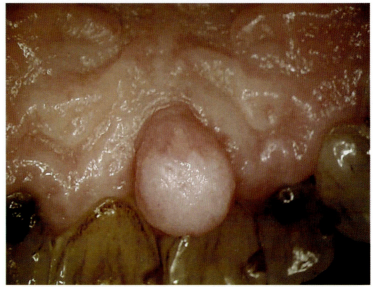

■ Figure **12.34**
Neurofibroma
Nodular mass of the anterior hard palate showing secondary ulceration. (Courtesy Dr. John Hall.)

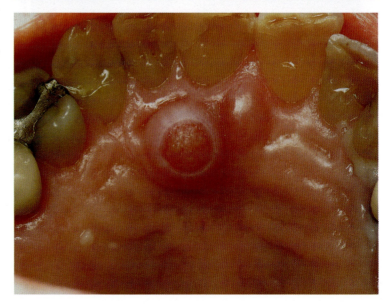

Figs. **12.35–12.38**

The term *neurofibromatosis* refers to a family of genetic disorders characterized by the development of tumors of the central and peripheral nervous systems. The most common form is **neurofibromatosis type I**, which is estimated to occur in one out of every 2500 to 3000 births. This disorder is caused by various mutations of the *NF1* gene on chromosome 17, which is responsible for the production of a tumor suppressor protein known as *neurofibromin*. Although the condition is inherited as an autosomal dominant trait, about half of affected patients have no family history and presumably represent new gene mutations.

Patients with this condition develop multiple neurofibromas on the skin and elsewhere throughout the body. The condition has widely variable expression; some individuals may have only a few tumors, whereas others have literally hundreds to thousands of lesions. A second common feature is the presence of multiple tan to brown macular skin lesions known as *café au lait spots*, so named because their color resembles that of coffee with milk. Similar freckle-like pigmentation *(Crowe sign)* also may be noted in the axilla or groin. Another frequent finding is the presence of pigmented spots on the iris, known as *Lisch nodules*. A variety of other problems can develop, including short stature, scoliosis, macrocephaly, hypertension, adrenal pheochromocytoma, central nervous system tumors (including optic glioma), and seizures. A feared complication is the development of malignancy—especially a malignant peripheral nerve sheath neoplasm, which is estimated to occur in as many as 5% of patients. Other potential malignancies associated with neurofibromatosis type I include leukemia, Wilms tumor, and rhabdomyosarcoma.

Oral manifestations have been described in as many as 72% to 92% of patients. The most common finding is enlargement of the fungiform papillae on the tongue, although the specificity of this finding for neurofibromatosis is unknown. This change may be subtle, but it has been reported in up to 50% of patients. Actual intraoral neurofibromas occur in only 25% to 37% of patients. Radiographic manifestations may include widening of the mandibular canal or foramina, increased bone density, increased size of the coronoid notch, and concavities of the mandibular ramus. Some patients with neurofibromatosis type I may present with unilateral facial and oral enlargement, which can mimic hemifacial hyperplasia.

Management of neurofibromatosis type I usually is directed toward prevention or treatment of its various complications. Individual neurofibromas that cause functional or cosmetic problems can be surgically removed. The average life span of affected patients is about 8 to 15 years less than that of the general population; this is mostly related to the increased risk for vascular disease and malignancy. The 5-year survival rate for malignant peripheral nerve sheath tumors in this condition ranges from 35% to 54%.

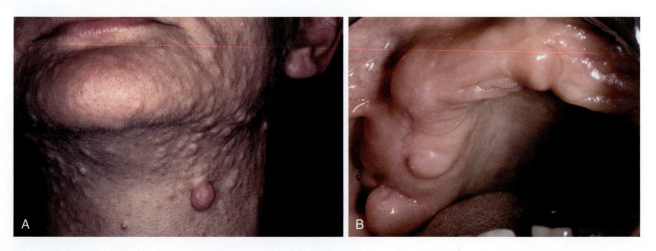

■ Figure **12.35**
Neurofibromatosis Type I
(A) Multiple neurofibromas appearing as soft, painless nodules and papules of the face and neck. (B) Pink nodules of the maxillary alveolar ridge representing intraoral neurofibromas.

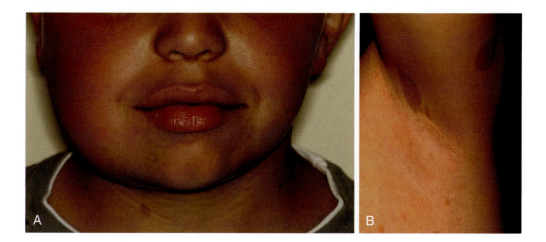

■ Figure **12.36**
Neurofibromatosis Type I
(A) Diffuse neurofibroma producing unilateral facial enlargement in a young boy. (B) Same patient showing café au lait pigmentation of the arm and axilla. (With appreciation to Dr. Terry Day.)

■ Figure **12.37**
Neurofibromatosis Type I
Axillary freckling (Crowe sign).

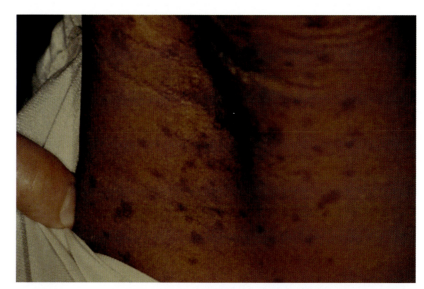

■ Figure **12.38**
Neurofibromatosis Type I
Rapidly enlarging ulcerated growth in a patient with neurofibromatosis type I. This was diagnosed as a malignant peripheral nerve sheath tumor.

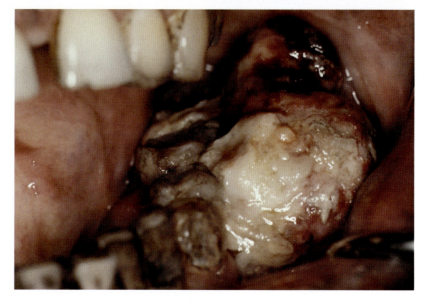

Figs. 12.39–12.42

The **multiple endocrine neoplasia** (MEN) syndromes are a group of autosomal dominant hereditary conditions characterized by tumors or hyperplasias of various tissues of neuroendocrine origin. MEN type 1 is caused by a mutation of the *MEN1* gene located on chromosome 11. Patients with this condition can develop a variety of tumors of the anterior pituitary gland, parathyroid gland, pancreas, and adrenal cortex. MEN type 2 encompasses a family of three disorders with mutations at various sites of the *RET* proto-oncogene on chromosome 10. All three of these disorders are characterized by the development of an aggressive thyroid tumor known as *medullary thyroid carcinoma* (MTC). In the first condition, known as *familial medullary thyroid carcinoma syndrome*, patients develop only MTC without an increased risk for other neuroendocrine tumors. Individuals with *MEN type 2A* develop MTC, adrenal pheochromocytoma (50% of patients), and primary hyperparathyroidism (15% to 25% of patients). *MEN type 2B* has important orofacial manifestations; therefore, the remainder of this discussion centers on this particular condition.

Although MEN type 2B is inherited as an autosomal dominant trait, approximately half of all cases have no family history and represent spontaneous new mutations. Affected patients exhibit a marfanoid body build with narrow, elongated limbs and muscle wasting. The face also appears narrow, with the presence of full, protuberant lips because of the proliferation of nerve bundles. Ocular manifestations may include ptosis, thickening, and eversion of the eyelids as well as subconjunctival neuromas. Multiple neuromas also typically develop along the anterior margin of the tongue and bilaterally at the commissures. These lesions appear as soft painless papules or nodules with a pink or slightly yellowish color. On occasion, neuromas also can occur on the gingiva or palate. A tendency for diastema formation also has been noted.

Pheochromocytomas of the adrenal gland develop in at least half of all patients with MEN type 2B. These tumors secrete catecholamines, which may produce a variety of symptoms such as sweating, diarrhea, headaches, heart palpitations, flushing, and severe hypertension. Another potential complication is ganglioneuromatosis of the gastrointestinal tract (40% of cases), which can result in abdominal distention, megacolon, diarrhea, or constipation.

The most significant manifestation of MEN type 2B is the development of MTC, which occurs in virtually all cases. This aggressive tumor arises from the parafollicular C cells of the thyroid gland, which are responsible for the production of calcitonin. Such tumors often develop very early in infancy or childhood and have a marked propensity for metastasis. Management of patients with MEN type 2B consists of early recognition and prophylactic thyroidectomy, which ideally should be performed before 1 year of age, before development and metastasis of MTC. The average age of death from this neoplasm is 21 years.

■ Figure **12.39**
Multiple Endocrine Neoplasia Type 2B
Young man with a history of medullary thyroid carcinoma and bilateral adrenal pheochromocytomas. Note the narrow face and full, protuberant lips.

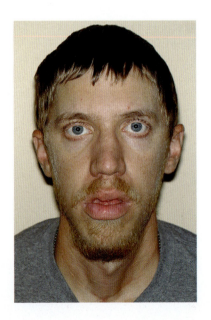

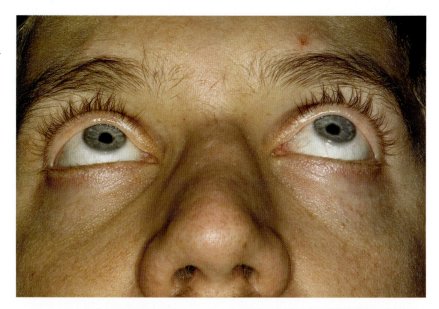

■ Figure **12.40**
Multiple Endocrine Neoplasia Type 2B
Same patient showing slight eversion of the upper eyelids.

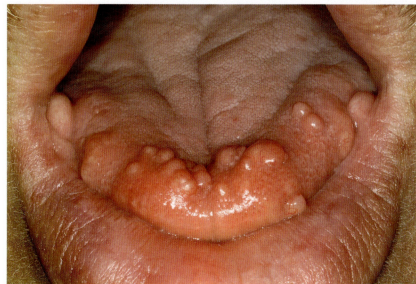

■ Figure **12.41**
Multiple Endocrine Neoplasia Type 2B.
Same patient showing multiple neuromas at the commissures and along the anterior margin of the tongue.

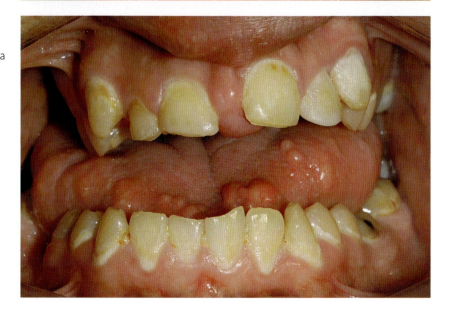

■ Figure **12.42**
Multiple Endocrine Neoplasia Type 2B.
Same patient showing midline diastema with a neuroma of the gingiva and incisive papilla area.

Melanotic Neuroectodermal Tumor of Infancy

Figs. **12.43 and 12.44**

The **melanotic neuroectodermal tumor of infancy** is a rare, locally aggressive tumor of neural crest origin that usually develops during the first year of life. The tumor has a striking predilection for the maxilla, which accounts for 62% of reported cases. Other reported sites include the skull, mandible, epididymis, testis, and brain. The tumor is composed of small neuroblastic cells as well as larger melanin-containing cells, which are responsible for the pigmentation observed clinically and pathologically.

The tumor develops most often in the anterior portion of the maxilla, where it appears as a rapidly growing mass that expands the alveolar ridge. Radiographic examination typically shows underlying bone destruction, which often is associated with displacement of the developing teeth. On occasion, the tumor results in a "sun ray" osteogenic reaction, which can mimic osteosarcoma.

The melanotic neuroectodermal tumor of infancy usually is treated surgically, either by curettage or local resection with 5-mm margins. Approximately 20% to 25% of cases will recur, usually within 6 months after treatment. Although most such tumors are considered to be benign, about 7% of reported cases have acted in a malignant fashion, resulting in metastasis and death. Malignant examples are more likely to arise in the skull and brain.

Granular Cell Tumor

Fig. **12.45**

The **granular cell tumor** is an uncommon mesenchymal neoplasm with a predilection for the oral cavity. Its name is derived from the presence of eosinophilic granules within the cytoplasm of the tumor cells. The most common site in the body for this tumor is the tongue, which accounts for one-third to one-half of all cases. The tumor also can be seen on the skin and at other oral mucosal sites. Because the cells often show an intimate relationship with adjacent skeletal muscle, the lesion originally was thought to be of muscular origin—hence the older term *granular cell myoblastoma*. However, current investigators agree that the lesion is most likely derived from Schwann cells.

The granular cell tumor is diagnosed most frequently in young to middle-aged adults, and it shows a 2 : 1 female predilection. It appears as a firm, painless, sessile nodule that is usually 2 cm or less in diameter. The patient often has been aware of the lesion for many months or years before diagnosis. The lesion may be pink, although a number of granular cell tumors will appear distinctly yellow, thus sometimes mimicking a lipoma. Some patients will develop multiple granular cell tumors.

The treatment for the granular cell tumor consists of local surgical excision. Recurrence is uncommon, even if the lesion is not entirely removed. Microscopically, some granular cell tumors will induce pseudoepitheliomatous hyperplasia of the overlying epithelium, which can mimic an invasive squamous cell carcinoma. It is important for the pathologist to be aware of this possibility to avoid a mistaken diagnosis of cancer.

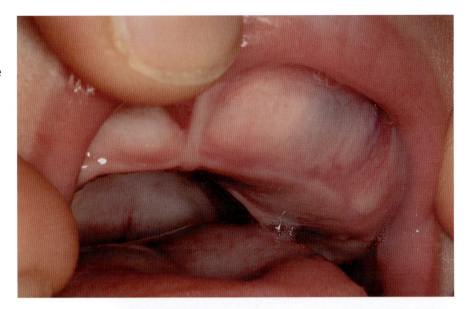

Figure **12.43**
Melanotic Neuroectodermal Tumor of Infancy
Infant with a bluish pigmented swelling of the anterior maxillary alveolar ridge.

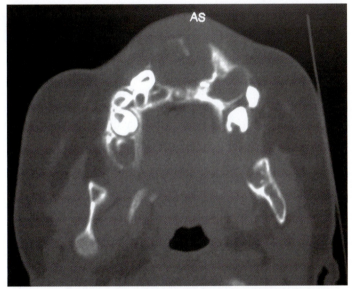

Figure **12.44**
Melanotic Neuroectodermal Tumor of Infancy
Axial computed tomography scan of same patient as in Fig. 12.43 showing a destructive radiolucent tumor of the anterior maxilla.

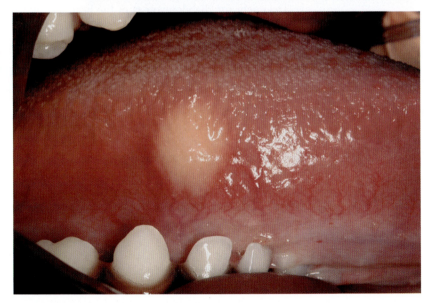

Figure **12.45**
Granular Cell Tumor
Four-year-old male with a slightly raised yellow nodule on the lateral border of the tongue. (With appreciation to Dr. Michael Tabor.)

Congenital Epulis

Fig. **12.46**

The **congenital epulis** is a rare tumor of uncertain histogenesis that is discovered almost exclusively on the alveolar ridge of a newborn. Although its microscopic appearance is somewhat similar to that of the granular cell tumor (discussed previously), it represents a distinct entity. Because occasional examples have also been reported on the tongue, some authors prefer the more generic name **congenital granular cell lesion** (avoiding the term *epulis*, which specifically implies a growth that develops on the gingiva or alveolar ridge).

The congenital epulis shows a striking predilection for females; this accounts for nearly 90% of cases. The lesion typically is noted at birth as a pink to red, polypoid, nodular mass of the anterior alveolar mucosa. On occasion, prenatal diagnosis can be made during fetal ultrasound examination. The tumor occurs two to three times more frequently on the maxillary ridge than the mandibular ridge. Most examples are less than 2 cm in diameter, although occasional examples can measure as large as 7.5 cm. In about 10% of cases, multiple tumors may develop.

The congenital epulis usually is treated by surgical excision, and the lesion has not been reported to recur. Interestingly, occasional examples have been documented to undergo complete regression without any treatment at all.

Rhabdomyoma

Fig. **12.47**

Rhabdomyomas are rare benign tumors of striated muscle; they can be divided into two major types: cardiac and extracardiac. Cardiac rhabdomyomas are hamartomatous lesions that may occur in the hearts of patients with tuberous sclerosis. Extracardiac rhabdomyomas are true neoplasms that are further subdivided into genital, adult, and fetal subtypes. Genital rhabdomyomas occur in the vagina and vulvar region of middle-aged females. However, the adult and fetal subtypes show a strong predilection for the head and neck region. The distinction between these last two subtypes is based primarily on the maturity of the skeletal muscle formed within the tumor.

Both adult and fetal rhabdomyomas occur more often in males (4:1 male-to-female ratio). The adult subtype is seen primarily in middle-aged and older adults, often being reported as a slowly enlarging mass in the pharynx, oral cavity, or larynx. Intraoral examples occur most frequently in the floor of mouth, soft palate, and base of the tongue. Tumor size can vary from small lesions less than 1 cm in diameter to large masses measuring up to 15 cm. Approximately 10% to 15% of patients with adult rhabdomyoma will have multifocal lesions. The fetal rhabdomyoma develops more frequently in children, although occasional examples also occur in adults. The most common locations are the face and periauricular region.

Treatment for rhabdomyomas of the head and neck typically consists of complete surgical excision. Recurrence has been reported in 16% to 27% of cases, although this may largely be due to incomplete removal.

Leiomyoma

Fig. **12.48**

A **leiomyoma** is a benign tumor of smooth muscle origin. As such, these tumors occur most often at sites that normally contain significant amounts of smooth muscle, such as the uterine wall, gastrointestinal tract, and skin (from the arrector pili muscles). Leiomyomas of the oral cavity are quite uncommon, mostly arising from smooth muscle in the walls of blood vessels. About 75% of oral smooth muscle tumors will have a combined vascular component and are known as *angiomyomas (vascular leiomyomas; angioleiomyomas)*. Other microscopic types include the *solid leiomyoma* and *epithelioid leiomyoma*. In addition, rare developmental tumor-like growths of smooth muscle (leiomyomatous hamartomas) also have been described in the oral cavity.

The lesion usually presents as a slow-growing, asymptomatic soft tissue mass, although occasional leiomyomas may be painful. Solid leiomyomas are typically normal in color, but angiomyomas may exhibit a bluish hue because of the associated vascularity. The tumor can develop anywhere in the mouth, including the lips, buccal mucosa, tongue, and palate. Extremely rare intraosseous examples also have been reported. Oral leiomyomatous hamartomas most frequently have been described in the anterior maxillary gingiva and incisive papilla region of infants and young children.

Oral leiomyomas are treated by local surgical excision. Recurrence is rare.

■ Figure **12.46**
Congenital Epulis

Newborn female with a pedunculated nodular mass of the anterior maxillary alveolar ridge. (Courtesy Dr. Larry Cunningham.)

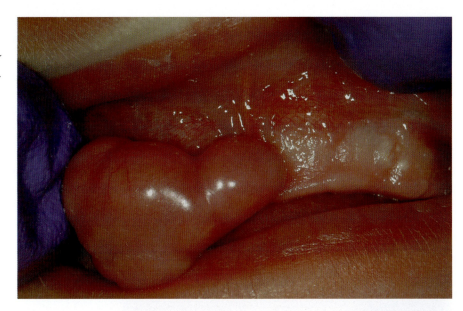

■ Figure **12.47**
Adult Rhabdomyoma

Nodular mass *(arrow)* in the right cheek. (With appreciation to Dr. Craig Little.)

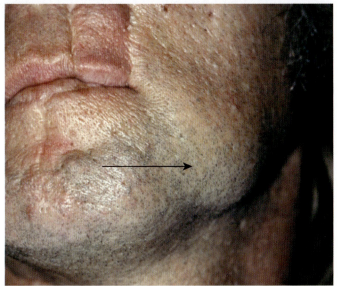

■ Figure **12.48**
Angiomyoma

Blue nodule on the upper lip vermilion. (Courtesy Dr. Michael Kolodychak.)

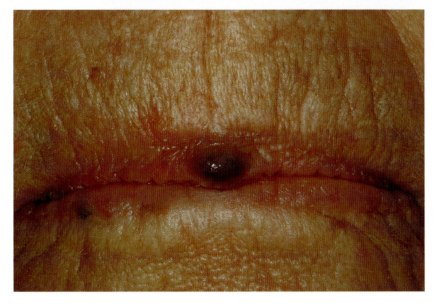

Osseous Choristoma

Fig. **12.49**

A **choristoma** is a developmental tumor-like growth of microscopically normal tissue in an abnormal location. The most common type of oral choristoma is composed of bone, cartilage, or both. Such lesions usually occur as nodular masses in the midline region, especially on the posterior dorsal tongue near the foramen cecum (almost 85% of cases). Lesions also may be seen within the mucosa of the palate. Infrequently, oral choristomas can be composed of other tissue types, such as glial tissue, gastrointestinal mucosa, or sebaceous glands.

An osseous or cartilaginous choristoma usually appears as a painless, slow-growing, hard mass that often appears pedunculated. Such lesions are diagnosed most frequently in the second and third decades of life, with a 3:1 female-to-male predilection. A choristoma that develops on the posterior dorsal tongue may be associated with dysphagia or a gagging sensation, but some patients may be unaware of its presence. Treatment consists of surgical removal, and the lesion should not recur.

Hemangioma and Vascular Malformations

Figs. **12.50 and 12.51**

Two major types of vascular anomalies have been identified: **vascular tumors** and **vascular malformations**. The most common vascular tumor is the *hemangioma of infancy*, which develops in about 5% of infants and shows a female predilection. This lesion usually appears within the first few weeks of life and is characterized by a rapid growth of endothelial cells over the next 3 to 12 months, followed by gradual involution over a period of 5 to 9 years. Approximately 60% of these lesions occur in the head and neck region, although documented intraoral examples are unusual. On the skin, this lesion often appears as a rubbery, red nodule ("strawberry" hemangioma) that shows a faster pace of enlargement than the infant's overall growth. As the lesion involutes and shrinks, the color will change to a dull purple. About 90% of infantile hemangiomas will show complete resolution by age 9, although up to 40% of lesions will show some residual evidence at the site, such as telangiectasia, atrophy, or scarring. Because most hemangiomas of infancy will involute, surgical excision rarely is warranted. For problematic examples, treatment with the beta blocker propranolol can be used to shrink the tumor. Systemic or intralesional corticosteroid therapy also sometimes is attempted.

In contrast to hemangiomas of infancy, vascular malformations are present from birth and persist throughout life. Such lesions can be classified on the basis of the predominant type(s) of vessel involved (capillary, venous, or arteriovenous) and the hemodynamic features (low-flow vs. high-flow). *Capillary malformations* ("port wine stains") are common lesions that are discussed separately. *Venous malformations* are low-flow anomalies that range from small, localized vascular dilatations to large, diffuse proliferations of blood vessels that may encompass multiple contiguous tissues or organs. Although such lesions are thought to be present from birth, sometimes they may not be immediately apparent. Venous malformations typically appear blue and are easily compressible. Such lesions usually grow proportionately with the patient, although increased vascular pressure can result in greater swelling. Because these anomalies are composed of dilated vessels with slow blood flow, secondary thrombosis and phlebolith formation can occur. *Arteriovenous malformations* are high-flow anomalies characterized by direct arterial and venous communication. They are present from birth but may not be noted until childhood or adult life. Because of the rapid flow of blood through the vessels, a bruit or thrill may be detected on clinical examination.

Treatment for venous malformations depends on the size and location of the lesion. Small, stable venous malformations may not require any treatment except observation. However, larger lesions that require treatment can be managed by a combination of sclerotherapy and surgical excision. Sclerotherapy attempts to induce fibrosis by the injection of sclerosing agents, such as sodium tetradecyl sulfate, into the lesion. Arteriovenous malformations are more difficult to manage because of the risk for significant bleeding. If surgical resection is deemed necessary, presurgical embolization of the feeding blood vessels usually is performed in an effort to reduce blood loss.

■ Figure **12.49**
Osseous Choristoma
Pedunculated mass at the junction of the hard and soft palate, which contained a central core of dense bone surrounded by fibrous connective tissue.

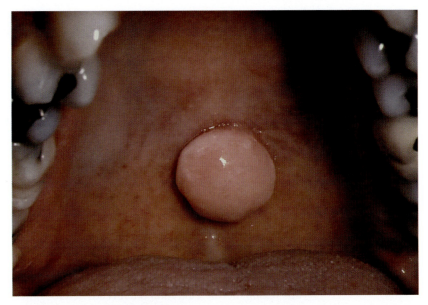

■ Figure **12.50**
Venous Vascular Malformation
Blue-purple mass of long duration on the upper lip.

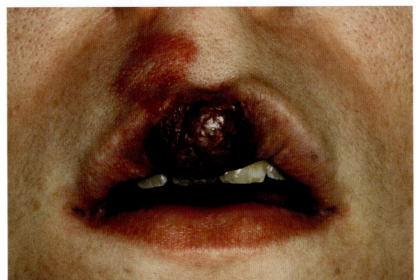

■ Figure **12.51**
Venous Vascular Malformation
Diffuse blue-purple lesion on the lower labial mucosa.

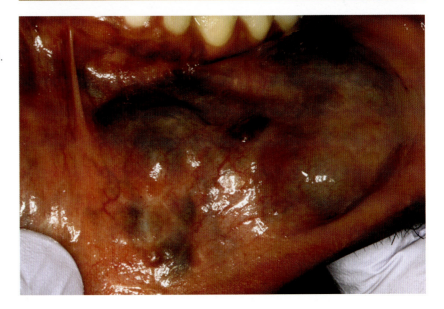

Figs. 12.52–12.54

In addition to vascular anomalies of the soft tissues, **intrabony vascular malformations** also can develop within the jaws. These intraosseous lesions can represent either low-flow venous malformations or high-flow arteriovenous proliferations. They usually are detected during the first three decades of life and occur three times more frequently in the mandible than in the maxilla. Some patients may present with mobility of teeth or gingival bleeding, although others can be totally asymptomatic. High-flow malformations can result in a bruit or pulsation on auscultation and palpation.

The radiographic presentation for intrabony vascular malformations is highly variable. Most examples result in a radiolucent defect, which can be unilocular, multilocular, or ill defined. If cortical expansion occurs, osteophytic changes can produce a "sunburst" appearance that may mimic osteosarcoma. Angiography is helpful to confirm the vascular nature of intrabony malformations.

Vascular malformations in the tooth-bearing regions create challenges in both diagnosis and management. Because of the rarity of such lesions, the clinician may not consider this possibility in the differential diagnosis for an intrabony radiolucency. Therefore, biopsy or tooth extraction might result in unexpected, severe, life-threatening hemorrhage, especially in the case of a high-flow arteriovenous malformation. For this reason, needle aspiration often is advised for initial assessment of any undiagnosed intrabony lesion before open biopsy is performed. Treatment of intrabony vascular malformations usually requires a team approach including an interventional radiologist as well as a head and neck surgeon. Prior to resection, endovascular embolization of feeding blood vessels often is performed to minimize blood loss during the surgical procedure.

Figure **12.52**
Intrabony Vascular Malformation
Panoramic radiograph of a high-flow vascular malformation that appears as an ill-defined loculated bony defect of the left body and ramus of the mandible. (Courtesy Dr. Chad Street.)

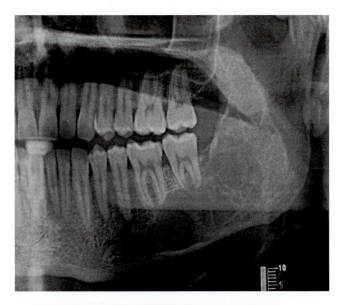

Figure **12.53**
Intrabony Vascular Malformation
Same patient as in Fig. 12.52 showing treatment of the lesion with coil embolization. (Courtesy Dr. Chad Street and Dr. Eric Carlson.)

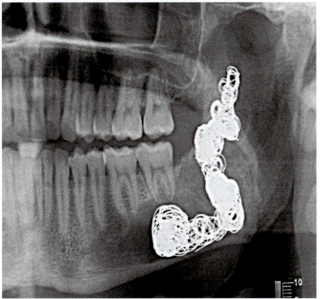

Figure **12.54**
Intrabony Vascular Malformation
Imaging study showing coil embolization, which was used as primary treatment of the lesion. (Courtesy Dr. Chad Street and Dr. Eric Carlson.)

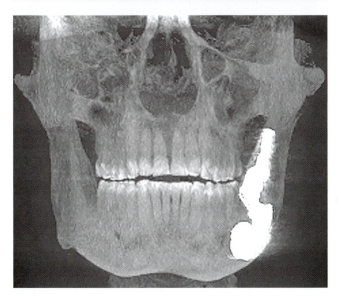

Fig. **12.55**

The **capillary vascular malformation** is the most common type of congenital vascular anomaly, occurring in 0.3% of newborns. Because of their deep purple color, such "birthmarks" often are called **port wine stains**. Capillary vascular malformations are not hereditary but are caused by somatic mosaic mutations of the *GNAQ* gene on chromosome 9. The most common location is the head and neck, although these lesions can occur anywhere on the skin.

Capillary vascular malformations are noted at birth as pink to red patches that gradually become deep red to purple with age. Most cases are unilateral in distribution, although some can develop bilaterally. Although the initial lesion is usually macular, many examples will become hypertrophic, thickened, and nodular later because of vascular ectasia. Intraoral mucosal involvement and underlying bony hypertrophy also may occur. Capillary malformations that involve the gingiva may make flossing or dental treatment difficult because of hemorrhage.

Early treatment of facial capillary vascular malformations with pulsed dye lasers can result in cosmetic improvement with a reduced risk for subsequent tissue hypertrophy. Surgical treatment can be attempted for cases that result in significant tissue hyperplasia.

Figs. **12.56 and 12.57**

Facial port wine vascular malformations sometimes may be associated with a more complex condition known as **Sturge-Weber syndrome**. In addition to the facial capillary malformation, Sturge-Weber syndrome also includes vascular malformations of the eye and cerebral leptomeninges. Similar to isolated capillary vascular malformations of the skin, this syndrome is not hereditary but is caused by a somatic mutation of the *GNAQ* gene. The prevalence of this condition is estimated at 1 in every 20,000 to 50,000 births.

The distribution of facial vascular malformations appears to follow the embryologic vasculature of the face rather than the trigeminal nerve. Therefore, the former term *encephalotrigeminal angiomatosis* for this condition is not accurate. Not all individuals with facial port wine stains will have Sturge-Weber syndrome. Studies have shown that infants with port wine vascular malformations involving the forehead or frontonasal region are at greatest risk for the syndrome.

Ipsilateral ocular vascular malformations may affect the eyelid, anterior chamber, cornea, choroid, and retina. Unilateral glaucoma is a frequent complication, being reported in 30% to 70% of patients. Severe choroidal involvement with retinal complications can result in vision loss. The most significant complications in Sturge-Weber syndrome arise from the cerebral vascular malformation of the leptomeninges (the inner two meningeal layers). Such lesions often are associated with seizure disorders, intellectual disability, and stroke-like episodes. Imaging studies of the brain may reveal "tramline" calcifications on the affected side.

The most important management issues for Sturge-Weber syndrome involve attempts to control the patient's seizure disorder and any ocular disease. If the patient's seizures are refractory to medical management, surgical therapy (e.g., hemispherectomy) may be attempted. Because antiseizure medications often will result in gingival hyperplasia, this tissue overgrowth may complicate attempts at dental care.

■ Figure **12.55**
Port Wine Capillary Vascular Malformation
Flat reddish purple lesion of the neck.

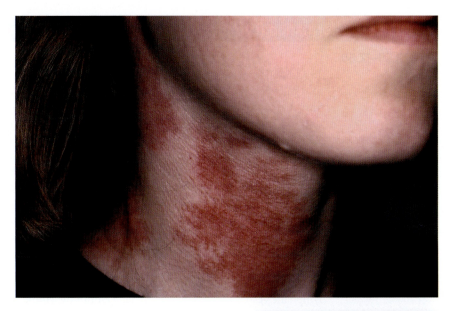

■ Figure **12.56**
Sturge-Weber Syndrome
Extensive port wine stain of the face, including the forehead region. The patient also had a seizure disorder and intellectual disability.

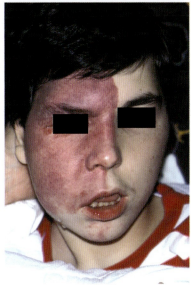

■ Figure **12.57**
Sturge-Weber Syndrome
This patient also had a mild capillary vascular malformation of the left soft palate, characterized by increased vascularity on this side.

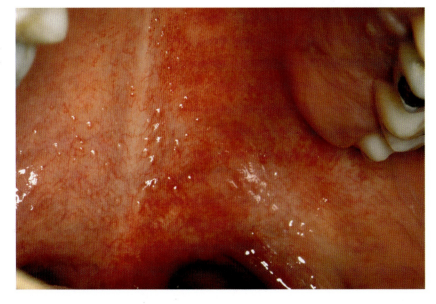

Figs. **12.58–12.60**

In addition to vascular malformations composed of blood vessels, developmental **lymphatic malformations** also may occur. Often known as *lymphangiomas*, lymphatic malformations are less common than their vascular counterparts, showing a prevalence ranging from 1.2 to 2.8 per 1000 births. From 50% to 75% of these lesions occur in the head and neck region. Approximately half of all cases are noted at birth, and 90% are detected by 2 years of age.

Lymphatic malformations can be composed of large, cyst-like lymphatic spaces *(macrocystic)*, smaller lymphatic channels *(microcystic)*, or a combination of both large and smaller vessels *(mixed)*. Macrocystic lymphatic malformations are more common in the neck, possibly because the looser surrounding tissue allows the vessels to expand. Such lesions, also known as *cystic hygromas*, occur more often in the posterior triangle than in the anterior triangle of the neck. They present as soft, fluctuant masses that can grow to a large size, sometimes resulting in difficulty with breathing or swallowing. Sometimes upper respiratory infection can lead to rapid enlargement of the swelling.

In contrast, intraoral lymphatic malformations usually are microcystic in nature. Such lesions are most common on the anterior two-thirds of the tongue, where they often result in macroglossia. Typically, the lymphatic vessels are located superficially within the connective tissue, producing a pebbly mucosal surface suggestive of a cluster of vesicles. This appearance sometimes is described as resembling tapioca pudding or a mass of frog eggs. Many of the surface blebs will be clear and translucent, whereas others may appear purple because of secondary hemorrhage or intermixed blood vessels.

Management of lymphatic malformations depends on the size, location, and symptoms associated with the lesion. Smaller stable lesions that do not cause cosmetic or functional problems may not require any specific treatment. Larger symptomatic lymphatic malformations can be managed by either surgery or sclerotherapy. However, total surgical removal can be difficult due to the diffuse nature of the vessels or their proximity to vital structures. Recurrence is common, especially for microcystic lesions in the oral cavity. Percutaneous sclerotherapy can be successful for many macrocystic lesions in the neck. In the United States, the most commonly used sclerosant drug is doxycycline, although other agents include sodium tetradecyl sulfate, alcohol, bleomycin, and OK-432 (outside the United States). The overall prognosis for lymphatic malformations is good, although sudden enlargement rarely may lead to airway obstruction and death.

■ Figure **12.58**
Lymphatic Malformation
Multiple translucent papules on the ventral surface of the tongue representing dilated lymphatic vessels. A few of the blebs appear purple due to hemorrhage or intermixed capillaries.

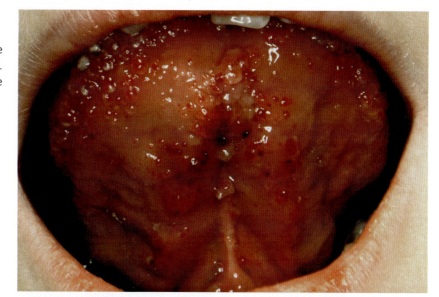

■ Figure **12.59**
Lymphatic Malformation
Mass composed of translucent papules on the dorsal tongue.

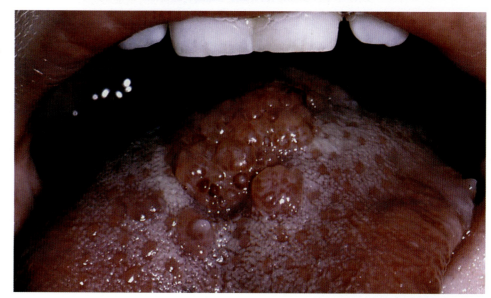

■ Figure **12.60**
Lymphatic Malformation
Child with a diffuse macrocystic lymphatic malformation of the neck and face.

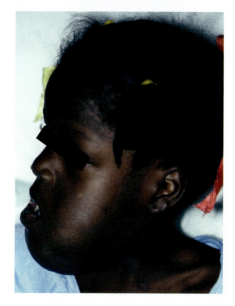

Soft tissue sarcomas comprise less than 1% of head and neck cancers. The most common of these malignancies is **rhabdomyosarcoma** (RMS), an aggressive neoplasm that shows skeletal muscle differentiation. This tumor is most common in children, accounting for about half of all soft tissue sarcomas in the pediatric population. In contrast, RMS accounts for only 2% to 5% of soft tissue sarcomas in adults. Four pathologic variants are recognized: embryonal, alveolar, spindle cell–sclerosing, and pleomorphic. The most common variant is embryonal RMS, which tends to occur in younger children during the first decade of life. Alveolar RMS is the second most common type and is seen most often in older children and young adults. These tumors are characterized by one of two chromosomal translocations that result in either a *PAX3-FOXO1* or *PAX7-FOXO1* fusion gene. Spindle cell–sclerosing RMS, which may occur in children or adults, can show one of several mutations, including the *NCOA2, VGLL2,* or *MYOD1* genes. Pleomorphic RMS is the rarest variant, usually being seen in patients older than 45 years of age.

Overall, approximately 35% of RMSs occur in the head and neck region. The tumor usually presents as a painless mass that may show rapid growth with infiltration into adjacent tissues. Common sites of occurrence include the paranasal sinuses, nasopharynx, parameningeal region, orbital region, and oral cavity. Treatment for RMS usually consists of a combination of chemotherapy, surgery, and radiation therapy. The 5-year survival rate for tumors in the head and neck region is 63%. However, survival is highly dependent on the age of the patient and microscopic subtype. For patients under the age of 10 years, the 5-year overall survival rate is 80%, whereas the survival rate drops to 46% for patients older than 10 years. This is likely related to the high proportion of embryonal RMS cases in younger patients, which have a significantly better prognosis than alveolar RMS. Therefore, genetic analysis plays a crucial role in distinguishing between embryonal and alveolar RMS. In addition, in the rarer spindle cell–sclerosing subtype of RMS, tumors showing *MYOD1* mutations are more aggressive and have a worse prognosis than tumors with *NCOA2* and *VGLL2* gene fusions.

■ Figure **12.61**
Rhabdomyosarcoma
Child with a bluish mass on the posterior mandibular alveolar mucosa. (Courtesy Dr. James Hargan.)

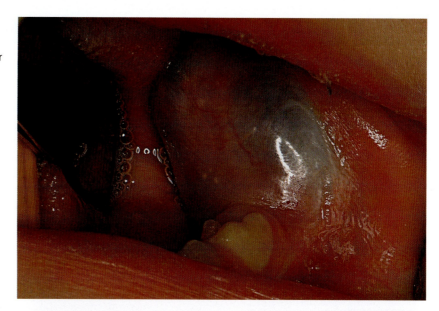

■ Figure **12.62**
Rhabdomyosarcoma
Rapidly growing mass of the right side of the face.

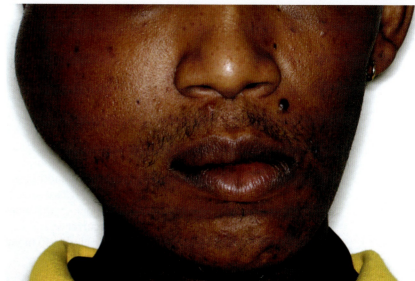

■ Figure **12.63**
Rhabdomyosarcoma
Intraoral photograph of same patient as in Fig. 12.62 showing an ulcerated mass of the buccal mucosa. The lesion was treated with chemotherapy and surgical resection, but the patient subsequently died from metastatic tumor.

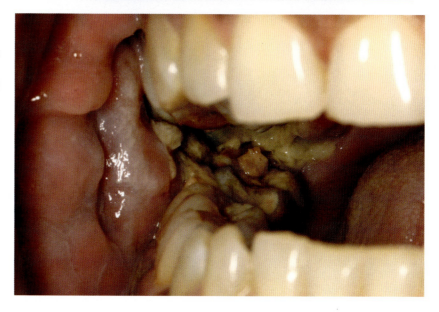

Leiomyosarcoma

Figs. **12.64 and 12.65**

Leiomyosarcoma is a malignant neoplasm that shows smooth muscle differentiation. Such tumors are diagnosed most frequently in the uterus and gastrointestinal tract—anatomic sites that normally have significant amounts of smooth muscle. However, because of the paucity of smooth muscle in the oral cavity, the mouth is a rare site for primary leiomyosarcoma.

Oral and maxillofacial leiomyosarcomas usually are seen in adults, but they can occur over a wide age range. Interestingly, the most common location is within the jawbones, accounting for approximately two-thirds of all cases. The maxilla and mandible are equally affected. The tumor typically presents as an enlarging mass, which may or may not be painful. Irregular radiolucent bone destruction often is noted with intrabony tumors. Rapidly enlarging tumors that involve soft tissues may result in ulceration of the overlying mucosal surface.

Treatment for oral leiomyosarcoma usually consists of wide surgical resection. For inoperable or metastatic tumors, palliative chemotherapy or radiation therapy may be attempted. The 5-year survival rate ranges from 55% to 62%.

Angiosarcoma

Fig. **12.66**

Angiosarcoma is a rare endothelial malignancy that may arise from blood or lymphatic vessels. Various risk factors include actinic damage, prior radiation therapy, chemical carcinogens (e.g., vinyl chloride), and chronic lymphedema (e.g., postmastectomy). Over half of all cases occur in the head and neck, with a predilection for the skin of the scalp and forehead. These dermatologic tumors usually occur in older adults and show a 2:1 male-to-female ratio. Angiosarcoma of the oral cavity is extremely rare.

Cutaneous angiosarcoma first appears as a bluish-purple lesion that may be mistaken for a simple bruise. Over time, however, the lesion will expand and become elevated, nodular, and possibly ulcerated. The tumor often may appear multifocal. Oral angiosarcoma has been reported most frequently on the gingiva.

Angiosarcoma is an aggressive malignancy that may be treated with surgery, radiation therapy, and chemotherapy. However, both local recurrence and distant metastases are common. The 5-year overall survival is 35% to 40%, with a median survival of 16 months. The 10-year survival rate drops to 14% to 21%.

■ Figure **12.64**
Leiomyosarcoma
Large ulcerated mass of the left buccal mucosa and vestibule.

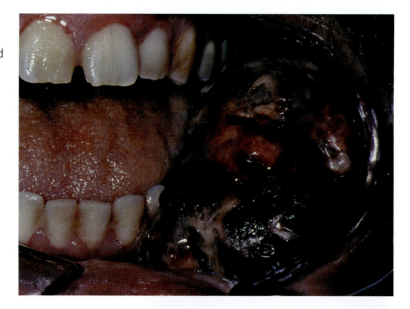

■ Figure **12.65**
Leiomyosarcoma
Axial computed tomography scan of same patient as in Fig. 12.64, showing a soft tissue mass with underlying bone destruction.

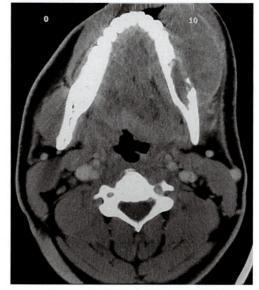

■ Figure **12.66**
Angiosarcoma
Slightly elevated blue-purple lesion on the scalp. (With appreciation to Dr. Terry Day.)

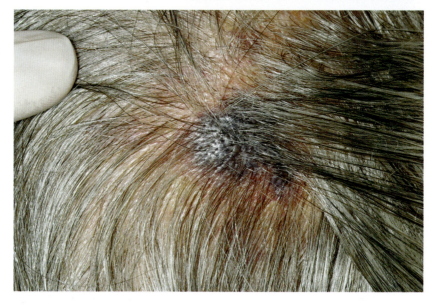

Figs. **12.67–12.69**

Kaposi sarcoma is an unusual vascular malignancy caused by a virus of the herpes family known as human herpesvirus 8 (HHV-8) or Kaposi sarcoma–associated herpesvirus (KSHV). Prior to the advent of the AIDS epidemic, Kaposi sarcoma was a rare malignancy, especially in the oral cavity. Currently, four major subtypes of Kaposi sarcoma are recognized: (1) classic, (2) endemic, (3) iatrogenic (transplant-associated), and (4) epidemic (AIDS-related). This discussion here centers primarily on the first three forms of the disease; AIDS-related Kaposi sarcoma is discussed in the section on HIV disease.

Classic Kaposi sarcoma is a slowly evolving disease seen primarily in older men of Mediterranean, Middle Eastern, and Eastern European background—presumably because countries in this region have a higher rate of KSHV/HHV-8 infection. Painless lesions first develop on the skin of the lower extremities, appearing as multiple blue-purple macules and plaques. Over a period of many years, these lesions gradually assume a more nodular morphology. However, only about 10% to 20% of patients will develop dissemination of tumor elsewhere in the body. Oral manifestations are rare, being seen most frequently on the hard palate.

Endemic Kaposi sarcoma occurs primarily in children and young adults in sub-Saharan Africa, also related to the high seroprevalence of KSHV/HHV-8 in this region. Two subtypes are identified. *African cutaneous Kaposi sarcoma* tends to occur in young adults, showing features similar to classic Kaposi sarcoma. However, patients often develop more aggressive disseminated tumors. *African lymphadenopathic Kaposi sarcoma* is a distinctly more aggressive process that occurs in young children, usually resulting in death within 2 to 3 years. This form of the disease is characterized by rapidly growing tumors that involve lymph nodes and internal organs.

Iatrogenic Kaposi sarcoma is seen with patients being treated with immunosuppressive therapy. This form occurs most frequently in individuals with solid-organ transplants who are being managed with immunosuppressive drugs (such as cyclosporine) to prevent organ rejection. It is estimated that iatrogenic Kaposi sarcoma develops in 0.5% of renal transplant patients.

Kaposi sarcoma is not curable, and treatment and prognosis depend on the clinical subtype and severity of the disease. Patients with classic Kaposi sarcoma may not require treatment because of the indolent nature of the lesions. Problematic individual tumors can be managed by radiation therapy, surgical excision, cryotherapy, or intralesional vinblastine injection. For patients with more widespread disease, a variety of systemic chemotherapeutic drugs may be used, including doxorubicin, paclitaxel, and interferon alpha. Iatrogenic Kaposi sarcoma in organ transplant patients can pursue an aggressive course, although tumor regression may occur if immunosuppressive therapy can be discontinued. For AIDS-related Kaposi sarcoma, immune reconstitution with combined antiretroviral therapy (cART) is the mainstay of treatment.

■ Figure **12.67**
Kaposi Sarcoma
Classic Kaposi sarcoma presenting as multiple purple macules and papules on the lower leg.

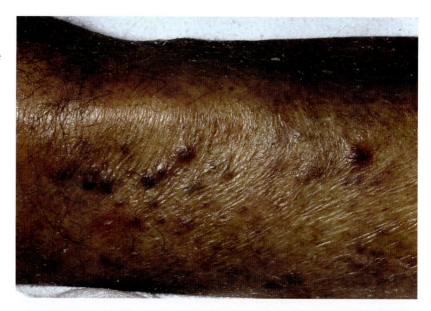

■ Figure **12.68**
Kaposi Sarcoma
Iatrogenic Kaposi sarcoma in a renal transplant patient who presented with diffuse purple nodular lesions on the maxillary alveolar ridge.

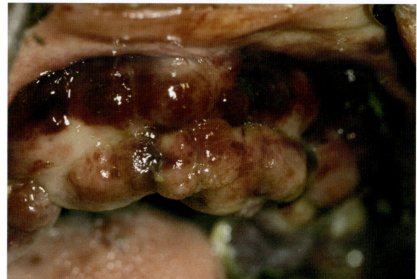

■ Figure **12.69**
Kaposi Sarcoma
Same patient as seen in Fig. 12.68, showing a row of purple nodules on the dorsal tongue.

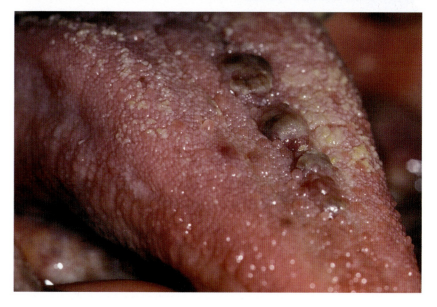

Figs. **12.70–12.72**

Metastatic tumors to the oral and maxillofacial region are uncommon, comprising only 1% to 2% of all malignancies diagnosed in this area. Most oral metastases arise from tumors located in the lower body, although it is difficult to explain how such lesions could metastasize to the head and neck, as ordinarily one would expect blood-borne tumors to be filtered out by the lungs. One theory that has been offered for such metastases involves the *Batson plexus*, a valveless venous plexus along the vertebral column that could allow retrograde extension of tumor cells that bypass the lungs. Oral metastases can occur either to bone or to soft tissue.

Soft tissue metastases can develop anywhere in the oral cavity, but the most common location is the gingiva; this accounts for slightly over half of all cases. A gingival metastasis often presents as an enlarging, ulcerated mass that may mimic one of the more common reactive gingival growths, such as a pyogenic granuloma or epulis granulomatosa. The tongue is the second most common location for oral metastases, accounting for about 22% of cases. These lesions may appear as either an ulcerated growth or a submucosal mass.

Metastatic tumors to the oral cavity are more common in men and usually occur in middle-aged and older patients. In men, the most common primary tumor sites are the lung, kidney, skin, gastrointestinal tract, and liver. For women, the most common primary site is the breast, followed by the female genital organs, kidney, and lung. Although a diagnosis of the primary tumor often is known already, it is important to emphasize that the oral lesion is the first sign of malignancy in 25% of patients. The prognosis for patients with oral metastases is very poor because tumor likely has spread to other body sites as well. Treatment usually is palliative in nature.

■ Figure **12.70**
Metastatic Thyroid Carcinoma
Patient with papillary thyroid carcinoma, which metastasized to the cervical lymph nodes at the angle of the mandible. (With appreciation to Dr. Terry Day.)

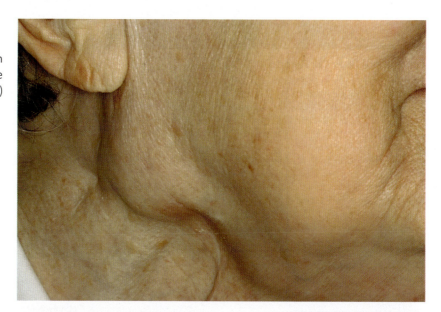

■ Figure **12.71**
Metastatic Lung Carcinoma
Ulcerated mass of the mandibular gingiva.

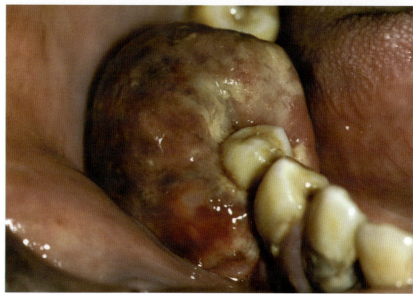

■ Figure **12.72**
Metastatic Renal Cell Carcinoma
Ulcerated mass of the edentulous mandibular alveolar ridge.

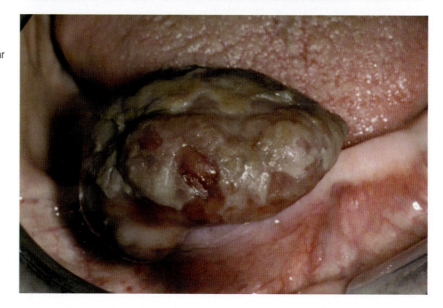

Bibliography

Fibroma and Giant Cell Fibroma

Brannon RB, Pousson RR. The retrocuspid papillae: a clinical evaluation of 51 cases. *J Dent Hyg.* 2003;77:180–184.

Gonsalves WC, Chi AC, Neville BW. Common oral lesions: part II. Masses and neoplasia. *Am Fam Physician.* 2007;75:509–512.

Houston GD. The giant cell fibroma: a review of 464 cases. *Oral Surg Oral Med Oral Pathol.* 1982;53:582–587.

Magnusson BC, Rasmusson LG. The giant cell fibroma: a review of 103 cases with immunohistochemical findings. *Acta Odontol Scand.* 1995;53: 293–296.

Savage NW, Monsour PA. Oral fibrous hyperplasias and the giant cell fibroma. *Aust Dent J.* 1985;30:405–409.

Weathers DR, Callihan MD. Giant cell fibroma. *Oral Surg Oral Med Oral Pathol.* 1974;37:374–384.

Oral Focal Mucinosis

Aldred MJ, Talacko AA, Ruljancich K, et al. Oral focal mucinosis: report of 15 cases and review of the literature. *Pathology.* 2003;35: 393–396.

Buchner A, Merrell PW, Leider AS, et al. Oral focal mucinosis. *Int J Oral Maxillofac Surg.* 1990;19:337–340.

Tomich CE. Oral focal mucinosis: a clinicopathologic and histochemical study of eight cases. *Oral Surg Oral Med Oral Pathol.* 1974;38: 714–724.

Epulis Fissuratum

Buchner A, Begleiter A, Hansen LS. The predominance of epulis fissuratum in females. *Quintessence Int.* 1984;15:699–702.

Canger EM, Celenk P, Kayipmaz S. Denture-related hyperplasia: a clinical study of a Turkish population group. *Braz Dent J.* 2009;20:243–248.

Coelho CMP, Zucoloto S, Lopes RA. Denture-induced fibrous inflammatory hyperplasia: a retrospective study in a school of dentistry. *Int J Prosthodont.* 2000;13:148–151.

Cutright DE. The histopathologic findings in 583 cases of epulis fissuratum. *Oral Surg Oral Med Oral Pathol.* 1974;37:401–411.

Inflammatory Papillary Hyperplasia

Bhaskar SN, Beasley JD III, Cutright DE. Inflammatory papillary hyperplasia of the oral mucosa: report of 341 cases. *J Am Dent Assoc.* 1970;81:949–952.

Budtz-Jørgensen E. Oral mucosal lesions associated with the wearing of removable dentures. *J Oral Pathol.* 1981;10:65–80.

Gual-Vaqués P, Jané-Salas E, Egido-Moreno S, et al. Inflammatory papillary hyperplasia: a systematic review. *Med Oral Patol Oral Cir Bucal.* 2017;22:e36–e42.

Salonen MAM, Raustia AM, Oikarinen KS. Effect of treatment of palatal inflammatory papillary hyperplasia with local and systemic antifungal agents accompanied by renewal of complete dentures. *Acta Odontol Scand.* 1996;54:87–91.

Leaflike Denture Fibroma

Neville BW, Damm DD, Allen CM, Chi AC. Epulis fissuratum. In: *Oral and Maxillofacial Pathology.* 4th ed. St. Louis: Elsevier; 2016:475–478.

Nikitakis NG, Brooks JK. Sessile nodule on the palate. Leaflike denture fibroma. *Gen Dent.* 2011;59:76–77.

Solitary Fibrous Tumor

Carlos R, de Andrade BA, Canedo NH, et al. Clinicopathologic and immunohistochemical features of five new cases of solitary fibrous tumor of the oral cavity. *Oral Surg Oral Med Oral Pathol Oral Radiol.* 2016;121:390–395.

O'Regan EM, Vanguri V, Allen CM, et al. Solitary fibrous tumor of the oral cavity: clinicopathologic and immunohistochemical study of 21 cases. *Head Neck Pathol.* 2009;3:106–115.

Smith MH, Islam NM, Bhattacharyya I, et al. STAT6 reliably distinguishes solitary fibrous tumors from myofibromas. *Head Neck Pathol.* 2017;doi:10.1007/s12105-017-0836-8. [Epub ahead of print].

Myofibroma

Abramowicz S, Simon LE, Kozakewich HP, et al. Myofibromas of the jaws in children. *J Oral Maxillofac Surg.* 2012;70:1880–1884.

Foss RD, Ellis GL. Myofibromas and myofibromatosis of the oral region: a clinicopathologic analysis of 79 cases. *Oral Surg Oral Med Oral Pathol Oral Radiol Endod.* 2000;89:57–65.

Lopes RN, Alves Fde A, Rocha AC, et al. Head and neck solitary infantile myofibroma: clinicopathological and immunohistochemical features of a case series. *Acta Histochem.* 2015;117:431–436.

Smith MH, Reith JD, Cohen DM, et al. An update on myofibromas and myofibromatosis affecting the oral regions with report of 24 new cases. *Oral Surg Oral Med Oral Pathol Oral Radiol.* 2017;124:62–75.

Fibromatosis

Fowler CB, Hartman KS, Brannon RB. Fibromatosis of the oral and paraoral region. *Oral Surg Oral Med Oral Pathol.* 1994;77:373–386.

Gnepp DR, Henley J, Weiss S, et al. Desmoid fibromatosis of the sinonasal tract and nasopharynx: a clinicopathologic study of 25 cases. *Cancer.* 1996;78:2572–2579.

Kruse AL, Luebbers HT, Grätz KW, et al. Aggressive fibromatosis of the head and neck: a new classification based on a literature review over 40 years (1968-2008). *Oral Maxillofac Surg.* 2010;14:227–232.

Vally IM, Altini M. Fibromatoses of the oral and paraoral soft tissues and jaws: review of the literature and report of 12 new cases. *Oral Surg Oral Med Oral Pathol.* 1990;69:191–198.

Pyogenic Granuloma

Bhaskar SN, Jacoway JR. Pyogenic granuloma—clinical features, incidence, histology, and result of treatment: report of 242 cases. *J Oral Surg.* 1966;24:391–398.

Cardoso JA, Spanemberg JC, Cherubini K, et al. Oral granuloma gravidarum: a retrospective study of 41 cases in southern Brazil. *J Appl Oral Sci.* 2013;21:215–218.

Daley TD, Nartey NO, Wysocki GP. Pregnancy tumor: an analysis. *Oral Surg Oral Med Oral Pathol.* 1991;72:196–199.

Gordón-Núñez MA, de Vasconcelos Carvalho M, Benevenuto TG, et al. Oral pyogenic granuloma: a retrospective analysis of 293 cases in a Brazilian population. *J Oral Maxillofac Surg.* 2010;68:2185–2188.

Epulis Granulomatosa

Ghadimi S, Chiniforush N, Najafi M, et al. Excision of epulis granulomatosa with diode laser in 8 years old boy. *J Lasers Med Sci.* 2015;6:92–95.

Leong R, Seng GF. Epulis granulomatosa: extraction sequelae. *Gen Dent.* 1998;46:252–255.

Peripheral Ossifying Fibroma

Childers ELB, Morton I, Fryer CE, et al. Giant peripheral ossifying fibroma: a case report and clinicopathologic review of 10 cases from the literature. *Head Neck Pathol.* 2013;7:356–360.

Cuisia ZE, Brannon RB. Peripheral ossifying fibroma—a clinical evaluation of 134 pediatric cases. *Pediatr Dent.* 2001;23:245–248.

Mergoni G, Meleti M, Magnolo S, et al. Peripheral ossifying fibroma: a clinicopathologic study of 27 cases and review of the literature with emphasis on histomorphologic features. *J Indian Soc Periodontol.* 2015;19:83–87.

Walters JD, Will JK, Hatfield RD, et al. Excision and repair of the peripheral ossifying fibroma: a report of 3 cases. *J Periodontol.* 2001;72:939–944.

Peripheral Giant Cell Granuloma

Giansanti JS, Waldron CA. Peripheral giant cell granuloma: review of 720 cases. *J Oral Surg.* 1969;17:787–791.

Katsikeris N, Kakarantza-Angelopoulou E, Angelopoulos AP. Peripheral giant cell granuloma: clinicopathologic study of 224 new cases and review of 956 reported cases. *Int J Oral Maxillofac Surg.* 1988;17:94–99.

Lester SR, Cordell KG, Rosebush MS, et al. Peripheral giant cell granulomas: a series of 279 cases. *Oral Surg Oral Med Oral Pathol Oral Radiol.* 2014;118:475–482.

Smith BR, Fowler CB, Svane TJ. Primary hyperparathyroidism presenting as a "peripheral" giant cell granuloma. *J Oral Maxillofac Surg.* 1988;46: 65–69.

Lipoma

Furlong MA, Fanburg-Smith JC, Childers ELB. Lipoma of the oral and maxillofacial region: site and subclassification of 125 cases. *Oral Surg Oral Med Oral Pathol Oral Radiol Endod.* 2004;98:441–450.

Manor E, Sion-Vardy N, Joshua BZ, et al. Oral lipoma: analysis of 58 new cases and review of the literature. *Ann Diagn Pathol.* 2011;15:257–261.

Studart-Soares EC, Costa FWG, Sousa FB, et al. Oral lipomas in a Brazilian population: a 10-year study and analysis of 450 cases reported in the literature. *Med Oral Patol Oral Cir Bucal.* 2010;15:e691–e696.

Schwannoma

Butler RT, Patel RM, McHugh JB. Head and neck schwannoma: 20-year experience of a single institution excluding cutaneous and acoustic sites. *Head Neck Pathol.* 2016;10:286–291.

Chi AC, Carey J, Muller S. Intraosseous schwannoma of the mandible: a case report and review of the literature. *Oral Surg Oral Med Oral Pathol Oral Radiol Endod.* 2003;96:54–65.

Colreavy MP, Lacy PD, Hughes J, et al. Head and neck schwannomas—a 10 year review. *J Laryngol Otol.* 2000;114:119–124.

Hoa M, Slattery WH 3rd. Neurofibromatosis 2. *Otolaryngol Clin N Am.* 2012;45:315–332.

Liu HL, Yu SY, Li GKH, et al. Extracranial head and neck schwannnomas: a study of the nerve of origin. *Eur Arch Otorhinolaryngol.* 2011;268:1343–1347.

Traumatic Neuroma

Jham BC, Costa NL, Batista AC, et al. Traumatic neuroma of the mandible: a case report with spontaneous remission. *J Clin Exp Dent.* 2014;6:e317–e320.

Lee EJ, Calcaterra TC, Zuckerbraun L. Traumatic neuromas of the head and neck. *Ear Nose Throat J.* 1998;77:670–676.

Sist TC Jr, Greene GW. Traumatic neuroma of the oral cavity: report of thirty-one new cases and review of the literature. *Oral Surg Oral Med Oral Pathol.* 1981;51:394–402.

Palisaded Encapsulated Neuroma

Chauvin PJ, Wysocki GP, Daley TD, et al. Palisaded encapsulated neuroma of oral mucosa. *Oral Surg Oral Med Oral Pathol.* 1992;73:71–74.

Koutlas IG, Scheithauer BW. Palisaded encapsulated ("solitary circumscribed") neuroma of the oral cavity: a review of 55 cases. *Head Neck Pathol.* 2010;4:15–26.

Magnusson B. Palisaded encapsulated neuroma (solitary circumscribed neuroma) of the oral mucosa. *Oral Surg Oral Med Oral Pathol Oral Radiol Endod.* 1996;82:302–304.

Neurofibroma

Campos MS, Fontes A, Marocchio LS, et al. Clinicopathologic and immunohistochemical features of oral neurofibroma. *Acta Odontol Scand.* 2012;70:577–582.

Ellis GL, Abrams AM, Melrose RJ. Intraosseous benign neural sheath neoplasms of the jaws: report of seven new cases and review of the literature. *Oral Surg Oral Med Oral Pathol.* 1977;44:731–743.

Marocchio LS, Oliveira DT, Pereira MC, et al. Sporadic and multiple neurofibromas in the head and neck region: a retrospective study of 33 years. *Clin Oral Investig.* 2007;11:165–169.

Neurofibromatosis

D'Ambrosio JA, Langlais RP, Young RS. Jaw and skull changes in neurofibromatosis. *Oral Surg Oral Med Oral Pathol.* 1988;66:391–396.

Ingham S, Huson SM, Moran A, et al. Malignant peripheral nerve sheath tumours in NF1: improved survival in women and in recent years. *Eur J Cancer.* 2011;47:2723–2728.

Lee L, Yan Y-H, Pharoah MJ. Radiographic features of the mandible in neurofibromatosis. A report of 10 cases and review of the literature. *Oral Surg Oral Med Oral Pathol Oral Radiol Endod.* 1996;81:361–367.

Neville BW, Hann J, Narang R, et al. Oral neurofibrosarcoma associated with neurofibromatosis type I. *Oral Surg Oral Med Oral Pathol.* 1991;72:456–461.

Shapiro SD, Abramovitch K, Van Dis ML, et al. Neurofibromatosis: oral and radiographic manifestations. *Oral Surg Oral Med Oral Pathol.* 1984;58:493–498.

Multiple Endocrine Neoplasia Type 2B

Callender GG, Rich TA, Perrier ND. Multiple endocrine neoplasia syndromes. *Surg Clin North Am.* 2008;88:863–895.

Carney JA. Familial multiple endocrine neoplasia: the first 100 years. *Am J Surg Pathol.* 2005;29:254–274.

Jasim S, Ying AK, Waguespack SG, et al. Multiple endocrine neoplasia type 2B with a RET proto-oncogene A883F mutation displays a more indolent form of medullary thyroid carcinoma compared with a RET M918T mutation. *Thyroid.* 2011;21:189–192.

MacIntosh RB, Shivapuja P-K, Krzemien MB, et al. Multiple endocrine neoplasia type 2B: maxillofacial significance in 5 cases. *J Oral Maxillofac Surg.* 2014;72:2498.e1–2498.e17.

Moline J, Eng C. Multiple endocrine neoplasia type 2: an overview. *Genet Med.* 2011;13:755–764.

Melanotic Neuroectodermal Tumor of Infancy

Azarisamani A, Petrisor D, Wright J, et al. Metastatic melanotic neuroectodermal tumor of infancy: report of a case and review of the literature. *J Oral Maxillofac Surg.* 2016;74:2431–2440.

Chaudhary A, Wakhlu A, Mittal N, et al. Melanotic neuroectodermal tumor of infancy: 2 decades of clinical experience with 18 patients. *J Oral Maxillofac Surg.* 2009;67:47–51.

Kruse-Lösler B, Gaertner C, Bürger H, et al. Melanotic neuroectodermal tumor of infancy: systematic review of the literature and presentation of a case. *Oral Surg Oral Med Oral Pathol Oral Radiol Endod.* 2006;102:204–216.

Rachidi S, Sood AJ, Patel KG, et al. Melanotic neuroectodermal tumor of infancy: a systematic review. *J Oral Maxillofac Surg.* 2015;73:1946–1956.

Granular Cell Tumor

Brannon RB, Anand PM. Oral granular cell tumors: an analysis of 10 new pediatric and adolescent cases and a review of the literature. *J Clin Pediatr Dent.* 2004;29:69–74.

Collins BM, Jones AC. Multiple granular cell tumors of the oral cavity: report of a case and review of the literature. *J Oral Maxillofac Surg.* 1995;53:707–711.

Mirchandani R, Sciubba JJ, Mir R. Granular cell lesions of the jaws and oral cavity: a clinicopathologic, immunohistochemical, and ultrastructural study. *J Oral Maxillofac Surg.* 1989;47:1248–1255.

Rejas RA, Campos MS, Cortes AR, et al. The neural histogenetic origin of the oral granular cell tumor: an immunohistochemical evidence. *Med Oral Patol Oral Cir Bucal.* 2011;16:e6–e10.

Congenital Epulis

Bhatia SK, Goyal A, Ritwik P, et al. Spontaneous regression of a congenital epulis in a newborn. *J Clin Pediatr Dent.* 2013;37:297–299.

Childers ELB, Fanburg-Smith JC. Congenital epulis of the newborn: 10 new cases of a rare oral tumor. *Ann Diagn Pathol.* 2011;15:157–161.

Damm DD, Cibull ML, Geissler RH, et al. Investigation into the histogenesis of congenital epulis of the newborn. *Oral Surg Oral Med Oral Pathol.* 1993;76:205–212.

Johnson KM, Shainker SA, Estroff JA, et al. Prenatal diagnosis of congenital epulis: Implications for delivery. *J Ultrasound Med.* 2017;36:449–451.

Lack EE, Worsham GF, Callihan MD, et al. Gingival granular cell tumors of the newborn (congenital "epulis"): a clinical and pathologic study of 21 patients. *Am J Surg Pathol.* 1981;5:37–46.

Rhabdomyoma

Cleveland DB, Chen SY, Allen CM, et al. Adult rhabdomyoma: a light microscopic, ultrastructural, virologic, and immunologic analysis. *Oral Surg Oral Med Oral Pathol.* 1994;77:147–153.

Kapadia SB, Meis JM, Frisman DM, et al. Adult rhabdomyoma of the head and neck: a clinicopathologic and immunophenotypic study. *Hum Pathol.* 1993;24:608–617.

Kapadia SB, Meis JM, Frisman DM, et al. Fetal rhabdomyoma of the head and neck: a clinicopathologic and immunophenotypic study of 24 cases. *Hum Pathol.* 1993;24:754–765.

Zhang GZ, Zhang GQ, Xiu JM, et al. Intraoral multifocal and multinodular adult rhabdomyoma: report of a case. *J Oral Maxillofac Surg.* 2012;70:2480–2485.

Leiomyoma

Damm DD, Neville BW. Oral leiomyomas. *Oral Surg Oral Med Oral Pathol.* 1979;47:343–348.

Freitas da Silva D, Fernandes IA, Wu A, et al. Oral leiomyomatous hamartoma of the anterior maxillary gingiva. *Clin Adv Periodontics.* 2016;6:190–194.

Liang H, Frederiksen NL, Binnie WH, et al. Intraosseous leiomyoma: systematic review and report of one case. *Dentomaxillofac Radiol.* 2003;32:285–290.

Liu Y, Li B, Li L, et al. Angioleiomyomas in the head and neck: a retrospective clinical and immunohistochemical analysis. *Oncol Lett.* 2014;8:241–247.

Osseous Choristoma

Chou L, Hansen LS, Daniels TE. Choristomas of the oral cavity: a review. *Oral Surg Oral Med Oral Pathol.* 1991;72:584–593.

Gorini E, Mullace M, Migliorini L, et al. Osseous choristoma of the tongue: a review of etiopathogenesis. *Case Rep Otolaryngol.* 2014;2014:373104. doi:10.1155/2014/373104.

Norris O, Mehra P. Chondroma (cartilaginous choristoma) of the tongue: report of a case. *J Oral Maxillofac Surg.* 2012;70:643–646.

Supiyaphun P, Sampatanakul P, Kerekhanjanarong V, et al. Lingual osseous choristoma: a study of eight cases and review of the literature. *Ear Nose Throat J.* 1998;77:312–318, 320, 325.

Hemangioma and Vascular Malformations

Adams DM, Lucky AW. Cervicofacial vascular anomalies. I. Hemangiomas and other benign vascular tumors. *Semin Pediatr Surg.* 2006;15:124–132.

Colletti G, Frigerio A, Giovanditto F, et al. Surgical treatment of vascular malformations of the facial bones. *J Oral Maxillofac Surg.* 2014;72: 1326.e1–1326.e18.

Fan X, Zhang Z, Zhang C, et al. Direct-puncture embolization of intraosseous arteriovenous malformation of jaws. *J Oral Maxillofac Surg.* 2002;60:890–896.

Fevurly RD, Fishman SJ. Vascular anomalies in pediatrics. *Surg Clin North Am.* 2012;92:769–800.

Greene AK. Management of hemangiomas and other vascular tumors. *Clin Plast Surg.* 2011;38:45–63.

Hogeling M. Propranolol for infantile hemangiomas: a review. *Curr Dermatol Rep.* 2012;1:179–185.

Huoh KC, Rosbe KW. Infantile hemangiomas of the head and neck. *Pediatr Clin North Am.* 2013;60:937–949.

Kaban LB, Mulliken JB. Vascular anomalies of the maxillofacial region. *J Oral Maxillofac Surg.* 1986;44:203–213.

Karim AB, Lindsey S, Bovino B, et al. Oral surgical procedures performed safely in patients with head and neck arteriovenous malformations: a retrospective case series of 12 patients. *J Oral Maxillofac Surg.* 2016;74:255.e1–255.e8.

Kwon EKM, Seefeldt M, Drolet BA. Infantile hemangiomas: an update. *Am J Clin Dermatol.* 2013;14:111–123.

Port Wine Vascular Malformation and Sturge-Weber Syndrome

Cerrati EW, O TM, Binetter D, et al. Surgical treatment of head and neck port-wine stains by means of a staged zonal approach. *Plast Reconstr Surg.* 2014;134:1003–1012.

Comi A. Current therapeutic options in Sturge-Weber syndrome. *Semin Pediatr Neurol.* 2015;22:295–301.

Dutkiewicz A-S, Ezzedine K, Mazereeuw-Hautier J, et al. A prospective study of risk for Sturge-Weber syndrome in children with upper facial port-wine stain. *J Am Acad Dermatol.* 2015;72:473–480.

Dymerska M, Kirkorian AY, Offermann EA, et al. Size of facial port-wine birthmark may predict neurologic outcome in Sturge-Weber syndrome. *J Pediatr.* 2017;188:205–209.

Lee JW, Chung HY, Cerrati EW, et al. The natural history of soft tissue hypertrophy, bony hypertrophy, and nodule formation in patients with untreated head and neck capillary malformations. *Dermatol Surg.* 2015;41:1241–1245.

Mantelli F, Bruscolini A, La Cava M, et al. Ocular manifestations of Sturge-Weber syndrome: pathogenesis, diagnosis, and management. *Clin Ophthalmol.* 2016;10:871–878.

Lymphatic Malformation

Lerat J, Mounayer C, Scomparin A, et al. Head and neck lymphatic malformation and treatment: clinical study of 23 cases. *Eur Ann Otorhinolaryngol Head Neck Dis.* 2016;133:393–396.

Nehra D, Jacobson L, Barnes P, et al. Doxycycline sclerotherapy as primary treatment of head and neck lymphatic malformations in children. *J Pediatr Surg.* 2008;43:451–460.

Perkins JA, Manning SC, Tempero RM, et al. Lymphatic malformations: review of current treatment. *Otolaryngol Head Neck Surg.* 2010;142:795–803.

Thomas DM, Wieck MM, Grant CN, et al. Doxycycline sclerotherapy is superior in the treatment of pediatric lymphatic malformations. *J Vasc Interv Radiol.* 2016;27:1846–1856.

Wiegand S, Elvazi B, Zimmermann AP, et al. Sclerotherapy of lymphangiomas of the head and neck. *Head Neck.* 2011;33: 1649–1655.

Rhabdomyosarcoma

Lee RJ, Lee KK, Lin T, et al. Rhabdomyosarcoma of the head and neck: impact of demographic and clinicopathologic factors on survival. *Oral Surg Oral Med Oral Pathol.* 2017;124:271–279.

Owosho AA, Huang S-C, Chen S, et al. A clinicopathologic study of head and neck rhabdomyosarcomas showing *FOXO1* fusion-positive alveolar and *MYOD1*-mutant sclerosing are associated with unfavorable outcome. *Oral Oncol.* 2016;61:89–97.

Smith MH, Atherton D, Reith JD, et al. Rhabdomyosarcoma, spindle cell/ sclerosing variant: a clinical and histopathological examination of this rare variant with three new cases from the oral cavity. *Head Neck Pathol.* 2017;doi:10.1007/s12105-017-0818-x. [Epub ahead of print].

Turner JH, Richmon JD. Head and neck rhabdomyosarcoma: a critical analysis of population-based incidence and survival data. *Otolaryngol Head Neck Surg.* 2011;145:967–973.

Leiomyosarcoma

Patel K, French C, Khariwala SS, et al. Intraosseous leiomyosarcoma of the mandible: a case report. *J Oral Maxillofac Surg.* 2013;71: 1209–1216.

Schütz A, Smeets R, Driemel O, et al. Primary and secondary leiomyosarcoma of the oral and perioral region – clinicopathological and immunohistochemical analysis of a rare entity with a review of the literature. *J Oral Maxillofac Surg.* 2013;71:1132–1142.

Sedghizadeh PP, Angiero F, Allen CM, et al. Post-irradiation leiomyosarcoma of the maxilla: report of a case in a patient with prior radiation treatment for retinoblastoma. *Oral Surg Oral Med Oral Pathol Oral Radiol Endod.* 2004;97:726–731.

Vilos GA, Rapidis AD, Lagogiannis GD, et al. Leiomyosarcomas of the oral tissues: clinicopathologic analysis of 50 cases. *J Oral Maxillofac Surg.* 2005;63:1461–1477.

Angiosarcoma

Albores-Saavedra J, Schwartz AM, Henson DE, et al. Cutaneous angiosarcoma. Analysis of 434 cases from the Surveillance, Epidemiology, and End Results Program, 1973-2007. *Ann Diagn Pathol.* 2011;15: 93–97.

Dettenborn T, Wermker K, Schulze H-J, et al. Prognostic features in angiosarcoma of the head and neck: a retrospective monocenter study. *J Craniomaxillofac Surg.* 2014;42:1623–1628.

Nagata M, Yoshitake Y, Nakayama H, et al. Angiosarcoma of the oral cavity: a clinicopathological study and a review of the literature. *Int J Oral Maxillofac Surg.* 2014;43:917–923.

Perez MC, Padhya TA, Messina JL, et al. Cutaneous angiosarcoma: a single-institution experience. *Ann Surg Oncol.* 2013;20:3391–3397.

Kaposi Sarcoma

Fatahzadeh M. Kaposi sarcoma: review and medical management update. *Oral Surg Oral Med Oral Pathol Oral Radiol.* 2012;113:2–16.

Hosseini-Moghaddam SM, Soleimanirahbar A, Mazzulli T, et al. Post renal transplantation Kaposi's sarcoma: a review of its epidemiology, pathogenesis, diagnosis, clinical aspects, and therapy. *Transpl Infect Dis.* 2012;14:338–345.

Radu O, Pantanowitz L. Kaposi sarcoma. *Arch Pathol Lab Med*. 2013;137:
  289–294.

Robey RC, Bower M. Facing up to the ongoing challenge of Kaposi's
  sarcoma. *Curr Opin Infect Dis*. 2015;28:31–40.

Schneider JW, Dittmer DP. Diagnosis and treatment of Kaposi sarcoma. *Am
  J Clin Dermatol*. 2017;18:529–539.

Metastatic Tumors to the Oral and Maxillofacial Soft Tissues

Hirshberg A, Shnaiderman-Shapiro A, Kaplan I, et al. Metastatic tumours to
  the oral cavity – pathogenesis and analysis of 673 cases. *Oral Oncol*.
  2008;44:743–752.

Irani S. Metastasis to the oral soft tissues: a review of 412 cases. *J Int Soc
  Prev Community Dent*. 2016;6:393–401.

Lim S-Y, Kim S-A, Ahn S-G, et al. Metastatic tumours to the jaws and oral
  soft tissues: a retrospective analysis of 41 Korean patients. *Int J Oral
  Maxillofac Surg*. 2006;35:412–415.

Hematologic Disorders

Figs. **13.1–13.4**

Lymphoid tissue is an important component of the body's defenses, and this tissue is commonly located within and adjacent to the oral cavity. In the posterior areas, it comprises the Waldeyer ring, including the palatine tonsils, adenoids, and subepithelial lymphoid tissue of the posterior lateral tongue (lingual tonsils), base of the tongue, and posterior oropharynx. Superficial lymphoid aggregates also can be found in the floor of the mouth and on the soft palate in some individuals. They may be solitary or multiple, and they may enlarge if presented with an antigenic challenge, such as an upper respiratory infection. In general, they are asymptomatic and normal in color, although some may appear slightly red, yellowish, or orange, depending on how superficially located or inflamed they might be. Fig. 13.1 illustrates a common location for lymphoid aggregates at the base of the uvula, and in this case, a yellowish hue can be appreciated.

In most instances, mild hyperplasia of oral and oropharyngeal lymphoid tissue can be diagnosed with reasonable certainty on a clinical basis, especially if the enlargement appears bilateral and symmetric. In such instances, biopsy usually is not required, although continued clinical follow-up still may be advisable. However, unusually large or asymmetric examples may necessitate biopsy to confirm the diagnosis, after which no additional treatment is necessary.

■ Figure **13.1**
Lymphoid Hyperplasia
Slightly yellow-orange papules with an intact, smooth surface mucosa, located on the right posterior lateral tongue.

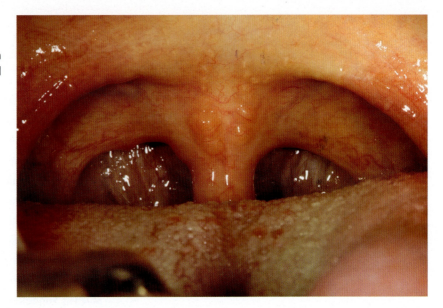

■ Figure 13.2
Lymphoid Hyperplasia
Multiple confluent slightly yellowish papules located on the posterior dorsal tongue.

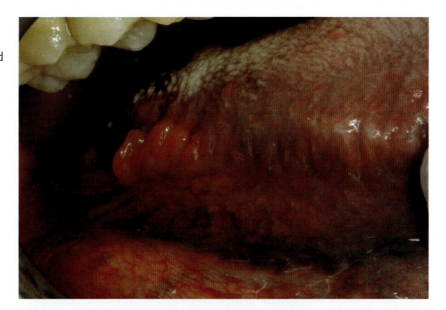

■ Figure 13.3
Lymphoid Hyperplasia
Slightly yellowish, sessile papules at the base of the uvula.

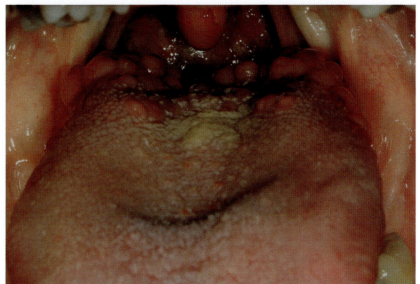

■ Figure 13.4
Lymphoid Hyperplasia
Pale papules in the anterior floor of the mouth.

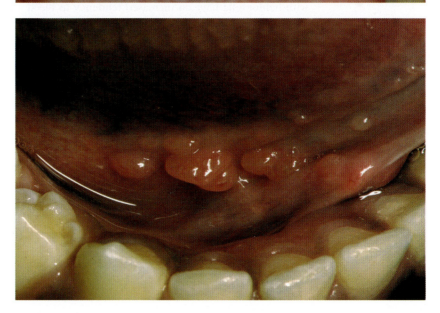

Thalassemia

Figs. **13.5 and 13.6**

Thalassemia represents a heritable hemolytic anemia that ranges in severity. Approximately 20% of the world's population carry at least one of the genes responsible for thalassemia; the high frequency of this disease primarily is attributed to antimalarial resistance conferred by erythrocyte alterations. Thalassemia mutations involve either the α-globin chain or β-globin chain of the hemoglobin molecule, resulting in α-thalassemia and β-thalassemia, respectively. Although a single mutation protects the individual from malaria, problems arise when both parents contribute abnormal globin genes. During normal hemoglobin synthesis, two α-globin chains bind with two β-globin chains. The quantities of the globin chains must be equal for normal hemoglobin synthesis to occur. When a mutation results in reduced or no production of one particular globin chain, the remaining globin chains cannot form a normal hemoglobin molecule. The accumulation of mutated globin chains alters the erythrocytes, allowing them to be identified as abnormal and subsequently destroyed by splenic macrophages. A microcytic, hypochromic anemia ensues, the severity of which depends on the number and type of globin chain mutations.

In more severely affected patients, anemia triggers a dramatic increase in hematopoiesis, most of which takes place in the marrow spaces. The hematopoietic precursor cells often undergo apoptosis, presumably caused by their molecular abnormality. As the hematopoietic cells multiply in the marrow spaces, the bone expands (sometimes resulting in "chipmunk facies") and the bony trabeculae are destroyed or thinned, causing a pattern of thin, widely spaced trabeculae in a radiolucent background. A lateral skull radiograph may show a "hair-on-end" appearance. Delayed growth and dental development also may be evident.

Patients with only one globin mutation may be relatively asymptomatic (thalassemia minor) and may require no treatment. Those who have two or more mutations will have a much more serious clinical presentation (thalassemia major), which requires treatment with multiple blood transfusions combined with iron chelation therapy. These patients typically have a markedly shortened life span. Prenatal testing is available for populations at risk for thalassemia, but significant public health issues often have to be addressed, including the expense of the testing and the dilemma of whether or not to terminate the pregnancy.

Hemophilia

Fig. **13.7**

Hemophilia is a term used to describe several heritable clotting disorders; a mutation in the gene responsible for a particular clotting factor clinically results in a reduced ability to form a blood clot. Patients with hemophilia have an increased tendency to bleed after minor trauma, including dental extractions, periodontal surgery, and subgingival scaling or curettage. The two most widely known forms of hemophilia are **hemophilia A** (factor VIII deficiency) and **hemophilia B** (factor IX deficiency; Christmas disease). Both of these conditions are inherited as X-linked recessive traits. As a result, most affected patients are males. It is estimated that approximately 1 in 5000 males have hemophilia A and 1 in 30,000 males have hemophilia B.

However, **von Willebrand disease** is the most common cause of coagulopathy. This condition is caused by a deficiency of a factor VIII transport molecule (von Willebrand factor). Von Willebrand factor also helps platelets to adhere to subendothelial connective tissue, and it facilitates platelet-to-platelet aggregation, helping to create a blood clot. This condition is thought to affect 1 in 800 to 1000 people, and it is inherited in a variety of patterns. Many patients have only mild signs and symptoms; often prolonged bleeding after tooth extraction leads to the initial diagnosis. Other potential signs include multiple episodes of epistaxis, easy bruising, and, in females, menorrhagia.

■ Figure **13.5**
Thalassemia
Expansile radiolucent change of the body of the mandible, with thinning of the cortical bone and residual wispy trabeculae. (Courtesy Dr. Andrew P. Wightman.)

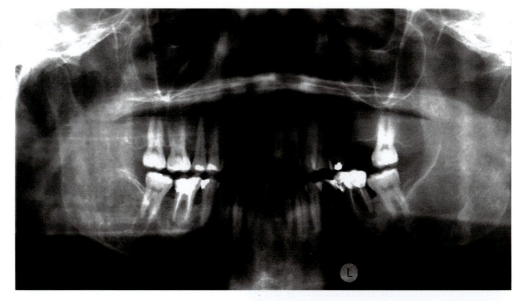

■ Figure **13.6**
Thalassemia
CT imaging showing the "cobweb-like" pattern of residual trabeculae. (Courtesy Dr. Andrew P. Wightman.)

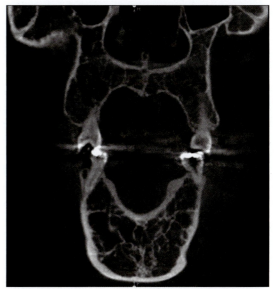

■ Figure **13.7**
Hemophilia B
Excessive gingival hemorrhage following gingival curettage in a patient with hemophilia B. The clinical features would be identical to those of someone afflicted with hemophilia A.

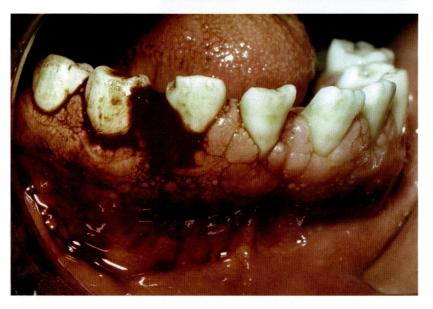

Plasminogen Deficiency

Fig. **13.8**

Plasminogen deficiency represents a rare autosomal recessive disorder that is characterized by mutation of the gene responsible for the production of plasminogen. Plasminogen normally circulates in the serum. With activation of the clotting cascade, plasminogen is enzymatically cleaved to form plasmin. Plasmin degrades fibrin in blood clots, thus preventing the clot from becoming too large.

This condition primarily affects mucosa, with oral mucosal lesions developing in approximately one-third of these patients. In addition, the conjunctival mucosa is involved in most patients, resulting in a condition called "ligneous conjunctivitis." Ligneous means "woody," and the fibrin deposits have a firm consistency. Laryngeal and vaginal mucosa also can be affected. Oral lesions may begin in childhood and are characterized by ulcerated areas of patchy gingival enlargement. The lesions have a creamy yellow-white appearance (characteristic of fibrin), with an irregular surface architecture. The severity of the lesions may fluctuate over time, and periodontitis is sometimes present.

Treatment is problematic because plasminogen replacement therapy is currently not available commercially. Investigations are hampered somewhat by the rarity of the condition. In general, the lesions can be controlled with agents that inhibit clot formation, such as topical heparin or systemic warfarin. The life span is essentially normal in most cases; moreover, postsurgical healing and intravascular coagulation do not seem to be altered significantly.

Neutropenia

Fig. **13.9**

Neutropenia is characterized by a reduction in the neutrophil count to less than 1500/mm², and this decrease can be caused by various factors that reduce production and/or increase destruction of neutrophils. Cytotoxic drugs, used for immune suppressive therapy or antineoplastic chemotherapy, often destroy neutrophils. Noncytotoxic medications may precipitate an immune-mediated destruction of neutrophils, and some autoimmune diseases may produce antineutrophil autoantibodies.

Other drugs, including some antibiotics, diuretics, and tranquilizers, can decrease production of neutrophils. Decreased production is also seen with myelophthisic anemias and with rare genetic conditions such as **cyclic neutropenia** or **congenital neutropenia**.

An increased prevalence of oral ulcers is typically seen, due to a reduced neutrophil count and the presence of large numbers of oral bacteria. These bacteria can infect the oral mucosa and induce oral ulcers due to the lack of neutrophils, perhaps assisted by minor trauma. These ulcers are often chronic, as long as the neutropenia persists. In cyclic neutropenia, there are 21-day cycles of oral ulcers that correspond to fluctuating numbers of neutrophils; the neutrophil nadir, which lasts 3 to 6 days, coincides with the onset of ulcers and fever.

Antibiotics are used to treat neutropenic ulcers, but the cause of the neutropenia ideally should be corrected. Optimal oral hygiene should be maintained to minimize oral bacteria. If an underlying cause cannot be eliminated, treatment with granulocyte colony-stimulating factor (G-CSF) may be necessary.

Thrombocytopenia

Fig. **13.10**

Thrombocytopenia refers to a reduction in blood platelet numbers (which normally range from 200,000 to 400,000/mm³). Platelets are produced in the hematopoietic marrow by megakaryocytes. Platelets play a critical role in the initial events of hemostasis, including the formation of a platelet plug, which functions to occlude the lumen of a blood vessel that has been disrupted. A significant drop in platelet numbers, therefore, will result in an increased tendency for bleeding. A variety of conditions may cause thrombocytopenia. These can be grouped as disorders that cause (1) a reduction in the production of platelets, (2) an increase in the destruction of platelets, and (3) increased sequestration of platelets in the spleen.

When platelet numbers fall to less than 100,000/mm³, patients may present with bleeding within the tissue following minor trauma, characterized by formation of petechiae (small hemorrhages). When platelet numbers drop to less than 10,000/mm³, epistaxis or significant bleeding from the gastrointestinal, pulmonary, or urinary tract may develop. Ecchymoses (medium-sized hemorrhages) and hematomas (large accumulations of extravasated blood) also may form, either spontaneously or with minor trauma. Fatal intracranial hemorrhage is another possible outcome.

■ Figure **13.8**
Plasminogen Deficiency
Characteristic chronically ulcerated gingivae with an irregular surface. (Courtesy Dr. Ken Rasenberger.)

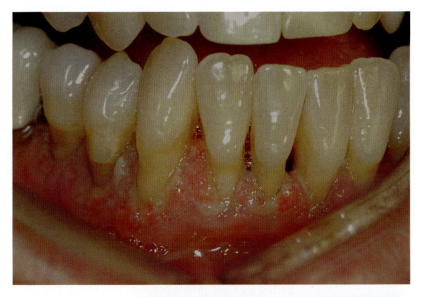

■ Figure **13.9**
Neutropenia
Ulcer of the left posterior buccal mucosa, probably secondary to minor dental trauma.

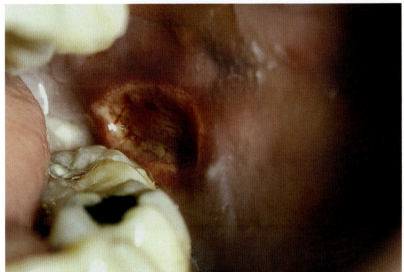

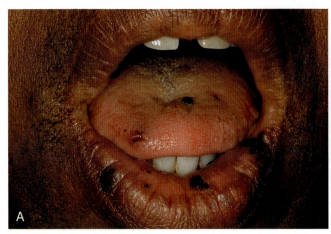

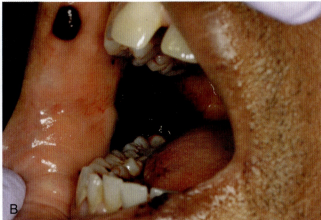

■ Figure **13.10**
Thrombocytopenia
Submucosal collections of extravasated blood (ecchymoses) are seen in (A), whereas a large collection of extravasated blood (hematoma) is seen in the right posterior region in (B). (Courtesy Dr. Louis M. Beto.)

Thrombotic thrombocytopenic purpura (TTP) is caused by a deficiency of a specific von Willebrand factor–cleaving enzyme (ADAMTS13). This results in abnormally large von Willebrand molecules, causing formation of microthrombi within the small blood vessels. Because so many platelets are incorporated into the microthrombi, the circulating platelet numbers drop significantly. **Immune ("idiopathic") thrombocytopenic purpura** (ITP) can be acute or chronic. Acute ITP usually occurs in childhood, often following a viral infection. Although severe thrombocytopenia develops, more than 90% of patients recover within 6 months. Chronic ITP occurs most often in young adult women due to autoimmune destruction of platelets in the spleen. Therefore, these patients may respond to splenectomy.

Leukemia

Fig. **13.11**

Leukemia represents a range of malignancies that arise from white blood cell precursors. Leukemias generally are classified according to precursor cell lineage (i.e., lymphocytic or myelomonocytic) and clinical course (i.e., acute or chronic). Thus, the four broad categories of leukemia include acute lymphoid leukemia, chronic lymphoid leukemia, acute myelomonocytic leukemia, and chronic myeloid leukemia. Numerous subtypes of leukemia are recognized under these four broad categories, with each subtype having a unique profile beyond the scope of this discussion.

Acute lymphoid leukemia usually is diagnosed in children between 3 and 6 years of age, whereas chronic lymphoid leukemia is identified in older adults. Acute myelomonocytic leukemia also typically is diagnosed in adults older than 60 years. Chronic myeloid leukemia generally is found in adults but over a wider age range. The clinical signs and symptoms that prompt a patient to seek medical attention often are related to myelophthisic anemia. Patients may present with fatigue or shortness of breath (secondary to anemia); fever, nonhealing wounds, and malaise (related to infection, secondary to neutropenia); or petechial hemorrhage or prolonged bleeding (secondary to thrombocytopenia).

Intraorally, oral mucosal pallor may signal anemia, nonhealing ulcers may reflect neutropenia, and petechial hemorrhages of the soft palate may identify thrombocytopenia. Leukemic cells occasionally form a soft tissue mass known as myeloid sarcoma. Gingival enlargement caused by infiltration of the soft tissues by myelomonocytic leukemia is a classic presentation; however, other intraoral sites occasionally may be affected.

Langerhans Cell Histiocytosis

Figs. **13.12 and 13.13**

Langerhans cell histiocytosis (LCH) is a relatively rare condition that many investigators believe represents a neoplastic proliferation of Langerhans cells (dendritic antigen-presenting immune cells). This condition has different presentations and biologic behaviors that seem to depend to a certain extent on the age at which the disease presents. Patients may be categorized with respect to single-organ or multi-organ involvement. Single-organ disease usually means only bone or skin. Multi-organ involvement is categorized by the degree of organ dysfunction as either low risk (skin, bone, lymph nodes, pituitary gland) or high risk (lung, liver, spleen, bone marrow).

Infants usually present with high-risk, multisystem LCH, characterized by a cutaneous papular rash that tends to involve the intertriginous areas and scalp. Hepatosplenomegaly also is frequently present. This form of LCH previously was termed *Letterer-Siwe disease*, and the prognosis generally is rather poor. Slightly older children also may present with multisystem disease, but this tends to be less aggressive. Involvement of bone will produce punched-out radiolucent lesions, whereas involvement of the pituitary gland may result in development of diabetes insipidus, due to destruction of cells that produce antidiuretic hormone. Exophthalmos (bulging of the eye) may occur if the lesional cells proliferate within the orbit. Previously this triad (lytic bone lesions, diabetes insipidus, and exophthalmos) was known as *Hand-Schüller-Christian disease*. In older children and adults, LCH usually presents as a solitary bone lesion (sometimes known as an *eosinophilic granuloma*), although multifocal sites can develop. In the jaws, this often is described as a noncorticated, circumscribed radiolucency that produces an appearance of "teeth floating in space" when it involves a tooth-bearing segment of the jaws. In addition, LCH may mimic chronic periodontitis. Infrequently, this condition can present as an oral soft tissue lesion that resembles oral squamous cell carcinoma due to the presence of ulceration and an irregular surface architecture.

Isolated jaw lesions can be treated with curettage, usually with a good prognosis; however, more extensive, multifocal jaw lesions may require low-dose radiation therapy or intralesional corticosteroid injections, depending on the accessibility of the lesions. Aggressive multi-organ disease in infants typically is treated with systemic chemotherapy, similar to that given for lymphoma.

■ Figure **13.11**
Leukemia

Diffuse severe enlargement of the gingivae. The blue-black color is probably related to submucosal extravasated blood. (With appreciation to Dr. Michael Tabor.)

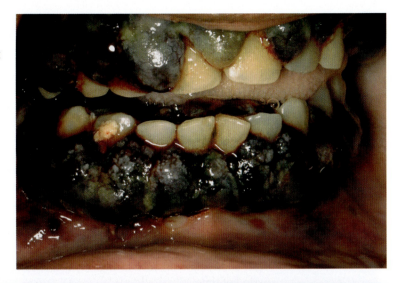

■ Figure **13.12**
Langerhans Cell Histiocytosis

Well-demarcated multifocal radiolucencies are seen, some of which mimic chronic periodontitis radiographically. (Courtesy Dr. Scott Price.)

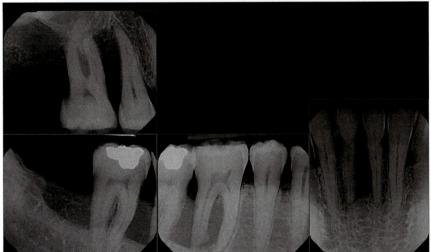

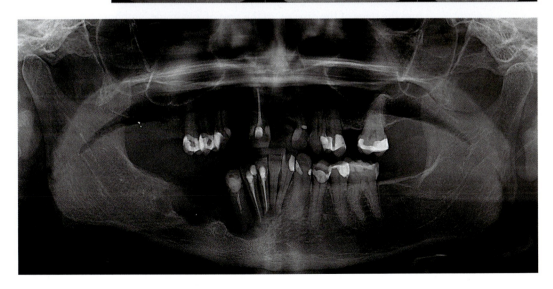

■ Figure **13.13**
Langerhans Cell Histiocytosis

Radiolucencies involving the right mandible and right anterior maxilla are present. Usually minimal or no expansion is present. (Courtesy Dr. Steven Anderson.)

The **non-Hodgkin lymphomas** represent a diverse group of malignancies that are derived primarily from cells that have differentiated along the lines of lymphocyte precursors. Approximately 90% of all lymphomas are non-Hodgkin lymphoma. These malignancies grow as solid masses, with 60% to 70% of non-Hodgkin lymphoma developing initially in the lymph nodes and the remainder developing in extranodal sites, including the oral soft tissues and within the jaws. The majority of these non-Hodgkin lymphomas (85% to 90%) are of B-lymphocyte differentiation, although some types are derived from T lymphocytes.

Most affected patients are adults, although non-Hodgkin lymphoma will occasionally occur in children. Those lesions arising in lymph nodes essentially have a clinical presentation identical to Hodgkin lymphoma (see next topic), with one or more firm to hard, nontender lymph nodes developing in the cervical region. Initially these lymph nodes are movable, but with time, the tumor extends beyond the capsule, resulting in lymph nodes that feel fixed to the surrounding tissue. Although most patients with non-Hodgkin lymphoma are otherwise asymptomatic, in some instances the malignancy is associated with systemic signs and symptoms, such as night sweats, fever, pruritus, fatigue, or unexplained weight loss in a short period of time.

When this malignancy develops in the oral soft tissues, the patient generally experiences a nontender, relatively ill-defined swelling that may range in consistency from boggy to firm. Common intraoral sites include the junction of the hard and soft palate and the buccal vestibule, although any anatomic region of the oral cavity may be affected, including the jaws. Secondary ulceration of the tumor mass may be seen.

A variety of benign and malignant lesions may have to be considered in the differential diagnosis. Palatal lymphomas often are mistaken for a palatal abscess, although the latter lesion is usually painful and no purulent drainage is identified when the tumor mass is incised. Palatal lymphomas also frequently mimic minor salivary gland tumors. Biopsy is required to make the diagnosis. Although routine hematoxylin and eosin–stained slides may show features consistent with non-Hodgkin lymphoma, immunohistochemical and cytogenetic testing of the tissue are needed to categorize the precise type of lymphoma. The most recent World Health Organization classification of non-Hodgkin lymphoma lists 65 different forms of this malignancy, with approximately one-third of these lymphoma types having been described in the oral region.

After the diagnosis is established, thorough medical evaluation is necessary to determine the extent, or stage, of the process. This typically includes a complete physical examination that is supplemented with positron emission tomography (PET) scans combined with computed tomography (CT) imaging.

Treatment for non-Hodgkin lymphoma varies widely, depending on the specific subtype of lymphoma and the stage of the disease. In the case of low-grade lymphomas, initial management may consist simply of watchful monitoring. For other forms of lymphoma, treatment options include radiation therapy (with or without chemotherapy), various chemotherapeutic regimens, and stem cell or allogeneic bone marrow transplantation. The type of treatment often is specifically tailored on the basis of the microscopic and immunohistochemical features of the tumor. For example, the most common form of non-Hodgkin lymphoma that affects the oral cavity is diffuse large B-cell lymphoma (DLBCL). This malignancy is typically treated with multidrug chemotherapy, combined with rituximab, which is a monoclonal antibody that is directed against CD20, a B-lymphocyte surface antigen. For patients with localized DLBCL, the prognosis is relatively good, with a 5-year survival rate of 80%. Of course, each of the various types of non-Hodgkin lymphoma has its own specific prognosis that is also dependent on the stage of the disease, as well as the age and general health of the patient.

■ Figure **13.14**
Non-Hodgkin Lymphoma

Multiple confluent lymph nodes that show advanced involvement with non-Hodgkin lymphoma. The swellings are nontender and feel firm and fixed upon palpation.

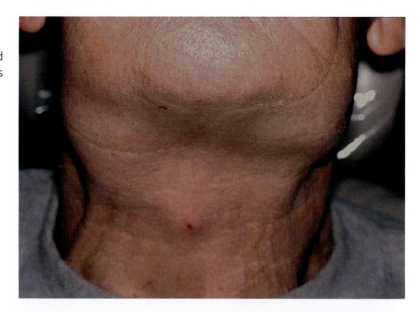

■ Figure **13.15**
Non-Hodgkin Lymphoma

A nontender, rubbery-firm swelling of the palatal mucosa.

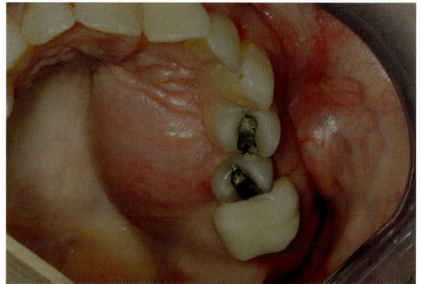

■ Figure **13.16**
Non-Hodgkin Lymphoma

An ulcerated mass of the posterior edentulous maxillary alveolar process. Although B-cell lymphomas tend to form masses, they can also develop secondary ulceration.

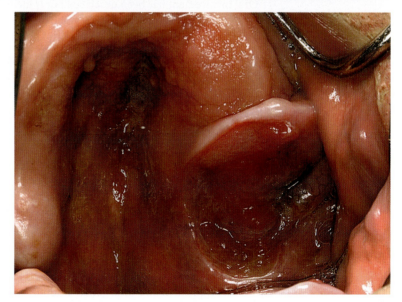

Hodgkin Lymphoma

Fig. **13.17**

Hodgkin lymphoma is a malignancy that primarily affects the lymph nodes and is derived from B lymphocytes. For many decades, there was debate as to whether this was truly a neoplastic disorder, and the term *Hodgkin disease* was used. Surprisingly, mutated B lymphocytes comprise only 1% to 3% of the cells in the involved lymph nodes, which is quite different than what is seen with non-Hodgkin lymphoma. Hodgkin lymphoma has been associated with Epstein-Barr virus (EBV) infection, but the precise etiology is unclear.

Hodgkin lymphoma has a bimodal epidemiologic pattern, with one incidence peak in the 2nd to 3rd decades of life and another peak in the 7th decade. The cervical lymph nodes are most commonly involved, although axillary, mediastinal, and inguinal lymph node regions also may be affected. Patients typically develop one or more enlarged, firm, nontender lymph nodes in a particular anatomic site. If the condition is not treated, the malignancy may spread to other lymph nodes in the contiguous anatomic region, and eventually to the spleen and other extralymphatic organs. Oral involvement is rare.

Patients with Hodgkin lymphoma may develop systemic signs and symptoms similar to non-Hodgkin lymphoma. Those with no additional signs or symptoms are designated "category A," whereas those with unexplained drenching night sweats, fever, unexplained weight loss, and/or generalized pruritus are designated "category B." Patients in category A tend to have a better prognosis than those in category B.

Mycosis Fungoides

Fig. **13.18**

Some non-Hodgkin lymphomas that are derived from T lymphocytes may have an affinity for skin involvement. As with B lymphocyte–derived lymphomas, these cutaneous T-cell lymphomas are a heterogeneous group. **Mycosis fungoides** is the most common cutaneous T-cell lymphoma. The name "mycosis fungoides" was designated in the 19th century, before the actual cause of the disease was known. Physicians at that time believed incorrectly that the skin changes seen in these patients were caused by a fungal infection.

This condition usually affects middle-aged or older adults and has a protracted course, often over a decade or more. It typically progresses through three stages: patch, plaque, and tumor stages. The patch stage presents as erythematous, scaly, macular areas on the skin, which may be mistaken for psoriasis. The plaque stage is characterized by erythematous, slightly elevated lesions, reflecting the proliferation of the neoplastic T lymphocytes in the epidermis and superficial dermis. As these cells continue proliferating, the tumor stage becomes evident. In addition, an aggressive end-stage process known as *Sezary syndrome* may develop, which is characterized by malignant T lymphocytes in the circulation. Exfoliative erythroderma develops in these patients, in addition to what essentially amounts to T-cell leukemia.

Oral involvement has been described but is identified in only a small percentage of reported cases. The lesions generally are described as erythematous patches or areas of ulceration involving the gingivae, palatal mucosa, or tongue in a patient with known mycosis fungoides.

NK/T-Cell Lymphoma, Nasal Type

Fig. **13.19**

NK/T-cell lymphoma, nasal type, is a malignancy that occurs most frequently in Asians and the indigenous populations of the Americas, particularly Central and South America. This tumor is also strongly associated with infection by Epstein-Barr virus (EBV).

Unlike many B-cell lymphomas, which tend to produce tumor masses, this T-cell lymphoma often will cause significant tissue destruction. Most affected patients are in the 5th to 6th decade of life when diagnosed. Nasal obstruction, pain, epistaxis, and nasal discharge are common initial presenting signs and symptoms. Approximately 40% of these patients have systemic signs and symptoms as well, such as unexplained weight loss, fever, night sweats, or pruritus. The malignancy usually grows rapidly, destroying the midfacial structures and producing an ulcerated tumor mass. At the initial presentation, most patients will have localized disease, but the tumor usually spreads quickly to other sites.

For many years, pathologists were puzzled as to the exact nature of this process, and various names have been applied in the past: lethal midline granuloma, polymorphic reticulosis, idiopathic midline destructive disease, and so on. Unlike most other lymphomas, which have a uniform, monomorphic population of tumor cells, this lesion seemed to be composed of a variety of different inflammatory cells. However, modern molecular methods have identified a clonal population of T lymphocytes within a background of other inflammatory cells attracted to the tumor area.

■ Figure **13.17**
Hodgkin Lymphoma
Enlargement of the right submandibular lymph nodes due to involvement with Hodgkin lymphoma. (Courtesy Dr. John Lovas.)

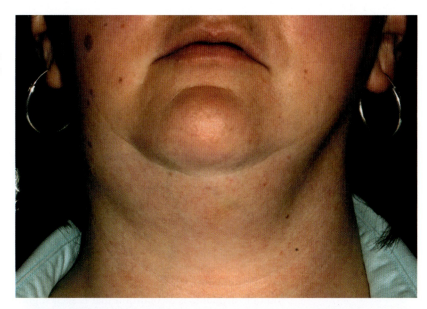

■ Figure **13.18**
Mycosis Fungoides
The erythematous change of the right maxillary buccal gingiva represents oral mucosal involvement by mycosis fungoides. The patient also had cutaneous lesions on her extremities.

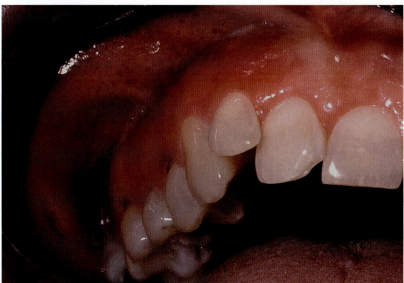

■ Figure **13.19**
NK/T-Cell Lymphoma
A destructive, ulcerative process, characteristic of many T-cell lymphomas.

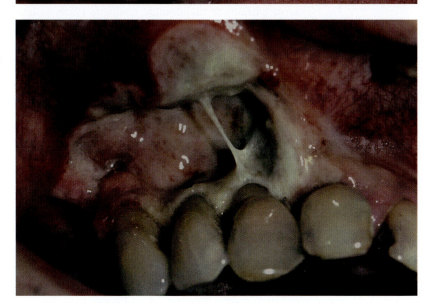

Figs. **13.20 and 13.21**

Multiple myeloma is a neoplastic proliferation of plasma cells and is the second most common hematologic malignancy after non-Hodgkin lymphoma. It represents approximately 1% of all cancers. One mutated plasma cell essentially gives rise to this malignancy, resulting in what is termed a "monoclonal" proliferation—in other words, a tumor that has developed from one mutated B lymphocyte that has the characteristics of a plasma cell. Because the plasma cells are monoclonal, they are capable of producing a single immunoglobulin component (which is completely nonfunctional). Sometimes an entire abnormal immunoglobulin protein is produced, and this is identified as a monoclonal gammopathy because so much of one type of immunoglobulin is present. The light-chain portion of the immunoglobulin molecule can be among the abnormal components produced by the lesional plasma cells, potentially resulting in a massive amount of light-chain protein circulating in the bloodstream. When this light-chain product spills over into the urine, it is known as *Bence Jones protein*. If this light-chain protein should be deposited in the soft tissues of the patient, it appears as an acellular, eosinophilic material called amyloid. A special stain called *Congo red* stains amyloid deposits, which have a characteristic apple-green birefringence when the tissue section is viewed with polarized light.

Multiple myeloma is a condition that is seen slightly more commonly in men than women, and most patients are older than 50 years, with the median age at diagnosis being approximately 69 years of age. For reasons that are unclear, it is seen twice as frequently in the black community, compared with the white population.

Because this tumor arises from a bone marrow precursor cell and begins growing within bone, the most common complaint is bone pain. Usually several bones of the skeleton are involved, and this may include the jaws. Sometimes the tumor cells displace the normal hematopoietic cells in the bone marrow, resulting in reduced production of granulocytes, platelets, and erythrocytes. In such cases a myelophthisic anemia is said to have developed, and patients may accordingly present with fever related to infection, prolonged bleeding, or fatigue accompanied by shortness of breath.

There are two main ways in which multiple myeloma may directly affect the oral region. First, the neoplastic plasma cells may proliferate within the jaws, producing either "punched-out" radiolucent areas or ragged radiolucencies. Second, if the malignant plasma cells produce significant amounts of light-chain protein, then this may be deposited in various anatomic sites as amyloid (described earlier), including the kidney and the soft tissues of the body, especially the tongue. Patients with tongue involvement will have an enlarged tongue, often with multiple submucosal nodular deposits and loss of function due to intramuscular amyloid deposition.

Treatment of multiple myeloma has evolved rapidly over the past 2 to 3 decades. Current chemotherapeutic regimens may include dexamethasone (a potent corticosteroid) combined with an alkylating agent (such as melphalan), a thalidomide analogue (such as lenalidomide), and a proteasome inhibitor (such as bortezomib). Stem cell transplantation also may be performed. The 5-year survival rate prior to 2000 averaged 40%, but this now has increased to 60% since 2010. Successful treatment still depends on the stage of disease, with more advanced disease having a poorer prognosis.

Fig. **13.22**

The **plasmacytoma** represents a monoclonal proliferation of neoplastic plasma cells at only one anatomic site; however, these lesions have the capability eventually to evolve into multiple myeloma. Plasmacytomas comprise only 5% of plasma cell neoplasms and can develop either within bone or in soft tissue, the latter being identified as extramedullary plasmacytoma. This lesion affects men approximately twice as frequently as women, and it is typically diagnosed approximately 10 years earlier than multiple myeloma. Solitary plasmacytoma of bone is found most commonly in the vertebrae, whereas the majority of extramedullary plasmacytomas affect the upper respiratory tract, including the oral cavity. For plasmacytoma of bone, bone pain is the often the presenting symptom, whereas extramedullary plasmacytoma will present as a soft tissue swelling.

The most common treatment is localized radiation therapy, but curettage and/or systemic chemotherapy also may be used. Initial control of the disease is typically seen, with nearly 95% showing apparent elimination of the tumor; however, this often is not a permanent cure. Regardless of the treatment, progression to multiple myeloma occurs for approximately 60% of patients whose plasmacytomas arise within bone. However, extramedullary plasmacytomas transform into multiple myeloma in only approximately 5% of cases.

■ Figure **13.20**
Multiple Myeloma
Relatively mild mandibular involvement by multiple myeloma, characterized by several "punched-out" radiolucencies. (Courtesy Dr. Phil Prickett.)

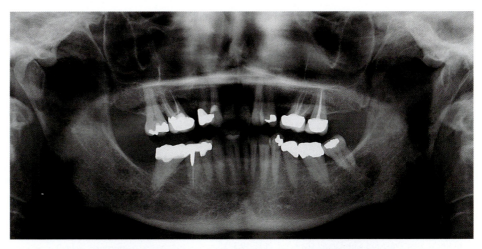

■ Figure **13.21**
Multiple Myeloma
A more advanced example of mandibular involvement by multiple myeloma, showing ragged and confluent radiolucencies with destruction of the cortical bone.

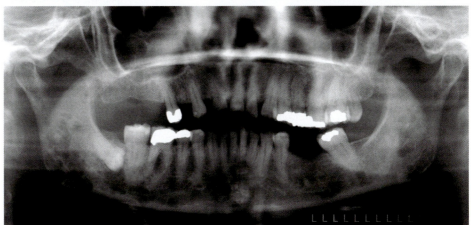

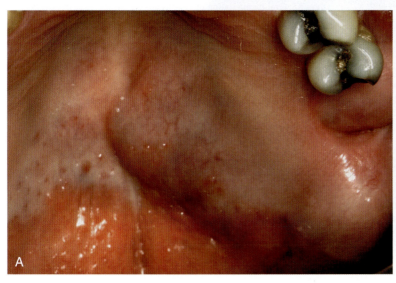

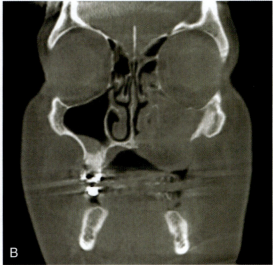

■ Figure **13.22**
Plasmacytoma
Nontender palatal swelling (A) representing a monoclonal proliferation of plasma cells that arose in the maxilla, occupying the left maxillary sinus and destroying bone in this area (B).

Bibliography

Lymphoid Hyperplasia

Jham BC, Binmadi NO, Scheper MA, et al. Follicular hyperplasia of the palate: case report and literature review. *J Craniomaxillofac Surg.* 2009;37:79–82.

Neville BW, Damm DD, Allen CM, Chi AC. Lymphoid hyperplasia. In: *Oral and Maxillofacial Pathology.* 4th ed. St. Louis: Elsevier; 2016:533–534.

Thalassemia

Hattab FN. Patterns of physical growth and dental development in Jordanian children and adolescents with thalassemia major. *J Oral Sci.* 2013;55:71–77.

Li C-K. New trend in the epidemiology of thalassemia. *Best Pract Res Clin Obstet Gynaecol.* 2017;39:16–26.

Shang X, Xu X. Update in the genetics of thalassemia: what clinicians need to know. *Best Pract Res Clin Obstet Gynaecol.* 2017;39:3–15.

Hemophilia

Castaman G, Linari S. Diagnosis and treatment of von Willebrand disease and rare bleeding disorders. *J Clin Med.* 2017;6:45–52.

Franchini M, Mannucci PM. Von Willebrand factor (Vonvendi®): the first recombinant product licensed for the treatment of von Willebrand disease. *Expert Rev Hematol.* 2016;9:825–830.

Kruse-Jarres R, Singleton TC, Leissinger CA. Identification and basic management of bleeding disorders in adults. *J Am Board Fam Med.* 2014;27:549–564.

Mistry T, Dogra N, Chauhan K, Shahani J. Perioperative considerations in a patient with hemophilia A: a case report and review of literature. *Anesth Essays Res.* 2017;11:243–245.

Paddock M, Chapin J. Bleeding diatheses. Approach to the patient who bleeds or has abnormal coagulation. *Prim Care.* 2016;43:637–650.

Peyvandi F, Garagiola I, Young G. The past and future of haemophilia: diagnosis, treatments, and its complications. *Lancet.* 2016;388:187–197.

Tamagond SB, Hugar SI, Patil A, et al. Christmas disease: diagnosis and management of a haemorrhagic diathesis following dentofacial trauma. *BMJ Case Rep.* 2015;2015:pii: bcr2014203790. doi:10.1136/bcr-2014-203790.

Plasminogen Deficiency

Conforti FM, Felice GD, Bernaschi P, et al. Novel plasminogen and hyaluronate sodium eye drop formulation for a patient with ligneous conjunctivitis. *Am J Health Syst Pharm.* 2016;73:556–561.

Celkan T. Plasminogen deficiency. *J Thromb Thrombolysis.* 2017;43:132–138.

Neering SH, Adyani-Fard S, Klocke A, et al. Periodontitis associated with plasminogen deficiency: a case report. *BMC Oral Health.* 2015;15:59–70.

Waschulewski IK, Gökbuget AY, Christiansen NM, et al. Immunohistochemical analysis of the gingiva with periodontitis of type I plasminogen deficiency compared to gingiva with gingivitis and periodontitis and healthy gingiva. *Arch Oral Biol.* 2016;72:75–86.

Neutropenias

Dale DC. How I diagnosis and treat neutropenia. *Curr Opin Hematol.* 2016;23:1–4.

Makaryan V, Zeidler C, Bolyard AA, et al. The diversity of mutations and clinical outcomes for ELANE-associated neutropenia. *Curr Opin Hematol.* 2015;22:3–11.

Okolo ON, Katsanis E, Yun S, et al. Allogeneic transplant in ELANE and MEFV mutation-positive severe cyclic neutropenia: review of prognostic factors for secondary severe events. *Case Rep Hematol.* 2017; Article ID 5375793.

Park MS, Tenenbaum HC, Dror Y, et al. Oral health comparison between children with neutropenia and healthy controls. *Spec Care Dentist.* 2014;34:12–18.

Sames E, Paterson H, Li C. Hydroxychloroquine-induced agranulocytosis in a patient with long-term rheumatoid arthritis. *Eur J Rheumatol.* 2016;3:91–92.

Thrombocytopenia

Abu-Hishmeh M, Sattar A, Zarlasht F, et al. Systemic lupus erythematosus presenting as refractory thrombotic thrombocytopenic purpura: a diagnostic and management challenge. A case report and concise review of the literature. *Am J Case Rep.* 2016;17:782–787.

Johnson B, Fletcher SJ, Morgan NV. Inherited thrombocytopenia: novel insights into megakaryocyte maturation, proplatelet formation and platelet lifespan. *Platelets.* 2016;27:519–525.

Lee E-J, Lee AI. Thrombocytopenia. *Prim Care Clin Office Pract.* 2016;43:543–557.

Larkin CM, Santos-Martinez M-J, Ryan T, et al. Sepsis-associated thrombocytopenia. *Thromb Res.* 2016;141:11–16.

Narayan N, Rigby S, Carlucci S. Sulfasalazine-induced immune thrombocytopenia in a patient with rheumatoid arthritis. *Clin Rheumatol.* 2017;36:477–479.

Sanchis-Picó C, Morales-Angulo C, García-Zornoza R. Haemorrhagic lesions in oral mucosa as the presentation of idiopathic thrombocytopenic purpura. *Acta Otorrinolaringol Esp.* 2015;66:e20–e21.

Leukemia

Inaba H, Greaves M, Mullighan CG. Acute lymphoblastic leukaemia. *Lancet.* 2013;381(9881).

Ferrara F, Schiffer CA. Acute myeloid leukaemia in adults. *Lancet.* 2013;381:484–495.

Apperly JF. Chronic myeloid leukaemia. *Lancet.* 2015;385:1447–1459.

Favaro-Francisconi C, Jardim-Caldas R, Oliveira-Martins LJ, et al. Leukemic oral manifestations and their management. *Asian Pac J Cancer Prev.* 2016;17:911–915.

Tamamyan G, Kadia T, Ravandi F, et al. Frontline treatment of acute myeloid leukemia in adults. *Crit Rev Oncol Hematol.* 2017;110:20–34.

Langerhans Cell Histiocytosis

Bezdjian A, Alarfaj AA, Varma N, et al. Isolated Langerhans cell histiocytosis bone lesion in pediatric patients: systematic review and treatment algorithm. *Otolaryngol Head Neck Surg.* 2015;153:751–757.

Divya KS. Oral manifestation of Langerhans cell histiocytosis mimicking inflammation. *Indian J Dent Res.* 2014;25:228–230.

El Demallawy D, Young JL, De Nanassy J, et al. Langerhans cell histiocytosis: a comprehensive review. *Pathology.* 2015;47:294–301.

Emile J-F, Abla O, Fraitag S, et al. Revised classification of histiocytoses and neoplasms of the macrophage-dendritic cell lineages. *Blood.* 2016;127:2672–2681.

Ferreira-Gonçalves C, Oliveira-Morais M, Gonçalves-Alencar RC, et al. Solitary Langerhans cell histiocytosis in an adult: case report and literature review. *BMC Res Notes.* 2016;9:19–24.

Haroche J, Cohen-Aubart F, Rollins BJ, et al. Histiocytoses: emerging neoplasia behind inflammation. *Lancet Oncol.* 2017;18:e113–e125.

Non-Hodgkin Lymphoma

Armitage JO, Gascoyne RD, Lunning MA, et al. Non-Hodgkin lymphoma. *Lancet.* published on-line January 30, 2017.

Mugnaini EN, Ghosh N. Lymphoma. *Prim Care Clin Office Pract.* 2016;43:661–675.

Perry AM, Diebold J, Nathwani BN, et al. Non-Hodgkin lymphoma in the developing world: review of 4539 cases from the International Non-Hodgkin Lymphoma Classification Project. *Haematologica.* 2016;101:1244–1250.

Sirsath NT, Lakshmaiah KC, Das U, et al. Primary extranodal non-Hodgkin's lymphoma of oral cavity - A single centre retrospective study. *J Cancer Res Ther.* 2014;10:945–950.

Hodgkin Lymphoma

Ali H, Naresh K, Aqel NM. Primary nodular lymphocyte predominant Hodgkin lymphoma of the palate: a rare incidence which was also associated with progressive transformation of germinal centres of cervical lymph node. *J Egypt Natl Canc Inst.* 2013;25:161–163.

Bröckelmann PJ, Angelopoulou MK, Vassilakopoulos TP. Prognostic factors in Hodgkin lymphoma. *Semin Hematol.* 2016;53:155–164.

Engert A, Raemaekers J. Treatment of early-stage Hodgkin lymphoma. *Semin Hematol.* 2016;53:165–170.

Gallamini A, Hutchings M, Ramadan S. Clinical presentation and staging of Hodgkin lymphoma. *Semin Hematol.* 2016;53:148–154.

Mathas S, Hartmann S, Küppers R. Hodgkin lymphoma: pathology and biology. *Semin Hematol.* 2016;53:139–147.

Ng AK, van Leeuwen FE. Hodgkin lymphoma: late effects of treatment and guidelines for surveillance. *Semin Hematol.* 2016;53:209–215.

Vassilakopoulos TP, Johnson PWM. Treatment of advanced-stage Hodgkin lymphoma. *Semin Hematol.* 2016;53:171–179.

Mycosis Fungoides

Bassuner J, Miranda RN, Emge DA, et al. Mycosis fungoides of the oral cavity: fungating tumor successfully treated with electron beam radiation and maintenance bexarotene. *Case Rep Dermatol Med.* 2016; Article ID 5857935.

Desai M, Liu S, Parker S. Clinical characteristics, prognostic factors, and survival of 393 patients with mycosis fungoides and Sézary syndrome in the southeastern United States: a single-institution cohort. *J Am Acad Dermatol.* 2015;72:276–285.

Furue M, Kadono T. New aspects of the clinicopathological features and treatment of mycosis fungoides and Sézary syndrome. *J Dermatol.* 2015;42:941–944.

Junkins-Hopkins JM. Aggressive cutaneous T-cell lymphomas. *Semin Diagn Pathol.* 2017;34:44–59.

Xu L, Pang H, Zhu J, et al. Mycosis fungoides staged by ^{18}F-flurodeoxyglucose positron emission tomography/computed tomography – case report and review of literature. *Medicine (Baltimore).* 2016;95(45):e5044.

NK/T-Cell Lymphoma, Nasal Type

Gru AA, Haverkos BH, Freud AG, et al. The Epstein-Barr virus (EBV) in T cell and NK cell lymphomas: time for a reassessment. *Curr Hematol Malig Rep.* 2015;10:456–467.

Kreisel FH. Hematolymphoid lesions of the sinonasal tract. *Head Neck Pathol.* 2016;10:109–117.

Makita S, Tobinai K. Clinical features and current optimal management of natural killer/T-cell lymphoma. *Hematol Oncol Clin North Am.* 2017;31:239–253.

Michot J-M, Mazeron R, Danu A, et al. Concurrent etoposide, steroid, high-dose ara-C, and platinum chemotherapy with radiation therapy in localized extranodal natural killer (NK)/T-cell lymphoma, nasal type. *Eur J Cancer.* 2015;51:2386–2395.

Pillai V, Tallarico M, Bishop MR, et al. Mature T- and NK-cell non-Hodgkin lymphoma in children and young adolescents. *Br J Haematol.* 2016;173:573–581.

Multiple Myeloma

Cardoso RC, Gerngross PJ, Hofstede TM, et al. The multiple oral presentations of multiple myeloma. *Support Care Cancer.* 2014;22:259–267.

Castillo JJ. Plasma cell disorders. *Prim Care Clin Office Pract.* 2016;43:677–691.

Kazandjian D. Multiple myeloma epidemiology and survival: a unique malignancy. *Semin Oncol.* 2016;43:676–681.

Moreau P, Rajkumar SV. Multiple myeloma – translation of trial results into reality. *Lancet.* 2016;388:111–113.

Scott K, Hayden PJ, Will A, et al. Bortezomib for the treatment of multiple myeloma. *Cochrane Database Syst Rev.* 2016;(4):Art. No.: CD010816,

Plasmacytoma

Amini B, Yellapragada S, Shah S, et al. State-of-the-art imaging and staging of plasma cell dyscrasias. *Radiol Clin N Am.* 2016;54:581–596.

Basile FG, Shi M, Sullivan M. Solitary plasmacytoma of the uvula. *Am J Hematol.* 2014;89:660–661.

Finsinger P, Grammatico S, Chisini M, et al. Clinical features and prognostic factors in solitary plasmacytoma. *Br J Haematol.* 2016;172:554–560.

14

Bone Pathology

Figs. **14.1–14.3**

The term **osteopetrosis** encompasses a family of rare, hereditary metabolic bone disorders that are characterized by markedly increased bone density. These conditions are related to defective function or differentiation of osteoclasts, which results in a decrease in the normal bone resorption process. A variety of gene mutations have been identified in these disorders, including both autosomal recessive and autosomal dominant inheritance patterns. Osteopetrosis shows a wide spectrum of clinical severity, and three major clinical patterns are recognized:

1. Autosomal recessive infantile ("malignant") type
2. Autosomal recessive intermediate type
3. Autosomal dominant adult ("benign") type

Autosomal recessive infantile osteopetrosis is the most severe form of the disease, and is usually diagnosed at birth or in early infancy. Although the bones are more densely mineralized, the brittle nature of this bone makes the patient subject to multiple pathologic fractures. Poor bone formation is associated with a variety of clinical manifestations, including macrocephaly, frontal bossing, exophthalmos, hypertelorism, micrognathia, and short stature. Because the normal marrow spaces are replaced by dense bone, patients typically develop secondary anemia with compensatory extramedullary hematopoiesis and associated hepatosplenomegaly. In addition, granulocytopenia increases the risk for various infections. Failure of normal bony resorption often causes narrowing of the skull foramina with compression of the exiting cranial nerves, which may result in blindness, deafness, and facial nerve paralysis. The denser bone in these patients is at greater risk for infection, and osteomyelitis of the jaws is a common complication following dental infections or extractions.

Radiographically, the bones will appear denser and more radiopaque, with loss of distinction between the normal cortical and cancellous bone. Parallel bands of dense bone can produce a "bone-within-bone" appearance. In the jaws, it may become more difficult to discern tooth roots against the background of denser bone. This dense bone also can lead to failure of tooth eruption.

Autosomal recessive intermediate osteopetrosis can result in similar, but milder, clinical manifestations. Patients with this subtype usually are not diagnosed at birth or infancy, but they may be identified later in childhood after the development of bony fractures.

Autosomal dominant adult osteopetrosis is the mildest form of the disease, which usually is not detected until adolescence or adulthood. Increased bone density primarily affects the axial skeleton, as opposed to the long bones. In many instances, the patient is asymptomatic and unaware of any problems. However, other patients will experience bone pain, fractures, and evidence of cranial nerve compression. Marrow failure is rare. Dental radiographs may reveal generalized increased bone density, which can make the mandible more susceptible to secondary infection or fracture.

Untreated autosomal recessive infantile osteopetrosis has a poor prognosis, with most patients dying within the first decade of life. Because multiple genetic forms of osteopetrosis exist, genetic testing is recommended to identify the specific mutation underlying the disease. Hematopoietic stem cell transplantation holds great promise for many affected children because it can prevent or reverse the bony manifestations; however, this approach does not work with some genetic subtypes of the disease. Also, identification of a suitable donor can be difficult, and bone marrow transplantation carries considerable risk. Calcium and vitamin D supplementation can be given for treatment of hypocalcemia and secondary hyperparathyroidism. Interferon gamma-1b may reduce bone mass and improve response to infections. Corticosteroid therapy also sometimes is employed to stimulate bone resorption and increase red blood cells. Appropriate antibiotic therapy is warranted for secondary osteomyelitis, and this may be supplemented with hyperbaric oxygen therapy.

Autosomal dominant adult osteopetrosis may not require any specific therapy, especially if it is discovered as an incidental finding. However, because jaw involvement can predispose the patient to secondary osteomyelitis, regular dental care is important to maintain a healthy dentition and to identify early signs of infection.

■ Figure **14.1**
Osteopetrosis
Young man with mandibular osteomyelitis and multiple cutaneous sinus tracts secondary to infantile osteopetrosis. (With appreciation to Dr. Dan Sarasin.)

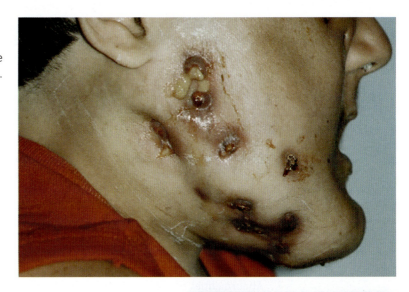

■ Figure **14.2**
Osteopetrosis
Cranial computed tomographic scan of the patient seen in Fig. 14.1. Note the thickening and dense sclerosis of the bone. (With appreciation to Dr. Dan Sarasin.)

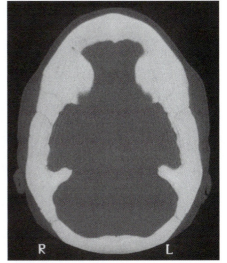

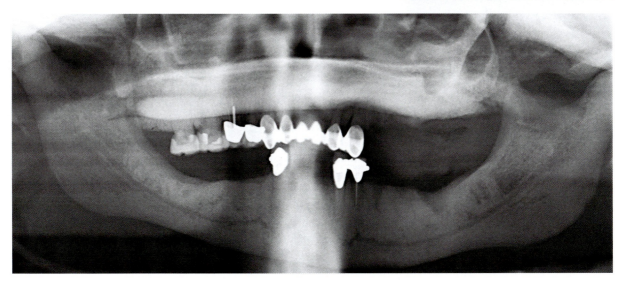

■ Figure **14.3**
Osteopetrosis
Diffuse sclerosis of the mandibular bone in a patient with adult osteopetrosis. (Courtesy Dr. Patrick Coleman.)

Cleidocranial Dysplasia

Figs. **14.4** and **14.5**

Cleidocranial dysplasia is a rare hereditary disorder that affects the formation of both bones and teeth. This autosomal dominant condition is caused by mutations in the *RUNX2 gene* (also known as *CBFA1*), which is responsible for the production of a protein involved in bone and tooth formation. Cleidocranial dysplasia is estimated to occur in 1 out of every 1,000,000 persons. As many as 40% of cases have no family history of the disorder and apparently represent new gene mutations.

As its name suggests, cleidocranial dysplasia is associated with defective formation of the clavicles and skull. The clavicles usually appear markedly hypoplastic or discontinuous; total absence of the clavicles is noted in about 10% of affected patients. As a result, the shoulders may exhibit a drooped appearance that can make the patient's neck appear longer. In addition, increased mobility often can allow the patient to approximate his or her shoulders anteriorly. The skull usually is enlarged with frontal and parietal bossing. The cranial sutures and fontanels typically show delayed closure and may remain open throughout life. Radiographic examination often reveals secondary centers of ossification in the suture lines, resulting in so-called Wormian bones.

Abnormalities of various other bones also may be identified, including pelvic anomalies, hypoplastic scapulae, brachydactyly, and scoliosis. Patients frequently are short in stature. Facial features include ocular hypertelorism with a broad base and depressed bridge of the nose. The paranasal sinuses may be absent or underdeveloped. Defective formation of the temporal bone and eustachian tube can result in hearing loss and susceptibility to recurring ear infections. Intraorally, many patients exhibit a narrow, high-arched palate, and there is an increased prevalence of cleft palate. The mandible may show coarse trabeculation, narrow rami, and slender coronoid processes with distal curvature. As the patient ages, mandibular prognathism can develop.

However, the most striking oral manifestation is the failure of eruption of most of the permanent dentition, which is associated with over-retention of the primary teeth. In addition, multiple unerupted supernumerary teeth frequently are present. It has been suggested that the failure of tooth eruption is related to the lack of secondary cementum formation on the roots, although this concept has been disputed by other studies.

Patients with cleidocranial dysplasia have a normal life expectancy. Dental management can be complex, often requiring extraction of retained primary teeth and any supernumerary teeth, followed by orthodontic-assisted eruption of impacted permanent teeth. Frequently, associated orthognathic surgery also is required. However, the success of therapy can vary, and appropriate prosthetic treatment may be required. Dental implants have been used successfully in some cases.

Focal Osteoporotic Bone Marrow Defect

Fig. **14.6**

The presence of hematopoietic bone marrow in the jaws is not unusual, although the distribution and amount of bone marrow can vary from patient to patient. On occasion, hematopoietic marrow is sufficient to produce a radiolucent defect that may be difficult to distinguish from other radiolucent bone lesions. Such lesions are known as **focal osteoporotic bone marrow defects**.

Marrow defects of the jaws are incidental, asymptomatic findings observed most frequently in the posterior mandible of adult females. Such lesions often are found in edentulous areas of the alveolar bone, possibly secondary to the growth of hematopoietic cells filling an extraction site. Radiographically, the lesion appears as a relative radiolucency that can range from several millimeters to several centimeters in diameter. The radiographic borders may appear well circumscribed on panoramic radiographs, although the lesion may be ill-defined on periapical films. Close examination often reveals faint bony trabeculation within the lesion, which can be a helpful clue to the diagnosis.

Most focal osteoporotic bone marrow defects can be diagnosed with reasonable confidence on a radiographic basis. However, if the diagnosis is uncertain, then biopsy sometimes is performed to rule out other bony lesions. The prognosis is excellent, and such isolated marrow spaces are not associated with systemic problems, such as generalized skeletal osteoporosis, anemia, or other hematologic disorders. However, displacement of dental implants into focal osteoporotic marrow defects rarely has been reported.

■ Figure **14.4**
Cleidocranial Dysplasia
This young man can approximate his shoulders because of the absence of his clavicles.

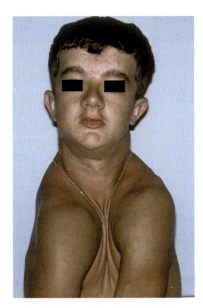

■ Figure **14.5**
Cleidocranial Dysplasia
Multiple unerupted and supernumerary teeth.

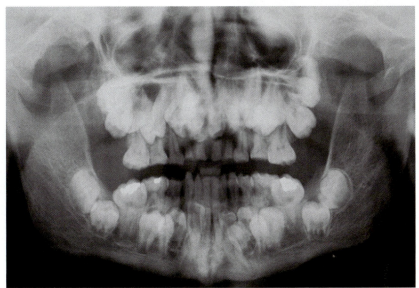

■ Figure **14.6**
Focal Osteoporotic Bone Marrow Defect
Decreased trabecular bone between the mandibular second bicuspid and first molar produces the appearance of a radiolucent defect. (Courtesy Dr. Michael Piepenbring.)

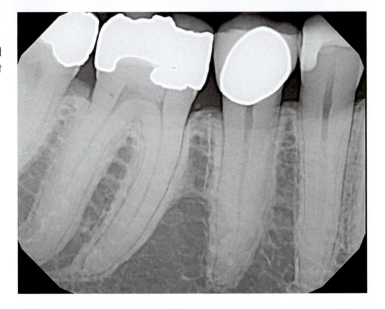

Figs. **14.7–14.10**

Idiopathic osteosclerosis is a term used to describe localized zones of increased bone density without a known cause. Such lesions are common in the jaws, with an overall estimated prevalence of 5%. Unlike condensing osteitis, there is no obvious source of inflammation, such as a nonvital tooth, that induces this bone formation. However, in some instances, it can be difficult to distinguish between these two lesions.

Idiopathic osteosclerosis of the jaws is seen primarily in the mandible, which accounts for approximately 90% of cases. Most examples occur in the region of the second premolar to second molar. The lesion often is discovered during the first through third decades of life as an incidental radiographic finding. Radiographs typically reveal a circumscribed, nonexpansile area of radiopacity between or beneath the tooth roots. Most examples measure from 2 mm to 2 cm in diameter, and no radiolucent rim should be present. Some patients can develop multiple lesions; in such cases, it may be prudent to rule out the possibility of osteomas associated with Gardner syndrome. Occasional examples occur around the crown of a developing tooth, impeding its eruption. On rare occasions, the dense bone can result in tooth movement or root resorption.

Once discovered, many cases of idiopathic osteosclerosis will remain stable without change. Examples discovered in children may slowly increase in size, becoming stable once the patient reaches maturity. In most instances, the diagnosis can be made radiographically with reasonable certainty, so that biopsy is not necessary. However, biopsy may be warranted for unusual cases where the diagnosis is uncertain (e.g., cases associated with root resorption, mild discomfort, or evidence of cortical expansion). Some cases of idiopathic osteosclerosis will diminish in size or disappear over time.

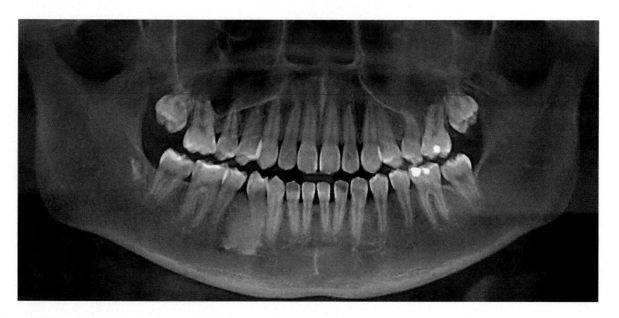

■ Figure **14.7**
Idiopathic Osteosclerosis
Dense, sclerotic bone is seen between and apical to the right mandibular bicuspids. (Courtesy Dr. Anthony Spina.)

■ Figure **14.8**
Idiopathic Osteosclerosis
A circumscribed radiopaque lesion is seen between the apices of the left mandibular second bicuspid and first molar. (Courtesy Dr. William R. Anderson.)

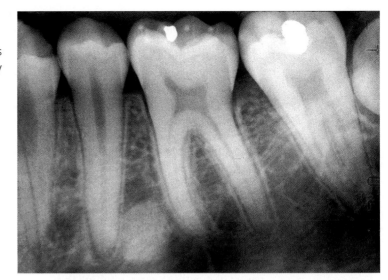

■ Figure **14.9**
Idiopathic Osteosclerosis
A well-defined zone of bone sclerosis is seen at the apex of the right mandibular first molar. This lesion has resulted in resorption of the tooth roots—an uncommon occurrence with idiopathic osteosclerosis. (Courtesy Dr. Jeff Laro.)

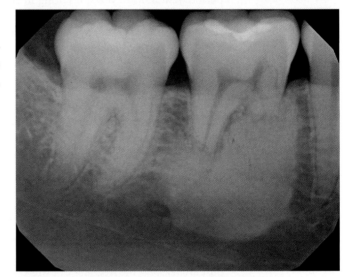

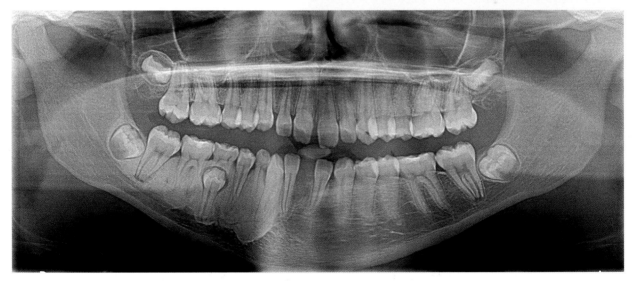

■ Figure **14.10**
Idiopathic Osteosclerosis
Diffuse sclerosis of the alveolar bone in the right mandible. (Courtesy Dr. Terry Ellis.)

Massive Osteolysis (Vanishing Bone Disease; Gorham Disease; Gorham-Stout Syndrome)

Fig. **14.11**

Massive osteolysis is a rare condition that results in the progressive destruction of one or more bones. The cause of this disease is unknown; various theories include trauma-induced proliferation of granulation tissue, accelerated osteoclastic activity mediated by interleukin-6, lymphatic vascular hyperplasia, and agenesis or abnormal function of thyroid C cells.

Massive osteolysis can occur at any age, but it is diagnosed most often in children and young adults. Approximately 30% of cases involve the craniofacial skeleton, with the mandible being the most common head and neck site. The involvement of multiple contiguous bones is not unusual. Patients with jaw involvement often present with pain, swelling, and tooth mobility, which might be mistaken initially for odontogenic infection. Displacement of the mandible or pathologic fracture eventually may occur. Radiographic examination reveals ill-defined radiolucent zones of bone destruction, which extend and worsen over time as more and more bone structure is dissolved. Microscopic examination of the resorbed bone usually reveals fibrosis and vascular hyperplasia consisting primarily of lymphatics.

The prognosis for this condition is highly unpredictable. Osseous destruction may continue over a period of months to years, resulting in complete loss of the affected bone(s). However, in some cases, the process can stabilize with only partial bone loss. Severe cases that involve the ribs, spine, or mandible can result in death secondary to airway obstruction, respiratory failure, chylothorax, and spinal cord compression. Various treatment approaches have included surgical resection, radiation therapy, bisphosphonates, denosumab, calcium, vitamin D, and chemotherapy. However, response to therapy is variable and often unsatisfactory.

Paget Disease of Bone (Osteitis Deformans)

Figs. **14.12 and 14.13**

Paget disease of bone is a disorder of bony metabolism that results in accelerated bone turnover. The cause of this disease is uncertain, although it may involve a combination of genetic and environmental factors. From 10% to 20% of patients have a family history of the disorder, half of whom will show mutations of the *SQSTM1* gene. Significant geographic differences are noted in the prevalence of Paget disease, with the highest rates seen in the United Kingdom and other populations of British descent. In the 1990s, radiographic examination showed an estimated prevalence as high as 2% in patients over the age of 55 years in the United Kingdom. However, the disease is rare in Scandinavia, India, and the Far East. For obscure reasons, the frequency of this condition appears to be declining rapidly in some populations, with prevalence rates that may be only 10% to 20% of that seen 20 to 30 years ago.

Paget disease of bone usually is diagnosed in patients over the age of 50 years, and most studies reveal a male predilection. Both monostotic and polyostotic forms of the disease can occur. The most commonly involved bones include the femur, spine, skull, sternum, and pelvis. Early disease is characterized by excessive osteoclastic resorption, which is followed in later stages by increased osteoblastic activity. Levels of serum alkaline phosphatase, a marker of osteoblastic activity, are significantly elevated and can be used to monitor the success of treatment.

The most common presenting symptom is bone pain, which is reported in approximately half of all cases. Accelerated remodeling eventually leads to bony expansion, deformation, and poor bone quality. Involvement of weight-bearing bones can result in bowing of the legs and alteration in gait. Pathologic fractures also may occur. Skull enlargement may cause an increase in circumference of the head, which classically is associated with the need for a larger hat size. In addition, bony enlargement of the skull may produce nerve compression, manifested clinically by deafness, vision impairment, and cranial nerve palsies. (It is speculated that Beethoven's hearing loss may have been related to Paget disease.) Secondary complications include congestive heart failure, aortic stenosis, and atherosclerosis.

Jaw involvement is reported in approximately 17% of patients, with a 2:1 maxilla-to-mandible ratio. Expansion of the alveolar bone may cause diastema formation between the teeth or tightening of dentures. Severe enlargement of the maxilla can lead to nasal obstruction, sinus obliteration, and a lion-like facial deformity known as *leontiasis ossea*. During early phases of the disease, the bone may appear less dense radiographically because of osteoclastic activity. However, over time, the bone develops patchy zones of sclerosis sometimes described as having a "cotton wool" appearance. In the jaws, hypercementosis of teeth may be seen.

Mild, asymptomatic Paget disease may not require any treatment. Patients with bone pain or more extensive involvement usually are treated with bisphosphonates, such as a single infusion of zoledronic

■ Figure **14.11**
Massive Osteolysis
Extensive destruction of almost the entire mandible. (Courtesy Dr. Mark Ludlow.)

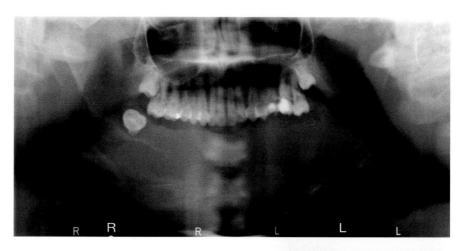

■ Figure **14.12**
Paget Disease of Bone
Radiograph showing new bone formation and enlargement of the skull with a "cotton wool" appearance. (Courtesy Dr. Reg Munden.)

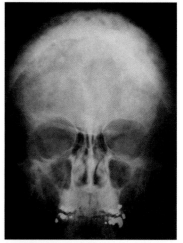

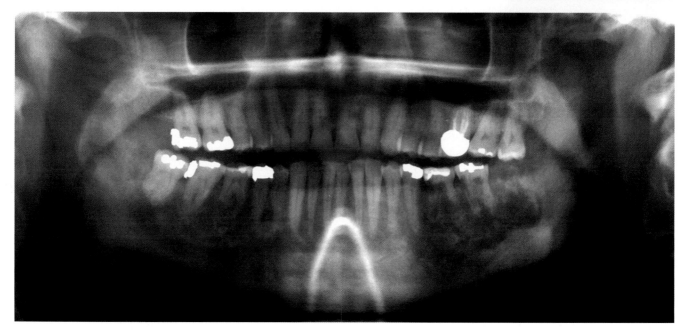

■ Figure **14.13**
Paget Disease of Bone
A 41-year-old male with diffuse radiopaque and radiolucent changes around the roots of the mandibular teeth. Biopsy and subsequent blood studies led to a diagnosis of early-onset Paget disease.

acid. The prognosis in most cases is excellent. However, malignant transformation into osteosarcoma or other sarcomas has been described in less than 1% of patients with Paget disease. These tumors have an extremely poor prognosis. An increased risk for the development of giant cell tumor of bone also is noted.

Central Giant Cell Granuloma

Figs. **14.14–14.17**

The **central giant cell granuloma** is an uncommon destructive lesion of the jaws comprised of osteoclast-like multinucleated giant cells. The cause of this lesion is unknown, and there is debate whether it represents a reactive process or a benign neoplasm. When initially described, the term *central giant cell "reparative" granuloma* was used because it was thought that the lesion might represent a response to local trauma-induced hemorrhage. However, there is no convincing evidence to support the idea that this represents a reparative process, especially in view of the destructive nature of these lesions. Although microscopic similarity exists, the central giant cell granuloma is thought to represent a different entity from *giant cell tumor* of extragnathic bones. However, rare examples of true giant cell tumor of bone have been reported in the jaws.

Central giant cell granulomas occur most often in children and young adults; more than 60% of cases are diagnosed before the age of 30 years. The lesion is seen twice as often in females than in males. Giant cell granulomas have a predilection for the anterior portions of the jaws, and approximately 70% of examples develop in the mandible. It is not unusual for mandibular lesions to cross the midline. Many cases are relatively nonaggressive, showing slow painless growth with little expansion. However, other lesions can demonstrate more rapid growth with significant expansion, cortical perforation, root resorption, and pain. Radiographic examination typically reveals a radiolucent zone of bone destruction that may be relatively well delineated, but without corticated borders. However, some cases can appear multilocular with a corticated peripheral margin. The size can range from small nonaggressive examples measuring less than 1 cm to large aggressive lesions that are more than 10 cm in diameter.

Microscopically, the lesion shows variable numbers of multinucleated giant cells in a background of mononuclear cells and hemorrhage. Because of the hemorrhagic nature of these lesions, they typically demonstrate a purplish brown color on gross examination, which can be a clue to the diagnosis at the time of biopsy. However, other hemorrhagic giant cell lesions can have a similar gross and microscopic appearance, such as the brown tumor of hyperparathyroidism. In addition, multiple giant cell granuloma-like lesions can occur in several genetic conditions, including cherubism (see next topic), Noonan-like/multiple giant cell lesion syndrome, Ramon syndrome, Jaffe-Campanacci syndrome, and neurofibromatosis type I.

The most common treatment for central giant cell granuloma of the jaws is thorough curettage, especially for smaller, less aggressive examples. However, recurrence is noted in approximately 20% of cases. Recurrent lesions may be managed by further curettage with peripheral ostectomy or by local resection. A variety of additional treatment modalities have been used for larger, more aggressive central giant cell granulomas in an attempt to minimize surgical morbidity, although the success rate has been inconsistent. These include subcutaneous interferon alpha-2a, intranasal calcitonin, antiresorptive medications (e.g., bisphosphonates or denosumab), and intralesional corticosteroid injections.

■ Figure **14.14**
Central Giant Cell Granuloma
Radiolucent lesion of the anterior mandible resulting in displacement of the teeth.

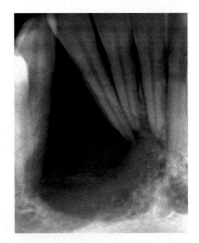

■ Figure **14.15**
Central Giant Cell Granuloma
Expansile radiolucent lesion of the midline anterior maxilla.

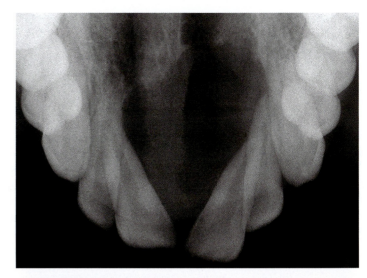

■ Figure **14.16**
Central Giant Cell Granuloma
Edentulous patient with an expansile mass of the left anterior maxilla. (With appreciation to Dr. Michael Tabor.)

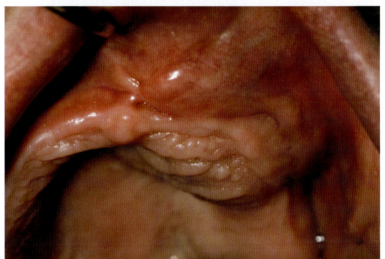

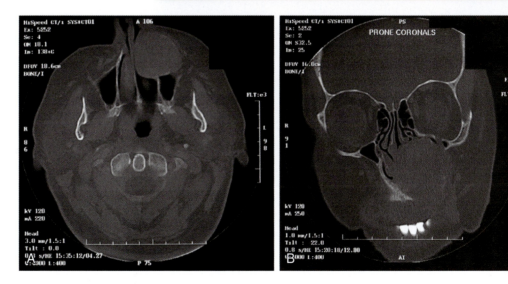

■ Figure **14.17**
Central Giant Cell Granuloma
Axial and coronal computed tomographic images of patient seen in Fig. 14.16, which demonstrate a solid mass extending into the maxillary sinus and the nasal cavity. (With appreciation to Dr. Michael Tabor.)

Cherubism is a rare hereditary disorder of the jaws that usually is caused by mutations of the *SH3BP2* gene. Affected patients have increased osteoclastic activity that results in expansile, lytic bone lesions, but it is uncertain why the disease primarily affects the jaws. Cherubism is inherited as an autosomal dominant trait, although some patients have no family history and appear to harbor new gene mutations. The disease shows variable clinical expressivity.

Cherubism often is diagnosed when the patient is 3 to 6 years of age, although milder examples of the disease may not be detected until later in childhood. Affected individuals present with painless bony expansion of the jaws with plump cheeks that resemble angelic cherubs, such as seen in Renaissance paintings. Cervical lymphadenopathy sometimes is noted, which may contribute to the swollen appearance. Milder examples may affect only the posterior mandible, but other cases will exhibit significant involvement throughout both jaws. In severe cases affecting the maxilla, upward tilting of the eyes and retraction of the lower eyelids can expose the inferior sclera, producing what has been described as an "eyes upturned to heaven" expression.

Radiographic examination of the jaws reveals bilateral, symmetrical, expansile radiolucencies that usually are multilocular. Patients with mild expression may show lesions only in the posterior mandibular molar/ramus region. However, individuals with more severe disease will show diffuse involvement throughout both jaws. Displacement of multiple developing teeth often is noted, as well as tooth impactions and root resorption. Microscopically, lesions of cherubism show a giant cell proliferation similar to that seen in the central giant cell granuloma. Laboratory results typically show normal levels of calcium and parathyroid hormone, which helps to rule out hyperparathyroidism.

Management of patients with cherubism can be challenging. In most cases, the lesions will improve after puberty and return to a more normal appearance during early adulthood (although less severe, residual radiographic changes may persist throughout life). Therefore, early surgical treatment during childhood usually is avoided, if possible. However, unusual aggressive examples may necessitate appropriate surgical intervention during active phases of the disease, such as curettage, resection, bone grafting, or recontouring. Dental management may include extraction of impacted teeth, orthodontic therapy, and prosthetic replacement of missing teeth. Medical treatment has been attempted in some patients with cherubism, including calcitonin, interferon, adalimumab, bisphosphonates, and tacrolimus. However, further study is needed to assess the usefulness of such medicines.

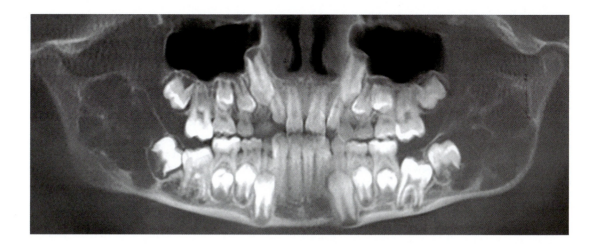

■ Figure **14.18**
Cherubism
Panoramic radiographic view of the jaws showing bilateral multilocular radiolucencies of the posterior mandible. (Courtesy Dr. Rob Naples.)

■ Figure **14.19**
Cherubism
A 7-year-old female with painless, symmetrical enlargement of the mandible and maxilla. (Courtesy Dr. Parish Sedghizadeh.)

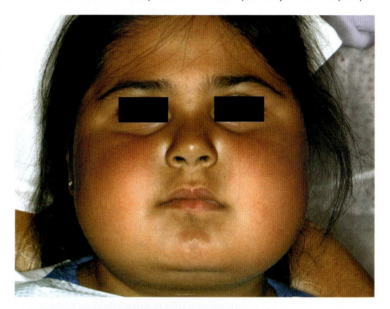

■ Figure **14.20**
Cherubism
Panoramic radiograph of patient seen in Fig. 14.19 showing diffuse multilocular changes in both jaws. (Courtesy Dr. Parish Sedghizadeh.)

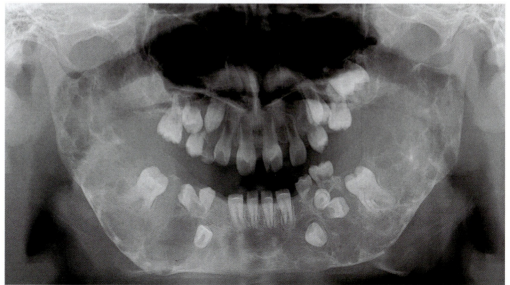

Aneurysmal Bone Cyst

Fig. **14.21**

The **aneurysmal bone cyst** is an uncommon destructive bony process that is most common in the long bones and vertebrae; only 2% of cases occur in the jaws. It is characterized by blood-filled cyst-like spaces that are surrounded by a giant cell proliferation similar to that seen in a central giant cell granuloma. Many aneurysmal bone cysts now are classified as neoplasms because of cytogenetic evidence of a translocation involving the *USP6* oncogene. However, other examples appear to represent a reactive process that develops after trauma or as a secondary phenomenon within a pre-existing bone lesion (such as a fibro-osseous lesion).

Aneurysmal bone cysts of the jaws occur most often during the first three decades of life; the mean age of occurrence is 21 years. The lesion is more common in the mandible than the maxilla, and the vast majority of cases develop in the posterior regions of the jaws. The most common clinical presentation is a rapidly expanding swelling of the involved bone. Some cases may be associated with pain or tooth mobility. Radiographically, the lesion can appear as either a unilocular or multilocular radiolucency with well-defined or ill-defined borders. Marked bony expansion is not unusual, which may result in a ballooned or "blow-out" distention of the overlying thin bony cortex. Because of the presence of multiple blood-filled cyst-like spaces in the lesion, the gross appearance has been described as resembling a "blood-soaked sponge."

Aneurysmal bone cysts of the jaws frequently are treated by enucleation and curettage, which may be supplemented with cryosurgery. However, *en bloc* resection may be required for more aggressive or recurrent examples. An estimated recurrence rate of 13% has been reported for aneurysmal bone cysts of the jaws.

Simple Bone Cyst (Traumatic Bone Cyst; Solitary Bone Cyst; Idiopathic Bone Cavity; Unicameral Bone Cyst)

Figs. **14.22 and 14.23**

The **simple bone cyst** is an empty or fluid-filled cavity that develops within bone. Despite its name, this lesion has no epithelial lining and does not represent a true cyst. The cause of simple bone cysts is uncertain. The synonymous term *traumatic bone cyst* is based on a theory that the lesion may arise secondary to a traumatic event that causes intrabony hemorrhage. If the intraosseous hematoma fails to organize and heal properly, then a pseudocystic cavity could remain within the bone. However, this concept has been questioned because a history of trauma frequently cannot be established. Another theory suggests that accumulation of interstitial fluid in bone leads to subsequent cavity formation. In some cases, simple bone cysts develop in association with a pre-existing fibro-osseous lesion.

Simple bone cysts can occur in almost any bone, including the jaws. Most examples are discovered in children, with peak prevalence during the second decade of life. No obvious sex predilection is noted for isolated simple bone cysts of the jaws. However, examples that occur secondary to cemento-osseous dysplasia usually are diagnosed in middle-aged adults, especially black women.

Simple bone cysts of the jaws usually occur in the mandible, often being discovered as an incidental finding on radiographic examination. However, some cases may produce a painless, bony expansion. The lesion often exhibits a relatively well-defined unilocular radiolucency, although some examples appear multilocular or ill defined. Many times, the radiolucency seems to scallop upward between the mandibular tooth roots. The overlying bony cortex may be thinned, especially in cases that cause expansion. Multifocal examples have been described, often in a background of florid cemento-osseous dysplasia.

Because a simple bone cyst cannot be diagnosed with certainty on a radiographic basis, surgical exploration and biopsy of any contents usually are recommended to rule out other possible diagnoses. Upon accessing the lesion, the surgeon may find serosanguineous fluid or the cavity may appear mostly empty. The mandibular neurovascular bundle sometimes is seen lying free within the bony cavity. After exploration, most simple bone cysts of the jaws will fill in with new bone formation and resolve over a period of 12 to 17 months. A low rate of recurrence (1% to 2%) has been reported in most studies. However, cases associated with cemento-osseous dysplasia have a much higher rate of persistence or recurrence.

■ Figure **14.21**
Aneurysmal Bone Cyst
Expansile and faintly multilocular lesion at the angle and ramus of the right mandible in a young child. (Courtesy Dr. Mojgan Ghazi.)

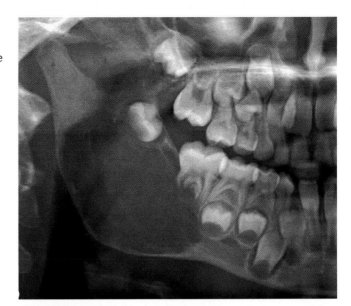

■ Figure **14.22**
Simple Bone Cyst
Radiolucent lesion of the left posterior mandibular molar region, which scallops up between the tooth roots. (With appreciation to Dr. Jensen Turner.)

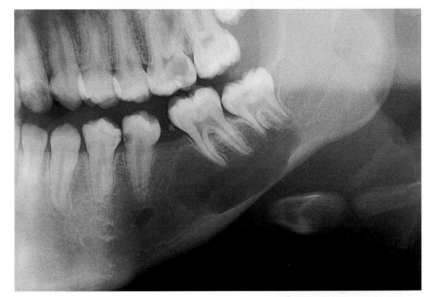

■ Figure **14.23**
Simple Bone Cyst
Young man with a well-circumscribed radiolucency of apical to the mandibular incisor teeth. Upon biopsy, an empty cavity was found. (Courtesy Dr. Paul Shirley.)

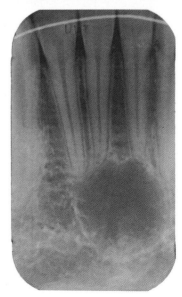

Figs. **14.24–14.27**

Fibrous dysplasia is a rare disorder of bone formation that is caused by a somatic activating mutation of the *GNAS* gene. The severity of the condition is determined by the timing of this postzygotic mutation during embryogenesis. If mutation occurs early in embryonic life, then progeny of the mutated cells may affect various developing tissues, including multiple bones (polyostotic fibrous dysplasia), melanocytes, and endocrine organs. More commonly, *GNAS* mutation occurs later in development, which results in localized disease affecting only a single bony site (monostotic fibrous dysplasia). The disease is characterized by replacement of the normal bone by fibrous connective tissue, which then exhibits the formation of new, immature bony trabeculae. Because of the combination of fibrous tissue and newly formed bone, fibrous dysplasia is classified as one of the benign fibro-osseous lesions.

Monostotic fibrous dysplasia can occur at any bony site, including the jaws. The maxilla is affected more often than the mandible. Maxillary lesions may involve adjacent bones of the zygoma or skull—a pattern known as *craniofacial fibrous dysplasia*. Fibrous dysplasia usually is noticed during the first two decades of life as a painless unilateral expansion with slow growth. Severe cases can produce significant facial asymmetry, tooth displacement, and malocclusion. Radiographs typically reveal a diffuse, ground-glass radiopacity with ill-defined margins. Maxillary lesions often result in obliteration of the maxillary sinus. On occasion, mandibular fibrous dysplasia shows a somewhat multilocular radiolucent appearance on panoramic films, although other dental radiographs typically will demonstrate a more classic ground-glass appearance. On rare occasions, the radiopaque pattern can resemble a fingerprint.

When more than one bony site is affected, the disease is referred to as polyostotic fibrous dysplasia. Some patients will show involvement of only a few bones, whereas others can have over half of the skeleton affected. Long bone lesions can result in pain, pathologic fractures, and bowing deformities. *McCune-Albright syndrome* refers to the combination of polyostotic fibrous dysplasia, irregular *café au lait* (coffee with milk) pigmentation of the skin, and various endocrine disturbances. This severe variant occurs more often in females, who may exhibit precocious puberty as well as other endocrinopathies (e.g., hyperthyroidism, hyperparathyroidism, hypercortisolism, excess growth hormone). When polyostotic bone lesions occur in combination with only *café au lait* spots on the skin, then the term *Jaffe-Lichtenstein syndrome* is used.

Mild craniofacial fibrous dysplasia may not require any specific treatment, although a biopsy usually is obtained to confirm the diagnosis. For patients with significant expansion and facial asymmetry, surgical recontouring of the affected bone can be performed. If possible, it usually is recommended that surgical management be delayed until later teenage years after the patient has stopped growing because early intervention may only stimulate the lesion to grow even faster. After recontouring, slow regrowth of the lesion can continue through adulthood, sometimes necessitating further bony "shave down" procedures. Orthodontic therapy and orthognathic surgery may be utilized to correct occlusal disharmonies.

In most cases, the prognosis for patients with fibrous dysplasia is excellent. However, rare examples of malignant transformation into osteosarcoma have been documented. Many of these malignancies developed in patients who were treated in the past with radiation therapy.

■ Figure **14.24**
Fibrous Dysplasia
Diffuse ground-glass radiopacity of the right posterior maxilla.

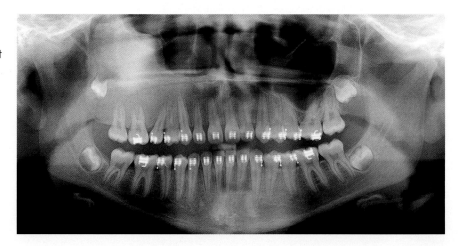

■ Figure **14.25**
Fibrous Dysplasia
Ground-glass radiopaque change that resembles a fingerprint.
(Courtesy Dr. Mark Freeland.)

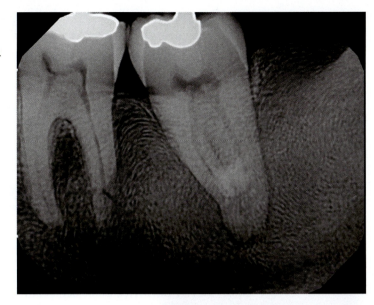

■ Figure **14.26**
Fibrous Dysplasia
Coronal computed tomographic image showing an expansile ground-glass radiopacity of the left maxilla with extension into the anterior maxillary sinus region.

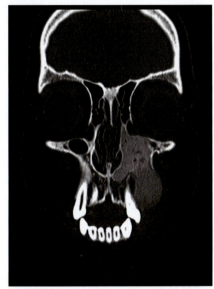

■ Figure **14.27**
Fibrous Dysplasia (Jaffe-Lichtenstein Syndrome)
Young man with polyostotic fibrous dysplasia. (A) A large area of *café au lait* pigmentation is seen on the calf. (B) Coronal computed tomographic image showing diffuse bony enlargement of the skull and maxilla.

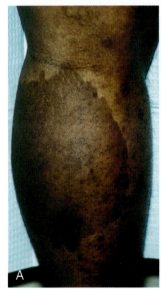
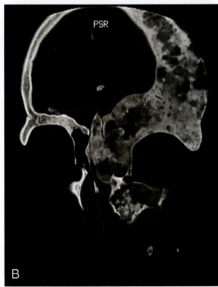

Cemento-Osseous Dysplasia (Osseous Dysplasia)

Cemento-osseous dysplasia is a fibro-osseous condition that occurs in the tooth-bearing areas of the jaws. Based on its frequent association with tooth roots, plus microscopic evidence showing production of both bone and a cementum-like product, it has been theorized that these lesions arise from cells of the periodontal ligament. Three different clinical patterns of cemento-osseous dysplasia are recognized, which vary in severity: (1) **periapical**, (2) **focal**, and (3) **florid**.

Periapical Cemento-Osseous Dysplasia (Periapical Cemental Dysplasia)

Figs. **14.28 and 14.29**

The most common and best recognized form of the disease is **periapical cemento-osseous dysplasia**. This condition shows a striking predilection for women, who outnumber men by more than a 10:1 margin. In addition, there is a strong predilection for blacks, who account for at least 70% of diagnosed cases. Most cases are discovered as incidental findings in young and middle-aged adults when radiographs are taken for other purposes. Rarely is the diagnosis made before the age of 20 years.

Early lesions classically present as multiple periapical radiolucencies associated with the roots of the anterior mandibular teeth. Some cases may occur as a radiolucency involving a single root apex, or multiple lesions may coalesce to form a single radiolucency encompassing several teeth. On occasion, additional lesions may be noted at the apices of the posterior teeth, which might be viewed as progression to the more "florid" end of the disease spectrum. Although the individual radiolucencies may resemble a periapical granuloma or periapical cyst, the associated teeth should be vital (unless they are nonvital for an unrelated reason). Over time, the lesions undergo central calcification, resulting in a mixed radiolucent/radiopaque appearance. Late-stage lesions become primarily radiopaque with a small radiolucent rim. Most lesions are nonexpansile and seldom exceed 1 cm in diameter.

Periapical cemento-osseous dysplasia rarely causes any problems. In most instances, the diagnosis can be made with reasonable certainty on a radiographic basis, so biopsy usually is not necessary. Recognition of this condition is important to avoid a mistaken diagnosis of pulpal/periapical disease and unnecessary root canal therapy.

Focal Cemento-Osseous Dysplasia

Fig. **14.30**

In **focal cemento-osseous dysplasia**, the patient develops a single lesion—most often at an extraction site in the posterior mandible. Like periapical cemento-osseous dysplasia, focal lesions are diagnosed most often in black women during the third through sixth decades of life. The lesion usually is discovered when radiographs are obtained for some other purpose. Early lesions appear as a well-defined radiolucency that may be difficult to distinguish from other lesions, such as a residual cyst. However, over time the lesion will develop a mixed radiolucent/radiopaque pattern, eventually becoming almost totally radiopaque in the later stages.

The diagnosis of focal cemento-osseous dysplasia often can be made with reasonable certainty based on the radiographic and clinical features. However, biopsy sometimes may be deemed necessary if other radiolucent/radiopaque lesions, such as a central ossifying fibroma, cannot be ruled out. These two fibro-osseous lesions may have similar microscopic features, although the surgical findings are helpful in distinguishing between them. Lesions of cemento-osseous dysplasia usually show a gritty, fragmented quality when biopsied, whereas central ossifying fibromas exhibit a more solid appearance, often shelling out cleanly as one or several large masses.

Focal cemento-osseous dysplasia usually has a good prognosis. However, late stage, densely sclerotic lesions occasionally can become secondarily infected, which may require surgical removal of the dead bone/cementum.

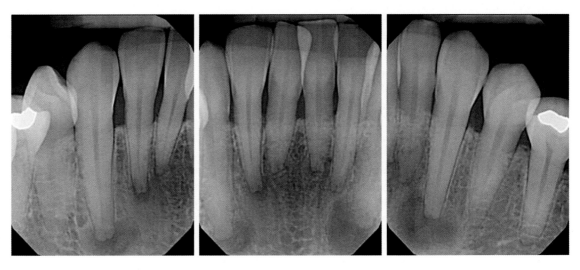

■ Figure **14.28**
Periapical Cemento-Osseous Dysplasia
Multiple radiolucencies involving the anterior mandibular teeth in a 50-year-old black female. (Courtesy Dr. Walker Pendarvis.)

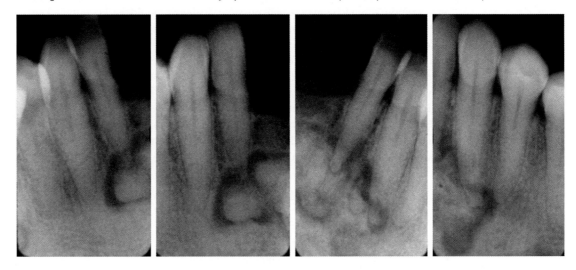

■ Figure **14.29**
Periapical Cemento-Osseous Dysplasia
Multiple confluent, late-stage lesions showing prominent central mineralization with a radiolucent border.

■ Figure **14.30**
Focal Cemento-Osseous Dysplasia
Well-circumscribed mixed radiolucent/radiopaque lesion in an extraction site of the left posterior mandible.

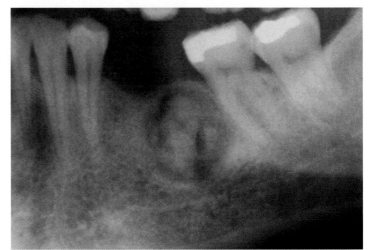

Figs. **14.31–14.34**

Florid cemento-osseous dysplasia represents the severe end of the cemento-osseous dysplasia spectrum. Patients develop multifocal lesions that may involve all four quadrants of the jaws. Mandibular disease usually is more significant and widespread than is maxillary involvement, sometimes resulting in confluent lesions apical to the entire dentition. Florid cemento-osseous dysplasia shows an even stronger predilection for black women, being diagnosed mostly in middle-aged and older patients.

Similar to other patterns of cemento-osseous dysplasia, florid lesions will demonstrate three radiographic phases in their evolution: radiolucent, mixed radiolucent/radiopaque, and almost totally radiopaque. Unfortunately, because of the avascular and widespread nature of the late-stage sclerotic lesions, patients have a significant risk for developing secondary osteomyelitis after dental infection or tooth extraction. In edentulous areas, segments of sclerotic, nonvital bone/cementum product may become exposed on the alveolar ridge as the surrounding alveolar bone undergoes resorption. Another potential complication is secondary simple bone cyst formation in association with one or more of these fibro-osseous lesions. Unlike isolated simple bone cysts seen in children, these bony cavities in patients with florid cemento-osseous dysplasia often do not resolve following surgical exploration.

The diagnosis of florid cemento-osseous dysplasia usually can be made on the basis of the radiographic and clinical features. Because of the risk for secondary infection in late-stage lesions, biopsy and surgical intervention should be avoided, if possible. Patients should be encouraged to maintain excellent oral hygiene to avoid any type of pulpal or periodontal disease that might introduce bacteria into the lesions. Secondary osteomyelitis in the setting of florid cemento-osseous dysplasia is difficult to manage because of the widespread and often confluent nature of the densely sclerotic mineralized product. Antibiotic therapy alone may not resolve the infection, and attempts at surgical resection of dead bone at one site may be followed by the spread of infection to adjacent lesions. However, saucerization and removal of sequestrating dead bone sometimes is required.

On rare occasions, patients with cemento-osseous dysplasia may develop tumor-like expansion of one or more lesions, a situation that has been termed *expansive osseous dysplasia*. Such lesions have been reported most often in the mandible of black females and may require surgical resection.

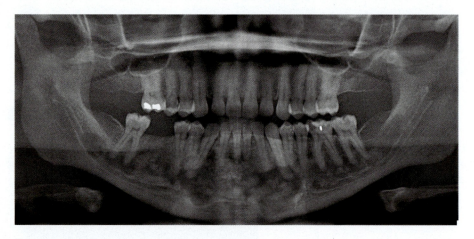

■ Figure **14.31**
Florid Cemento-Osseous Dysplasia
Multiple confluent radiolucent and radiopaque lesions at the apices of the mandibular teeth. (Courtesy Dr. James Sutton.)

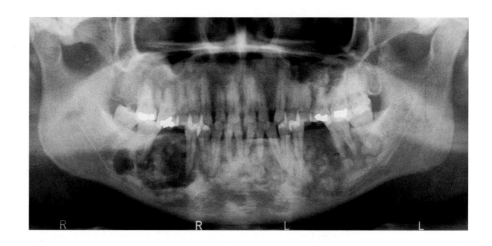

■ Figure **14.32**
Florid Cemento-Osseous Dysplasia
Multiple radiolucent and radiopaque lesions throughout the body of the mandible. Milder maxillary involvement also appears to be present. (Courtesy Dr. Tom McDonald.)

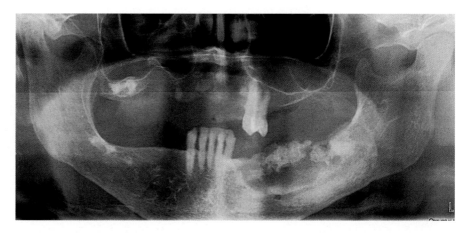

■ Figure **14.33**
Florid Cemento-Osseous Dysplasia
A segment of sequestrating bone and cementum is seen in the left mandible. Additional smaller lesions are present in the right posterior maxilla and mandible. (Courtesy Dr. Robert Crooks.)

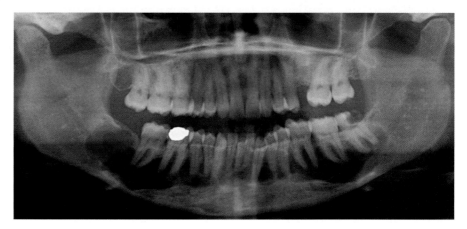

■ Figure **14.34**
Florid Cemento-Osseous Dysplasia
Extensive secondary simple bone cyst formation has resulted in a diffuse radiolucent defect around the mandibular teeth. (Courtesy Dr. Laura Summers.)

Figs. **14.35–14.38**

The **central ossifying fibroma** is an uncommon neoplasm that often was confused with focal cemento-osseous dysplasia prior to the separation of these two entities in the 1990s. The tumor occurs most frequently in young adult females, and the body of the mandible is typically affected. Clinically, swelling is a characteristic presenting sign. Because these lesions typically cause no pain or tenderness, they often are identified when the patient has routine dental radiographs taken. Radiographic examination shows a well-defined unilocular radiolucency with varying amounts of calcification within the lesion. As the tumor enlarges, root resorption and movement of the teeth may occur, as well as thinning and outward bowing of the cortical plate.

These lesions are characterized microscopically by a well-circumscribed, cellular proliferation of plump spindle-shaped cells set in a moderately collagenous background. Occasionally a well-developed capsule is present. Varying amounts of mineralized product can be found throughout the lesional tissue, and the mineralized component may resemble bony trabeculae or spherules of cementum.

Treatment consists of surgical enucleation, which usually is accomplished easily because the tumor is demarcated from the surrounding bone. Recurrence is uncommon, with the average recurrence rate of reported cases in the literature being slightly more than 10%. If multiple central ossifying fibromas are identified in a patient, this should trigger an investigation to rule out the relatively rare condition known as *hyperparathyroidism–jaw tumor syndrome*.

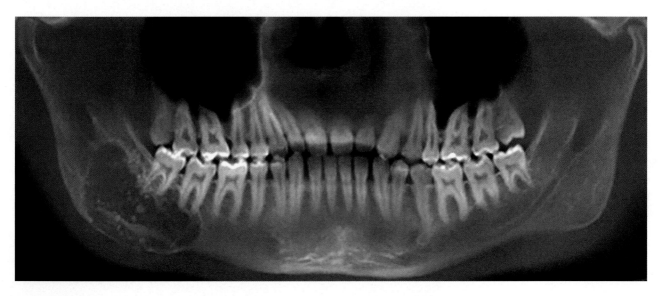

■ Figure **14.35**
Central Ossifying Fibroma
A demarcated expansile radiolucency that contains scattered radiopacities is noted in the right posterior mandible. The expansion has produced marked thinning of the inferior border of the mandible.

■ Figure 14.36
Central Ossifying Fibroma
This demarcated radiolucency of the right body of the mandible also contains a few mineralized flecks. The lesion has caused resorption of the inferior border of the mandible. (Courtesy Dr. Richard Marks.)

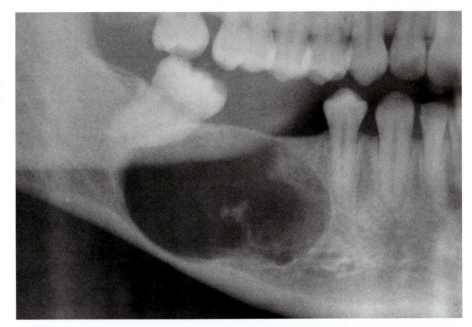

■ Figure 14.37
Central Ossifying Fibroma
Gross photograph of the lesion seen in Fig. 14.36. The well-developed capsule of this lesion often results in a potato-like tumor mass.

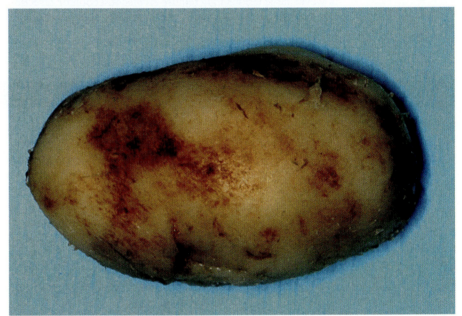

■ Figure 14.38
Central Ossifying Fibroma
The cut surface of the tumor seen in Fig. 14.37 reveals a solid mass with a yellow-white color.

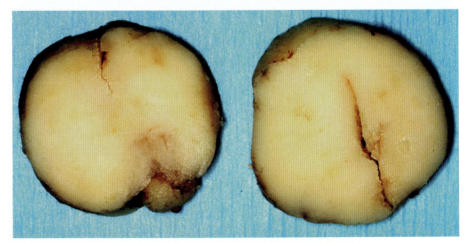

Juvenile Ossifying Fibroma

Figs. **14.39 and 14.40**

The **juvenile ossifying fibroma** is a relatively rare neoplasm that, as the name implies, usually develops in younger patients, typically in the first or second decades of life. In the jaws, the most common site for this lesion is the maxilla, although other craniofacial bones may be affected. Based on their microscopic features, two forms of this lesion have been described: *trabecular* and *psammomatoid*. The psammomatoid variant tends to develop in the cranial bones, and the trabecular variant seems to favor the jaws. Jaw lesions may exhibit relatively rapid enlargement. Radiographs show a unilocular radiolucency initially, but as the lesion grows, a multilocular appearance may develop. Eventually the cortical bone becomes thinned as the lesion expands. Computed tomographic (CT) imaging shows varying degrees of intralesional calcification in some lesions, a feature that is consistently associated with the trabecular form of the tumor. In other lesions, CT imaging identifies a "ground-glass" pattern, and this is related to the psammomatoid variant. Both types of juvenile ossifying fibroma have well-defined borders.

The trabecular pattern of juvenile ossifying fibroma is characterized by a loosely cellular spindle-cell proliferation with delicate trabeculae of woven bone and scattered benign multinucleated giant cells. The psammomatoid pattern exhibits rounded acellular calcifications set in a cellular fibroblastic background.

Treatment consists of curettage or surgical excision, with the extent of the surgery dependent on the size and anatomic site of the tumor. For small lesions, thorough curettage is often adequate treatment; however, large lesions may require *en bloc* resection or resection with reconstruction. Recurrence rates in some series have been reported to be as high as 30% to 50%.

Osteoma

Fig. **14.41**

The **osteoma** infrequently involves the jaws, although adjacent anatomic sites, such as the bones of the sinuses, may be affected. In the jaws, the mandibular body and condylar region are favored sites. This lesion is usually asymptomatic unless it develops in a location where swelling can be detected or its growth impinges on other anatomic structures. The osteoma is usually identified in adults, often as an incidental finding when obtaining imaging studies for other reasons. The tumor appears as a demarcated radiodensity on radiographic examination. Microscopically, these lesions consist of a benign proliferation of dense vital lamellar bone. In some instances, the distinction between an osteoma and an exostosis can be difficult to make and somewhat arbitrary.

If treatment is necessary, conservative surgical removal is typically curative. If multiple osteomas are noted in the craniofacial bones, then the possibility of Gardner syndrome must be considered (see next topic).

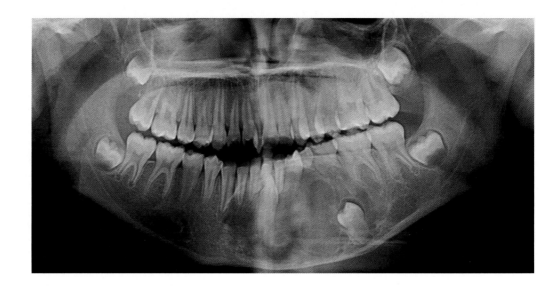

■ Figure 14.39
Juvenile Ossifying Fibroma
This multilocular expansile radiolucency with focal calcification extends from the right mandibular canine region to the left mandibular first molar region. (Courtesy Dr. David Bender.)

■ Figure 14.40
Juvenile Ossifying Fibroma
This coronal computed tomographic image shows the same lesion that is depicted in Fig. 14.39. Marked expansion is evident, as well as areas of mineralization within the tumor. (Courtesy Dr. David Bender.)

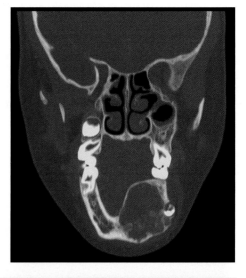

■ Figure 14.41
Osteoma
This demarcated, uniformly dense radiopacity is associated with the surface of the mandibular posterior cortical bone. (Courtesy Dr. Chuck Hobart.)

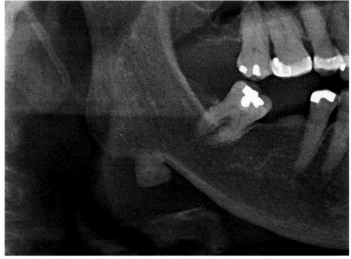

Figs. **14.42–14.44**

Gardner syndrome represents a small proportion of the *familial adenomatous polyposis (FAP)* spectrum of genetic mutations, all of which are caused by mutations of the *adenomatous polyposis coli (APC)* tumor suppressor gene. The resulting condition is characterized by the development at a relatively early age of precancerous lesions (adenomatous polyps) of the colon. The polyps often number in the hundreds, and if allowed to persist, they eventually transform to adenocarcinoma of the colon. The mutated *APC* gene is inherited in an autosomal dominant fashion, with a high degree of penetrance and variable gene expression. In most cases, a family history of Gardner syndrome is present, although 20% to 30% appear to be new mutations of the *APC* gene.

Patients affected by Gardner syndrome, in addition to the colonic polyps, develop multiple osteomas that primarily involve the craniofacial bones. The osteomas generally begin developing in the second decade of life. The presence of the osteomas involving the jaws often will initiate an evaluation to rule out Gardner syndrome. Other signs include increased numbers of epidermoid cysts, impacted and supernumerary teeth, odontomas, and development of locally aggressive fibrous neoplasms, which are known as desmoid tumors. Congenital hypertrophy of the retinal pigment epithelium is an ophthalmologic finding that occurs sporadically as an isolated brown macule on the retina. Patients with four or more of these retinal spots are very likely to have Gardner syndrome.

Treatment of Gardner syndrome primarily consists of genetic counseling and colectomy. Approximately half of these patients develop adenocarcinoma of the colon before 30 years of age, so complete colectomy at a relatively young age is often advised. If this is not performed, nearly 100% of patients will develop colon cancer by age 50. Approximately 20% of these patients develop desmoid tumors, primarily in the abdominal region. These aggressive fibrous growths are poorly demarcated and frequently recur after surgical excision, although they do not metastasize. Radiation therapy has been used to manage nonresectable tumors. Even though they are not considered to be malignant, these neoplasms often have a pronounced impact on the patient's quality of life. Removal of epidermoid cysts and osteomas may be considered if these are associated with significant cosmetic or functional concerns.

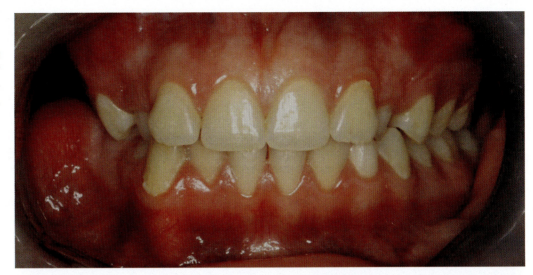

■ Figure 14.42
Gardner Syndrome
The smooth-surfaced nodule in the right posterior mandibular region is bony hard, representing an osteoma. (Courtesy Dr. Jason Sheikh.)

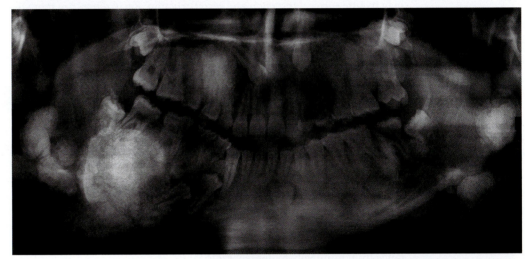

■ Figure 14.43
Gardner Syndrome
A panoramic radiograph of the patient depicted in Fig. 14.42, showing the prominent demarcated radiopaque osteoma in the right posterior mandibular region, as well as numerous additional osteomas involving the maxilla and other mandibular areas. (Courtesy Dr. Molly Cohen.)

■ Figure 14.44
Gardner Syndrome
This axial computed tomographic image of the same patient seen in Figs. 14.42 and 14.43 depicts numerous osteomas involving the mandible. (Courtesy Dr. Molly Cohen.)

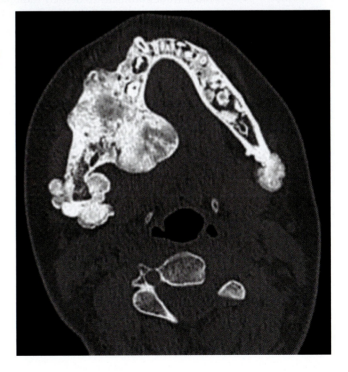

Desmoplastic Fibroma

Figs. **14.45 and 14.46**

The **desmoplastic fibroma** is a rare neoplasm of fibroblastic differentiation that is considered to be benign but locally aggressive. This tumor arises in bone, and a soft tissue counterpart, *aggressive fibromatosis*, is also recognized. Usually these lesions are identified in young adults, and the mandible is the most commonly affected bone, although this tumor may also develop in the femur, pelvic bones, radius, and tibia. Radiographically, the desmoplastic fibroma presents as a radiolucency that initially may be unilocular, but as the tumor grows, an expansile, multilocular appearance develops, often with thinning or perforation of the cortical bone. The margins of the lesion may be demarcated, but indistinct margins are also frequently noted, presumably because of the infiltrative nature of the neoplasm.

The histopathologic features of the desmoplastic fibroma typically consist of a proliferation of bland fibroblastic cells that are arranged in fascicles and set in a densely collagenous background. Mitotic figures are sparse or absent.

The management of this process essentially consists of surgical excision, the extent of which depends on the size and anatomic site of the tumor. Small lesions may be treated with curettage, but large lesions may require surgical resection and reconstruction. Recurrences are more likely with conservative surgical approaches because of the infiltrative nature of this neoplasm.

Osteoblastoma

Fig. **14.47**

The **osteoblastoma** is a rare benign tumor of bone that is significant because it may be mistaken histopathologically for osteosarcoma. Osteoblastomas are found most frequently in the spine, although the jaws also may be involved. This tumor typically presents in younger individuals, usually in the second or third decade of life. Most osteoblastomas develop within the medullary cavity the jaw, but periosteal osteoblastomas have been reported. Pain or tenderness is a common initial symptom, and swelling is often a presenting sign. Although most of these lesions are unilocular radiolucencies, the radiographic features can be somewhat diverse. The variation is seen in the degree of intralesional calcification that may be present, which can range from minimally to densely radiopaque. The radiographic margins of the tumor also may vary, with some lesions being well demarcated, and others ill defined.

Histopathologically, this neoplasm is characterized by plump osteoblastic cells that line interlacing trabeculae of lesional osteoid or woven bone. Most osteoblastomas have scattered benign multinucleated giant cells and a rather prominent vascular pattern. Mitoses are usually not prominent, and no evidence of necrosis or invasion of adjacent normal tissue should be seen.

Treatment consists of surgical excision, which may range from aggressive curettage to *en bloc* resection, depending on the size and anatomic location of the tumor. Recurrence is uncommon.

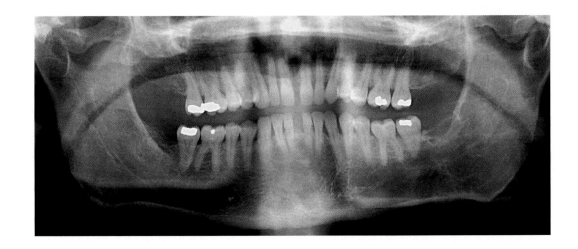

■ Figure **14.45**
Desmoplastic Fibroma
A rather poorly demarcated, multilocular radiolucency is noted in the left posterior mandible. (Courtesy Dr. Jonathan Bailey.)

■ Figure **14.46**
Desmoplastic Fibroma
This axial computed tomographic image of the patient depicted in Fig. 14.45 shows a poorly defined radiolucency with a modest degree of expansion and perforation of the lingual cortex of the mandible. (Courtesy Dr. Jonathan Bailey.)

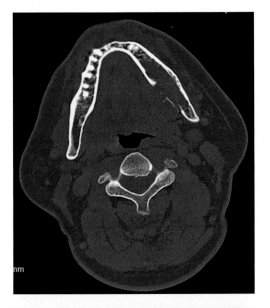

■ Figure **14.47**
Osteoblastoma
This sagittal computed tomographic image shows a large, demarcated mixed radiolucent/radiopaque tumor of the anterior maxilla. (Courtesy Dr. Michael Zetz.)

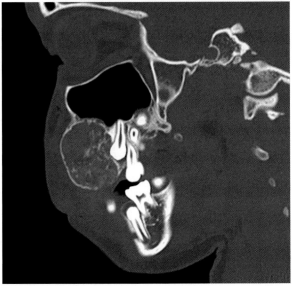

Figs. **14.48–14.50**

The **cementoblastoma** is a rare, somewhat controversial, benign neoplasm that is considered to be a bone tumor by some authorities, and an odontogenic tumor by others. This lesion has some histopathologic features in common with osteoblastoma, and cementoblastoma has been known to be misinterpreted as osteosarcoma as well. Like osteoblastoma, the cementoblastoma tends to occur in younger individuals, with the majority being diagnosed before 30 years of age. Pain and swelling are often the initial presenting complaints. Most cementoblastomas develop in the mandible, particularly in the permanent first molar region, although examples in the maxilla and in the deciduous dentition have been described.

The radiographic features of the cementoblastoma may, at times, be virtually pathognomonic for this tumor. These features include the fusion of a circumscribed radiopaque mass to the resorbed root of a tooth, with a uniform, radiolucent rim surrounding the radiopaque mass. Cementoblastomas that are identified early in their development may not have all of these diagnostic findings.

Microscopically, the cementoblastoma is composed of interlacing trabeculae and sheets of mineralized tissue that resemble cementum. This material is fused to the resorbed root of the affected tooth. The mineralized trabeculae are lined by plump cells that some investigators believe represent cementoblasts. The trabeculae at the periphery of the cementoblastoma often are oriented perpendicular to the outer surface in a radiating pattern.

Treatment consists of enucleation, although sometimes this requires sacrifice of the tooth that is fused to the cementoblastoma. If the tumor is fused to the root of a multirooted tooth, some clinicians have described amputation of the affected root and enucleation of the associated cementoblastoma in conjunction with endodontic treatment of the remaining unaffected pulp canals. This allows the tooth to remain in place. Recurrence of the cementoblastoma following enucleation is possible if the entire lesion is not removed. One large series and literature review reported an overall recurrence rate of 22%.

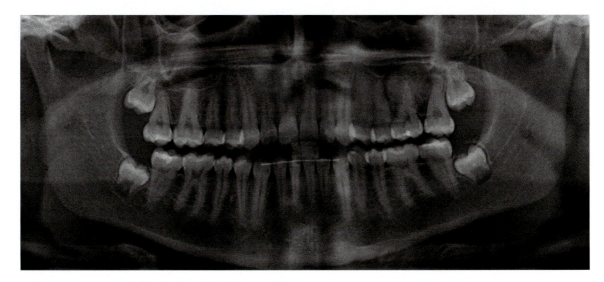

■ Figure 14.48
Cementoblastoma
This panoramic radiograph demonstrates a radiopaque lesion with a radiolucent rim associated with the roots of the left maxillary first molar. (Courtesy Dr. Louis M. Beto.)

■ Figure 14.49
Cementoblastoma
The tooth and its associated tumor, depicted in Fig. 14.48, show characteristic fusion of the lesion to the roots of the affected tooth. (Courtesy Dr. Louis M. Beto.)

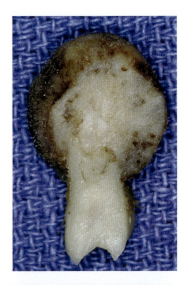

■ Figure 14.50
Cementoblastoma
This panoramic radiograph shows a large developing cementoblastoma in the left posterior mandible of a 9-year-old male. Expansion of the inferior border of the mandible is evident.

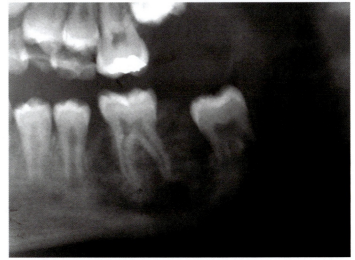

Figs. **14.51–14.59**

Osteosarcoma is a relatively rare bone malignancy that sometimes develops in the jaws. Most osteosarcomas originate within the medullary cavity of the bone, but a small percentage can arise from the periosteal surface. Although the mean age of patients with osteosarcoma of the long bones is approximately 18 to 24 years, osteosarcoma of the jaws occurs, on average, about 10 to 15 years later. Patients typically complain of pain and/or swelling of the jaw, although paresthesia or loosening of the teeth also may be present. Radiographically, osteosarcoma is characterized by an ill-defined, expansile radiolucency with variable amounts of radiopacity. Expansion or destruction of the cortical bone is often seen. When the tumor grows into the adjacent soft tissue, radiographs may identify radiating calcifications, a pattern that has been described as resembling a "sunburst." This finding is noted in about 25% of osteosarcomas of the jaw. If the tumor is adjacent to teeth, it is common for the lesion to invade the periodontal ligament space, producing marked widening of the space and destruction of the lamina dura. The roots of the teeth may show evidence of resorption, resulting in a pointed or "spiked" appearance.

The microscopic features of osteosarcoma can be diverse, but areas of the tumor should show some degree of osteoid (immature bone) production by the neoplastic cells. Some osteosarcomas, especially of the jaws, will produce abundant cartilage in the tumor; however, areas that show definitive production of osteoid by the tumor cells indicate a diagnosis of chondroblastic osteosarcoma, not chondrosarcoma.

Treatment of osteosarcoma has been evolving over the past few decades, and the prognosis has improved significantly. When treating long-bone osteosarcomas, preoperative chemotherapy is usually given prior to wide resection of the malignancy. However, this protocol appears to have equivocal results for osteosarcoma of the jaws. Radiation therapy does not appear to be effective. Radical surgical excision, followed by reconstruction, seems to be the best approach for these lesions currently. The prognosis of osteosarcoma of the jaws depends on the stage of the tumor, the age of the patient at the time of diagnosis, the size of the tumor, and whether the tumor is identified microscopically at the resection margins. A better prognosis is associated with early stage disease, a younger age at diagnosis, small tumor size, and the absence of tumor at the resection margins. Overall disease-specific 5-year survival is approximately 60% to 70% in most recent series of cases, although patients may develop recurrences beyond the 5-year period.

■ Figure **14.51**
Osteosarcoma

This large bony hard mass of the anterior mandible extends both facially and lingually. The surface exhibits areas of ulceration and telangiectasia. (With appreciation to Dr. Charles Ferguson.)

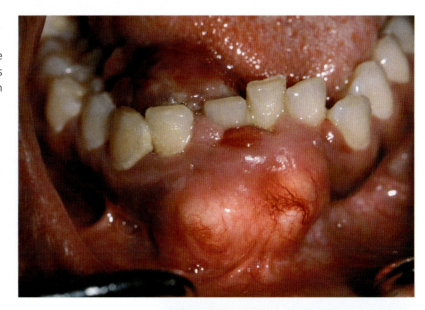

■ Figure **14.52**
Osteosarcoma

Periapical radiograph of the patient depicted in Fig. 14.51, showing the characteristic widening of the periodontal ligament space and loss of lamina dura that may be seen with osteosarcoma of the jaws. (With appreciation to Dr. Charles Ferguson.)

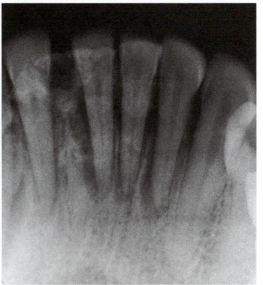

■ Figure **14.53**
Osteosarcoma

A large, ulcerated tumor mass engulfing the right posterior mandibular teeth. (With appreciation to Dr. Terry Day.)

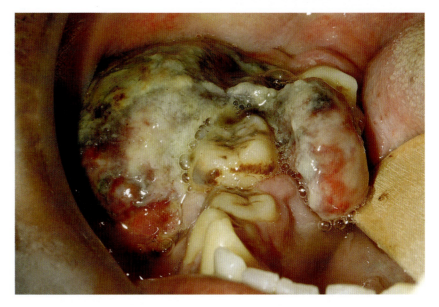

■ Figure **14.54**
Osteosarcoma
Panoramic radiograph of the same patient depicted in Fig. 14.53, showing a large, ill-defined radiolucency of the right posterior mandible, with thinning of the inferior border. (Courtesy Dr. Tom Rollar.)

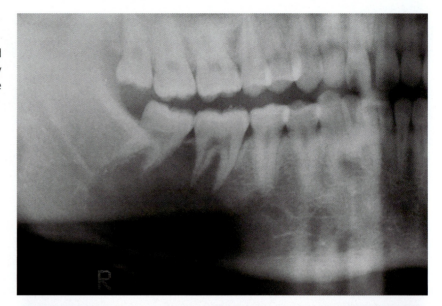

■ Figure **14.55**
Osteosarcoma
An ulcerated nodule involving the left posterior palatal alveolar process. (Courtesy Dr. Steven Bengtson.)

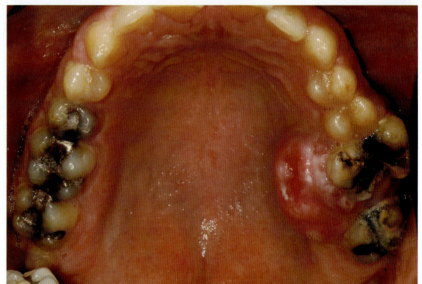

■ Figure **14.56**
Osteosarcoma
A periapical radiograph of the same patient depicted in Fig. 14.55, showing an ill-defined, mixed radiolucent/radiopaque lesion in the left posterior maxilla. (Courtesy Dr. Steven Bengtson.)

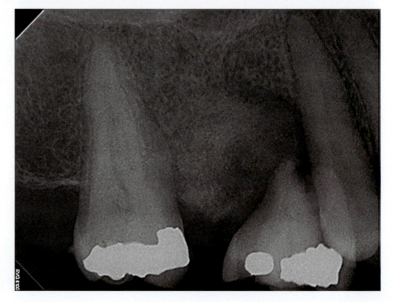

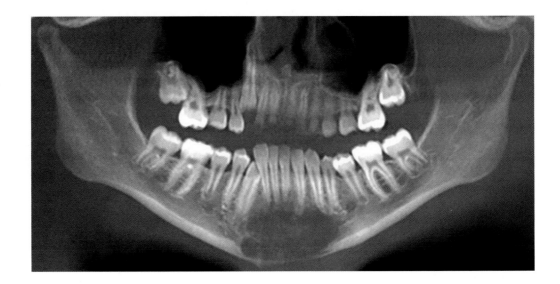

■ Figure **14.57**
Osteosarcoma
A large, poorly defined radiolucency involving the anterior mandible and causing thinning and destruction of the inferior border of the mandible. (Courtesy Dr. Alexander Balaci.)

■ Figure **14.58**
Osteosarcoma
A coronal computed tomographic image of the same patient depicted in Fig. 14.57, showing intralesional calcification, as well as thinning and destruction of the inferior and left cortical plate. (Courtesy Dr. Alexander Balaci.)

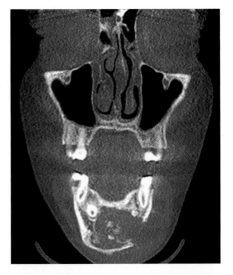

■ Figure **14.59**
Osteosarcoma
A sagittal computed tomographic image of the same patient depicted in Fig. 14.57, showing intralesional calcification, as well as perforation of the facial cortical plate. Radiating mineralized areas are seen within the bulging tumor mass, suggesting a "sun-ray" pattern. (Courtesy Dr. Alexander Balaci.)

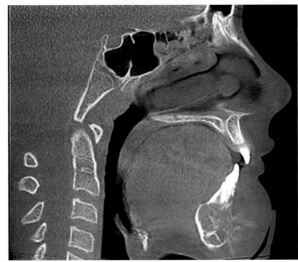

Ewing Sarcoma

Fig. **14.60**

Ewing sarcoma is a rare malignancy that generally arises within bone. Currently it is thought that this tumor differentiates along the lines of mesenchymal stem cells that have a neural component. Classic Ewing sarcoma is the most common entity in what is known as the Ewing family of tumors, which all share certain cytogenetic features. Ewing sarcoma typically affects younger individuals, and most patients are between 5 and 30 years of age at the time of diagnosis. Usually the long bones are involved, but the tumor may develop in the pelvis, spine, or ribs. Very rarely, this malignancy may occur in the jaws. Pain, tenderness, or swelling may be present, and systemic signs and symptoms, such as fever, weight loss, fever, or anemia, may evolve. Early in its course, this tumor may be difficult to detect on plain radiographs because the changes in the medullary bone can be subtle. After the lesion perforates the cortical bone, development of an "onion-skin" pattern may be evident on the surface of the bone, although this is seen more often with long bone lesions.

Histopathologically, Ewing sarcoma is often referred to as a "small blue-cell tumor," which is a descriptive term that applies to a variety of poorly differentiated malignancies. Sheets of small, rounded cells, each with a nucleus that occupies most of the cytoplasm, characterize this malignancy. Immunohistochemical and cytogenetic studies are required to make a definitive diagnosis.

Treatment consists of multiagent chemotherapy combined with surgery and/or radiation therapy. The prognosis has been improving over the past few decades, and factors that appear to improve the prognosis include being less than 15 years old at the time of diagnosis and having localized disease. One study has suggested that Ewing sarcoma of the jaws may also have a slightly better prognosis compared to other sites.

Chondrosarcoma

Figs. **14.61 and 14.62**

Chondrosarcoma represents a very uncommon malignancy of cartilaginous differentiation that occurs primarily in middle-aged or older adults. Most chondrosarcomas arise in the bones of the pelvis and shoulder girdle, but occasionally the jaws may be affected. Conventional chondrosarcomas are slow-growing tumors, and signs and symptoms generally include swelling that may be accompanied by pain. The radiographic features are similar to osteosarcoma, in that the neoplasm is expansile, has ill-defined margins, and presents as a radiolucency with varying degrees of radiopacity. Widening of the periodontal ligament of the teeth adjacent to the tumor also may be seen.

Microscopically, conventional chondrosarcoma is characterized by an infiltrative proliferation of atypical cartilage or chondroid, with no evidence of osteoid production by the tumor cells. Depending on the degree of cytologic atypia, mitotic activity, and necrosis, these lesions may be assigned a description, ranging from low grade to high grade. Low-grade chondrosarcomas often appear quite bland, and most examples of "chondroma" of the jaws later prove to be low-grade chondrosarcoma, based on their tendency to recur locally. High-grade chondrosarcomas are usually more aggressive, with increased potential for metastasis.

Treatment of chondrosarcoma is very similar to that of osteosarcoma, although unlike osteosarcoma, chemotherapy does not play a role in the management of this malignancy. Wide surgical excision without neck dissection is generally used to treat this tumor. Most gnathic chondrosarcoma-related deaths are caused by uncontrollable recurrent disease, rather than distant metastases. The 5-year survival rate is typically reported to be between 80% and 90%, although 10-year disease-specific survival drops to around 70%.

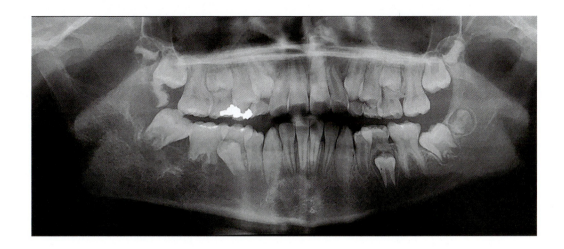

■ Figure **14.60**
Ewing Sarcoma
This panoramic radiograph shows an ill-defined, "moth-eaten" pattern of bone destruction with displacement and resorption of the teeth in the right posterior mandible of this young patient. (Courtesy Dr. Mojgan Ghazi.)

■ Figure **14.61**
Chondrosarcoma
A large hard mass involving the left posterior lingual mandible of a middle-aged female.

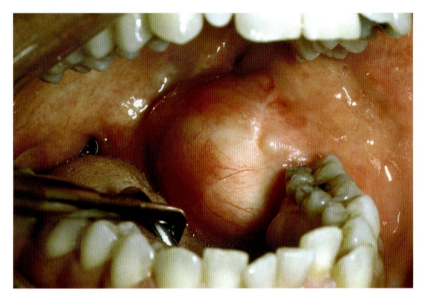

■ Figure **14.62**
Chondrosarcoma
This panoramic radiograph of the same patient depicted in Fig. 14.61 shows an ill-defined, expansile mixed radiopaque/radiolucent lesion involving the left posterior mandible.

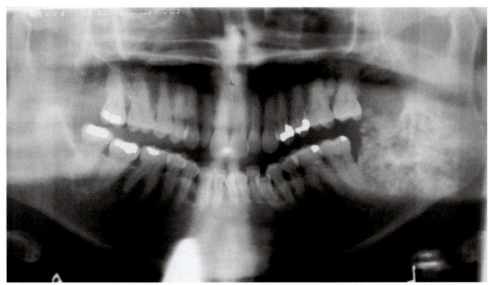

Figs. **14.63–14.65**

Mesenchymal chondrosarcoma is a rare malignancy of cartilaginous differentiation that tends to occur in a younger age group, compared to conventional chondrosarcoma, with the majority of patients being younger than 30 years of age. The ribs and jaws are among the more common sites of involvement of this tumor, although a significant percentage also may develop in the soft tissues. Pain, paresthesia, and swelling are among the more common complaints related to mesenchymal chondrosarcoma of the jaws. Radiographically, the lesion typically presents as a poorly demarcated radiolucency that may have radiopaque flecks.

This tumor is characterized histopathologically by a proliferation of small undifferentiated cells with minimal cytoplasm. Interspersed among these undifferentiated cells are islands of hyaline cartilage that are produced by the tumor. Immunohistochemical studies are often used to confirm the diagnosis.

Unfortunately, compared to conventional chondrosarcoma, the prognosis for mesenchymal chondrosarcoma is significantly worse, partly because of its greater ability to metastasize. Treatment of this malignancy consists of surgical resection, often combined with multiagent chemotherapy. Patients who present with metastatic disease have a poorer prognosis, as do patients who have evidence of tumor at the margins of their resection. The overall 5-year survival rate for gnathic mesenchymal chondrosarcoma is generally in the range of 50% to 60%, although this figure may continue to decline over time because of local recurrence or delayed metastases.

■ Figure **14.63**
Mesenchymal Chondrosarcoma
An ulcerated mass of the left posterior hard palate. (Courtesy Dr. Terry Day.)

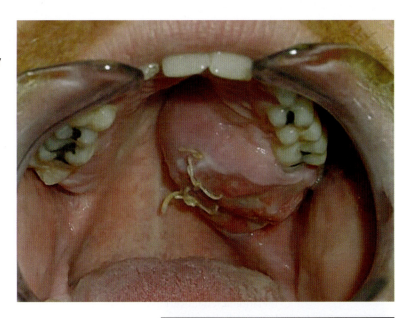

■ Figure **14.64**
Mesenchymal Chondrosarcoma
A coronal computed tomographic image of the same patient depicted in Fig. 14.62 showing tumor filling the left maxillary sinus. A few radiopaque foci are noted within the tumor. (Courtesy Dr. Terry Day.)

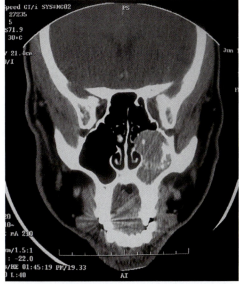

■ Figure **14.65**
Mesenchymal Chondrosarcoma
A periapical radiograph showing an ill-defined radiolucency that has caused resorption and splaying of the premolar roots. (Courtesy Dr. Michael Robinson.)

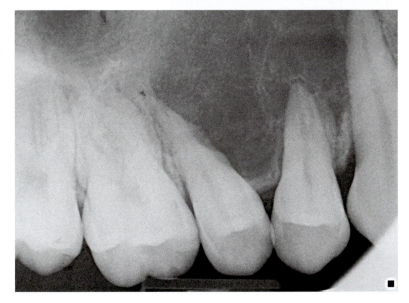

Figs. **14.66–14.69**

Metastatic tumors to the jaws occasionally occur, and these lesions may represent dissemination of malignancy that originated from virtually any anatomic site in the body. The most likely route of dissemination is by way of *Batson paravertebral plexus* of veins, which have no valves, allowing the blood (and any tumor emboli) to flow cephalically when intraabdominal pressure is increased. The mean age of affected patients is typically in the sixth decade of life. The metastatic deposits may present clinically in a variety of ways, with the lesions potentially causing swelling, ulceration, hemorrhage, pain, paresthesia, numbness, or loosening of teeth in the area. Radiographically, these lesions generally present as a radiolucency with ill-defined margins, although in some instances, metastatic tumors may induce an osteoblastic response and appear radiopaque. This latter finding is most often seen with metastatic adenocarcinoma of the prostate. When the metastatic lesion is near the apex of a tooth, it may be mistaken for a periapical inflammatory process. In approximately 20% to 25% of cases, the metastatic deposit is the first indication that the patient is suffering from malignancy, and an evaluation to identify the primary tumor is then initiated.

The microscopic findings are as diverse as the various primary tumor sources. As a result, metastatic disease histopathologically may have microscopic features of squamous cell carcinoma, renal cell carcinoma, melanoma, adenocarcinoma from any one of various glandular organs (e.g., breast, thyroid, prostate), hepatocellular carcinoma, and so on, depending on the primary tumor type.

In most cases, treatment of metastatic disease to the jaws is palliative. The majority of patients with metastasis to the jaws succumb to their disease within 1 to 2 years after diagnosis.

■ Figure **14.66**
Metastatic Adenocarcinoma of the Lung
This panoramic radiograph shows a large, ill-defined radiolucency of the right posterior mandible. Following biopsy of this lesion, further workup of the patient revealed the primary lung tumor. (Courtesy Dr. Martin Steed.)

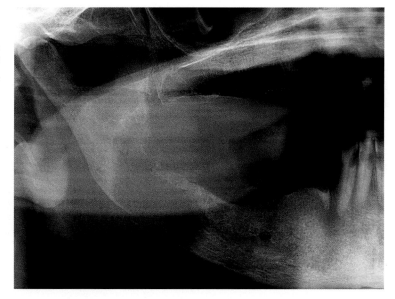

■ Figure **14.67**
Metastatic Melanoma

A periapical radiograph of the anterior maxilla shows an ill-defined radiolucency that easily could be mistaken for pulpal/periapical disease. Biopsy revealed metastatic melanoma. (Courtesy Dr. Cornelious Slaton.)

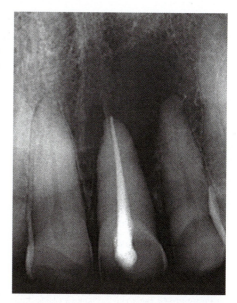

■ Figure **14.68**
Metastatic Thyroid Carcinoma

A prominent swelling is evident in the left posterior mandibular region in a patient with documented thyroid carcinoma. (With appreciation to Dr. Terry Day.)

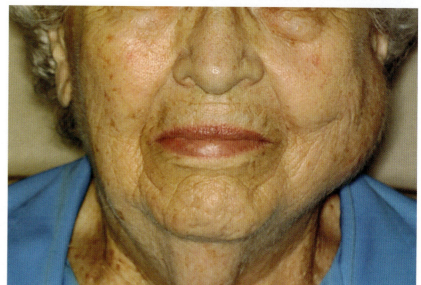

■ Figure **14.69**
Metastatic Thyroid Carcinoma

A panoramic radiograph of the same patient depicted in Fig. 14.68 identifies a large, ill-defined radiolucency of the left ramus of the mandible. The lesion has thinned and perforated the cortical bone. (With appreciation to Dr. Terry Day.)

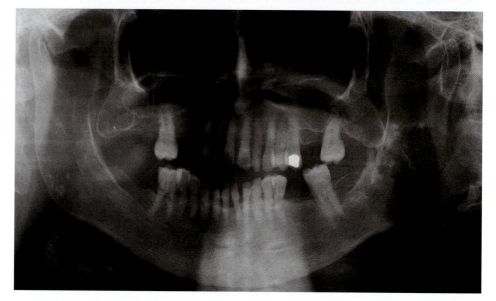

Bibliography

Osteopetrosis

Bollerslev J, Henriksen K, Nielsen MF, et al. Autosomal dominant osteopetrosis revisited: lessons from recent studies. *Eur J Endocrinol.* 2013;169:R39–R57.

Oğütcen-Toller M, Tek M, Sener I, et al. Intractable bimaxillary osteomyelitis in osteopetrosis: review of the literature and current therapy. *J Oral Maxillofac Surg.* 2010;68:167–175.

Sobacchi C, Schulz A, Coxon FP, et al. Osteopetrosis: genetics, treatment and new insights into osteoclast function. *Nat Rev Endocrinol.* 2013;9:522–536.

Wu CC, Econs MJ, DiMeglio LA, et al. Diagnosis and management of osteopetrosis: consensus guidelines from the osteopetrosis working group. *J Clin Endocrinol Metab.* 2017;102:3111–3123.

Cleidocranial Dysplasia

Bufalino A, Paranaíba LMR, Gouvêa AF, et al. Cleidocranial dysplasia: oral features and genetic analysis of 11 patients. *Oral Dis.* 2012;18: 184–190.

D'Alessandro G, Tagariello T, Piana G. Cleidocranial dysplasia: etiology and stomatognathic and craniofacial abnormalities. *Minerva Stomatol.* 2010;59:117–127.

Farrow E, Nicot R, Wiss A, et al. Cleidocranial dysplasia: a review of clinical, radiological, genetic implications and a guidelines proposal. *J Craniofac Surg.* 2017 Nov 17;doi:10.1097/SCS.0000000000004200. [Epub ahead of print].

Roberts T, Stephen L, Beighton P. Cleidocranial dysplasia: a review of the dental, historical, and practical implications with an overview of the South African experience. *Oral Surg Oral Med Oral Pathol Oral Radiol.* 2013;115:46–55.

Focal Osteoporotic Bone Marrow Defect

Barker BF, Jensen JL, Howell FV. Focal osteoporotic marrow defects of the jaws. *Oral Surg Oral Med Oral Pathol.* 1974;38:404–413.

Lee SC, Jeong CH, Im HY, et al. Displacement of dental implants into the focal osteoporotic bone marrow defect: a report of three cases. *J Korean Assoc Oral Maxillofac Surg.* 2013;39:94–99.

Makek M, Lello GE. Focal osteoporotic bone marrow defects of the jaws. *J Oral Maxillofac Surg.* 1986;44:268–273.

Idiopathic Osteosclerosis

MacDonald-Jankowski DS. Idiopathic osteosclerosis in the jaws of Britons and of the Hong Kong Chinese: radiology and systematic review. *Dentomaxillofac Radiol.* 1999;28:357–363.

Petrikowski CG, Peters E. Longitudinal radiographic assessment of dense bone islands of the jaws. *Oral Surg Oral Med Oral Pathol Oral Radiol Endod.* 1997;83:627–634.

Sisman Y, Ertas ET, Ertas H, et al. The frequency and distribution of idiopathic osteosclerosis of the jaw. *Eur J Dent.* 2011;5:409–414.

Tolentino Ede S, Gusmão PH, Cardia GS, et al. Idiopathic osteosclerosis of the jaw in a Brazilian population: a retrospective study. *Acta Stomatol Croat.* 2014;48:183–192.

Massive Osteolysis

Al-Jamali J, Glaum R, Kassem A, et al. Gorham-Stout syndrome of the facial bones: a review of pathogenesis and treatment modalities and report of a case with a rare cutaneous manifestations. *Oral Surg Oral Med Oral Pathol Oral Radiol.* 2012;114:e23–e29.

Gataa IS, Nader NH, Abdallah DT. Massive craniofacial Gorham disease treated successfully by cisplatin and 5-fluorouracil with ten years of follow-up: a case report and literature review. *J Oral Maxillofac Surg.* 2016;74:1774–1782.

Gondivkar SM, Gadbail AR. Gorham-Stout syndrome: a rare clinical entity and review of literature. *Oral Surg Oral Med Oral Pathol Oral Radiol Endod.* 2010;109:e41–e48.

Kim MK, Hong JR, Kim SG, et al. Fatal progression of Gorham disease: a case report and review of the literature. *J Oral Maxillofac Surg.* 2015;73:2352–2360.

Paget Disease of Bone

Al-Rashid M, Ramkumar DB, Raskin K, et al. Paget disease of bone. *Orthop Clin North Am.* 2015;46:577–585.

Tan A, Ralston SH. Clinical presentation of Paget's disease: evaluation of a contemporary cohort and systematic review. *Calcif Tissue Int.* 2014;95:385–392.

Tuck SP, Layfield R, Walker J, et al. Adult Paget's disease of bone: a review. *Rheumatology (Oxford).* 2017;56:2050–2059.

Valenzuela EN, Pietschmann P. Epidemiology and pathology of Paget's disease of bone – a review. *Wien Med Wochenschr.* 2017;167:2–8.

Central Giant Cell Granuloma

da Silva NG, Carreira AS, Pedreira EN, et al. Treatment of central giant cell lesions using bisphosphonates with intralesional corticosteroid injections. *Head Face Med.* 2012;8:23.

DeLange J, van den Akker HP. Clinical and radiological features of central giant-cell lesions of the jaw. *Oral Surg Oral Med Oral Pathol Oral Radiol Endod.* 2005;99:464–470.

Naidu A, Malmquist MP, Denham CA, et al. Management of central giant cell granuloma with subcutaneous denosumab therapy. *J Oral Maxillofac Surg.* 2014;72:2469–2484.

Tabrizi R, Fardisi S, Zamiri B, et al. Can calcitonin nasal spray reduce the risk of recurrence of central giant cell granuloma of the jaws? A double-blind clinical trial. *Int J Oral Maxillofac Surg.* 2016;45:756–759.

Whitaker SB, Waldron CA. Central giant cell lesions of the jaws: a clinical, radiologic and histopathologic study. *Oral Surg Oral Med Oral Pathol.* 1993;75:199–208.

Cherubism

Machado RA, Pontes HA, Pires FR, et al. Clinical and genetic analysis of patients with cherubism. *Oral Dis.* 2017;23:1109–1115.

Redfors M, Jensen JL, Storhaug K, et al. Cherubism: panoramic and CT features in adults. *Dentomaxillofac Radiol.* 2013;42:20130034. doi:10.1259/dmfr.20130034.

Stoor P, Suomalainen A, Kemola M, et al. Craniofacial and dental features in six children with cherubism. *J Craniofac Surg.* 2017;28:1806–1811.

Aneurysmal Bone Cyst

Henriques AC, Carvalho Mde V, Miguel MC, et al. Clinical pathological analysis of nine cases of aneurysmal bone cyst of the jaws in a Brazilian population. *Eur Arch Otorhinolaryngol.* 2012;269:971–976.

Motamedi MH, Behroozian A, Azizi T, et al. Assessment of 120 maxillofacial aneurysmal bone cysts: a nationwide quest to understand this enigma. *J Oral Maxillofac Surg.* 2014;72:1523–1530.

Motamedi MH, Navi F, Eshkevari PS, et al. Variable presentations of aneurysmal bone cysts of the jaws: 51 cases treated during a 30-year period. *J Oral Maxillofac Surg.* 2008;66:2098–2103.

Sun ZJ, Zhao YF, Yang RL, et al. Aneurysmal bone cysts of the jaws: analysis of 17 cases. *J Oral Maxillofac Surg.* 2010;68:2122–2128.

Simple Bone Cyst

Martins-Filho PR, Santos Tde S, Araújo VL, et al. Traumatic bone cyst of the mandible: a review of 26 cases. *Braz J Otorhinolaryngol.* 2012;78:16–21.

Peacock ME, Krishna R, Gustin JW, et al. Retrospective study on idiopathic bone cavity and its association with cementoosseous dysplasia. *Oral Surg Oral Med Oral Pathol Oral Radiol.* 2015;119:e246–e251.

Suei Y, Taguchi A, Nagasaki T, et al. Radiographic findings and prognosis of simple bone cyst of the jaws. *Dentomaxillofac Radiol.* 2012;39:65–71.

Suei Y, Taguchi A, Tanimoto K. Simple bone cyst of the jaws: evaluation of treatment outcome by review of 132 cases. *J Oral Maxillofac Surg.* 2007;65:918–923.

Fibrous Dysplasia

Akintoye SO, Boyce AM, Collins MT. Dental perspectives in fibrous dysplasia and McCune-Albright syndrome. *Oral Surg Oral Med Oral Pathol Oral Radiol.* 2013;116:e149–e155.

MacDonald-Jankowski D. Fibrous dysplasia: a systematic review. *Dentomaxillofac Radiol.* 2009;38:196–215.

Ricalde P, Magliocca KR, Lee JS. Craniofacial fibrous dysplasia. *Oral Maxillofac Surg Clin North Am.* 2012;24:427–441.

Waldron CA, Giansanti JS. Benign fibro-osseous lesions of the jaws. I. Fibrous dysplasia of the jaws. *Oral Surg Oral Med Oral Pathol.* 1973;35:190–201.

Cemento-Osseous Dysplasia

Alsufyani NA, Lam EWN. Cemento-osseous dysplasia of the jaw bones: key radiographic features. *Dentomaxillofac Radiol.* 2011;40:141–146.

Fenerty S, Shaw W, Verma R, et al. Florid cemento-osseous dysplasia: review of an uncommon fibro-osseous lesion of the jaw with important clinical implications. *Skeletal Radiol.* 2017;46:581–590.

Kawai T, Hiranuma H, Kishino M, et al. Cemento-osseous dysplasia of the jaws in 54 patients: a radiographic study. *Oral Surg Oral Med Oral Pathol Oral Radiol Endod.* 1999;87:107–114.

MacDonald-Jankowski DS. Focal cemento-osseous dysplasia: a systematic review. *Dentomaxillofac Radiol.* 2008;37:350–360.

Neville BW, Albenesius RJ. The prevalence of benign fibro-osseous lesions of periodontal ligament origin in black women: a radiographic survey. *Oral Surg Oral Med Oral Pathol.* 1986;62:340–344.

Raubenheimer EJ, Noffke CE, Boy SC. Osseous dysplasia with gross jaw expansion: a review of 18 lesions. *Head Neck Pathol.* 2016;10:437–443.

Su L, Weathers DR, Waldron CA. Distinguishing features of focal cemento-osseous dysplasias and cemento-ossifying fibromas. I. A pathologic spectrum of 316 cases. *Oral Surg Oral Med Oral Pathol Oral Radiol Endod.* 1997;84:301–309.

Ossifying Fibroma

Abramovitch K, Rice DD. Benign fibro-osseous lesions of the jaws. *Dent Clin North Am.* 2016;60:167–193.

Ahmad M, Gaalaas L. Fibro-osseous and other lesions of bone in the jaws. *Radiol Clin North Am.* 2018;56:91–104.

Mainville GN, Turgeon DP, Kauzman A. Diagnosis and management of benign fibro-osseous lesions of the jaws: a current review for the dental clinician. *Oral Dis.* 2017;23:440–450.

Parfitt J, Harris M, Wright JM, et al. Tumor suppressor gene mutation in a patient with a history of hyperparathyroidism–jaw tumor syndrome and healed generalized osteitis fibrosa cystica: a case report and genetic pathophysiology review. *J Oral Maxillofac Surg.* 2015;73:194.e1–194.e9.

Su L, Weathers DR, Waldron CA. Distinguishing features of focal cemento-osseous dysplasias and cemento-ossifying fibromas I. A pathologic spectrum of 316 cases. *Oral Surg Oral Med Oral Pathol Oral Radiol Endod.* 1997;84:301–309.

Woo S-B. Central cemento-ossifying fibroma: primary odontogenic or osseous neoplasm? *J Oral Maxillofac Surg.* 2015;73:S87–S93.

Juvenile Ossifying Fibroma

Aboujaoude S, Aoun G. Juvenile trabecular ossifying fibroma of the maxilla: a case report. *Med Arch.* 2016;70:470–472.

Barrena-López C, Bollar-Zabala A, Úrculo-Bareño E, et al. Cranial juvenile psammomatoid ossifying fibroma: case report. *J Neurosurg Pediatr.* 2016;17:318–323.

Becker M, Stefanelli S, Rougemont A-L, et al. Non-odontogenic tumors of the facial bones in children, and adolescents: role of multiparametric imaging. *Neuroradiology.* 2017;59:327–342.

Han J, Hu L, Zhang C, et al. Juvenile ossifying fibroma of the jaw: a retrospective study of 15 cases. *Int J Oral Maxillofac Surg.* 2016;45:368–376.

Maria A, Sharma Y, Malik M. Juvenile ossifying fibroma of mandible: a case report. *J Maxillofac Oral Surg.* 2013;12:447–450.

Owosho AA, Hughes MA, Prasad JL, et al. Psammomatoid and trabecular juvenile ossifying fibroma: two distinct radiologic entities. *Oral Surg Oral Med Oral Pathol Oral Radiol.* 2014;118:732–738.

Osteoma

Dell'Aversana-Orabona G, Salzano G, Iaconetta G, et al. Facial osteomas: fourteen cases and a review of literature. *Eur Rev Med Pharmacol Sci.* 2015;19:1796–1802.

Manjunatha BS, Das N, Sutariya R, et al. Peripheral osteoma of the body of mandible. *BMJ Case Rep.* 2013;doi:10.1136/bcr-2013-009857.

Sanchez-Burgos R, González Martín-Moro J, Arias-Gallo J, et al. Giant osteoma of the ethmoid sinus with orbital extension: craniofacial approach and orbital reconstruction. *Acta Otorhinolaryngol Ital.* 2013;33:431–434.

Tavares de Souza N, Lopes-Cavalcante RC, Aparecida de Albuquerque-Cavalcante M, et al. An unusual osteoma in the mandibular condyle and the successful replacement of the temporomandibular joint with a custom-made prosthesis: a case report. *BMC Res Notes.* 2017;10:727.

Gardner Syndrome

Agrawal D, Newaskar V, Shrivastava S, et al. External manifestations of Gardner's syndrome as the presenting clinical entity. *BMJ Case Rep.* 2014;doi:10.1136/bcr-2013-200293.

Cristofaro MG, Giudice A, Amantea M, et al. Gardner's syndrome: a clinical and genetic study of a family. *Oral Surg Oral Med Oral Pathol Oral Radiol.* 2013;115:e1–e6.

Dahl NA, Sheil A, Knapke S, et al. Gardner fibroma: clinical and histopathologic implications of germline APC mutation association. *J Pediatr Hematol Oncol.* 2016;38:e154–e157.

de Marchis ML, Tonelli F, Quaresmini D, et al. Desmoid tumors in familial adenomatous polyposis. *Anticancer Res.* 2017;37:3357–3366.

Guignard N, Cartier C, Crampette L, et al. Gardner's syndrome presenting with a fibromatous tumour of the parotid. *Eur Ann Otorhinolaryngol Head Neck Dis.* 2016;133:357–359.

Herford AS, Stoffella E, Tandon R. Osteomas involving the facial skeleton: a report of 2 cases and review of the literature. *Oral Surg Oral Med Oral Pathol Oral Radiol.* 2013;115:e1–e6.

Li W, Zhou T, Li Q, et al. Intestinal perforation during chemotherapeutic treatment of intra-abdominal desmoid tumor in patients with Gardner's syndrome: report of two cases. *World J Surg Oncol.* 2016;14:178.

Turina M, Pavlik CM, Heinimann K, et al. Recurrent desmoids determine outcome in patients with Gardner syndrome: a cohort study of three generations of an APC mutation-positive family across 30 years. *Int J Colorectal Dis.* 2013;28:865–872.

Desmoplastic Fibroma

Ferri A, Leporati M, Corradi D, et al. Huge desmoplastic fibroma of the paediatric mandible: surgical considerations and follow-up in three cases. *J Craniomaxillofac Surg.* 2013;41:367–370.

Oliveira-Gondak R, Brum-Corrêa M, Vieira da Costa M, et al. Maxillary desmoplastic fibroma with initial symptoms suggestive of sinusitis. *Oral Surg Oral Med Oral Pathol Oral Radiol.* 2013;116:e510–e513.

Ramírez-Skinner H, Vargas A, Solar A, et al. Desmoplastic fibroma of the mandible in a pediatric patient: a case report of resection and reconstruction with a six-year follow-up. *J Oral Maxillofac Surg.* 2017;75:1568.e1–1568.e10.

Woods TR, Cohen DM, Islam MN, et al. Desmoplastic fibroma of the mandible: a series of three cases and review of literature. *Head Neck Pathol.* 2015;9:196–204.

Osteoblastoma

Barlow E, Davies AM, Cool WP, et al. Osteoid osteoma and osteoblastoma: novelhistological and immunohistochemical observations as evidence for a single entity. *J Clin Pathol.* 2013;66:768–774.

Harrington C, Accurso BT, Kalmar JR, et al. Aggressive osteoblastoma of the maxilla: a case report and review of the literature. *Head Neck Pathol.* 2011;5:165–170.

Kashikar S, Steinle M, Reich R, et al. Epithelioid multinodular osteoblastoma of the mandible: a case report and review of literature. *Head Neck Pathol.* 2016;10:182–187.

Shah S, Kim J-E, Huh K-H, et al. Recurrent osteoblastoma of the maxilla. *Dentomaxillofac Radiol.* 2013;42:20100263.

Strobel K, Merwald M, Huellner M, et al. Osteoblastoma of the mandible mimicking osteosarcoma in FDG PET/CT imaging. *Clin Nucl Med.* 2013;38:143–144.

Yalcinkaya U, Doganavsargil B, Sezak M, et al. Clinical and morphological characteristics of osteoid osteoma and osteoblastoma: a retrospective single-center analysis of 204 patients. *Ann Diagn Pathol.* 2014;18:319–325.

Cementoblastoma

Abrahams JM, McClure SA. Pediatric odontogenic tumors. *Oral Maxillofacial Surg Clin N Am.* 2016;28:45–58.

Brannon RB, Fowler CB, Carpenter WM, et al. Cementoblastoma: an innocuous neoplasm? A clinicopathologic study of 44 cases and review of the literature with special emphasis on recurrence. *Oral Surg Oral Med Oral Pathol Oral Radiol Endod.* 2002;93:311–320.

Monti LM, Moraes-Souza AM, Pires-Soubhia AM, et al. Cementoblastoma: a case report in deciduous tooth. *Oral Maxillofac Surg.* 2013;17:145–149.

Urs AB, Singh H, Rawat G, et al. Cementoblastoma solely involving maxillary primary teeth - a rare presentation. *J Clin Pediatr Dent.* 2016;40:147–151.

Osteosarcoma

Anderson ME. Update on survival in osteosarcoma. *Orthop Clin North Am.* 2016;47:283–292.

Baumhoer D, Brunner P, Eppenberger-Castori S, et al. Osteosarcomas of the jaws differ from their peripheral counterparts and require a distinct treatment approach. Experiences from the DOESAK Registry. *Oral Oncol.* 2014;50:147–153.

Ferrari D, Codecà C, Battisti N, et al. Multimodality treatment of osteosarcoma of the jaw: a single institution experience. *Med Oncol.* 2014;31:171.

Gibbs J, Henderson-Jackson E, Bui MM. Bone and soft tissue pathology. Diagnostic and prognostic implications. *Surg Clin North Am.* 2016;96:915–962.

Green JT, Mills AM. Osteogenic tumors of bone. *Semin Diagn Pathol.* 2014;31:21–29.

Gutowski CJ, Basu-Mallick A, Abraham JA. Management of bone sarcoma. *Surg Clin North Am.* 2016;96:1077–1106.

Lee RJ, Arshi A, Schwartz HC, et al. Characteristics and prognostic factors of osteosarcoma of the jaws. A retrospective cohort study. *JAMA Otolaryngol Head Neck Surg.* 2015;141:470–477.

Purgina B, Lai CK. Distinctive head and neck bone and soft tissue neoplasms. *Surg Pathol Clin.* 2017;10:223–279.

Singer SR, Creanga AG. Diagnostic imaging of malignant tumors in the orofacial region. *Dent Clin North Am.* 2016;60:143–165.

Stewart BD, Reith JD, Knapik JA, et al. Bone- and cartilage-forming tumors and Ewing sarcoma: an update with a gnathic emphasis. *Head Neck Pathol.* 2014;8:454–462.

White SM. Malignant lesions in the dentomaxillofacial complex. *Radiol Clin N Am.* 2018;56:63–76.

Chondrosarcoma

Gutowski CJ, Basu-Mallick A, Abraham JA. Management of bone sarcoma. *Surg Clin North Am.* 2016;96:1077–1106.

MacIntosh RB, Khan F, Waligora BM. Chondrosarcoma of the temporomandibular disc: behavior over a 28-Year observation period. *J Oral Maxillofac Surg.* 2015;73:465–474.

Qasem SA, DeYoung BR. Cartilage-forming tumors. *Semin Diagn Pathol.* 2014;31:10–20.

Singer SR, Creanga AG. Diagnostic imaging of malignant tumors in the orofacial region. *Dent Clin North Am.* 2016;60:143–165.

Stewart BD, Reith JD, Knapik JA, et al. Bone- and cartilage-forming tumors and Ewing sarcoma: an update with a gnathic emphasis. *Head Neck Pathol.* 2014;8:454–462.

White SM. Malignant Lesions in the dentomaxillofacial complex. *Radiol Clin N Am.* 2018;56:63–76.

Mesenchymal Chondrosarcoma

Frezza AM, Cesari M, Baumhoer D, et al. Mesenchymal chondrosarcoma: prognostic factors and outcome in 113 patients. A European Musculoskeletal Oncology Society study. *Eur J Cancer.* 2015;51: 374–381.

Pelliteri PK, Ferlito A, Fagan JJ, et al. Mesenchymal chondrosarcoma of the head and neck. *Oral Oncol.* 2007;43:970–975.

Singh RK, Varshney S, Bist SS, et al. Mesenchymal chondrosarcoma of the mandible: a rare malignant tumor. *Ear Nose Throat J.* 2014;93:E18.

Tsuda Y, Ogura K, Hakozaki M, et al. Mesenchymal chondrosarcoma: a Japanese Musculoskeletal Oncology Group (JMOG) study on 57 patients. *J Surg Oncol.* 2017;115:760–767.

Ewing Sarcoma

Choi E-YK, Gardner JM, Lucas DR, et al. Ewing sarcoma. *Semin Diagn Pathol.* 2014;31:39–47.

Grevener K, Haveman LM, Ranft A, et al. Management and outcome of Ewing sarcoma of the head and neck. *Pediatr Blood Cancer.* 2016;63:604–610.

Ko E, Brouns EREA, Korones DN, et al. Primary Ewing sarcoma of the anterior mandible localized to the midline. *Oral Surg Oral Med Oral Pathol Oral Radiol.* 2013;115:e46–e50.

Owosho AA, Ko E, Rosenberg HI, et al. Primary Ewing family of tumors of the jaw has a better prognosis compared to tumors of extragnathic sites. *J Oral Maxillofac Surg.* 2016;74:973–981.

Metastatic Tumors to the Jaws

Corrêa-Pontes FS, Paiva-Fonseca F, Souza de Jesus S, et al. Nonendodontic lesions misdiagnosed as apical periodontitis lesions: series of case reports and review of literature. *J Endod.* 2014;40:16–27.

Hirshberg A, Berger B, Allon I, et al. Metastatic tumors to the jaws and mouth. *Head Neck Pathol.* 2014;8:463–474.

Kolokythas A, Miloro MB, Olsson AB, et al. Metastatic pancreatic adenocarcinoma to the mandibular condyle: a rare clinical presentation. *J Oral Maxillofac Surg.* 2014;72:83–88.

Owosho AA, Xu B, Kadempour A, et al. Metastatic solid tumors to the jaw and oral soft tissue: a retrospective clinical analysis of 44 patients from a single institution. *J Craniomaxillofac Surg.* 2016;44:1047–1053.

Torregrossa VR, Faria KM, Bicudo MM, et al. Metastatic cervical carcinoma of thejaw presenting as periapical disease. *Int Endod J.* 2016;49:203–211.

15

Odontogenic Cysts and Tumors

Figs. **15.1–15.4**

Tooth enamel is formed by ameloblasts, a specialized layer of cells on the inner aspect of the enamel organ epithelium. After enamel formation is completed, this epithelium remains as a thin layer of cells (known as the *reduced enamel epithelium*), which surrounds the crown of the unerupted tooth. If the tooth fails to erupt, then fluid may accumulate between this epithelium and the crown of the tooth, forming what is known as a **dentigerous cyst**. This lesion is the most common developmental cyst of odontogenic origin, comprising 17% to 20% of cysts in the jaws.

Logically, dentigerous cysts are most common around teeth that frequently are impacted. The most common site is the mandibular third molar, which accounts for 65% to 75% of all cases. Other less frequent locations include the maxillary canine, the maxillary third molar, and the mandibular second premolar. Dentigerous cysts rarely develop around deciduous teeth. Although they can occur at any age, most examples are diagnosed in teenagers and young adults. There is a slight male predilection.

Most dentigerous cysts are discovered during routine radiographic examination or when a radiograph is obtained to investigate failure of a tooth to erupt. The lesion typically appears as a well-circumscribed unilocular radiolucency with a corticated rim surrounding the crown of the unerupted tooth. Dentigerous cysts associated with mandibular premolars sometimes occur beneath nonvital primary molars. It is theorized that periapical inflammation from the primary tooth causes separation of the reduced enamel epithelium from the crown of the developing premolar, resulting in what has been termed an *inflammatory dentigerous cyst.*

A small dentigerous cyst can be difficult to distinguish radiographically from a hyperplastic dental follicle, but if the radiolucent space measures greater than 3 to 4 mm in diameter, a cyst should be suspected. On rare occasions, dentigerous cysts can grow to a large size, resulting in displacement of the impacted tooth, resorption of adjacent tooth roots, and clinical evidence of expansion. However, large pericoronal radiolucencies should be viewed with greater suspicion because they often represent one of the more aggressive odontogenic lesions, such as odontogenic keratocyst or ameloblastoma. Microscopically, most dentigerous cysts are lined by stratified squamous epithelium, which typically is attached to the tooth at the cemento-enamel junction. The lining also may include scattered mucous cells, especially in larger cysts.

Dentigerous cysts usually are treated by enucleation of the cyst in conjunction with removal of the associated tooth. In cases where the tooth roots are intimately associated with the mandibular nerve, coronectomy can be performed rather than total tooth removal. For particularly large cysts, initial biopsy and marsupialization can be considered, allowing decompression and shrinkage of the lesion before subsequent total enucleation. Finally, in situations where salvage of the tooth is desired and deemed feasible, cyst removal and orthodontic-assisted tooth eruption can be considered.

Upon removal, any significant pericoronal radiolucent lesion should be submitted for biopsy to confirm the diagnosis, because even a small "dentigerous" lesion sometimes is proven to be an early ameloblastoma or odontogenic keratocyst on microscopic examination. Also, rare examples of squamous cell carcinoma and intraosseous mucoepidermoid carcinoma may arise from dentigerous cyst linings.

■ Figure **15.1**
Dentigerous Cyst
A 14-year-old female with a small radiolucency surrounding the crown of the right mandibular second molar. Such a lesion would be difficult to distinguish from a hyperplastic dental follicle. (Courtesy Dr. Laura Summers.)

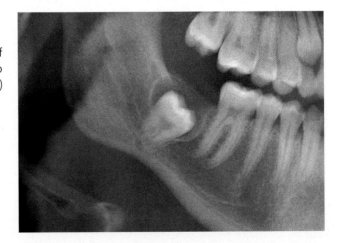

■ Figure **15.2**
Dentigerous Cyst
Gross specimen showing a saclike structure attached to the tooth at the cemento-enamel junction.

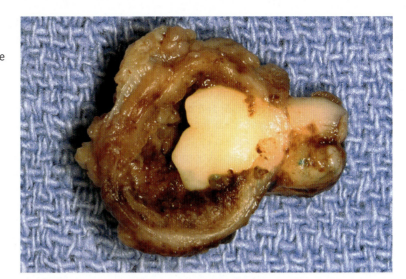

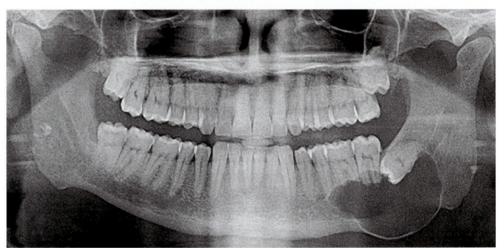

■ Figure **15.3**
Dentigerous Cyst
Large radiolucency associated with a mesioangular impacted left mandibular third molar. (Courtesy Dr. Jason Ford.)

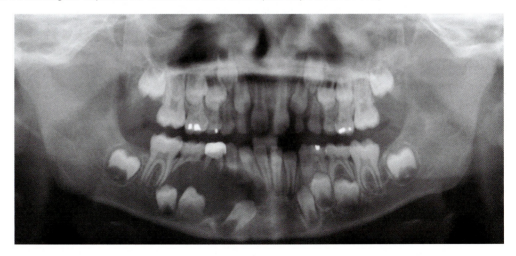

■ Figure **15.4**
"Inflammatory" Dentigerous Cyst
Radiolucency associated with the nonvital right mandibular primary first molar and unerupted right mandibular first bicuspid. (Courtesy Dr. Michael Nichols.)

Eruption Cyst (Eruption Hematoma)

Fig. **15.5**

The **eruption cyst** can be considered a variant of the dentigerous cyst that occurs in the soft tissue overlying an erupting tooth. Similar to its intrabony counterpart, it is caused by separation of the reduced enamel epithelium and dental follicular tissues from the crown of the tooth. The lumen of the cyst may contain mostly clear fluid or secondary hemorrhage—hence, the term **eruption hematoma**.

Eruption cysts almost always are diagnosed before the age of 12 years, which corresponds to the most active period of tooth eruption. There is a male predilection, which ranges from 1.4:1 to 2:1 in different series. Eruption cysts occur most frequently in association with the incisor and molar teeth of either the primary or permanent dentition. The lesion appears as a translucent and often bluish dome-shaped swelling on the alveolar mucosa. On occasion, more than one lesion will develop.

Most eruption cysts do not require any treatment because the lesion will rupture and resolve on its own as the tooth erupts through the surface. However, if eruption appears to be impeded by the lesion, then the cyst can be unroofed to release the fluid and expose the tooth crown. The tooth should then be able to erupt on its own accord.

Buccal Bifurcation Cyst (Inflammatory Collateral Cyst; Paradental Cyst)

Figs. **15.6 and 15.7**

The **buccal bifurcation cyst** is an uncommon inflammatory odontogenic cyst of uncertain pathogenesis. Because some examples develop in association with a *cervical enamel extension* on the buccal aspect of the associated tooth, it has been speculated that this enamel projection could interfere with a proper periodontal ligament attachment in the furcation area. As the tooth proceeds to eruption, inflammation in the perifollicular tissues may then induce cyst formation on the buccal aspect of the tooth. The simple term *paradental cyst* sometimes is used interchangeably with buccal bifurcation cyst. However, because this term often is used in reference to lesions found along the distal and distobuccal aspect of third molars, distinction from an inflamed dentigerous cyst can be difficult and somewhat arbitrary.

Buccal bifurcation cysts occur most frequently along the buccal aspect of the mandibular first molar, although some cases may involve the second molar. Cysts associated with first molars typically occur between the ages of 5 and 9 years, whereas examples occurring with second molars develop later toward early teenage years. The patient often notices a tender swelling along the buccal aspect of the molar, which may be in the process of erupting. Periodontal probing often reveals a deep pocket in the area. Examination of plain radiographs usually shows a cupped-out unilocular radiolucent lesion surrounding the roots of the involved tooth. Computed tomography imaging will demonstrate the characteristic buccal location of the lesion, with tipping of the tooth roots toward the lingual cortex. As many as one-fourth to one-third of patients will have bilateral lesions.

Buccal bifurcation cysts usually can be treated successfully by enucleation and curettage of the cystic lining. Some surgeons may elect to use bone grafting material at the surgical site. Importantly, however, the associated tooth does not need to be extracted. Following surgery, the site usually heals well without any further sequelae. Several papers even have described successful resolution of individual cases using daily irrigation with saline and hydrogen peroxide, or without any treatment at all.

■ Figure **15.5**
Eruption Cyst
Infant with a blue swelling of the anterior maxillary alveolar mucosa overlying an unerupted primary central incisor. (Courtesy Dr. Michael Day.)

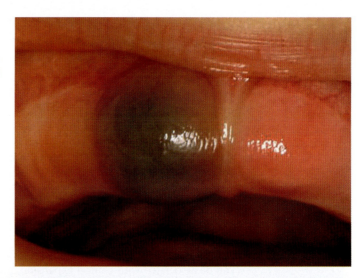

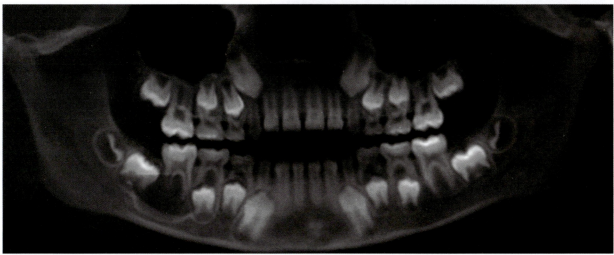

■ Figure **15.6**
Buccal Bifurcation Cyst
Panoramic radiograph showing a cupped-out radiolucency associated with the roots of the right mandibular first molar. (Courtesy Dr. Kenneth Blais.)

■ Figure **15.7**
Buccal Bifurcation Cyst
Axial and coronal computed tomography images of patient seen in Fig. 15.6. Note the location of the radiolucency on the buccal aspect of the tooth. (Courtesy Dr. Kenneth Blais.)

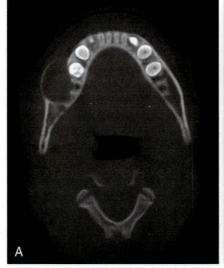

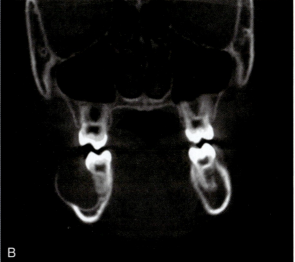

Figs. **15.8–15.11**

The **odontogenic keratocyst** is a relatively common developmental odontogenic cyst that represents approximately 10% to 14% of all jaw cysts. It is defined by its characteristic microscopic features, which include basilar nuclear palisading and the production of keratin (primarily in the form of parakeratin). Based on its potentially aggressive behavior and molecular findings, there has been controversy in recent years over whether this lesion should be classified as a cyst or a tumor (**keratocystic odontogenic tumor**). Both terms currently are being used, although the most recent World Health Organization classification system supports designation as a cyst.

The odontogenic keratocyst occurs over a wide age range, with a peak prevalence in the second to fourth decades of life. There is a slight male predilection, with a male:female ratio of 3:2. The lesion is most common in the molar/ramus region of the mandible, which accounts for half of all cases. A small odontogenic keratocyst typically appears as well-circumscribed unilocular radiolucency that is discovered incidentally on radiographic examination. Advanced lesions may assume a multilocular appearance, which can be associated with clinical expansion and thinning of the overlying bony cortex. From a differential diagnosis standpoint, the odontogenic keratocyst can mimic a variety of other odontogenic cysts and tumors. In 25% to 40% of cases, the lesion will be associated with the crown of an unerupted tooth, thereby resembling a dentigerous cyst. Sometimes a cyst will occur at the site where a tooth fails to develop, producing a lesion formerly known as a *primordial cyst*. Small examples between roots of teeth can be mistaken for lateral periodontal cysts. Odontogenic keratocysts sometimes develop in the midline maxillary region in older patients, and thus these lesions can be confused with nasopalatine duct cysts. Finally, lesions located beneath tooth roots can mimic periapical cysts.

The diagnosis of odontogenic keratocyst is important for three reasons: (1) they have potential for significant growth; (2) they have a high recurrence rate (estimated at 20% to 25%); and (3) sometimes they are associated with the nevoid basal cell carcinoma syndrome. Most odontogenic keratocysts are treated by enucleation and curettage. If the diagnosis is known or suspected at the time of surgery, peripheral ostectomy can be performed to reduce the recurrence risk. Some surgeons advocate the usage of Carnoy solution to cauterize the bony cavity (although the use of Carnoy solution currently is not allowed by many hospitals). Large odontogenic keratocysts sometimes are treated initially by cystotomy and insertion of a drainage tube, which can promote shrinkage of the lesion and fibrous thickening of the cyst wall before subsequent total removal. In rare instances, particularly large cysts may require resection and bone grafting. Regardless of the size of the lesion or treatment modality, continued clinical follow-up of the patient is necessary because of the high recurrence potential of the odontogenic keratocyst. Because recurrences may not be manifested until 10 years or more, long-term monitoring is important. In addition, any patient with an odontogenic keratocyst should be evaluated clinically to rule out the possibility of the nevoid basal cell carcinoma syndrome (see next topic).

■ Figure **15.8**
Odontogenic Keratocyst
(A) Well-circumscribed radiolucency of the right mandibular ramus associated with the crown of the developing third molar. (B) Radiograph taken 6 months later, which shows shrinkage of the lesion following insertion of a polyethylene tube *(arrow)*. (Courtesy Dr. Brad Gregory.)

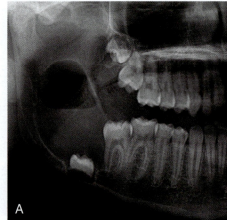
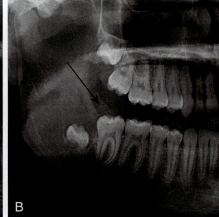

■ Figure **15.9**
Odontogenic Keratocyst

Well-circumscribed radiolucency of the left posterior mandible at the site of a missing third molar. (Courtesy Dr. Gregg Jowers.)

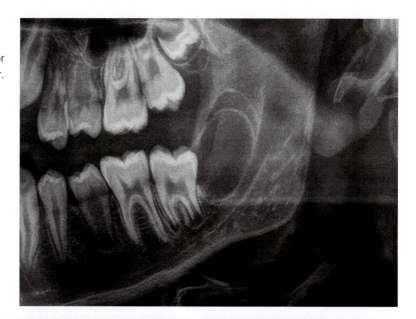

■ Figure **15.10**
Odontogenic Keratocyst

(A) Radiolucency between and apical to the roots of the maxillary central incisors, which could be mistaken for a nasopalatine duct cyst. (B) Radiolucency between and apical to the roots of the maxillary left canine and first bicuspid. (Courtesy Dr. Patrick Coleman and Dr. Edward Marshall.)

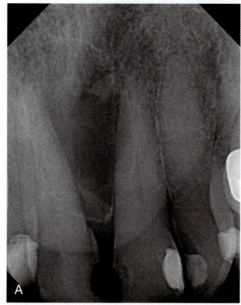
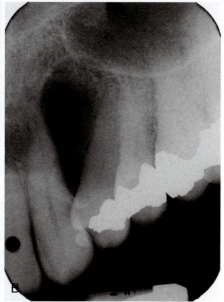

■ Figure **15.11**
Odontogenic Keratocyst

Large multilocular lesion of the left posterior body and ramus of mandible. (Courtesy Dr. Jason Rosetti.)

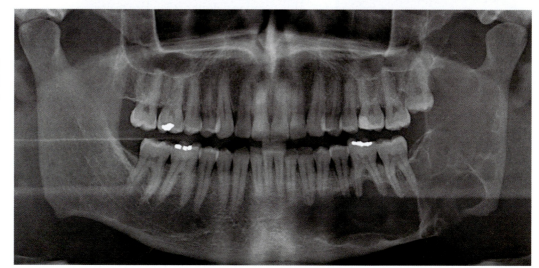

Figs. **15.12–15.20**

The **nevoid basal cell carcinoma syndrome (Gorlin syndrome)** is an uncommon autosomal dominant hereditary disorder that is caused by mutation of *patched (PTCH1)*, a tumor suppressor gene located on chromosome 9. Although the frequency of this condition may vary depending the particular population being studied, the overall prevalence is estimated at 1 in 60,000 individuals. Approximately 35% to 50% of affected patients have no family history and represent new gene mutations. Individuals with this disorder may exhibit a wide variety of clinical manifestations, including a greatly increased risk for developing multiple basal cell carcinomas of the skin.

The most common and significant oral manifestation of the nevoid basal cell carcinoma syndrome is the tendency to develop odontogenic keratocysts, which occur in up to 90% of affected patients. Because these cysts usually begin to form during childhood, their presence is often the first sign that can lead to the diagnosis. The development of more than one odontogenic keratocyst is strongly suggestive of the disorder.

Multiple basal cell carcinomas typically develop, often beginning before the patient is 20 years of age. However, there is great variation in the numbers of these skin cancers; some patients may develop only a few tumors, whereas others have literally hundreds of such lesions that develop over a lifetime. Basal cell carcinomas tend to occur most often in areas of actinic damage, although patients also can develop tumors in areas that are infrequently exposed to sunlight. A significant racial variation also is noted with respect to development of these skin cancers. Approximately 90% of white patients with this syndrome will exhibit formation of basal cell carcinomas, whereas only about 40% of black patients will develop these lesions. Another common skin manifestation is the presence of pitting defects on the palms and soles, which occur in 65% to 85% of patients. On rare occasions, basal cell carcinomas can develop at the base of these pits.

Patients with Gorlin syndrome often exhibit a characteristic facies with frontal and temporoparietal bossing, mild hypertelorism, and mild mandibular prognathism. A common finding on skull radiographs is the presence of calcifications along the falx cerebri and tentorium cerebelli. Chest films often reveal the presence of bifid, fused, or splayed ribs. Other skeletal anomalies may include kyphoscoliosis, spina bifida occulta, and shortened metacarpals. A variety of other abnormalities also occur with increased frequency, such as cleft lip/palate, pectus excavatum, ovarian fibromas, cardiac fibromas, medulloblastoma, and meningioma.

The jaw cysts in patients with Gorlin syndrome are treated in a similar fashion as isolated odontogenic keratocysts. Close periodic radiographic monitoring is necessary to evaluate for possible recurrences or development of new cysts in other areas. Early recognition of this syndrome is important so that patients can be counseled to avoid excessive ultraviolet light, which can trigger development of the skin cancers. Because the basal cell carcinomas in patients with Gorlin syndrome have a lower mutational load and increased genomic stability in comparison to sporadic basal cell carcinomas, they often exhibit a less aggressive clinical course. However, the morbidity associated with the development of multiple tumors can be considerable. Also, occasional deaths secondary to aggressive tumors extending to the base of the skull or other vital structures have been documented. Individual basal cell carcinomas can be surgically removed. Intermittent therapy with vismodegib has shown promise in the management of basal cell carcinomas in patients with this condition.

■ Figure **15.12**
Nevoid Basal Cell Carcinoma Syndrome
Multiple odontogenic keratocysts in the mandibular rami and in the midline maxillary region. (Courtesy Dr. James Strider.)

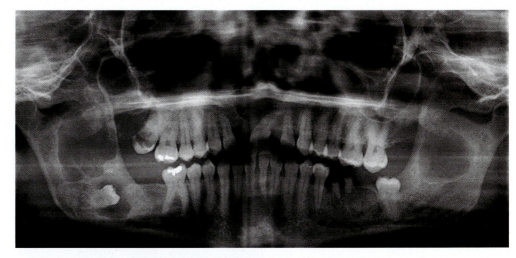

■ Figure **15.13**
Nevoid Basal Cell Carcinoma Syndrome
Multiple odontogenic keratocysts of the mandible and left posterior maxilla. (Courtesy Dr. Leslie Heffez.)

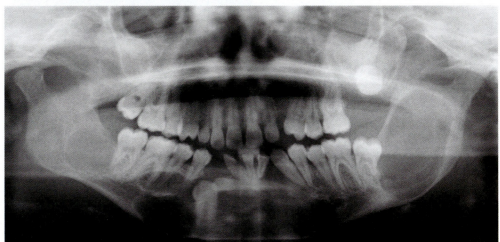

■ Figure **15.14**
Nevoid Basal Cell Carcinoma Syndrome
Extensive radiolucencies throughout the mandible and posterior maxilla, which represent multiple odontogenic keratocysts.

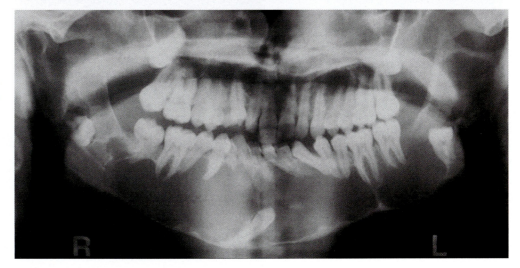

■ Figure **15.15**
Nevoid Basal Cell Carcinoma Syndrome
Aspiration of an odontogenic keratocyst revealing creamy keratinaceous fluid.

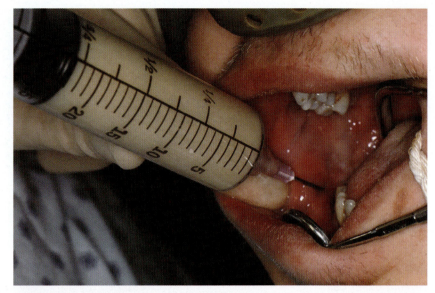

■ Figure **15.16**
Nevoid Basal Cell Carcinoma Syndrome
Pitting defects on the sole of the foot.

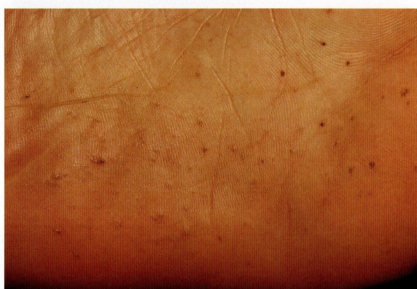

■ Figure **15.17**
Nevoid Basal Cell Carcinoma Syndrome
Erythematous, scaly lesion on the foot, which represents a basal cell carcinoma.

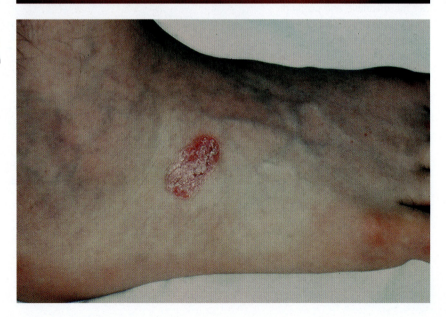

■ Figure **15.18**
Nevoid Basal Cell Carcinoma Syndrome
Extensive scarring changes of the face and scalp secondary to removal of multiple basal cell carcinomas.

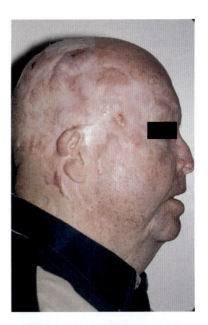

■ Figure **15.19**
Nevoid Basal Cell Carcinoma Syndrome
Coronal computed tomography image showing calcification in the midline falx cerebri region. (Courtesy Dr. Steven Anderson.)

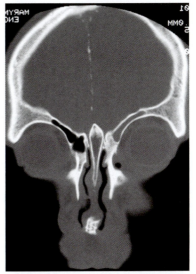

■ Figure **15.20**
Nevoid Basal Cell Carcinoma Syndrome
Chest radiograph showing the presence of bifid ribs *(arrow)*. (Courtesy Dr. Steven Anderson.)

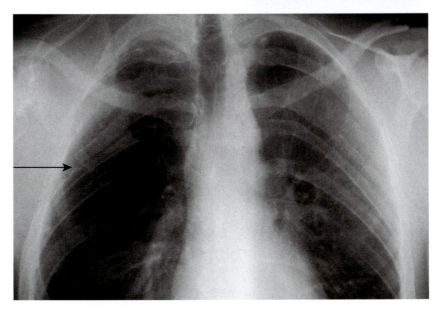

Fig. **15.21**

The odontogenic keratocyst is well recognized for its unique microscopic features, which include a palisaded cuboidal/columnar basal cell layer and the ability to produce parakeratin, in which epithelial nuclei are retained. However, other odontogenic cysts without basilar palisading may produce exclusively orthokeratin, in which the nuclei are lost. Because these cysts are biologically different from odontogenic keratocysts, they are placed into their own separate category and known as **orthokeratinized odontogenic cysts**.

The orthokeratinized odontogenic cyst is diagnosed most frequently in young adults and it shows a 2:1 male-to-female ratio. It has a predilection for the posterior areas of the jaws, and approximately 75% of examples occur in the mandible. The lesion usually appears as a unilocular radiolucency, although occasional examples can be multilocular. From one-half to two-thirds of cases are associated with an impacted tooth, thereby mimicking a dentigerous cyst. Size can range from small cysts less than 1 cm in diameter to larger lesions measuring over 7 cm in greatest dimension. A rare example of a patient with multiple orthokeratinized odontogenic cysts has been reported.

Orthokeratinized odontogenic cysts can be treated by enucleation and curettage. The risk for recurrence is estimated at 2%, which is much lower than the recurrence potential for the odontogenic keratocyst. In addition, the orthokeratinized odontogenic cyst has not been associated with the nevoid basal cell carcinoma syndrome.

Lateral Periodontal Cyst (Botryoid Odontogenic Cyst)

Figs. **15.22 and 15.23**

The **lateral periodontal cyst** is a developmental type of odontogenic cyst that is thought to arise from remnants of dental lamina epithelium. This cyst exhibits characteristic microscopic features that it shares with its soft tissue counterpart, the gingival cyst of the adult (see next topic). As its name implies, the lateral periodontal cyst typically occurs between the roots of two teeth. However, it must be distinguished from other cysts and tumors that might arise between tooth roots, such as lateral radicular cyst, odontogenic keratocyst, and early ameloblastoma.

Although the lateral periodontal cyst is "developmental" in nature, it does not develop in children but usually is seen in middle-aged and older adults in the fourth through seventh decades of life. Approximately 75% of cases occur in the mandible, with a marked predilection for the premolar-canine-lateral incisor area. Maxillary examples also tend to occur in the same tooth region. The lateral periodontal cyst often is discovered as an incidental finding on radiographic examination, although some cases may produce slight clinical expansion. The lesion usually appears as a well-circumscribed unilocular radiolucency adjacent to the tooth roots. On occasion, displacement of the roots may be seen, but obvious root resorption is rarely noted. The adjacent teeth are typically vital (unless root canal therapy has been performed for unrelated reasons). Lateral periodontal cysts also can develop in edentulous areas of alveolar bone. In addition, rare patients with multiple lateral periodontal cysts have been reported.

Occasional examples of this lesion will have a multicystic growth pattern, sometimes presenting as a somewhat multilocular radiolucency. The term **botryoid odontogenic cyst** is used for such lesions because their gross appearance may resemble a small cluster of grapes.

The lateral periodontal cyst is treated by local enucleation or curettage, which usually can be accomplished without damage to the adjacent teeth. Recurrence of simple lateral periodontal cysts is rare. However, botryoid odontogenic cysts have a more significant recurrence risk, which has been estimated as high as 21.7%. Therefore, more aggressive surgical management, such as peripheral ostectomy, may be considered for botryoid examples.

■ Figure **15.21**
Orthokeratinized Odontogenic Cyst
Unilocular radiolucency associated with the mesioangular impacted mandibular left third molar. (Courtesy Dr. Jeffrey Simmons.)

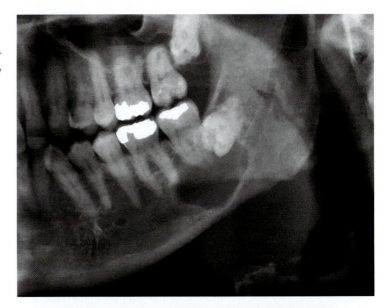

■ Figure **15.22**
Lateral Periodontal Cyst
A corticated, unilocular radiolucency is seen between the roots of the mandibular lateral incisor and canine.

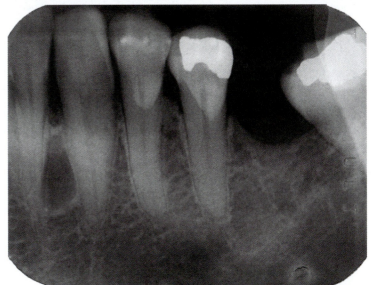

■ Figure **15.23**
Lateral Periodontal Cyst (Botryoid Type)
Slightly multilocular radiolucency between the roots of the right mandibular canine and first bicuspid. (With appreciation to Dr. Artur Aburad de Carvalhosa.)

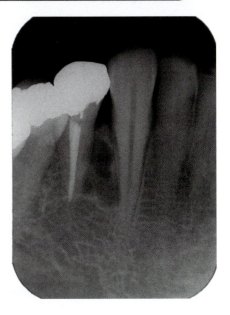

Gingival Cyst of the Adult

Figs. **15.24 and 15.25**

The **gingival cyst of the adult** is an uncommon developmental cyst that arises from remnants of dental lamina epithelium within the gingival soft tissues. It represents a soft tissue counterpart of the lateral periodontal cyst.

Like the lateral periodontal cyst, the gingival cyst of the adult mostly occurs in middle-aged and older adults. It has a predilection for the mandibular premolar-canine-lateral incisor region, which accounts for 60% to 75% of all cases. Maxillary examples also tend to occur in the same tooth region. The lesion almost always develops on the facial aspect of the gingiva rather than the lingual surface. On occasion, gingival cysts of the adult can occur in edentulous areas of the alveolar ridge.

Clinically, this cyst usually presents as a dome-shaped, painless swelling that may appear somewhat blue or translucent because of its fluid contents. Most examples are 5 mm or less in size. On occasion, underlying cupping resorption of the alveolar bone can be observed at the time of surgery. In fact, some examples may be partially within soft tissue and partially within bone, which could raise an argument over whether they should be classified as a lateral periodontal cyst. However, because these two lesions really represent the same entity, this becomes a moot point.

Treatment for the gingival cyst of the adult consists of local conservative excision. The prognosis is excellent and the lesion should not be expected to recur.

Gingival Cyst of the Newborn

Fig. **15.26**

Gingival cysts of the newborn are tiny keratin-filled cysts commonly observed on the alveolar ridge in newborn infants. These developmental anomalies are thought to arise from remnants of dental lamina epithelium within the gingival soft tissues. The term *Bohn nodules* sometimes is applied to these lesions, although that name also has been used for similar tiny developmental cysts that occur along the junction of the hard and soft palate.

If close, detailed examination of the oral cavity is performed, gingival cysts of the newborn are common lesions that have been described in over half of infants in some studies. They appear as asymptomatic white or yellowish–white papules on the alveolar surface. No treatment is warranted because the lesions disappear on their own accord within the first couple of months of life, presumably secondary to rupture and contact with the mucosal surface.

■ Figure **15.24**
Gingival Cyst of the Adult
Slightly blue, translucent swelling of the facial gingiva between the right mandibular lateral incisor and canine.

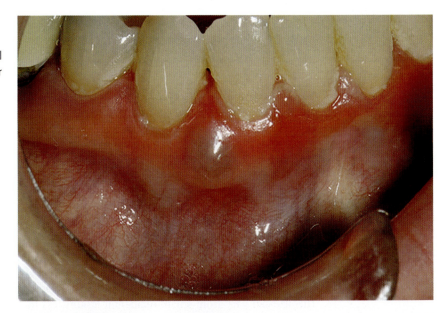

■ Figure **15.25**
Gingival Cyst of the Adult
Small, bluish swelling of the facial gingiva of the right mandibular canine.

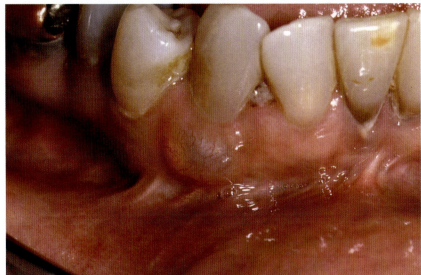

■ Figure **15.26**
Gingival Cysts of the Newborn
Multiple yellowish papules on the anterior maxillary facial gingiva of a newborn infant. (Courtesy Dr. Beatriz Aldape and Dr. Rana Alshagroud.)

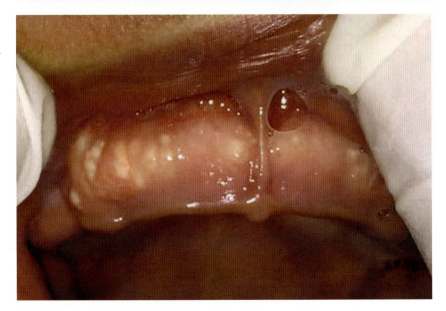

Calcifying Odontogenic Cyst (Calcifying Cystic Odontogenic Tumor; Dentinogenic Ghost Cell Tumor; Gorlin Cyst)

Figs. **15.27–15.30**

Originally described by Gorlin and colleagues in 1962, the **calcifying odontogenic cyst** is a rare lesion of odontogenic origin that can show a variety of clinicopathologic patterns. The basic microscopic features resemble a cystic ameloblastoma, but the lesion also includes the presence of characteristic ghost cells, calcifications, and, oftentimes, a dentinoid product. Because most lesions in this spectrum grow primarily in a cyst-like fashion, it usually is classified as one of the odontogenic cysts. However, some authors recommend classification as a tumor on the basis of its genetic features and because some examples grow in a solid, tumorlike fashion (**dentinogenic ghost cell tumor**). About 20% of cases are associated with adjacent odontoma formation. Rare examples also have been reported in combination with other odontogenic tumors, such as adenomatoid odontogenic tumor, ameloblastic fibroma, and ameloblastoma.

The mean age at diagnosis is 30 years and most cases are found in the second through the fourth decades of life. Although calcifying odontogenic cysts can develop anywhere in the jaws, almost two-thirds of cases are seen in the incisor-canine region. The lesion occurs in the maxilla and mandible with equal frequency. In about one-third of cases, the lesion is associated with an impacted tooth, most often a canine. The size can vary from small, incidental lesions less than 1 cm in diameter to large, expansile growths measuring as great as 12 cm. Radiographically, the lesion usually appears as a well-circumscribed unilocular radiolucency, which may or may not show evidence of central calcifications or adjacent odontoma formation. Larger examples may appear multilocular.

From 5% to 17% of cases occur peripherally in the gingival soft tissues, appearing as a sessile or pedunculated growth. The mean age for peripheral calcifying odontogenic cysts (51 years) is significantly older than for intraosseous examples, with a bimodal peak prevalence in the second and sixth to eighth decades of life. They are more likely to occur in the mandibular arch (65%) than the maxillary arch (35%). Peripheral lesions also appear more often as solid tumor-like growths microscopically ("peripheral dentinogenic ghost cell tumor").

In spite of its basic microscopic resemblance to ameloblastoma, the calcifying odontogenic cyst usually can be treated by enucleation and curettage with a good prognosis. Recurrence has been reported in less than 5% of cases, and peripheral examples appear to have a similarly good outcome. Rare examples of malignant transformation have been reported (*ghost cell odontogenic carcinoma*), which have an unpredictable behavior.

■ Figure **15.27**
Calcifying Odontogenic Cyst
Well-circumscribed mixed radiolucency/radiopacity located between the roots of the right mandibular lateral incisor and canine. (Courtesy Dr. Elliott Maxwell.)

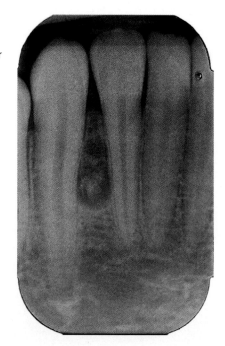

■ Figure **15.28**
Calcifying Odontogenic Cyst
Computed tomography image showing an expansile radiolucency of the right mandible. (With appreciation to Dr. Martin Steed.)

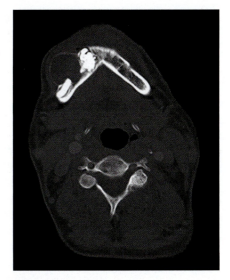

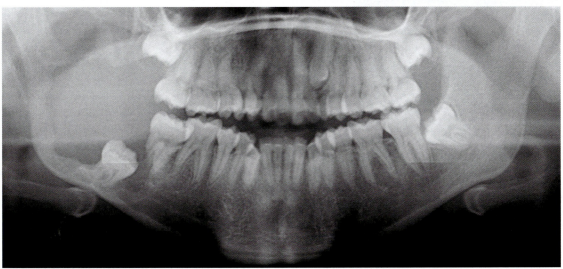

■ Figure **15.29**
Calcifying Odontogenic Cyst
Large radiolucency of the right mandibular ramus associated with an impacted third molar. (Courtesy Dr. Antonia Kolokythas.)

■ Figure **15.30**
Peripheral Calcifying Odontogenic Cyst
Nodular mass of the lingual mandibular gingiva with secondary ulceration. (Courtesy Dr. Mark Anderson.)

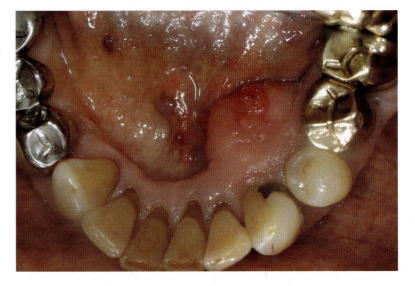

Glandular Odontogenic Cyst (Sialo-Odontogenic Cyst)

Fig. **15.31**

The **glandular odontogenic cyst** is a rare developmental cyst of odontogenic origin that microscopically shows glandular features. Its resemblance to salivary tissue, including mucous cells and glandlike spaces, is considered evidence of the pluripotentiality of odontogenic epithelium. Additionally, this cyst frequently includes microscopic features similar to the lateral periodontal cyst, suggesting that these two lesions are related entities.

The glandular odontogenic cyst occurs most often in middle-aged adults, with a mean age at diagnosis of 48 years. Nearly 75% of cases occur in the mandible, most often in the anterior region. It is not unusual for anterior mandibular lesions to cross the midline. The size of the lesion can vary from small unilocular cysts less than 1 cm in diameter to large multilocular lesions that extend from the molar region on one side of the mandible to the opposite molar region. Larger glandular odontogenic cysts often result in clinical evidence of expansion, thinning of the overlying cortical plate, and displacement of teeth. On rare occasions, pain or paresthesia can be produced by larger cysts.

Most examples of glandular odontogenic cyst are treated initially by enucleation or curettage. However, this cyst is known for its recurrence potential, which has been estimated at 22% to 30%. Therefore, continued long-term clinical and radiographic follow-up are important. Some surgeons have recommended *en bloc* resection for larger, more aggressive glandular odontogenic cysts.

Carcinoma in Odontogenic Cysts

Figs. **15.32 and 15.33**

On rare occasions, a primary intraosseous squamous cell carcinoma will appear to arise from the lining of a pre-existing odontogenic cyst. Such malignant transformation has been reported to develop most frequently from either a periapical or residual periapical cyst. Carcinoma also can arise from other types of odontogenic cysts—especially dentigerous cysts, odontogenic keratocysts, and orthokeratinized odontogenic cysts. Although such malignancies may occur over a wide age range, they are seen most often in middle-aged and older patients. The mean patient age in several studies has ranged from 52 to 60 years. Men are affected twice as often as women.

The most common presenting symptoms include pain and swelling. However, early carcinomas can be totally asymptomatic, being discovered as incidental radiographic findings suggestive of a benign cystic process. Such early lesions may appear as well-circumscribed unilocular radiolucencies. However, more advanced lesions often demonstrate irregular bone destruction that may include cortical perforation and ragged tooth resorption.

Treatment for these carcinomas typically requires wide local resection of the involved portion of the jaw, as well as selective lymph node dissection. Adjunctive radiation therapy often is warranted. Because few series are reported, accurate assessment of prognosis is difficult. However, one series reported an overall 2-year survival rate of 62%, with the 5-year survival rate dropping to 38%.

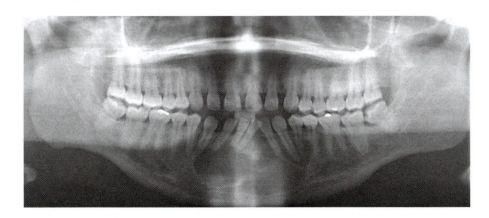

■ Figure **15.31**
Glandular Odontogenic Cyst
Loculated radiolucency in the anterior mandible, which has displaced roots of teeth. (Courtesy Dr. Taylor McGuire.)

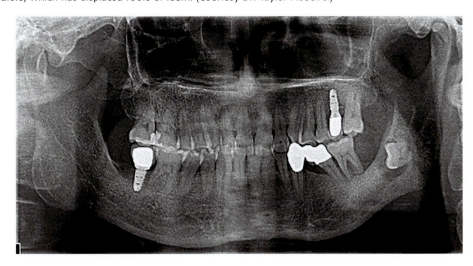

■ Figure **15.32**
Carcinoma Arising in an Odontogenic Cyst
A small radiolucency around the crown of the impacted left mandibular third molar, which revealed a carcinoma arising in a dentigerous cyst lining. (Courtesy Dr. Chris Jo.)

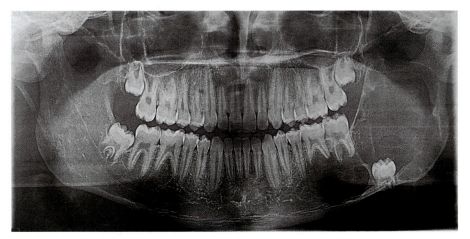

■ Figure **15.33**
Carcinoma Arising in an Odontogenic Cyst
Large multilocular radiolucency of the left posterior body and ramus of the mandible in a 15-year-old male. (Courtesy Dr. Alessandra Schmitt.)

Figs. **15.34–15.45**

The **ameloblastoma** is considered to be the second-most common odontogenic tumor, exceeded in frequency only by odontomas (although many oral and maxillofacial pathologists consider the odontoma to be an odontogenic hamartoma, rather than a true neoplasm). Nevertheless, this neoplasm is still a rather uncommon entity when compared to other nonodontogenic lesions of the oral cavity. Ameloblastomas arise from odontogenic epithelium that primarily is associated with two sources: odontogenic epithelial rests that remain in the jaws following completion of odontogenesis and the lining of odontogenic cysts. Although the term *ameloblastoma* refers to the resemblance of the lesional cells to ameloblasts, which are responsible for the deposition of enamel, this tumor has no hard tissue component. Molecular genetic analysis of the lesional cells has identified certain genes (e.g., the amelogenin gene) that are typically found in normal ameloblasts. The ameloblastoma is considered to be a benign but locally aggressive neoplasm that usually is confined to bone. However, without treatment such tumors can achieve grotesque proportions.

Ameloblastomas can be seen at virtually any age, from the first to the ninth decade of life, although the mean age in most large series of cases is generally between 30 and 40 years. The sex ratio is essentially equal. Mandibular lesions account for 80% to 85% of cases, whereas maxillary lesions comprise 15% to 20% of these tumors. Approximately 2% of ameloblastomas occur in the soft tissue, and these peripheral ameloblastomas are discussed in a separate section later in the text. Clinically, ameloblastomas may produce swelling of the jaw or may be discovered upon routine radiographic examination. At times, the swelling can become large enough to be noticeable extraorally. Patients infrequently may complain of tenderness, pain, paresthesia, or numbness. If the tumor produces significant intraoral swelling, then secondary surface ulceration may result, although this is unusual.

The radiographic appearance of ameloblastoma can vary considerably, depending on the duration and the growth pattern of the tumor. In the early phase of an ameloblastoma, a unilocular radiolucency is characteristically identified. As the neoplasm continues to grow, it may continue to have a unilocular appearance, or it may develop scalloped borders and a multilocular growth pattern. Larger lesions will typically cause thinning of the cortical plates and expansion of the jaw. Desmoplastic ameloblastoma is a histopathologically distinct form of the tumor, which may have a dissimilar radiographic appearance from routine ameloblastoma. Although some desmoplastic ameloblastomas may have a typical multilocular pattern, others can present as a mixed radiolucent and radiopaque lesion, similar to a fibro-osseous process.

Ameloblastomas are known for having a variety of histopathologic patterns, although most of these patterns seem to have little or no impact on the biologic behavior of the tumor. (One possible exception is the unicystic ameloblastoma, which is discussed later.) Follicular, acanthomatous, basal cell, plexiform, granular cell, and desmoplastic patterns are seen in most solid, multilocular ameloblastomas. Most of these patterns have a common feature, namely, the presence of columnar cells with hyperchromatic nuclei at the periphery of the tumor islands and strands. The nuclei are typically oriented away from the basement membrane, with clearing of the basal cytoplasm. This feature may be more difficult to identify in desmoplastic ameloblastoma, but it can usually be found, sometimes after obtaining multiple deeper sections of the tumor.

The management of ameloblastoma can be controversial, although most surgeons agree that this tumor demands a certain degree of respect due to its locally aggressive biologic behavior. Although ameloblastoma does not invade cortical bone, it can expand and thin such bone over a period of years. Studies have shown that invasion of the tumor into the adjacent cancellous bone is common, and the invasive front may extend 5 to 7 mm beyond the apparent radiographic boundary of the tumor. Simple curettage has historically been associated with recurrence rates as high as 90% in some series. Most authorities recommend resection of the lesion with a 1- to 2-cm margin. Sometimes this can be accomplished with an *en bloc* resection, but in some cases, segmental resection is necessary, followed by either immediate or delayed reconstruction. Maxillary ameloblastomas usually require a more aggressive surgical approach because the bone in this region is relatively thin and therefore more readily destroyed by the invading tumor. In addition, recurrence of a maxillary ameloblastoma is worrisome because of the potential for the tumor to extend superiorly to the base of the skull where it could become unresectable and eventually fatal. Infrequently, radiation therapy has been used as either primary or adjunctive therapy for lesions that are not amenable to surgical excision, although the results of this treatment have been mixed.

The prognosis for ameloblastomas that are treated with these guidelines is generally good, although recurrence is still possible. Monitoring the patient for at least 10 years after treatment is often recommended, but rare cases of recurrences that develop after 20 years or longer have been documented.

Text continued on p. 436.

■ Figure **15.34**
Ameloblastoma
A well-defined, unilocular radiolucency associated with the crown of an impacted third molar, simulating a dentigerous cyst. (Courtesy Dr. Doug Oliver.)

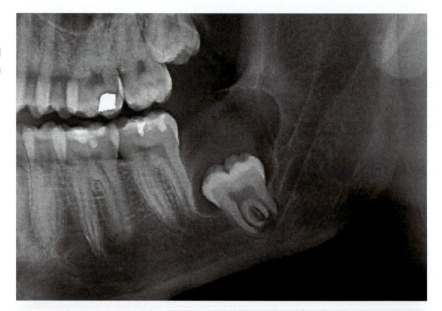

■ Figure **15.35**
Ameloblastoma
Swelling of the right posterior mandible. (With appreciation to Dr. Michael Tabor.)

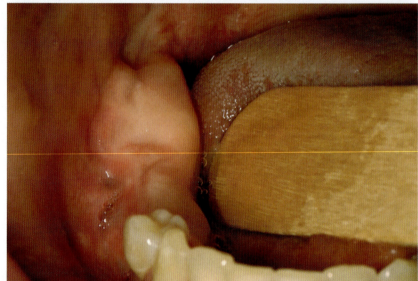

■ Figure **15.36**
Ameloblastoma
Panoramic radiograph of patient seen in Fig. 15.35 demonstrating a multilocular, expansile radiolucency of the right posterior mandible. (With appreciation to Dr. Michael Tabor.)

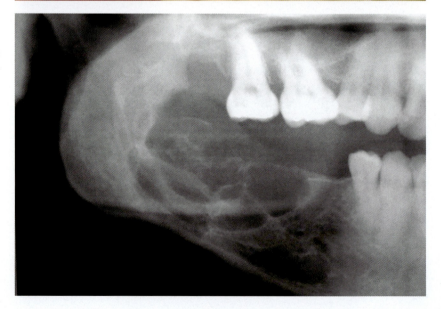

Ameloblastoma

A unilocular radiolucency is present in the right anterior mandible. Such a lesion could easily be mistaken for a lateral periodontal cyst. (Courtesy Dr. Mark Baker.)

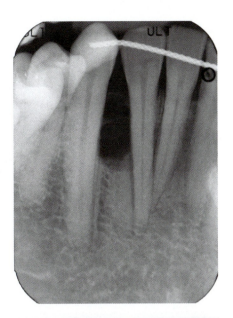

■ Figure **15.38**
Ameloblastoma

A unilocular radiolucency between the roots of the left mandibular first and second molars, with associated root resorption of #19. (Courtesy Dr. Mark Lawhon.)

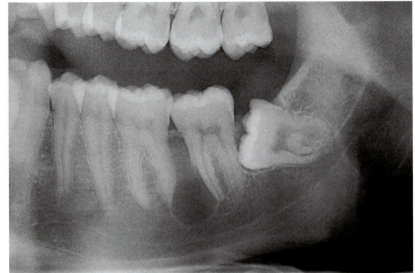

■ Figure **15.39**
Ameloblastoma

Same patient as Fig. 15.38, showing significant increase in size of this lesion 1 year later, with marked resorption of the roots of #18 and #19. (Courtesy Dr. Mark Lawhon.)

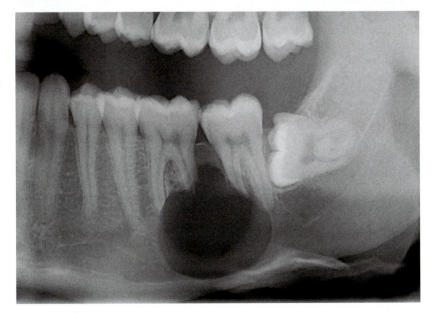

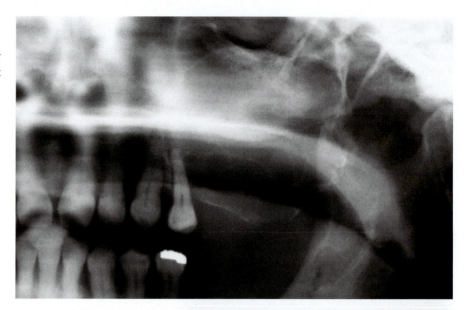

Figure 15.40
Ameloblastoma
A large radiolucency of the left posterior maxilla, noted on panoramic radiographic examination. (Courtesy Dr. Derek Dunlap.)

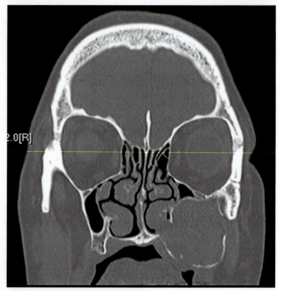

Figure 15.41
Ameloblastoma
Computed tomography imaging of same patient seen in Fig. 15.40, which demonstrates that this lesion fills the left maxillary sinus and encroaches upon the nasal cavity. (Courtesy Dr. Derek Dunlap.)

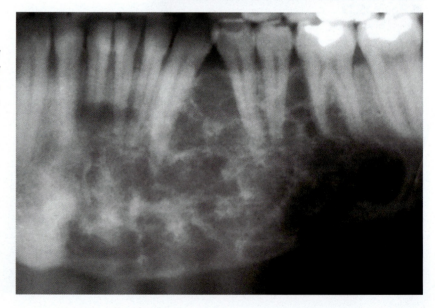

Figure 15.42
Desmoplastic Ameloblastoma
An extensive multilocular expansile radiolucency with areas of radiopacity involving the left body and symphysis of the mandible. Microscopically, this represented a desmoplastic ameloblastoma. (Courtesy Dr. Denise Clark.)

■ Figure 15.43
Ameloblastoma
The growth potential of ameloblastoma is demonstrated by the massive tumor affecting the mandible of this 24-year-old male. (Courtesy Dr. Timothy Bartholomew.)

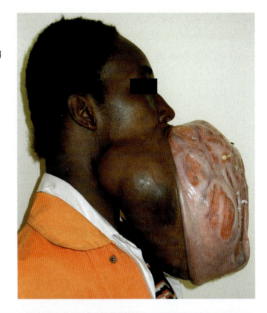

■ Figure 15.44
Ameloblastoma
Same patient as Fig. 15.43, showing lateral and antero-posterior radiographic views of the tumor. (Courtesy Dr. Timothy Bartholomew.)

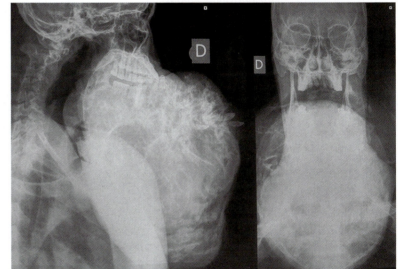

■ Figure 15.45
Ameloblastoma
Resection of a mandibular ameloblastoma (A) and accompanying radiograph of the same lesion (B). (Courtesy Dr. Mary Richardson.)

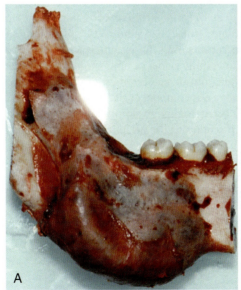 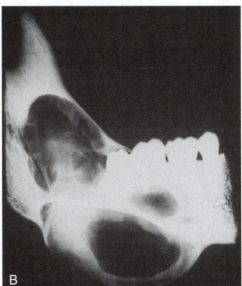

Unicystic Ameloblastoma

Figs. **15.46 and 15.47**

Unicystic ameloblastoma denotes a group of ameloblastomas that are characterized microscopically by a single cystic cavity lined by ameloblastic epithelium. The definition of this lesion has evolved over the decades, and currently three different subtypes are recognized, based on their histopathologic features: luminal, intraluminal, and intramural. The luminal type shows a thin cyst-like ameloblastic lining only. A cystic lining is seen in the intraluminal type, in addition to ameloblastic proliferation into the lumen of the lesion. A similar cystic lining is seen in the intramural type, although invasive cords and islands of ameloblastic cells extend from this lining into the connective tissue wall. Because different definitions of this process have been applied over the years in the literature, assessment of the frequency of these lesions and their biologic behavior can be challenging. More recent reviews of this process seem to indicate that the luminal and intraluminal subtypes have a less aggressive biologic behavior, but the intramural subtype behaves essentially the same as a solid or multicystic ameloblastoma. Unicystic ameloblastomas tend to occur in a younger age group, compared to solid multilocular ameloblastomas, with the mean age often occurring during the second decade of life. This lesion is frequently associated with an impacted tooth, mimicking a dentigerous cyst radiographically.

Some investigators have suggested that the precise diagnosis of the particular subtype of unicystic ameloblastoma requires a coordinated evaluation of the radiographic, clinical, and histopathologic findings. The latter aspect is particularly important, because an incisional biopsy of a large radiolucency may not be representative of the entire lesion. The pathologist may incorrectly assume that the diagnosis is unicystic ameloblastoma with a luminal growth pattern, when in fact other areas may show mural infiltration by the tumor. For this reason, examination of multiple areas of the entire lesion is necessary to assess whether intramural involvement by the neoplastic cells is present.

Accurate classification is important because the treatment and prognosis depend on which subtype of unicystic ameloblastoma is present. Luminal and intraluminal types may be treated with aggressive curettage, and a low rate of recurrence is typically reported for lesions treated in this manner. However, the intramural type requires more aggressive management, similar to that of solid, multilocular ameloblastoma, as described in the preceding topic.

Peripheral Ameloblastoma

Fig. **15.48**

When an ameloblastoma develops in soft tissue, the term **peripheral ameloblastoma** is applied, although the designation *extraosseous ameloblastoma* also may be used. Approximately 2% of ameloblastomas present in this fashion, and the tumor usually is found in the gingivae of adults. However, rare examples have been described in the buccal mucosa. The lesion typically presents as a slow-growing, asymptomatic, sessile nodule, and no radiographic evidence of its origin from the underlying bone should be identified. Occasionally, a slight cupping out or saucerization of the underlying bone may be evident, although no evidence of a distinct intraosseous component should be present. The clinical differential diagnosis usually includes more commonly occurring gingival nodules, such as fibroma, peripheral ossifying fibroma, or pyogenic granuloma. Microscopically, the peripheral ameloblastoma appears identical to its intraosseous counterpart.

The peripheral ameloblastoma is much less aggressive than ameloblastoma that develops within bone. Generally, simple conservative excision is performed, and the reported recurrence rate ranges from 10% to 20%. However, additional conservative surgery typically results in eradication of the tumor.

■ Figure **15.46**
Unicystic Ameloblastoma
A large, well-defined, unilocular radiolucency in the left posterior mandible in a teenager. (Courtesy Dr. Antonia Kolokythas.)

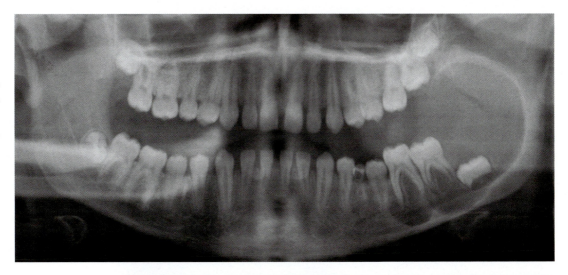

■ Figure **15.47**
Unicystic Ameloblastoma
A well-defined radiolucency extending into the ramus and associated with the crown of an impacted right mandibular second molar. (Courtesy Dr. Robert Coles.)

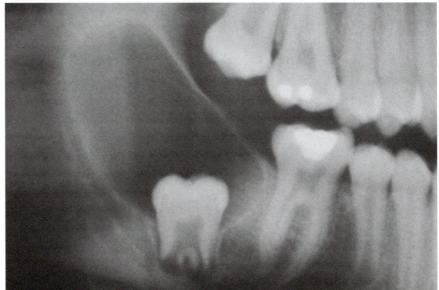

■ Figure **15.48**
Peripheral Ameloblastoma
A smooth-surfaced, sessile nodule of the right mandibular buccal attached gingiva.

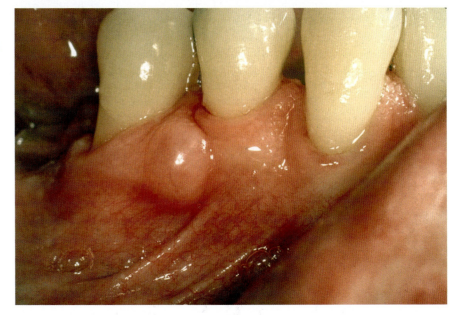

Ameloblastic Carcinoma

Figs. **15.49 and 15.50**

Ameloblastic carcinoma is a rare malignancy that can develop from a pre-existing ameloblastoma, or it may arise *de novo* from other sources of odontogenic epithelium. This malignancy develops over a wide age range, from the first to the ninth decades of life, although the median age is generally in the fifth to sixth decade. Males are affected slightly more often than females in most series, and similar to ameloblastoma, most of these lesions develop in the posterior mandible. Patients often present with pain, swelling, dysphagia, and trismus, but ulceration, loosening of the teeth, and hemorrhage also can be noted. Radiographically, ameloblastic carcinoma usually exhibits features of most intraosseous malignancies, such as expansion, destruction of cortical bone, irregular and ragged margins, tooth resorption, or pathologic fracture.

Histopathologically, the ameloblastic carcinoma vaguely resembles ameloblastoma, in that the cells at the periphery of the tumor islands often exhibit palisading of their nuclei. Other features are more characteristic of malignancy, such as enlarged, pale-staining nuclei with an increased nuclear/cytoplasmic ratio, variation in nuclear and cellular size and shape, increased mitotic activity, and varying degrees of necrosis.

Treatment consists of wide to radical surgical excision in most cases, depending on the size of the lesion and the clinical presence of nodal metastases. The prognosis varies with the stage of disease, although overall 5-year survival is usually reported to be between 60% and 70%.

Clear Cell Odontogenic Carcinoma

Fig. **15.51**

Clear cell odontogenic carcinoma is a rare odontogenic malignancy that was first described in the literature in 1985 as *clear cell odontogenic tumor*. Since then, approximately 100 cases have been documented, and the malignant nature of this lesion has been confirmed. Most of these tumors develop in the posterior mandible of middle-aged adults, and a female predilection is found. Patients usually present with a complaint of swelling that has been present and enlarging for many months. Pain eventually develops, although it may not be an early feature. Less commonly, tooth mobility, hemorrhage, or ulceration may be seen. Radiographically, the lesion can present as an expansile, ill-defined radiolucency or as a multilocular radiolucency that may mimic ameloblastoma.

The histopathologic features often bear some resemblance to ameloblastoma, showing invasive islands and cords of epithelial cells with some degree of nuclear palisading of the cells at the periphery of the islands; however, lesional cells with clearing of their cytoplasms represent a prominent component of the tumor. Other clear cell malignancies, such as metastatic renal cell carcinoma, may need to be ruled out. A characteristic *EWSRI-ATF1* gene rearrangement can be identified in the majority of these tumors. However, this finding also is associated with hyalinizing clear cell carcinoma, a salivary gland malignancy that typically develops in the oral soft tissues.

Treatment consists of wide surgical excision with assured clear margins. If clinically indicated, neck dissection may be appropriate. Resected tumors with positive margins often recur, although metastasis is relatively uncommon, primarily affecting the cervical lymph nodes and lungs. The 5-year survival for patients with clear cell odontogenic carcinoma is generally reported to be in the range of 80% to 90%.

■ Figure **15.49**
Ameloblastic Carcinoma

A large, ulcerated, erythematous mass with an irregular surface involving the right mandible. (With appreciation to Dr. Kelley Lybrand.)

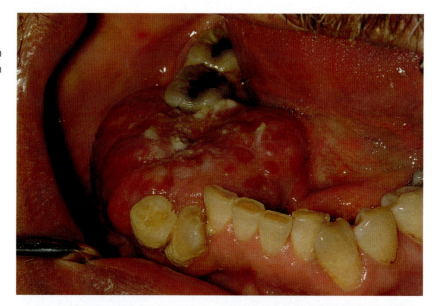

■ Figure **15.50**
Ameloblastic Carcinoma

Panoramic radiograph of patient seen in Fig. 15.49, showing a multilocular, expansile radiolucency of the right posterior mandible, with root resorption and thinning of the inferior border of the mandible. The anterior aspect of the lesion appears poorly demarcated, consistent with malignancy. (With appreciation to Dr. Kelley Lybrand.)

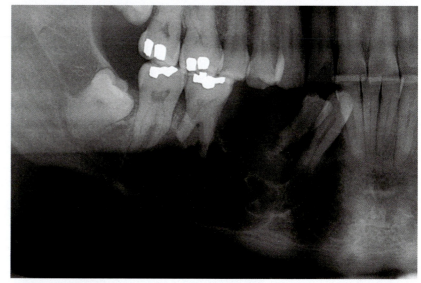

■ Figure **15.51**
Clear Cell Odontogenic Carcinoma

A multilocular radiolucency with ill-defined margins in several areas, simulating periapical inflammatory disease. (Courtesy Dr. John Werther.)

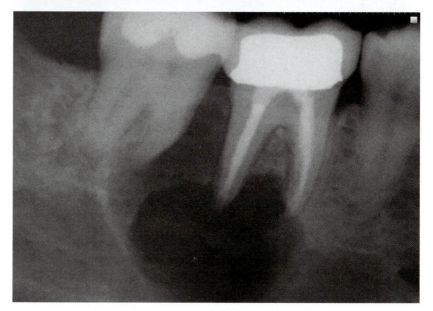

Figs. **15.52–15.55**

The **adenomatoid odontogenic tumor** (AOT) is a very uncommon benign lesion that tends to occur in a younger age group, with most being identified in the second or third decades of life. Although the term *adenoameloblastoma* was used originally for this tumor, this name has been abandoned because, unlike ameloblastoma, the AOT has a very unaggressive biologic behavior. In contrast to many other odontogenic neoplasms, the AOT is found most frequently in the maxilla, anterior to the molar teeth. Females are affected more often than males. In many cases, the lesion is identified upon routine radiographic examination, although sometimes local swelling is noted. AOT rarely has been described within the gingival soft tissue, presenting as a small nodule on the facial aspect in the maxillary anterior region. Radiographically, the AOT presents as a unilocular radiolucency that may or may not be associated with the crown of an impacted tooth. Those that are related to an impacted tooth could be mistaken for a dentigerous cyst, although the radiolucent process often extends apically beyond the cemento-enamel junction. In addition, scattered radiopaque flecks sometimes can be identified in these tumors.

Histopathologically, the AOT exhibits a well-developed capsule. The lesional cells are characterized by clusters of spindle-shaped cells and basaloid cells that are arranged in interlacing trabeculae. Scattered throughout the lesion are duct-like structures, from which the term "adenomatoid" (resembling a glandular tumor) is derived. Droplet-like calcifications may also be seen histopathologically in some lesions.

Treatment consists of simple enucleation. The encapsulated nature of the lesion undoubtedly accounts for the ease of its complete removal, and it rarely recurs.

■ Figure **15.52**
Adenomatoid Odontogenic Tumor
A unilocular expansile radiolucency is noted in the right anterior maxilla, associated with the crown of the unerupted lateral incisor. A few radiopaque flecks are seen in the superior aspect of the lesion. (Courtesy Dr. Drane Oliphant.)

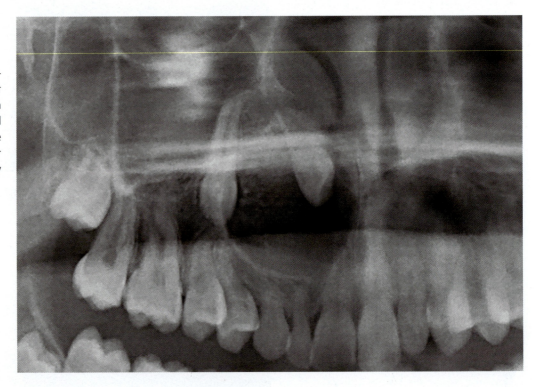

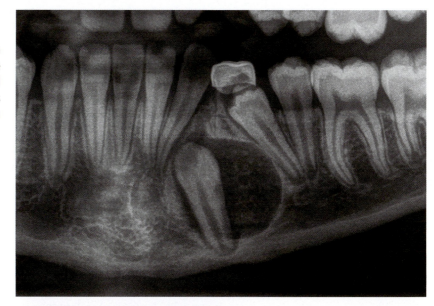

■ Figure 15.53
Adenomatoid Odontogenic Tumor
A well-defined, unilocular radiolucency is seen in association with the impacted left mandibular canine tooth. The radiolucency extends apically beyond the cemento-enamel junction. Radiopaque flecks also are seen within the lesion. (Courtesy Dr. Sarah Proulx.)

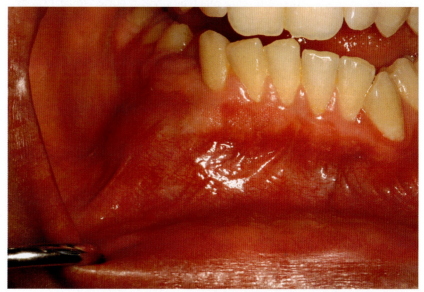

■ Figure 15.54
Adenomatoid Odontogenic Tumor
Prominent buccal expansion is noted in the right mandibular canine area. (With appreciation to Dr. Michael Tabor.)

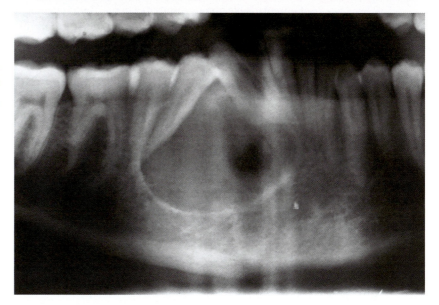

■ Figure 15.55
Adenomatoid Odontogenic Tumor
A panoramic radiograph of the patient seen in Fig. 15.54, which shows marked splaying of the roots of the right mandibular canine and first premolar caused by a well-defined unilocular radiolucent lesion. (With appreciation to Dr. Michael Tabor.)

Calcifying Epithelial Odontogenic Tumor (Pindborg Tumor)

Figs. **15.56 and 15.57**

Also known as the *Pindborg tumor* (named after the Danish oral pathologist who first described it), the **calcifying epithelial odontogenic tumor** (CEOT) is a rare benign neoplasm of the jaws that is thought to arise from the stratum intermedium of the enamel organ. The lesion can be found over a wide age range, with the mean age in the fifth decade in most series, and no sex predilection. Often the CEOT is detected on routine radiographic evaluation, presenting as a well-demarcated unilocular or multilocular radiolucency that tends to develop central opacities with the increasing age of the patient. Frequently the tumor is found in association with the crown of an impacted tooth. Clinical signs usually consist of swelling. Even less commonly, peripheral CEOT may develop in the gingival soft tissues, and rare examples of multifocal CEOT involving the jaws also have been described.

Microscopically, the CEOT is characterized by nests, sheets, and strands of polygonal cells with abundant eosinophilic cytoplasm. Deposits of tumor-associated amyloid should be evident upon staining with the Congo red method. Calcifications are reported in fewer than half of these lesions, and some of the foci of mineralization may exhibit a pattern of concentric rings, a finding that has been described as *Liesegang ring calcification*.

Treatment consists of conservative excision, as this neoplasm is much less aggressive than ameloblastoma. The recurrence rate typically is reported to be 15%, and seems to be associated with those lesions that have been treated with simple curettage. Recurrences are usually managed readily with re-excision. Very rare examples of malignant CEOT have been described.

Squamous Odontogenic Tumor

Fig. **15.58**

The **squamous odontogenic tumor** (SOT) is a very rare benign odontogenic neoplasm that is significant because it may be mistakenly diagnosed as squamous cell carcinoma by the pathologist who is unaware of this entity. The SOT may arise from the epithelial rests of Malassez, which is suggested by its frequent location between the roots of two adjacent teeth, or from rests of dental lamina. Often this lesion is identified upon routine radiographic examination of an adult patient, although sometimes tooth mobility or mild discomfort in the area of the lesion may be appreciated. If swelling is present, it is generally modest. Radiographically, this tumor often is characterized by an interradicular radiolucency that may have a triangular shape. Rare multifocal examples have been described.

Histopathologically, numerous discrete islands of bland squamous cells are found within a background of unremarkable fibrous connective tissue. Both squamous cell carcinoma and acanthomatous ameloblastoma could be considered in the microscopic differential diagnosis of this tumor; however, no evidence of nuclear or cellular atypia should be present, nor should there be palisading of the nuclei at the periphery of the tumor islands. Occasionally, foci of reactive squamous epithelial proliferation that resemble SOT can be seen arising from the lining of an inflamed odontogenic cyst, although these microscopic findings are not considered to be neoplastic. The term *squamous odontogenic tumor-like proliferations* has been applied to this phenomenon.

Treatment of the SOT consists of thorough curettage or conservative excision. Recurrences have been reported, although these can be managed by additional excision. A definitive recurrence rate is not available because this tumor is so rare. One acceptable example of malignant transformation of SOT has been reported.

■ Figure **15.56**
Calcifying Epithelial Odontogenic Tumor

An occlusal radiograph shows a demarcated expansile radiolucency with central radiopacities in association with several impacted mandibular teeth. (Courtesy Dr. James Lemon.)

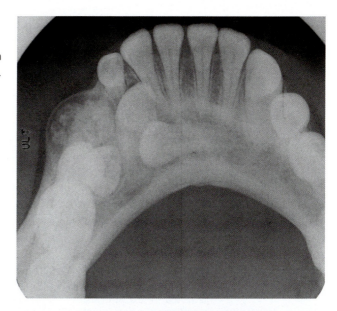

■ Figure **15.57**
Calcifying Epithelial Odontogenic Tumor

A demarcated unilocular radiolucency is noted in association with the crown of the impacted, displaced mandibular right third molar. (Courtesy Dr. George Arquitt.)

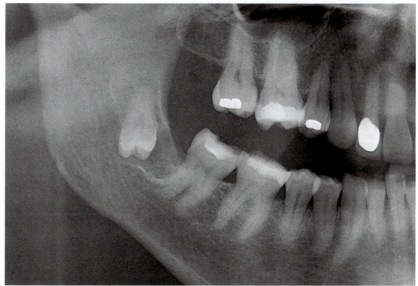

■ Figure **15.58**
Squamous Odontogenic Tumor

A somewhat triangular interradicular radiolucency is present between the maxillary canine and first premolar teeth. (From Haghighat K, Kalmar JR, Mariotti AJ: Squamous odontogenic tumor: diagnosis and management. *J Periodontol.* 202;73:653–656.)

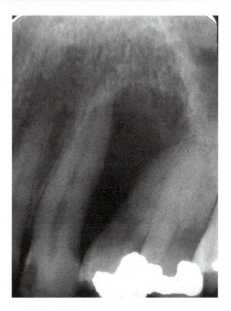

Ameloblastic Fibroma

Fig. **15.59**

The **ameloblastic fibroma** represents a benign mixed odontogenic epithelial/ectomesenchymal neoplasm. This tumor is generally identified in the first 2 decades of life, and failure of tooth eruption may trigger radiographic examination that discloses a well-defined radiolucency associated with an impacted tooth in the posterior mandible, where approximately 80% of these lesions are found. Usually the radiolucency is unilocular, although larger lesions may have a multilocular pattern. Swelling is sometimes present as well, particularly with large lesions. Rare examples of ameloblastic fibroma developing in the gingival soft tissues also have been reported.

Histopathologically, the ameloblastic fibroma is characterized by nests and strands of odontogenic epithelium that resembles dental lamina, and the strands of epithelium are set in a background of myxoid connective tissue that resembles dental papilla. Some cases have been diagnosed incorrectly as ameloblastoma because the pathologist was not familiar with the significance of the ectomesenchymal component of this lesion.

Management of the ameloblastic fibroma is conservative excision. Although recurrence is possible, it appears to be an uncommon event, with most series reporting recurrence rates of less than 18%. If recurrence is noted, re-excision using a more aggressive surgical approach may be appropriate. Some investigators have noted that multiple recurrences of this tumor potentially may contribute to the development of the rare ameloblastic fibrosarcoma (see next topic).

Ameloblastic Fibrosarcoma

Figs. **15.60 and 15.61**

The **ameloblastic fibrosarcoma** is a very rare odontogenic malignancy that may occur *de novo*, although one-third of these tumors seem to evolve from an ameloblastic fibroma (see preceding topic). Several reported cases have developed after unsuccessful attempts to treat a recurrent ameloblastic fibroma or ameloblastic fibro-odontoma. Whether the repeated surgeries are responsible for the malignant transformation or the tumor was inherently more aggressive, and thus more likely to recur, is unknown. Also, the possibility that reports of such cases are more likely to be documented and published in the dental/medical literature (so-called publication bias) cannot be excluded. Males are reported to be affected more often than females, and, like ameloblastic fibroma, the lesions are usually found in the posterior mandible. The mean age at diagnosis of this tumor is approximately a decade later than that of ameloblastic fibroma. Patients often present with signs and symptoms that suggest malignancy, including pain, paresthesia, swelling, loosening of the teeth, and/or ulceration. Radiographs show an ill-defined radiolucency with ragged margins in most instances.

Histopathologically, the neoplasm has a biphasic pattern, similar to ameloblastic fibroma; however, the ectomesenchymal component appears hypercellular and exhibits significant nuclear and cytologic atypia of the lesional cells, usually with pronounced mitotic activity. In most cases, the epithelial component appears rather unremarkable; however, a few examples have been reported in which both the epithelial and the ectomesenchymal components have undergone malignant transformation, resulting in an *ameloblastic carcinosarcoma*.

Treatment consists of radical surgical excision, with radiation therapy and/or neck dissection as indicated for certain cases, depending on the clinical presentation. Accurate 5-year survival rates are difficult to determine because of the rarity of this neoplasm, although mortality seems to be associated more with uncontrolled local disease rather than widespread metastasis.

■ Figure **15.59**
Ameloblastic Fibroma
This large radiolucency with scalloped margins is associated with three impacted teeth in the right posterior mandible of a young patient. (Courtesy Dr. Susie Lin.)

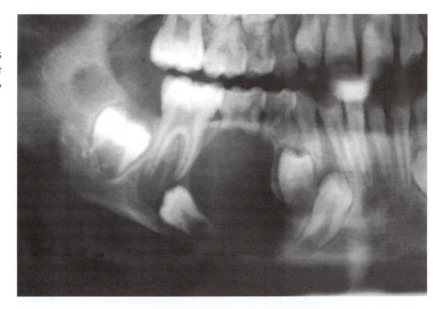

■ Figure **15.60**
Ameloblastic Fibrosarcoma
This large, ulcerated, fungating tumor mass is seen in the right posterior mandible. (Courtesy Dr. Sam McKenna.)

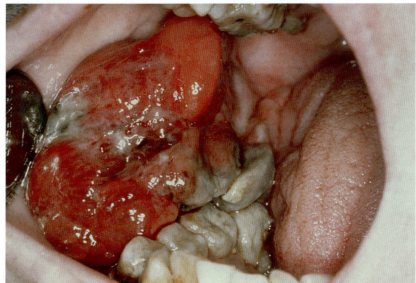

■ Figure **15.61**
Ameloblastic Fibrosarcoma
Panoramic radiograph of the lesion seen in Fig. 15.60, which shows a destructive multilocular radiolucency of the right posterior mandible. An impacted molar tooth is noted near the inferior border of the mandible. (Courtesy Dr. Sam McKenna.)

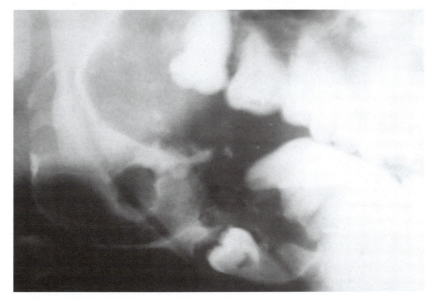

Ameloblastic Fibro-Odontoma

Figs. **15.62 and 15.63**

The **ameloblastic fibro-odontoma** (AFO) is defined as a mixed odontogenic tumor that represents a combination of an ameloblastic fibroma with an odontoma. The AFO is a somewhat controversial lesion, in that some authorities would prefer to classify this process as a developing odontoma (see next two topics). Although this may be the case in some instances, there are examples of this tumor that appear to have such a significant amount of ameloblastic fibroma-like tissue that it would be highly unlikely for such a lesion to completely differentiate into an odontoma. The AFO is typically diagnosed in the first and second decades of life, presenting as a swelling that is associated with the failure of a posterior tooth to erupt. The lesion is seen more often in the mandible than the maxilla, and males are affected more frequently than females. Radiographically, a well-demarcated radiolucency with varying degrees of central opacity overlies an impacted tooth, usually a molar.

Microscopically, this biphasic tumor consists of an ameloblastic fibroma component in conjunction with an odontoma, usually a complex odontoma (see next topic).

Conservative surgical excision or thorough curettage is generally used to manage these lesions, and a review of the reported cases with adequate follow-up found a recurrence rate of slightly less than 8%. In each of the recurrent tumors, inadequate initial excision was described as the reason for recurrence.

Complex Odontoma

Fig. **15.64**

Odontomas are the most common of the odontogenic tumors, and many authorities consider these to be hamartomas, and not true neoplasms. The **complex odontoma** develops most frequently in the posterior quadrants of the jaws, and is often discovered radiographically during the first or second decade of life, when the patient is evaluated for failure of eruption of a posterior tooth. Occasionally, swelling is the presenting sign. Radiographs typically show a well-demarcated radiolucency with varying degrees of central radiopacity, usually overlying an impacted tooth.

Histopathologically, the complex odontoma is characterized by a haphazard mixture of odontogenic soft and hard tissues. Even though tooth-like structures are not formed, the odontogenic components maintain their normal relationship with each other; that is, ameloblasts are associated with enamel matrix, and dental papilla is associated with developing dentin. The entire lesion is surrounded by a connective tissue capsule, similar to a dental follicle.

Simple enucleation of the complex odontoma is typically curative, although large lesions may require reconstructive procedures after removal.

■ Figure **15.62**
Ameloblastic Fibro-Odontoma
A well-defined radiolucency with central radiopacity overlies an impacted right mandibular second molar tooth in a 7-year-old male. (Courtesy Dr. Lee Moore.)

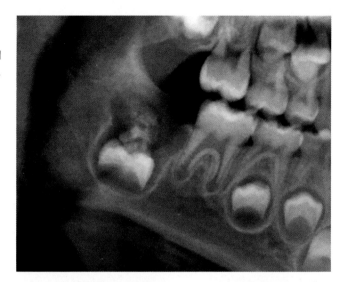

■ Figure **15.63**
Ameloblastic Fibro-Odontoma
An expansile, well-defined radiolucency is seen in the left posterior mandible overlying an impacted left mandibular third molar tooth, which is displaced distally. Radiopaque flecks are associated with the crown of the impacted tooth. (Courtesy Dr. Dominick Adornato.)

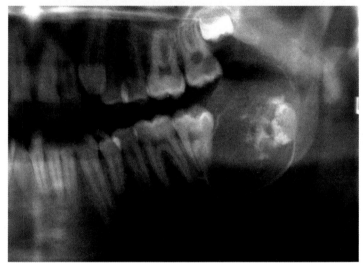

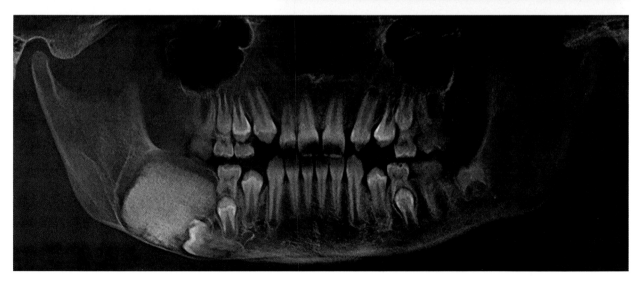

■ Figure **15.64**
Complex Odontoma
A large demarcated radiolucency with prominent central opacity overlies the crown of the right mandibular first molar, which is displaced toward the inferior border of the mandible. (Courtesy Dr. Samer Joudeh.)

Figs. **15.65–15.68**

The **compound odontoma** clinically presents in a similar fashion as the complex odontoma, although the former tends to occur more frequently in the anterior segments of the jaws. Failure of eruption of one of the maxillary anterior permanent teeth in a child is often seen with this lesion. Radiographically, a unilocular radiolucency is evident, with the central aspect occupied by variable numbers of small, malformed tooth-like structures. Less frequently, odontomas may present in the gingival soft tissues. Histopathologically, the compound odontoma differs from its complex counterpart, in that the odontogenic hard and soft tissues are neatly arranged in the form of small, malformed teeth.

As with the complex odontoma, enucleation is curative. Recurrence would not be expected with either type of odontoma.

■ Figure **15.65**
Compound Odontoma
A demarcated radiolucency with central radiopaque structures that resemble small, malformed teeth. The lesion is forming between the roots of two anterior teeth. (Courtesy Dr. James Wilson.)

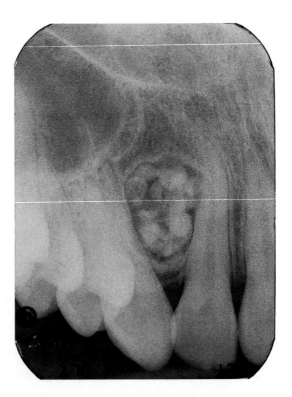

■ Figure **15.66**
Compound Odontoma
An appearance that is similar to the previous image is noted, although the odontoma overlies the crown of an impacted maxillary incisor tooth in this case.

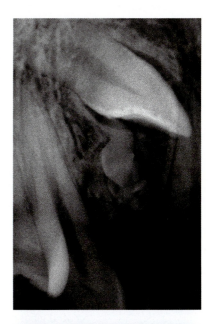

■ Figure **15.67**
Compound Odontoma
Cluster of small, malformed teeth between the mandibular lateral incisor and canine. (Courtesy Dr. James Moore.)

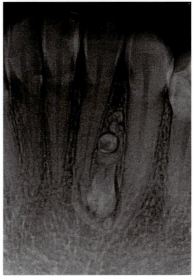

■ Figure **15.68**
Compound Odontoma
Small, malformed tooth-like structures that comprise the hard tissue component of a compound odontoma.

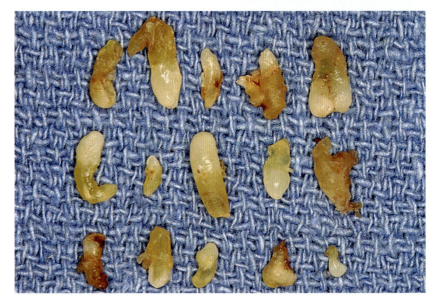

Central Odontogenic Fibroma

Figs. **15.69 and 15.70**

The **central odontogenic fibroma** (COF) represents an uncommon benign neoplasm of odontogenic ectomesenchymal differentiation. Women are affected more frequently than men by almost a 2:1 margin, and the tumor occurs equally in the both jaws. However, in the maxilla the COF develops in the anterior segment, whereas mandibular lesions are more frequently found in the molar region. By definition, this tumor develops within the jaws, typically presenting as a unilocular radiolucency that may produce some swelling. Larger examples may have a multilocular radiographic appearance. Radiopaque flecks have been described in fewer than 15% of these neoplasms. Maxillary lesions often will cause a cleft or groove to develop on the palatal mucosa that overlies the tumor. Resorption of the adjacent tooth roots is frequently evident, in addition to spreading of the roots by the tumor.

The histopathologic features of the COF can be variable, with some being composed of bland fibrous connective tissue that is characterized by plump fibroblastic cells set in a loose to relatively dense collagenous background. Nests and strands of bland odontogenic epithelium are scattered sparsely throughout this form of the lesion. Other COFs may be composed of rather cellular connective tissue in association with abundant cords and nests of odontogenic epithelium. Calcifications of various types, such as dentinoid or cementum-like mineralizations, are more likely to be associated with this form of COF. Very infrequently, central giant cell granuloma-like areas may be found in this tumor.

Treatment consists of thorough curettage or conservative excision, and recurrence rates are generally low in most reported series of cases.

Peripheral Odontogenic Fibroma

Fig. **15.71**

The **peripheral odontogenic fibroma** (POF) is an uncommon benign tumor of ectomesenchymal differentiation that develops in the soft tissues of the gingivae. Clinically this lesion is identical to the far more common *peripheral ossifying fibroma*, presenting as a slow-growing, smooth-surfaced, firm gingival nodule that may be ulcerated. However, no particular distinguishing clinical feature is evident.

Histopathologically, the POF is characterized by a cellular proliferation of fibrous connective tissue that is associated with bland nests and strands of odontogenic epithelium. Calcifications are sometimes scattered throughout the lesion.

Treatment consists of conservative excision, and most reports describe a recurrence rate in the range of 20% to 30%, although the number of reported cases with adequate follow-up is relatively small, and may be skewed toward those lesions that recur.

■ Figure **15.69**
Central Odontogenic Fibroma
A palatal depression overlying a central odontogenic fibroma is seen in this patient. (Courtesy Dr. Michael Poth.)

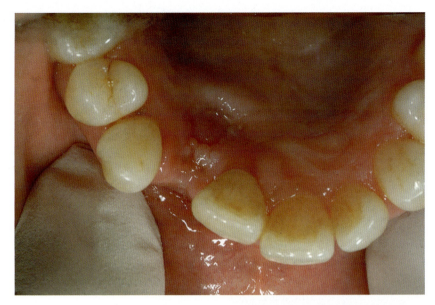

■ Figure **15.70**
Central Odontogenic Fibroma
A periapical radiograph of the same patient seen in Fig. 15.69 reveals a demarcated, somewhat multilocular radiolucency. (Courtesy Dr. Michael Poth.)

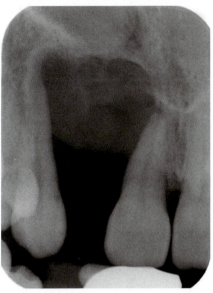

■ Figure **15.71**
Peripheral Odontogenic Fibroma
A smooth-surfaced nodule of normal color is present on the labial aspect of the right maxillary anterior gingivae. (Courtesy Dr. John Russo.)

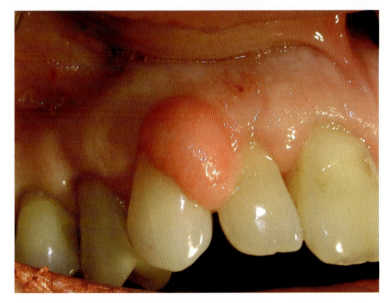

Figs. **15.72 and 15.73**

The **odontogenic myxoma** represents an uncommon neoplasm of odontogenic ectomesenchymal differentiation. Although myxomas may develop at various soft tissue sites, the only intraosseous location seems to be the jaws; therefore, the assumption is that these tumors are of odontogenic origin. This tumor is diagnosed most frequently in the second to fourth decades of life, and the mandible is affected more often than the maxilla in most reported series of patients. No significant sex predilection is seen. Swelling is the most common sign, identified in over half of these patients in most series. Pain is also associated with these lesions, typically occurring in approximately one-third of the cases. The odontogenic myxoma may also be discovered when routine dental radiographs are obtained, and when the tumor is small, a unilocular radiographic appearance often is seen. With larger examples, a multilocular pattern is more frequently found, with an internal trabecular configuration that has been described as a honeycomb pattern, a soap bubble pattern, or sometimes as fine "cobweb-like" trabeculae coursing through the lesion.

Histopathologically, the odontogenic myxoma is a paucicellular proliferation of loose connective tissue with haphazardly arranged spindled or stellate-shaped cells set in abundant ground substance. In some lesions, rests of bland odontogenic epithelium may be seen. Often the lesional tissue will invade between the trabeculae of adjacent cancellous bone.

Treatment of the odontogenic myxoma requires complete removal of the lesional tissue, and because of its tendency to invade the cancellous bone, the surgical procedures used to treat this lesion are often similar to those used for ameloblastoma. The recurrence rates of the odontogenic myxoma typically range from 10% to 30% in most reported series of patients. Higher recurrence rates are generally reported when this lesion is treated with curettage, rather than excision with a 1.0- to 1.5-cm margin.

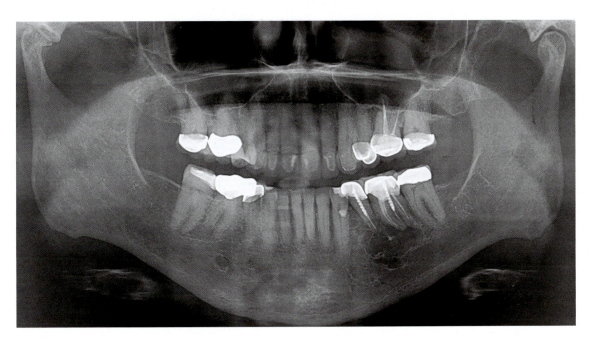

■ Figure **15.72**
Odontogenic Myxoma
A multilocular radiolucency in the left body of the mandible, associated with the apices of the endodontically treated premolar and molar. (Courtesy Dr. Mark Spinazze.)

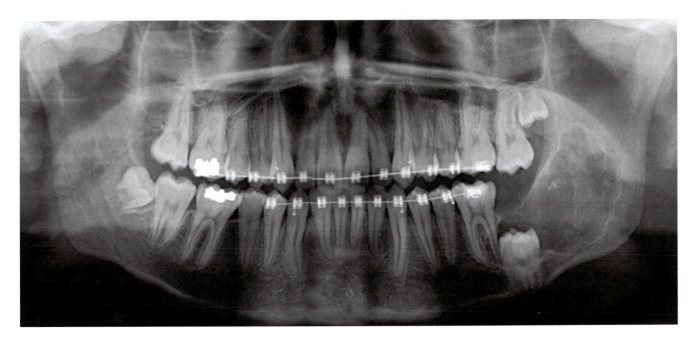

■ Figure **15.73**
Odontogenic Myxoma
A large multilocular radiolucency is associated with an impacted left mandibular second molar and extends into the left ramus of the mandible. (Courtesy Dr. Antonia Kolokythas.)

Bibliography

Dentigerous Cyst

Henien M, Sproat C, Kwok J, et al. Coronectomy and dentigerous cysts: a review of 68 patients. *Oral Surg Oral Med Oral Pathol Oral Radiol.* 2017;123:670–674.

Lin HP, Wang YP, Chen HM, et al. A clinicopathologic study of 338 dentigerous cysts. *J Oral Pathol Med.* 2013;42:462–467.

Yao L, Xu X, Ren M, et al. Inflammatory dentigerous cyst of mandibular first premolar associated with endodontically treated primary first molar: a rare case report. *Eur J Paediatr Dent.* 2015;16:201–204.

Zhang LL, Yang R, Zhang L, et al. Dentigerous cyst: a retrospective clinicopathological analysis of 2082 dentigerous cysts in British Columbia, Canada. *Int J Oral Maxillofac Surg.* 2010;39:876–882.

Eruption Cyst

Aguiló L, Cibrián R, Bagán JV, et al. Eruption cysts: retrospective clinical study of 36 cases. *ASDC J Dent Child.* 1998;65:102–106.

Bodner L, Goldstein J, Sarnat H. Eruption cysts: a clinical report of 24 new cases. *J Clin Pediatr Dent.* 2004;28:183–186.

Şen-Tunç E, Açikel H, Şaroğlu-Sönmez I, et al. Eruption cysts: a series of 66 cases with clinical features. *Med Oral Patol Oral Cir Bucal.* 2017;22:e228–e232.

Buccal Bifurcation Cyst

Levarek RE, Wiltz MJ, Kelsch RD, et al. Surgical management of the buccal bifurcation cyst: bone grafting as a treatment adjunct to enucleation and curettage. *J Oral Maxillofac Surg.* 2014;72:1966–1973.

Philipsen HP, Reichart PA, Ogawa I, et al. The inflammatory paradental cyst: a critical review of 342 cases from a literature survey, including 17 new cases from the author's files. *J Oral Pathol Med.* 2004;33:147–155.

Pompura JR, Sàndor GKB, Stoneman DW. The buccal bifurcation cyst: a prospective study of treatment outcomes in 44 sites. *Oral Surg Oral Med Oral Pathol Oral Radiol Endod.* 1997;83:215–221.

Shohat I, Buchner A, Taicher S. Mandibular buccal bifurcation cyst: enucleation without extraction. *Int J Oral Maxillofac Surg.* 2003;32:610–613.

Odontogenic Keratocyst

Brannon RB. The odontogenic keratocyst—a clinicopathologic study of 312 cases. Part I: clinical features. *Oral Surg Oral Med Oral Pathol.* 1976;42:54–72.

Chrcanovic BR, Gomez RS. Recurrence probability for keratocystic odontogenic tumors: an analysis of 6427 cases. *J Craniomaxillofac Surg.* 2017;45:244–251.

Finkelstein MW, Hellstein JW, Lake KS, et al. Keratocystic odontogenic tumor: a retrospective analysis of genetic, immunohistochemical and therapeutic features. Proposal of a multicenter clinical survey tool. *Oral Surg Oral Med Oral Pathol Oral Radiol.* 2013;116:75–83.

Li T-J. The odontogenic keratocyst: a cyst, or a cystic neoplasm? *J Dent Res.* 2011;90:133–142.

Myoung H, Hong S-P, Hong S-D, et al. Odontogenic keratocyst: review of 256 cases for recurrence and clinicopathologic parameters. *Oral Surg Med Oral Pathol Oral Radiol Endod.* 2001;91:328–333.

Speight P, Devilliers P, Li T-J, et al. Odontogenic keratocyst. In: El-Naggar AK, Chan JK, Grandis JR, et al, eds. *WHO Classification of Head and Neck Tumours.* 4th ed. Lyon: IARC; 2017:235–236.

Nevoid Basal Cell Carcinoma Syndrome

Bree AF, Shah MR; BCNS Colloquium Group. Consensus statement from the first international colloquium on basal cell nevus syndrome (BCNS). *Am J Med Genet A.* 2011;155:2091–2097.

Carlson ER, Oreadi D, McCoy JM. Nevoid basal cell carcinoma syndrome and the keratocystic odontogenic tumor. *J Oral Maxillofac Surg.* 2015;73:S77–S86.

Chiang A, Jaju PD, Batra P, et al. Genomic stability in syndromic basal cell carcinoma. *J Invest Dermatol.* 2017;doi:10.1016/j.jid.2017.09.048.

Gorlin RJ. Nevoid basal cell carcinoma (Gorlin) syndrome. *Genet Med.* 2004;6:530–539.

Solis DC, Kwon GP, Ransohoff KJ, et al. Risk factors for basal cell carcinoma among patients with basal cell nevus syndrome. Development of a basal cell nevus syndrome patient registry. *JAMA Dermatol.* 2017;153:189–192.

Orthokeratinized Odontogenic Cyst

Cheng YS, Liang H, Wright J, et al. Multiple orthokeratinized odontogenic cysts: a case report. *Head Neck Pathol.* 2015;9:153–157.

Dong Q, Pan S, Sun LS, et al. Orthokeratinized odontogenic cyst: a clinicopathologic study of 61 cases. *Arch Pathol Lab Med.* 2010;134:271–275.

MacDonald-Jankowski DS. Orthokeratinized odontogenic cyst: a systemic review. *Dentomaxillofac Radiol.* 2010;39:455–467.

Lateral Periodontal Cyst

Chrcanovic BR, Gomez RS. Gingival cyst of the adult, lateral periodontal cyst, and botryoid odontogenic cyst: an updated systematic review. *Oral Dis.* 2017 Nov 20; doi:10.1111/odi.12808. [Epub ahead of print].

Cohen D, Neville B, Damm D, et al. The lateral periodontal cyst: a report of 37 cases. *J Periodontol.* 1984;55:230–234.

Santos PP, Freitas VS, Freitas Rde A, et al. Botryoid odontogenic cyst: a clinicopathologic study of 10 cases. *Ann Diagn Pathol.* 2011;15:221–224.

Siponen M, Neville BW, Damm DD, et al. Multifocal lateral periodontal cysts: a report of 4 cases and review of the literature. *Oral Surg Oral Med Oral Pathol Oral Radiol Endod.* 2011;111:225–233.

Gingival Cyst of the Adult

Bell RC, Chauvin PJ, Tyler MT. Gingival cyst of the adult: a review and report of eight cases. *J Can Dent Assoc.* 1997;63:533–535.

Chrcanovic BR, Gomez RS. Gingival cyst of the adult, lateral periodontal cyst, and botryoid odontogenic cyst: an updated systematic review. *Oral Dis.* 2017 Nov 20;doi:10.1111/odi.12808. [Epub ahead of print].

Giunta JL. Gingival cysts in the adult. *J Periodontol.* 2002;73:827–831.

Nxumalo TN, Shear M. Gingival cyst in adults. *J Oral Pathol Med.* 1992;21:309–313.

Gingival Cyst of the Newborn

Cataldo E, Berkman M. Cysts of the oral mucosa in newborns. *Am J Dis Child.* 1968;116:44–48.

Fromm A. Epstein's pearls, Bohn's nodules and inclusion cysts of the oral cavity. *J Dent Child.* 1967;34:275–287.

Monteagudo B, Labandeira J, Cabanillas M, et al. Prevalence of milia and palatal and gingival cysts in Spanish newborns. *Pediatr Dermatol.* 2012;29:301–305.

Paula JDR, Dezan CC, Frossard WTG, et al. Oral and facial inclusion cysts in newborns. *J Clin Pediatr Dent.* 2006;31:127–129.

Calcifying Odontogenic Cyst

Chrcanovic BR, Gomez RS. Peripheral calcifying cystic odontogenic tumour and peripheral dentinogenic ghost cell tumor: an updated systematic review of 117 cases reported in the literature. *Acta Odontol Scand.* 2016;74:591–597.

Hong SP, Ellis GL, Hartman KS. Calcifying odontogenic cyst: a review of ninety-two cases with reevaluation of their nature as cysts or neoplasms, the nature of the ghost cells and subclassification. *Oral Surg Oral Med Oral Pathol.* 1991;72:56–64.

Ledesma-Montes C, Gorlin RJ, Shear M, et al. International collaborative study on ghost cell odontogenic tumours: calcifying cystic odontogenic tumour, dentinogenic ghost cell tumour and ghost cell odontogenic carcinoma. *J Oral Pathol Med.* 2008;37:302–308.

Yukimori A, Oikawa Y, Morita KI, et al. Genetic basis of calcifying cystic odontogenic tumors. *PLoS ONE.* 2017;12(6):e0180224.

Glandular Odontogenic Cyst

Chrcanovic BR, Gomez RS. Glandular odontogenic cyst: an updated analysis of 169 cases reported in the literature. *Oral Dis.* 2017 Jul 26;doi:10.1111/odi.12719. [Epub ahead of print].

Fowler CB, Brannon RB, Kessler HP, et al. Glandular odontogenic cyst: analysis of 46 cases with special emphasis on microscopic criteria for diagnosis. *Head Neck Pathol.* 2011;5:364–375.

Gardner DG, Kessler HP, Morency R, et al. The glandular odontogenic cyst: an apparent entity. *J Oral Pathol.* 1988;17:359–366.

Kaplan I, Anavi Y, Hirshberg A. Glandular odontogenic cyst: a challenge in diagnosis and treatment. *Oral Dis.* 2008;14:575–581.

Carcinoma in Odontogenic Cysts

Bodner L, Manor E, Shear M, et al. Primary intraosseous squamous cell carcinoma arising in an odontogenic cyst – a clinicopathologic analysis of 116 reported cases. *J Oral Pathol Med.* 2011;40:733–738.

Borrás-Ferreres J, Sánchez-Torres A, Gay-Escoda C. Malignant changes developing from odontogenic cysts: a systematic review. *J Clin Exp Dent.* 2016;8:e622–e628.

Chaisuparat R, Coletti D, Kolokythas A, et al. Primary intraosseous odontogenic carcinoma arising in an odontogenic cyst or de novo: a clinicopathologic study of six new cases. *Oral Surg Oral Med Oral Pathol Oral Radiol Endod.* 2006;101:196–202.

Lukandu OM, Micha CS. Primary intraosseous squamous cell carcinoma arising from keratocystic odontogenic tumor. *Oral Surg Oral Med Oral Pathol Oral Radiol.* 2015;120:e204–e209.

Ameloblastoma

Bilodeau EA, Collins BM. Odontogenic cysts and neoplasms. *Surg Pathol.* 2017;10:177–222.

Kennedy WR, Werning JW, Kaye FJ, et al. Treatment of ameloblastoma and ameloblastic carcinoma with radiotherapy. *Eur Arch Otorhinolaryngol.* 2016;273:3293–3297.

Milman T, Ying G-S, Pan W, et al. Ameloblastoma: 25 Year experience at a single institution. *Head Neck Pathol.* 2016;10:513–520.

Parmar S, Al-Qamachi L, Aga H. Ameloblastomas of the mandible and maxilla. *Curr Opin Otolaryngol Head Neck Surg.* 2016;24:148–154.

Unicystic Ameloblastoma

Arora S. Unicystic ameloblastoma: a perception for the cautious interpretation of radiographic and histological findings. *J Coll Physicians Surg Pak.* 2015;25:761–764.

Lau SL, Samman N. Recurrence related to treatment modalities of unicystic ameloblastoma: a systematic review. *Int J Oral Maxillofac Surg.* 2006;35:681–690.

Samuel S, Mistry FK, Chopra S, et al. Unicystic ameloblastoma with mural proliferation: conservative or surgical approach? *BMJ Case Rep.* 2014;doi:10.1136/bcr-2014-206273.

Singh T, Wiesenfeld D, Clement J, et al. Ameloblastoma: demographic data and treatment outcomes from Melbourne, Australia. *Aust Dent J.* 2015;60:24–29.

Peripheral Ameloblastoma

Chhina S, Rathore AS. Peripheral ameloblastoma of gingiva with cytokeratin 19 analysis. *BMJ Case Rep.* 2015;doi:10.1136/bcr-2015-210227.

Filizzola AI, Bartholomeu-dos-Santos TC, Pires FR. Ameloblastomas: clinicopathological features from 70 cases diagnosed in a single oral pathology service in an 8-year period. *Med Oral Patol Oral Cir Bucal.* 2014;19:e556–e561.

Lascane NA, Sedassari BT, Alves Fde A, et al. Peripheral ameloblastoma with dystrophic calcification: an unusual feature in non-calcifying odontogenic tumors. *Braz Dent J.* 2014;25:253–256.

Saghravanian N, Salehinejad J, Ghazi N, et al. A 40-year retrospective clinicopathological study of ameloblastoma in Iran. *Asian Pac J Cancer Prev.* 2016;17:619–623.

Ameloblastic Carcinoma

Fitzpatrick SG, Hirsch SA, Listinsky CM, et al. Ameloblastic carcinoma with features of ghost cell odontogenic carcinoma in a patient with suspected Gardner syndrome. *Oral Surg Oral Med Oral Pathol Oral Radiol.* 2015;119:e241–e245.

Gunaratne DA, Coleman HG, Lim L, et al. Ameloblastic carcinoma. *Am J Case Rep.* 2015;16:415–419.

Lee RJ, Tong EL, Patel R, et al. Epidemiology, prognostic factors, and management of malignant odontogenic tumors: an analysis of 295 cases. *Oral Surg Oral Med Oral Pathol Oral Radiol.* 2015;120:616–621.

Loyola AM, Cardoso SV, de Faria PR, et al. Ameloblastic carcinoma: a Brazilian collaborative study of 17 cases. *Histopathol.* 2016;69:687–701.

Martínez-Martínez M, Mosqueda-Taylor A, Carlos R, et al. Malignant odontogenic tumors: a multicentric Latin American study of 25 cases. *Oral Dis.* 2014;20:380–385.

Matsushita Y, Fujita S, Yanamoto S, et al. Spindle cell variant of ameloblastic carcinoma: a case report and literature review. *Oral Surg Oral Med Oral Pathol Oral Radiol.* 2016;121:e54–e61.

Clear Cell Odontogenic Carcinoma

Ginat DT, Villaflor V, Cipriani NA. Oral cavity clear cell odontogenic carcinoma. *Head Neck Pathol.* 2016;10:217–220.

Kalsi AS, Williams SP, Shah KA, et al. Clear cell odontogenic carcinoma: a rare neoplasm of the maxillary bone. *J Oral Maxillofac Surg.* 2014;72:935–938.

Loyola AM, Cardoso SV, de Faria PR, et al. Clear cell odontogenic carcinoma: report of 7 new cases and systematic review of the current knowledge. *Oral Surg Oral Med Oral Pathol Oral Radiol.* 2015;120:483–496.

Yancoskie AE, Sreekantaiah C, Jacob J, et al. EWSR1 and ATF1 rearrangements in clear cell odontogenic carcinoma: presentation of a case. *Oral Surg Oral Med Oral Pathol Oral Radiol.* 2014;118:e115–e118.

Adenomatoid Odontogenic Tumor

Adisa AO, Lawal AO, Effiom OA, et al. A retrospective review of 61 cases of adenomatoid odontogenic tumour seen in five tertiary health facilities in Nigeria. *Pan African Med J.* 2016;24:102. doi:10.11604/pamj.2016.24.102.9400.

de Matos FR, Nonaka CF, Pinto LP, et al. Adenomatoid odontogenic tumor: retrospective study of 15 cases with emphasis on histopathologic features. *Head Neck Pathol.* 2012;6:430–437.

Ide F, Muramatsu T, Ito Y, et al. An expanded and revised early history of the adenomatoid odontogenic tumor. *Oral Surg Oral Med Oral Pathol Oral Radiol.* 2013;115:646–651.

Naidu A, Slater LJ, Hamao-Sakamoto A, et al. Adenomatoid odontogenic tumor with peripheral cemento-osseous reactive proliferation: report of 2 cases and review of the literature. *Oral Surg Oral Med Oral Pathol Oral Radiol.* 2016;122:e86–e92.

Philipsen HP, Khongkhunthiang P, Reichart PA. The adenomatoid odontogenic tumour: an update of selected issues. *J Oral Pathol Med.* 2016;45:394–398.

Calcifying Epithelial Odontogenic Tumor

Azevedo R, Mosqueda-Taylor A, Carlos R, et al. Calcifying epithelial odontogenic tumor (CEOT): a clinicopathologic and immunohistochemical study and comparison with dental follicles containing CEOT-like areas. *Oral Surg Oral Med Oral Pathol Oral Radiol.* 2013;116:759–768.

Chen Y, Wang TT, Gao Y, et al. A clinicopathologic study on calcifying epithelial odontogenic tumor: with special reference to Langerhans cell variant. *Diagn Pathol.* 2014;9:37.

Munteanu C, Pirici D, Stepan AE, et al. Maxillary calcifying epithelial odontogenic tumor with sinus and buccal vestibule extension: a case report and immunohistochemical study. *Diagn Pathol.* 2016;11:134.

Rydin K, Sjöström M, Warfvinge G. Clear cell variant of intraosseous calcifying epithelial odontogenic tumor: a case report and review of the literature. *Oral Surg Oral Med Oral Pathol Oral Radiol.* 2016;122:e125–e130.

Shetty SJ, Pereira T, Desai RS. Peripheral clear cell variant of calcifying epithelial odontogenic tumor: case report and review of the literature. *Head Neck Pathol.* 2016;10:481–485.

Zhang A, Chaw SY, Talacko AA, et al. Central calcifying epithelial odontogenic tumour in the posterior maxilla: a case report. *Aust Dent J.* 2016;61:381–385.

Squamous Odontogenic Tumor

Badni M, Nagaraja A, Kamath VV. Squamous odontogenic tumor: a case report and review of the literature. *J Oral Maxillofac Pathol.* 2012;16:113–117.

Brierley DJ, Hunter KD. Odontogenic tumours. *Diagn Histopathol.* 2015;21:370–379.

Elmuradi S, Mair Y, Suresh L, et al. Multicentric squamous odontogenic tumor: a case report and review of the literature. *Head Neck Pathol.* 2017;11:168–174.

Verhelst PJ, Grosjean L, Shaheen E, et al. Surgical management of an aggressive multifocal squamous odontogenic tumor. *J Oral Maxillofac Surg.* 2017 Jul 21;doi:10.1016/j.joms.2017.07.153. [Epub ahead of print]; pii: S0278-2391(17)30948-5.

Ameloblastic Fibroma

Buchner A, Vered M. Ameloblastic fibroma: a stage in the development of a hamartomatous odontoma or a true neoplasm? Critical analysis of 162 previously reported cases plus 10 new cases. *Oral Surg Oral Med Oral Pathol Oral Radiol.* 2013;116:598–606.

Chen Y, Li T-J, Gao Y, et al. Ameloblastic fibroma and related lesions: a clinicopathologic study with reference to their nature and interrelationship. *J Oral Pathol Med.* 2005;34:588–595.

Cohen DM, Bhattacharyya I. Ameloblastic fibroma, ameloblastic fibro-odontoma, and odontoma. *Oral Maxillofac Surg Clin North Am.* 2004;16:375–384.

Darling MR, Daley TD. Peripheral ameloblastic fibroma. *J Oral Pathol Med.* 2006;35:190–192.

Melo Lde A, Barros AC, Sardinha Sde C, et al. Ameloblastic fibroma: a rare case report with 7-year follow-up. *Srp Arh Celok Lek.* 2015;143:190–194.

Nelson BL, Folk GS. Ameloblastic fibroma. *Head Neck Pathol.* 2009;3:51–53.

Ameloblastic Fibro-Odontoma

Abrahams JM, McClure SA. Pediatric odontogenic tumors. *Oral Maxillofacial Surg Clin N Am.* 2016;28:45–58.

Boxberger NR, Brannon RB, Fowler CB. Ameloblastic fibro-odontoma: a clinicopathologic study of 12 cases. *J Clin Pediatr Dent.* 2011;35:397–404.

Buchner A, Kaffe I, Vered M. Clinical and radiological profile of ameloblastic fibro-odontoma: an update on an uncommon odontogenic tumor based on a critical analysis of 114 cases. *Head Neck Pathol.* 2013;7:54–63.

Chrcanovic BR, Gomez RS. Ameloblastic fibrodentinoma and ameloblastic fibro-odontoma: an updated systematic review of cases reported in the literature. *J Oral Maxillofac Surg.* 2017;75:1425–1437.

Cohen DM, Bhattacharyya I. Ameloblastic fibroma, ameloblastic fibro-odontoma, and odontoma. *Oral Maxillofac Surg Clin North Am.* 2004;16:375–384.

Gantala R, Gotoor SG, Kumar RV, et al. Ameloblastic fibro-odontoma. *BMJ Case Rep.* 2015;doi:10.1136/bcr-2015-209739.

Martínez Martínez M, Romero CS, Piña AR, et al. Pigmented ameloblastic fibro-odontoma: clinical, histological, and immunohistochemical profile. *Int J Surg Pathol.* 2015;23:52–60.

Nelson BL, Thompson LDR. Ameloblastic fibro-odontoma. *Head Neck Pathol.* 2014;8:168–170.

Ameloblastic Fibrosarcoma

Carlos-Bregni R, Mosqueda-Taylor A, Meneses-Garcia A. Ameloblastic fibrosarcoma of the mandible: report of two cases and review of the literature. *J Oral Pathol Med.* 2001;30:316–320.

Gilani SM, Raza A, Al-Khafaji BM. Ameloblastic fibrosarcoma: a rare malignant odontogenic tumor. *Eur Ann Otorhinolaryngol Head Neck Dis.* 2014;131:53–56.

Mohsenifar Z, Behrad S, Abbas FM. Epithelial dysplasia in ameloblastic fibrosarcoma arising from recurrent ameloblastic fibroma in a 26-year-old Iranian man. *Am J Case Rep.* 2015;16:548–553.

Pourdanesh F, Mohamadi M, Moshref M, et al. Ameloblastic fibrosarcoma of the mandible with distant metastases. *J Oral Maxillofac Surg.* 2015;73:2067.e1–2067.e7.

Compound Odontoma

Cohen DM, Bhattacharyya I. Ameloblastic fibroma, ameloblastic fibro-odontoma, and odontoma. *Oral Maxillofac Surg Clin North Am.* 2004;16:375–384.

Erdogan Ö, Keceli O, Öztunc H, et al. Compound odontoma involving the four quadrants of the jaws: a case report and review of the literature. *Quintessence Int.* 2014;45:341–344.

Machado C de V, Henriques Knop LA, Barreiros Siquara da Rocha MC, et al. Impacted permanent incisors associated with compound odontoma. *BMJ Case Rep.* 2015;doi:10.1136/bcr-2014-208201.

Tuczyńska A, Bartosik D, Abu-Fillat Y, et al. Compound odontoma in the mandible - case study and literature review. *Dev Period Med.* 2015;19:484–489.

Complex Odontoma

Arora A, Donald PM. Complex odontomas hindering eruption of maxillary permanent teeth: a radiological perspective. *BMJ Case Rep.* 2016;doi:10.1136/bcr-2016-216797.

Bereket C, Çakır-Özkan N, Şener İ, et al. Complex and compound odontomas: analysis of 69 cases and a rare case of erupted compound odontoma. *Niger J Clin Pract.* 2015;18:726–730.

Dagrus K, Purohit S, Manjunatha BS. Dentigerous cyst arising from a complex odontoma: an unusual presentation. *BMJ Case Rep.* 2016;doi:10.1136/bcr-2016-214936.

Sun L, Sun Z, Ma X. Multiple complex odontoma of the maxilla and the mandible. *Oral Surg Oral Med Oral Pathol Oral Radiol.* 2015;120:e11–e16.

Central Odontogenic Fibroma

Eversole LR. Odontogenic fibroma, including amyloid and ossifying variants. *Head Neck Pathol.* 2011;5:335–343.

Handlers JP, Abrams AM, Melrose RJ, et al. Central odontogenic fibroma: clinicopathologic features of 19 cases and review of the literature. *J Oral Maxillofac Surg.* 1991;49:46–54.

Mosqueda-Taylor A, Martínez-Mata G, Carlos-Bregni R, et al. Central odontogenic fibroma: new findings and report of a multicentric collaborative study. *Oral Surg Oral Med Oral Pathol Oral Radiol Endod.* 2011;112:349–358.

Tosios KI, Gopalakrishnan R, Koutlas IG. So-called hybrid central odontogenic fibroma/central giant cell lesion of the jaws. A report on seven additional cases, including an example in a patient with cherubism, and hypotheses on the pathogenesis. *Head Neck Pathol.* 2008;2:333–338.

Upadhyaya JD, Cohen DM, Islam MN, et al. Hybrid central odontogenic fibroma with giant cell granuloma-like lesion: a report of three additional cases and review of the literature. *Head Neck Pathol.* Published on-line 2017 August 7;doi:10.1007/s12105-017-0845-7.

Peripheral Odontogenic Fibroma

Alaeddini M, Salehizadeh S, Baghaii F, et al. A retrospective analysis of peripheral odontogenic fibroma in an Iranian population. *J Oral Maxillofac Surg.* 2010;68:2099–2103.

Buchner A, Merrell PW, Carpenter WM. Relative frequency of peripheral odontogenic tumors: a study of 45 new cases and comparison with studies from the literature. *J Oral Pathol Med.* 2006;35:385–391.

Reddy SV, Medikonda SK, Konda A, et al. A rare benign odontogenic neoplasm: peripheral odontogenic fibroma. *BMJ Case Rep.* 2014;doi:10.1136/bcr-2013-201065.

Ritwik P, Brannon RB. Peripheral odontogenic fibroma: a clinico-pathologic study of 151 cases and review of the literature with special emphasis on recurrence. *Oral Surg Oral Med Oral Pathol Oral Radiol Endod.* 2010;110:357–363.

Truschnegg A, Acham S, Kiefer BA, et al. Epulis: a study of 92 cases with special emphasis on histopathological diagnosis and associated clinical data. *Clin Oral Invest.* 2016;20:1757–1764.

Odontogenic Myxoma

Hammad HM, Hasen YM, Odat A-AM, et al. Odontogenic myxoma with diffuse calcifications: a case report and review of a rare histologic feature. *Oral Surg Oral Med Oral Pathol Oral Radiol.* 2016;122:e116–e124.

Kawase-Koga Y, Saijo H, Hoshi K, et al. Surgical management of odontogenic myxoma: a case report and review of the literature. *BMC Research Notes.* 2014;7:214.

Lahey E, Woo S-B, Park H-K. Odontogenic myxoma with diffuse calcifications: a case report and review of the literature. *Head Neck Pathol.* 2013;7:97–102.

Murphy C, Hayes R, McDermott M, et al. Odontogenic myxoma of the maxilla: surgical management and case report. *Ir J Med Sci.* 2017;186:243–246.

Titinchi F, Hassan BA, Morkel JA, et al. Odontogenic myxoma: a clinicopathological study in a South African population. *J Oral Pathol Med.* 2016;45:599–604.

Dermatologic Diseases

Ectodermal Dysplasia

Figs. **16.1 and 16.2**

Approximately 170 different, well-defined, heritable conditions make up the group of disorders that fall under the heading of **ectodermal dysplasia**. These disorders are characterized by either aplasia or hypoplasia of ectodermally derived anatomic structures, including the skin and its appendages, nails, and teeth. Any of the various types of inheritance patterns may be associated with ectodermal dysplasia, depending on the particular type. One of the more common and widely known examples is X-linked hypohidrotic ectodermal dysplasia. These patients typically have reduced numbers of sweat glands (thus, hypohidrotic); fine, sparse hair; oligodontia with conically shaped anterior teeth; and saddle nose deformity. Other features that may be evident include reduced eyebrow and eyelash hairs; brittle, dystrophic nails; fine skin creases at the lateral aspect of the eyes; and midface hypoplasia.

Because of the reduction in eccrine sweat glands and subsequent decreased sweat production, these patients are often intolerant to warm temperatures. The reduction in the number of teeth and the shape of the teeth results in both functional and aesthetic problems.

Genetic counseling is appropriate for these patients and their families. Management of the dental problems can be difficult, requiring the expertise of prosthodontists and, potentially, implant specialists. Fixed and removable appliances, as well as overdentures, can be fabricated. For older children, dental implant placement may enhance restorative possibilities.

White Sponge Nevus

Fig. **16.3**

White sponge nevus is a benign heritable process that is caused by any one of a variety of mutations of the genes responsible for production of either keratin type 4 or 13. This uncommon autosomal dominant disorder is characterized by white plaques affecting the oral mucosa, although nasal, vaginal, esophageal, and anal mucosa also may be affected.

The oral lesions often are detected in the first or second decade of life, usually presenting as bilateral thick, white plaques involving the buccal mucosa. These lesions typically have blending, indistinct margins, unlike leukoplakia, which usually exhibits sharply demarcated margins. Other oral mucosal sites can also be affected, including the labial mucosa, lingual mucosa, floor of the mouth, and palate. Typically the lesions are asymptomatic, although they may be susceptible to superimposed candidiasis, which could result in some degree of irritation. A family history of the problem may be present, but this is not absolutely necessary for diagnosis because the affected patient may have acquired a new gene mutation.

Biopsy of the lesions shows a thick, superficial layer of parakeratin and increased thickness of the spinous layer, usually with clearing of the cytoplasm of the spinous cells. High-power examination of the spinous cells often shows perinuclear eosinophilic condensation of keratin tonofilaments, which is a characteristic feature. Frequently, this finding is more evident upon examination of a Papanicolaou-stained exfoliative cytologic preparation.

Treatment is generally not necessary because of the benign nature of the condition. However, the clinician should be aware of white sponge nevus to avoid confusion with leukoplakia, which is a potentially malignant process.

■ Figure **16.1**
Ectodermal Dysplasia
Sparse scalp hair with absence of eyelashes and eyebrow hair in a patient affected by X-linked hypohidrotic ectodermal dysplasia. (Courtesy Dr. Marco T. Padilla.)

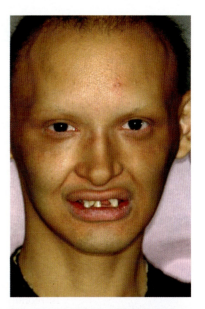

■ Figure **16.2**
Ectodermal Dysplasia
Same patient as Fig. 16.1, showing a reduced number of teeth with a conical crown shape. (Courtesy Dr. Marco T. Padilla.)

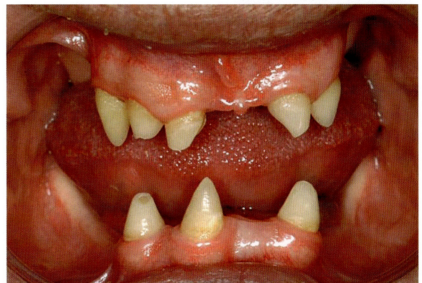

■ Figure **16.3**
White Sponge Nevus
Diffuse white plaques found bilaterally on the buccal mucosa.

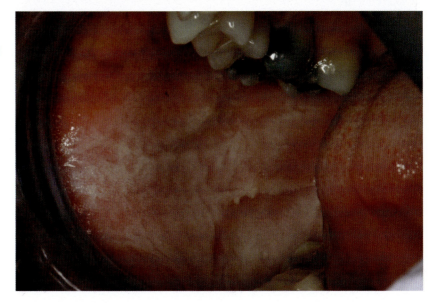

Figs. **16.4–16.6**

Pachyonychia congenita is a small group of conditions that are considered to be part of the spectrum of ectodermal dysplasias. This rare disorder is caused by mutation of one of several specific keratin genes, including *keratin 6a, 6b, 16, or 17*. In the past, pachyonychia congenita was subdivided into the Jackson-Lawler type and the Jadassohn-Lewandowsky type; however, modern genetic analysis now reveals that classification that is based on the specific genetically altered keratin is more accurate and appropriate. Most patients who have prominent oral lesions show mutations of *keratin 6a*, although the other mutations may also have some degree of oral involvement.

In many instances, the cutaneous lesions are the most prominent aspect of this condition, with alterations in the appearance of the nails being most prominent. Due to the accumulation of keratin under the nail bed, the nails develop a tubular configuration at a very early age. Eventually this deformity may lead to loss of the nail. Thick, callus-like lesions form on the palmar and plantar surfaces, and the plantar lesions may become fissured and painful. The plantar changes are particularly symptomatic, presumably due to the development of blisters that form beneath the thickened keratin layer. Accumulation of keratin within the hair follicles results in a pattern of cutaneous punctate papules.

Intraorally, white plaques tend to develop on the lateral and dorsal aspects of the tongue, although other areas that are subject to chronic frictional trauma, such as the palate, buccal mucosa, and alveolar mucosa, may develop similar keratoses. Patients who have *keratin 17* mutations tend to present with neonatal teeth; however, the keratotic oral mucosal changes are not seen as frequently in these individuals.

As with white sponge nevus, the oral lesions of pachyonychia congenita are harmless and require no treatment. Management of the nail, palmar, and plantar lesions can be challenging. Removal of infected nails may be necessary, and attempts at reducing the degree of keratin accumulation have to be continuous. Retinoids may help in this process, but the side effects of these medications sometimes limit their use. Genetic counseling is appropriate for patients with this condition, and prenatal diagnosis can be accomplished by genetic analysis of chorionic villus samples.

■ Figure **16.4**
Pachyonychia Congenita
Thickened, fissured hyperkeratosis of the plantar skin in an affected patient.

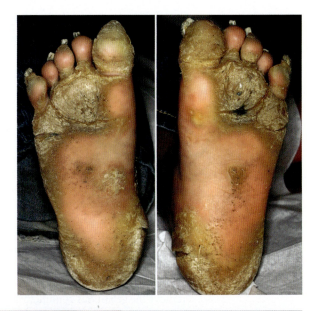

■ Figure **16.5**
Pachyonychia Congenita
Tubular, arched toenails and fingernails are the result of increased inappropriate keratin production.

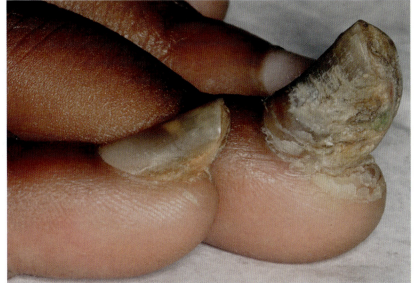

■ Figure **16.6**
Pachyonychia Congenita
Subtle white plaques are noted on the buccal mucosa of this patient, although a range of severity may be present.

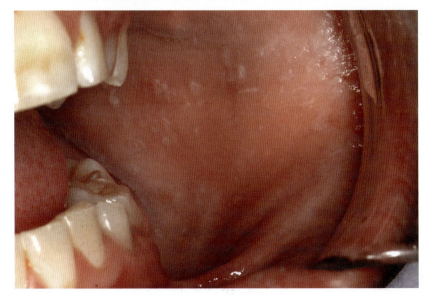

Figs. **16.7 and 16.8**

Hereditary benign intraepithelial dyskeratosis (HBID) represents a very rare heritable autosomal dominant condition that affects the oral and conjunctival mucosa. HBID was initially described in an isolated population of the Haliwa-Saponi Native American people in the northeastern area of North Carolina in the United States. A handful of affected individuals who do not appear to have a relation to this group also have been reported. The causative genetic alteration continues to be debated.

Lesions typically begin to develop in childhood, presenting as gelatinous or granular plaques with pronounced vascularity involving the bulbar conjunctiva. Occasionally the plaques can grow over the cornea, obstructing vision. Irritation may be associated with the ocular lesions, and some patients report seasonal variation in their severity.

Oral lesions usually present as asymptomatic thickened white plaques of the buccal and labial mucosae, floor of the mouth, and tongue. Microscopically these lesions show marked acanthosis and parakeratosis with dyskeratotic changes, including a "cell-within-a-cell" pattern within the lesional epithelium.

No treatment is typically necessary for this benign condition, particularly with respect to the oral lesions. Artificial tears may provide some relief for patients who develop ocular irritation, but attempts to remove the gelatinous conjunctival plaques may result in recurrence. However, significant visual impairment is relatively uncommon.

Fig. **16.9**

Hereditary mucoepithelial dysplasia is a rare autosomal dominant condition that also may occur sporadically. This condition is characterized by epithelial cells that do not develop normally, although the precise mechanism for this disrupted development is unclear. Skin, hair, and mucosal tissues may be affected, with atypical cells being found histopathologically, although these do not have any premalignant potential. Because the mucosal epithelial cells appear atypical microscopically, Papanicolaou-stained cytologic preparations (Pap smears) of the uterine cervical mucosa may be interpreted as showing cancer or precancerous changes, and hysterectomy has been performed inappropriately in some cases.

Clinically these patients have alopecia (reduced hair) affecting the scalp, eyebrows, and eyelashes, and the hair that is present appears coarse. Conjunctival erythema, corneal erosions, cataracts, and nystagmus may be present, and patients often have impaired vision. A rash often develops in the perineal region of affected infants. Pulmonary complications tend to develop later in life and include disruption of the alveoli, recurrent pneumonia, pulmonary fibrosis, and pneumothorax.

Oral mucosal changes consist primarily of a striking bright red appearance of the palatal mucosa, primarily affecting the anterior hard palate. The gingivae and tongue also may be affected, to a lesser extent. Despite the erythema, the lesions are essentially asymptomatic. Other mucosal surfaces, including the previously mentioned vaginal mucosa, may be affected.

Genetic counseling is an important aspect of managing this condition, and women should alert their healthcare providers to the presence of this disorder so that their Pap smear is not misinterpreted. Periodic reevaluation for pulmonary complications is appropriate as these patients age.

■ Figure **16.7**
Hereditary Benign Intraepithelial Dyskeratosis
Thickened white appearance of the buccal mucosa. (Courtesy Dr. Alice Curran.)

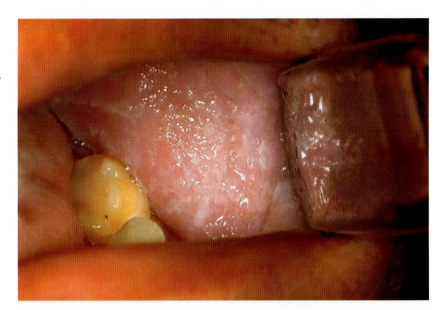

■ Figure **16.8**
Hereditary Benign Intraepithelial Dyskeratosis
Gelatinous plaque of the bulbar conjunctiva of the left eye. (Courtesy Dr. Valerie Murrah.)

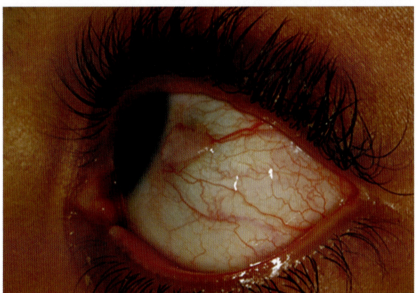

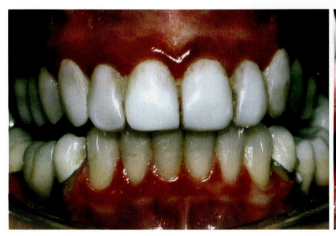
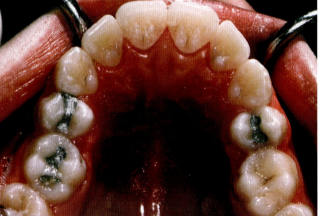

■ Figure **16.9**
Hereditary Mucoepithelial Dysplasia
Striking red appearance of the attached gingivae and the anterior portion of the hard palate mucosa.

Dyskeratosis congenita also is considered to be one of the ectodermal dysplasias. This rare condition is caused by mutation of any one of nine different genes that are responsible for producing telomerase and its associated factors, which are necessary for maintaining the length of chromosomal telomeres. Telomeres are found on the ends of chromosomes, and normally with each cell division, they tend to shorten. Telomerase activity adds some of that length back, but eventually the telomeres become too short and the cell undergoes senescence, as eventually the entire organism does. One of the genes that is responsible for maintaining the length of the telomeres is *DKC1*. Because *DKC1* was the first mutation that was identified in dyskeratosis congenita, and this mutation was inherited as an X-linked recessive disorder, the assumption was that all cases of dyskeratosis congenita were inherited in this fashion. It is now known that the other mutations that can cause this disorder can have either autosomal dominant or recessive inheritance patterns.

The characteristic features of dyskeratosis congenita begin to appear, on average, around 8 years of age. Oral leukoplakia, nail dystrophy (including loss of nails), and reticular hyperpigmentation and hypopigmentation of the skin of the back and trunk comprise a triad of features that are associated with this disorder. The increased risk of oral squamous cell carcinoma is very high, with the median age of diagnosis being 32 years. Cutaneous squamous cell carcinoma rates are elevated, as well as gastrointestinal cancers. Bone marrow failure, so-called myelodysplastic syndrome, is also common, and these patients are at risk of developing acute myelomonocytic leukemia. In addition, these patients will have increased risk of pulmonary fibrosis, probably as a result of degeneration of the lining epithelial cells of the lungs, with replacement by a fibroblastic response. Approximately 10% to 15% of individuals with dyskeratosis congenita will die due to pulmonary fibrosis.

The diagnosis of dyskeratosis congenita can be made based on the triad of characteristic clinical features, although these may not be present in every patient. In such cases, molecular genetic studies can identify shortened telomeres, which are typically less than the first percentile in length.

Management of this disorder is challenging. Genetic counseling is certainly appropriate. Bone marrow transplant may be helpful in reducing the risk of hematopoietic malignancies, but the conditioning regimen prior to the transplant itself may result in tissue damage that leads to complications such as pulmonary fibrosis.

Xeroderma Pigmentosum

Fig. **16.12**

Xeroderma pigmentosum is a rare autosomal recessive disorder that is characterized by extreme sensitivity of the skin to ultraviolet light exposure. Affected patients are susceptible to sunburns caused by minimal sun exposure and by the development of numerous cutaneous malignancies at a very early age, often beginning in the first decade of life. The condition is caused by mutation of any one of seven different genes that participate in nucleotide excision repair of DNA. When cutaneous keratinocytes are exposed to ultraviolet light, damage to the normal DNA structure will occur. Without recognition, excision, and repair of this damaged DNA, keratinocyte mutations may result, a process that leads to a greatly increased risk for malignancy.

The cutaneous changes are often first noticed when an affected child is first exposed to sunlight, resulting in a severe sunburn after a small amount of time. Basal cell and squamous cells carcinomas often develop in the first decade of life, and melanoma typically presents in the second decade. Variation in the color of the skin (poikiloderma) appears as areas with variable amounts of melanin pigmentation. Cataract formation and other ocular disorders, dwarfism, gonadal hypoplasia, and neurologic degeneration also may be seen. An increased risk of squamous cell carcinoma of the anterior tongue has been described in these patients.

No cure for xeroderma pigmentosum exists. Patients who avoid all ultraviolet light (sunlight) exposure will have delayed onset of their cutaneous malignancies. Early tumors can be excised, followed by skin grafting from nonexposed areas of skin. Death is usually related to complications of cutaneous squamous cell carcinoma or metastatic melanoma.

■ Figure **16.10**
Dyskeratosis Congenita
The tongue appears atrophic and exhibits focal areas of leukoplakia.

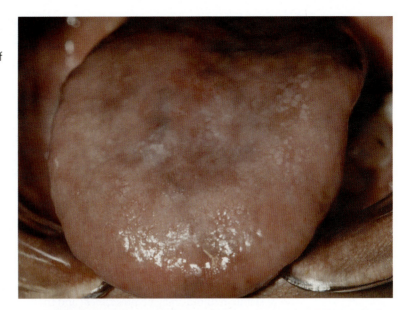

■ Figure **16.11**
Dyskeratosis Congenita
The absence of fingernails is one of several cutaneous manifestations of this disorder.

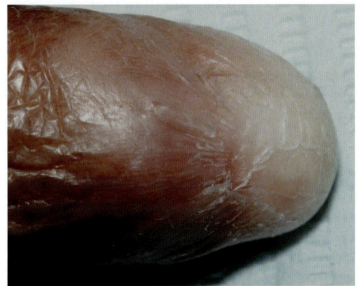

■ Figure **16.12**
Xeroderma Pigmentosum
This 21-year-old patient has had several procedures to remove cutaneous malignancies and actinic keratoses from his facial skin.

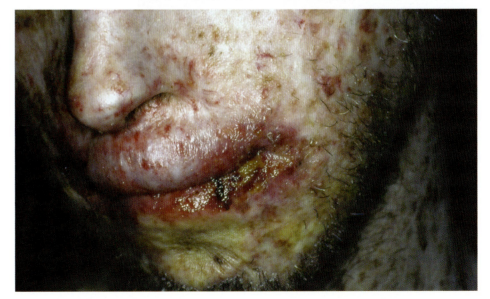

Darier Disease

Figs. **16.13 and 16.14**

Darier disease, also known as *keratosis follicularis*, is an autosomal dominant condition that is caused by mutation of the *ATP2A2* gene. This gene encodes for sarco/endoplasmic reticulum ATPase type 2 (SERCA2), which is a calcium pump associated with the endoplasmic reticulum. Although this disorder may be seen in families, as many as 50% of cases may represent new mutations. Currently, the mechanism by which the altered calcium metabolism causes the changes seen in the surface epithelium is unknown.

Cutaneous lesions of Darier disease usually are noticed during childhood, appearing as erythematous to brown papules that are sometimes so numerous that they coalesce. The facial skin, as well as the skin of the trunk and chest, may be affected preferentially. Accumulations of keratin can become malodorous at times.

Oral lesions present as white, flat-topped papules that may be sparse; however, they can be so numerous that they produce a cobblestone texture. The hard palate and attached gingivae are typically affected.

The cutaneous lesions tend to be uncomfortable in warm temperatures or humid environments, so minimizing these situations is desirable. Treatment is directed at reducing the amount of keratin. This can be done by removing the accumulating keratin with mild abrasion or by use of keratolytic agents. Alternatively, systemic retinoids may be prescribed, and these seem to limit keratin production. However, care must be exercised with respect to side effects of retinoids.

Warty Dyskeratoma

Fig. **16.15**

Warty dyskeratoma, also known as *localized Darier disease*, is a very uncommon lesion that can develop on either the skin or oral mucosa. The cause is unknown, although the microscopic features are very similar to those of Darier disease.

Intraorally, the condition is characterized by the development of a small papule, typically less than 5 mm in diameter, on the keratinized mucosa of the palate or attached gingiva. The papule may show a central white, keratotic plug, although this plug may be sloughed out, leaving a red central area. The lesion is generally asymptomatic. The diagnosis is established by excisional biopsy, which is curative.

■ Figure **16.13**
Darier Disease
Confluent erythematous papules and erosions characterize the cutaneous lesions of this condition.

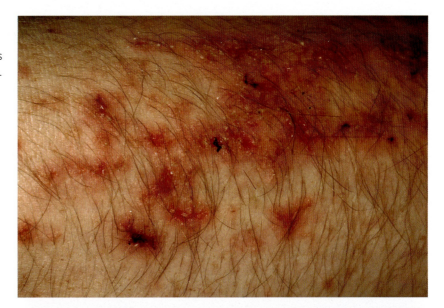

■ Figure **16.14**
Darier Disease
Numerous umbilicated papules affect the hard palate and attached gingivae.

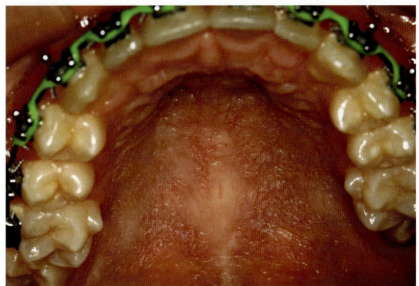

■ Figure **16.15**
Warty Dyskeratoma
A solitary papule with a central erythematous erosion that develops after its keratin plug is lost. (Courtesy Dr. Jeff Barnes.)

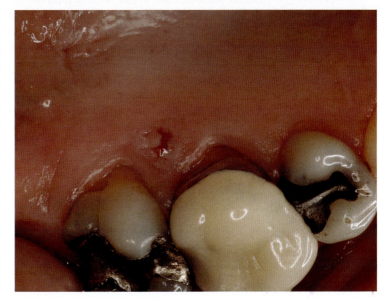

Fig. **16.16**

Peutz-Jeghers syndrome is an autosomal dominant condition that is caused by mutation of a tumor suppressor gene, *STK11*, which encodes for a serine/threonine kinase. Affected individuals have polyps that form primarily in the small intestine, but these do not undergo malignant transformation. Because the polyps may become relatively large, intussusception (the sliding of a proximal segment of bowel into a distal segment) can cause significant problems due to potential ischemic necrosis of the involved bowel, resulting in rupture, spillage of contents, and peritonitis. However, these patients do have an increased incidence of cancer affecting the gastrointestinal tract (although the polyps do not appear to undergo malignant transformation), ovary, breast, and male and female reproductive tract.

In many cases, the oral lesions are the first indication of the disorder. Brown macular lesions that resemble freckles develop on the skin around body orifices, such as the mouth, nose, genitals, and anus. The lesions can also extend intraorally to involve the buccal mucosa and tongue; the fingers also can be affected.

These patients and their families should receive genetic counseling. In addition, periodic evaluation to monitor for the development of intussusception, as well as malignancy, is recommended.

Hereditary Hemorrhagic Telangiectasia

Figs. **16.17 and 16.18**

Hereditary hemorrhagic telangiectasia, also known as *Osler-Weber-Rendu* syndrome, is an uncommon autosomal dominant condition that is caused by mutation of either one of two genes, although the clinical presentation of both mutations is quite similar. HHT1 is caused by mutation of the *endoglin (ENG)* gene (located on chromosome 9). On the other hand, HHT2 is caused by mutation of *activin receptor-like kinase-1 (ALK1; ACVRL1)* gene, which is located on chromosome 12. These mutations result in the development of multiple superficial vascular malformations involving the nasal mucosa and other mucosal surfaces. Often the diagnosis of this disorder is suggested by a history of frequent epistaxis. Further evaluation may identify additional family members who are affected.

The oral lesions are characterized by multiple, flat to slightly elevated, red lesions that are usually 1 to 2 mm in diameter, described as mat-like telangiectasias. Upon diascopy (pressing a clean glass slide against the lesion), blanching of the lesion should be easily demonstrated, as the blood in the lesional vessels is pushed into the surrounding vasculature. The oral lesions are usually seen on the lips, labial mucosa, buccal mucosa, and tongue, but any intraoral site may be affected.

Although these small telangiectatic collections do not present any problems with respect to dental care, laser ablation of the more cosmetically problematic lesions could be considered. More importantly, a significant percentage of these patients, particularly those with HHT1, have been shown to have pulmonary or cerebral vascular shunts, which may predispose them to cerebral abscess formation. To prevent this from happening, some investigators have recommended that prophylactic antibiotics be given prior to dental procedures that cause bacteremia.

■ Figure **16.16**
Peutz-Jeghers Syndrome
Multiple lentigines, ranging from brown to black in color, are often found in a periorificial pattern, although the oral mucosa is frequently affected as well. (Courtesy Dr. Asadur Jorge Tchekmedyian.)

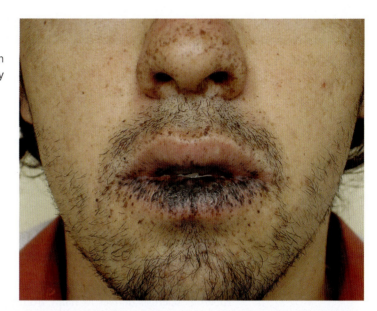

■ Figure **16.17**
Hereditary Hemorrhagic Telangiectasia
These erythematous papules and macules on the dorsal tongue represent focal superficial collections of small blood vessels.

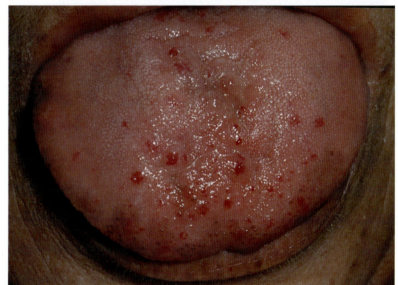

■ Figure **16.18**
Hereditary Hemorrhagic Telangiectasia
Vascular lesions are noted on this patient's hard palate.

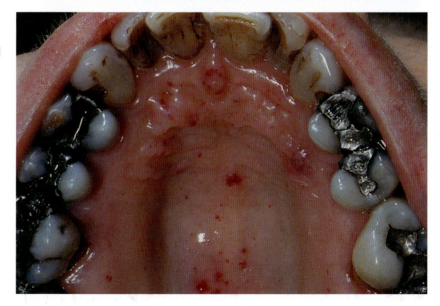

Figs. **16.19–16.21**

Tuberous sclerosis is an uncommon autosomal dominant condition that is caused by mutations associated with either one of two tumor suppressor genes—*TSC1* and *TSC2*—which are found on chromosomes 9 and 16, respectively. Mutation of either of these genes results in a characteristic pattern of clinical findings, including intellectual disability, a variety of hamartomatous growths, and seizure disorders. The hamartomatous growths are thought to be induced by disruption of a tumor suppressor pathway that no longer functions normally. Patients with the *TSC2* mutation seem to have a more severe presentation.

Angiofibromas of the facial skin are one of the more common lesions seen in tuberous sclerosis, presenting as multiple small (1 to 3 mm) papules that develop primarily on the perinasal skin, especially in the nasolabial folds. Similar smooth-surfaced papules, termed *periungual fibromas*, may be found on the skin adjacent to the nails. *Shagreen patches* are superficial connective tissue hamartomas that produce velvety areas of the skin, and their name is derived from the polishing cloths made from shark skin that have this designation. Small, ovoid areas of hypopigmentation, termed *ash leaf spots*, are seen commonly in tuberous sclerosis and are best visualized by using a Wood (ultraviolet) lamp. Other characteristic hamartomas associated with tuberous sclerosis include angiomyolipoma of the kidney and cardiac rhabdomyoma.

Tuberous sclerosis derives its name from the dense, potato-like hamartomatous growths of the brain that are often identified at autopsy of an affected individual. Other central nervous system findings include seizure disorders, experienced by many of these patients, and intellectual disability, found in approximately one-third.

Oral manifestations may include fibrous papules of anterior facial gingiva, although other oral sites, such as the tongue, lips, palate, and buccal mucosa also may be affected. The gingival enlargement that has been reported in these patients is probably caused by treatment of their associated seizure disorder with phenytoin in most cases. Radiolucencies of the jaws may also develop, and upon biopsy, these typically contain dense fibrous connective tissue. Pitting enamel defects are also relatively common in these patients, especially on the facial aspect of the permanent anterior teeth.

Genetic counseling is recommended for patients and families affected by this disorder. Prenatal genetic testing for the responsible mutations can be used for family planning, if desired. Management of the seizure disorder of the tuberous sclerosis patient is important, although monitoring for other potential associated problems is necessary as well.

■ Figure **16.19**
Tuberous Sclerosis
The papules involving the midfacial skin represent angiofibromas. (Courtesy Dr. Alfredo Aguirre.)

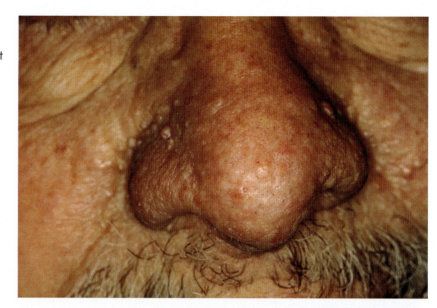

■ Figure **16.20**
Tuberous Sclerosis
Periungual fibromas are a characteristic finding in this condition.

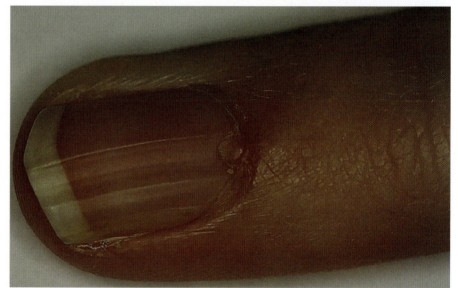

■ Figure **16.21**
Tuberous Sclerosis
Multiple papules and nodules may occasionally affect the oral mucosa. (Courtesy Dr. Alfredo Aguirre.)

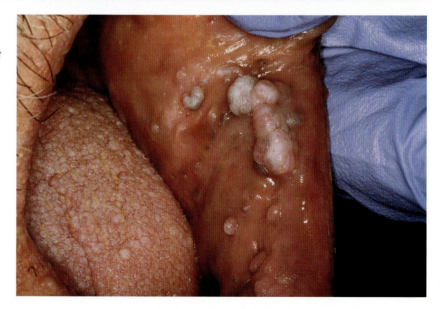

Multiple hamartoma syndrome, also known as *Cowden syndrome*, is a rare autosomal dominant disorder that was named after the first patient who was identified with this condition. The condition is caused by mutation of the *PTEN (phosphatase and tensin homologue deleted on chromosome 10)* gene, which has overlapping features with other disorders associated with mutations of this gene, including Proteus-like syndrome, Bannayan-Riley-Ruvalcaba syndrome, and Lhermitte-Duclos disease (a hamartomatous tumor of the cerebellum). Although several different benign tumors and hamartomas develop in this syndrome, the most important aspect is that an increased incidence of various malignancies is seen, including breast carcinoma, follicular carcinoma of the thyroid, ovarian and endometrial carcinoma, and gastrointestinal adenocarcinoma.

Mucocutaneous manifestations are among the most common signs of this disorder, developing in the first or second decade of life. Hair follicle hamartomas called *trichilemmomas* occur as multiple small papules on the facial skin around the eyes, nose, and mouth. Oral *fibroepithelial polyps* are very common, affecting the labial mucosa, buccal mucosa, dorsal tongue, and gingivae. Small superficial keratotic plaques, called *acral keratoses*, can affect the dorsal surface of the hands, and palmar keratoses also can develop.

A variety of benign tumors also may develop, such as lipomas, angiomas, polyps of the gastrointestinal tract and urethra, thyroid adenomas, and central nervous system tumors such as meningioma.

The diagnosis is based on the clinical presentation and necessitates identification of a certain number of features that have been designated as major and minor criteria. Currently, genetic testing for this disorder, although often performed, is not completely reliable as a diagnostic tool, primarily because the *PTEN* mutation cannot be detected in all patients who otherwise have a well-documented diagnosis of this condition.

Management includes genetic counseling of patients and their families. Treatment of the benign tumors and hamartomas may be performed on an as-needed basis. Careful monitoring of these patients for malignancies is mandatory, and some investigators have recommended prophylactic mastectomy for affected women due to the high risk of their developing breast cancer.

■ Figure **16.22**
Multiple Hamartoma Syndrome
Multiple papules involving the keratinized and non-keratinized mucosa. (Courtesy Dr. Lynn Wallace.)

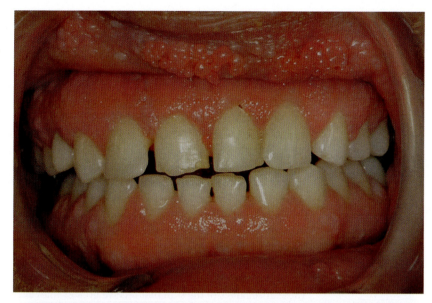

■ Figure **16.23**
Multiple Hamartoma Syndrome
Multiple papules of the dorsal tongue. (Courtesy Dr. Lynn Wallace.)

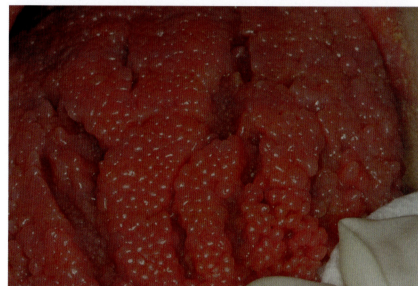

■ Figure **16.24**
Multiple Hamartoma Syndrome
Multiple papules of the hard palate. (Courtesy Dr. Lynn Wallace.)

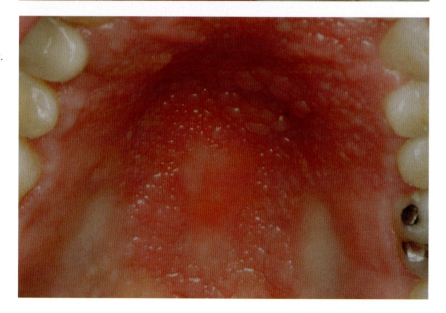

Figs. **16.25 and 16.26**

Epidermolysis bullosa (EB) refers to a group of uncommon inherited disorders that are all characterized by mutation of at least one of the various surface epithelial cell attachment mechanisms. Sometimes the affected target is related to epithelial cell–to–epithelial cell attachment and, in other instances, to epithelial cell–to–connective tissue attachment. All forms of EB have some degree of fragility of the skin. Some forms of the condition are rather mild and merely constitute a nuisance (e.g., EB simplex type), whereas other forms are lethal or severely debilitating (such as EB junctional type). At least 44 different subtypes of EB have been described, and these are distributed among four major groups, most having either an autosomal dominant or autosomal recessive inheritance pattern. In addition, there is a rare acquired autoimmune blistering disorder, known as *EB acquisita*, that is nonhereditary. Discussion will center on the dystrophic group because these have the most relevance to the oral region. Both autosomal dominant and autosomal recessive dystrophic EB have mutations in the *COL7A1* gene, which is responsible for production of type VII collagen. The phenotypic expression appears to reflect the degree to which the mutation disrupts the production of normal type VII collagen.

Patients with dominant dystrophic EB will develop vesicles and bullae with relatively minor injury. These affect areas of the skin that receive greater than average trauma, such as the fingers, elbows, or knees. The blisters rupture and eventually heal with scarring. Over a period of years, the nails are typically lost as a result of repeated injury. Oral vesicles and bullae may also occur, and it is not unusual for the buccal vestibule to be reduced in depth due to adhesions that develop after the bullae rupture. However, this condition is usually not life threatening.

In contrast, recessive dystrophic EB is a more serious blistering disorder. Affected patients develop bullae with minimal trauma, both on the skin and intraorally. Management of this condition requires minimizing any type of frictional trauma to the skin, although it is virtually impossible to prevent bullae from forming. Treating the denuded cutaneous lesions after the bullae have ruptured is challenging due to secondary bacterial contamination, and scarring is characteristic after healing. Eventual development of cutaneous squamous cell carcinoma in these areas is common. The fingers and toes become encased in scar tissue as well, after multiple episodes of bulla formation, healing, and development of adhesions. This results in the so-called mitten deformity of the hands.

Oral vesicles and bullae may develop when the patient ingests any food that has any resistance to chewing and swallowing. Routine toothbrushing results in stripping of the gingival epithelium, and, as a result of decreased oral hygiene and a soft diet that is often rich in carbohydrates, the rate of dental caries is markedly increased. Microstomia and ankyloglossia result after multiple episodes of perioral and intraoral blistering, with subsequent scarring, contracture, and adhesions.

The approach to management depends on the type of EB. Genetic counseling is generally appropriate. Recessive dystrophic EB is one of the more challenging forms of this condition, typically requiring input from various medical specialists, dental specialists, nurses, and physical therapists. Topical fluoride treatments and a soft, noncariogenic diet should be instituted from a young age. If dental restorative procedures are necessary, they should be carried out in an atraumatic fashion, if possible.

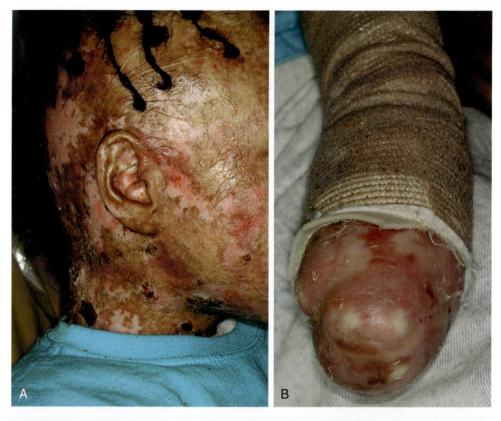

■ Figure 16.25
Epidermolysis Bullosa

(A) Multiple areas of scarring develop after healing of blisters associated with the autosomal recessive form of epidermolysis bullosa. Secondary hypopigmentation and hyperpigmentation is evident. (B) So-called mitten deformity of the hand, a result of multiple episodes of blistering and scarring of the fingers. Typically the bones of the fingers are incorporated within the mass of tissue. (With appreciation to Dr. Michelle Ziegler.)

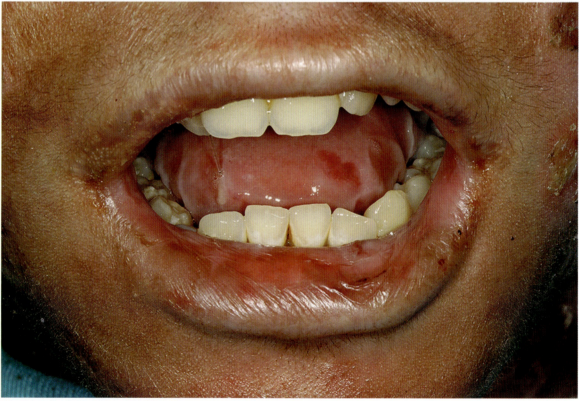

■ Figure 16.26
Epidermolysis Bullosa

Same patient as Fig. 16.25, showing oral and perioral erosions and shallow ulcerations. (With appreciation to Dr. Michelle Ziegler.)

Figs. **16.27–16.30**

Although several different types of **pemphigus** have been described, the only one that exhibits significant oral mucosal involvement is **pemphigus vulgaris**. These rare autoimmune disorders are characterized by production of antibodies that are directed against the desmosomal components known as desmoglein 1 and desmoglein 3. Desmoglein 3 is a critical part of the desmosomal attachment mechanism that binds one epithelial cell to another. As a result of this antibody attack on the desmosomes, the surface epithelial cells detach from one another, and an intraepithelial blister is produced clinically. Because this is an intraepithelial process, the roof of the blister is quite thin and fragile.

Pemphigus vulgaris mostly affects adults, although there are reports of the disease in childhood. In most cases the oral mucosa is the first site of involvement. The blisters can develop on virtually any oral mucosal surface, although they are short-lived and rupture very soon after forming, leaving red erosions and shallow ulcers with ragged margins. These lesions tend to migrate, healing in one area and developing in another, and usually they are painful. Eventually the blisters begin to form on the skin, where they tend to form flaccid bullae that rupture within a few hours to days, leaving raw, erythematous erosions and crusts.

The diagnosis is made by examining a biopsy sample from the perilesional area microscopically and identifying the intraepithelial clefting that usually develops just above the basal cell layer. Confirmation of the diagnosis is done by performing direct immunofluorescence studies on a biopsy taken from adjacent normal-appearing mucosa, submitted in Michel solution. Serum also may be submitted for indirect immunofluorescence studies or enzyme-linked immunosorbent assay (ELISA) testing if the patient is at a tertiary care center that performs these tests.

Prior to the development of modern immunosuppressive therapy, pemphigus patients typically died of complications of their disease, such as dehydration, infection, and electrolyte imbalance. With treatment today, approximately 90% of these patients will experience remission and control of their disease. Treatment generally consists of systemic corticosteroids that are given with another immune-modulating drug (a so-called steroid-sparing agent) to reduce the dose of corticosteroid while still controlling the patient's lesions. These steroid-sparing agents include azathioprine, mycophenolate mofetil, methotrexate, cyclophosphamide, and others. Cases that do not respond to this therapy may be treated with rituximab or intravenous immunoglobulin (IVIg). However, complications of the immunosuppressive treatment may result in death, usually from infection. In the past, 60% to 90% of these patients died of this disease; with modern immunosuppressive regimens, the mortality rate is 5% to 10%.

■ Figure **16.27**
Pemphigus Vulgaris
Partially collapsed bulla on the skin.

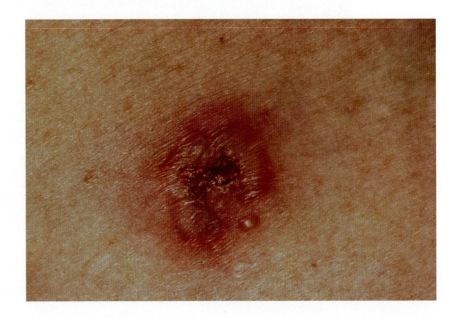

■ Figure **16.28**
Pemphigus Vulgaris
Ragged erosions of the buccal mucosa.

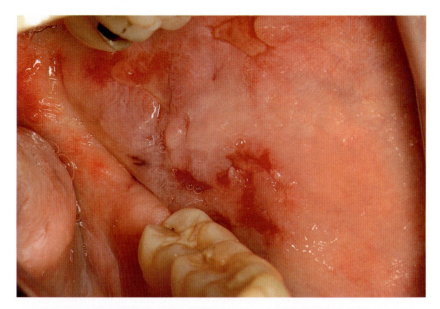

■ Figure **16.29**
Pemphigus Vulgaris
Erythema and ulceration of the palatal mucosa.

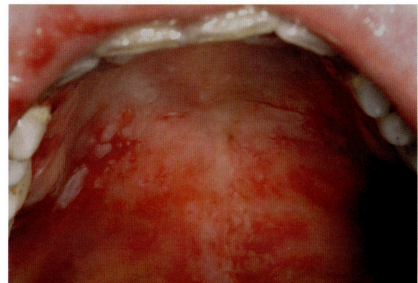

■ Figure **16.30**
Pemphigus Vulgaris
Erosions of the mandibular buccal attached gingiva.

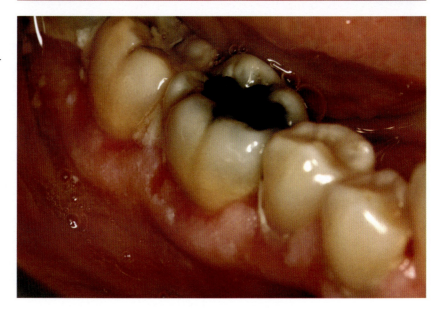

Figs. **16.31–16.34**

Paraneoplastic pemphigus is a rare immune-mediated condition that generally seems to be triggered by the presence of a malignant lymphoreticular process, most commonly lymphocytic lymphoma or leukemia. Benign lymphoid proliferations, such as Castleman disease, as well as cancers other than lymphoreticular malignancies, also may be responsible. Although this is an autoimmune process, similar to pemphigus vulgaris, there is a much greater number of antibodies that are directed against many different antigenic targets of the oral, respiratory, and genital mucosa, as well as the skin. Cytotoxic T lymphocytes also may play a role in some instances. As a result, the presentation of this disease is much more severe than pemphigus vulgaris. Paraneoplastic pemphigus may have overlapping clinical features with pemphigus, pemphigoid, erythema multiforme, and lichen planus.

Affected patients may exhibit erythematous lichenoid cutaneous papules, vesicles, and bullae; severe conjunctivitis that may lead to scarring; and pulmonary symptoms related to bronchiolitis obliterans. A variety of oral lesions can develop, including hemorrhagic crusting of the vermilion zone of the lips, widespread shallow ulcerations preceded by vesicles and bullae, and areas of erythema with lichenoid striae. Typically the patient has already been diagnosed with lymphoma or leukemia, but in one-third of the reported cases, the appearance of paraneoplastic pemphigus resulted in discovery of the neoplasm.

The diagnosis of paraneoplastic pemphigus is often delayed because the patient is usually receiving aggressive chemotherapy for a lymphoreticular malignancy, and this treatment impairs the patient's ability to fight infection. Consequently, paraneoplastic pemphigus is frequently mistaken for a viral or bacterial infection, and it is only after weeks of futile antibiotic treatment and negative culture results that the correct diagnosis is entertained and confirmed. Biopsy of perilesional tissue may show a lichenoid mucositis that is combined with both intraepithelial clefting and subepithelial clefting. Although direct immunofluorescence may show characteristic features of antibody deposition within the tissue, indirect immunofluorescence using rat bladder epithelium as a substrate is considered a more definitive diagnostic test. This should identify diagnostic patterns of intraepithelial and basement membrane deposition of autoantibodies that are circulating in the patient's serum.

If the condition is caused by a benign tumor, such as Castleman disease or thymoma, surgical excision sometimes results in remission of the paraneoplastic pemphigus. Management of cases associated with malignancy can be very challenging because the immunosuppressive therapy that is necessary to control the abnormal antibody production may also allow the patient's tumor to recur. The additional reduction in the patient's immune status will increase the risk for serious infections as well. The prognosis generally is considered to be poor, with some series reporting a 90% mortality rate for these patients.

■ Figure **16.31**
Paraneoplastic Pemphigus
Bullae involving the palmar surface of the hand.

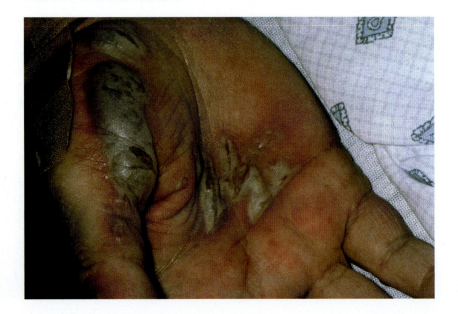

■ Figure **16.32**
Paraneoplastic Pemphigus
Cicatrizing conjunctivitis with ulceration and hemorrhagic crusting of the periocular skin.

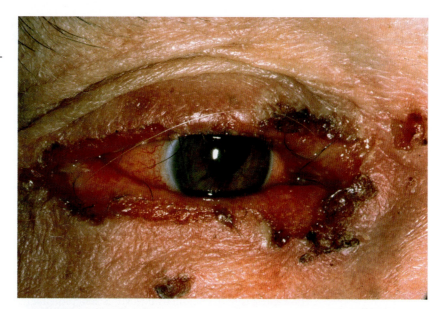

■ Figure **16.33**
Paraneoplastic Pemphigus
Ulceration and hemorrhagic crusting of the vermilion zone of the lips.

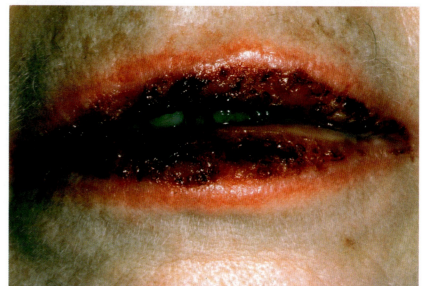

■ Figure **16.34**
Paraneoplastic Pemphigus
Erosions and ulcerations with adjacent white lichenoid striae of the dorsal and lateral tongue.

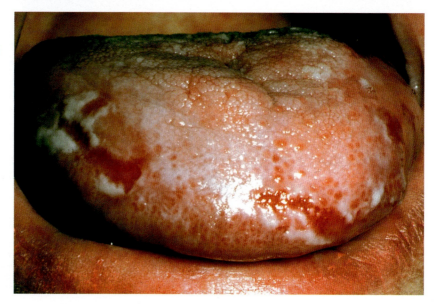

Mucous Membrane Pemphigoid

Figs. **16.35–16.38**

Mucous membrane pemphigoid (MMP), also known as cicatricial (scarring) pemphigoid, is a group of autoimmune disorders that are characterized by the formation of vesicles and bullae, mostly involving the mucosal surfaces (oral, conjunctival, laryngeal, nasal, vaginal). Approximately 20% of these patients may have cutaneous lesions as well. This disorder is caused by the production of autoantibodies that are directed against any one of several antigenic targets that comprise the basement membrane of the mucosa. The anatomic sites and severity of the disease are often dependent on which component of the basement membrane is targeted by the antibody attack.

Most patients who develop MMP are older adults, and children are rarely affected. Individuals may notice vesicles or bullae developing on the oral mucosa, particularly the gingiva and palate, although any oral site may be affected. The blisters rupture within several hours, leaving an irregularly shaped, shallow ulceration with smooth borders. As some lesions heal, others will develop at other sites. Intraoral scarring is usually not a prominent feature.

Although the oral ulcers are painful and annoying, the most significant complication of this condition is conjunctival involvement, which may lead to blindness if not identified early and treated appropriately. The earliest sign of conjunctival MMP is subepithelial fibrosis, a process that requires identification by an ophthalmologic slit-lamp microscopic examination. With continued lesional activity, the fibrosis causes disruption of the various glands that lubricate the surface of the eye, causing significant dryness. This leads to conjunctival inflammation, and scarring (synechiae) can form between the bulbar (globe of the eye) and the palpebral (eyelid lining) conjunctiva. Eventually blindness ensues.

The diagnosis is established by identifying a subepithelial cleft upon examination of perilesional mucosa using routine light microscopy. In addition, adjacent normal mucosa should be submitted in Michel solution for direct immunofluorescence studies, which should confirm a linear band of immunoreactants (usually C3 and IgG) at the basement membrane zone. Once the diagnosis is established, referral of the patient for ophthalmologic examination is appropriate, and this should be repeated every 6 months.

MMP may respond to a variety of treatments, and this may reflect the fact that this process is probably a variety of different diseases with a common immunopathologic feature. Treatment is initially driven by the presence of ocular involvement, which typically requires systemic immunosuppressive therapy. If there are oral lesions only, then treatment is based on how extensive they are. With limited disease, topical corticosteroids may adequately control the problem. With more extensive disease, medications such as systemic corticosteroids, dapsone, mycophenolate mofetil, or other immune suppressive and immune modulating drugs, such as rituximab, may be appropriate.

■ Figure **16.35**
Mucous Membrane Pemphigoid

Intact bullae and vesicles involving the soft palate mucosa. A shallow ulcer with an erythematous periphery is adjacent to the bullae, representing an area where the roof of the bulla has been lost.

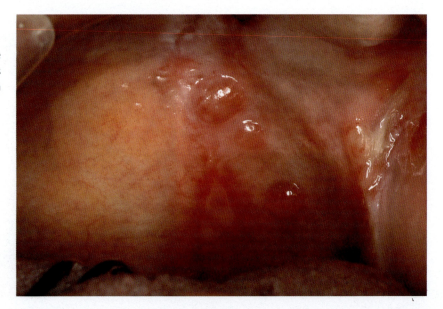

■ Figure **16.36**
Mucous Membrane Pemphigoid
Relatively mild example presenting as erythematous gingivae, the so-called desquamative gingivitis pattern.

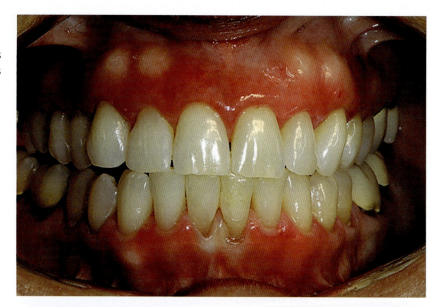

■ Figure **16.37**
Mucous Membrane Pemphigoid
A more severe example of gingival involvement, probably exacerbated by bacterial plaque accumulation.

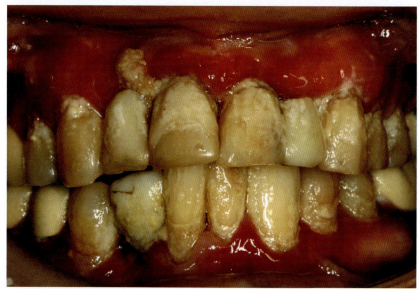

■ Figure **16.38**
Mucous Membrane Pemphigoid
Involvement of the conjunctival mucosa, demonstrating a band of scar tissue between the bulbar and palpebral conjunctiva (symblepharon formation).

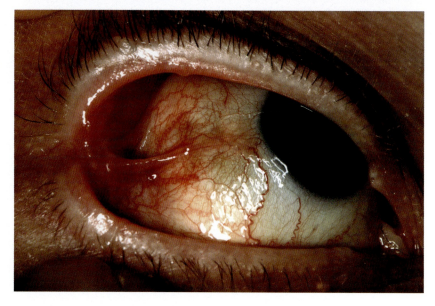

Figs. **16.39–16.42**

Erythema multiforme is an uncommon mucocutaneous disease that is most likely immune mediated, although the precise pathogenetic mechanisms are unclear. Antecedent herpesvirus or mycoplasma infections are often described, and perhaps these somehow trigger the condition. Less commonly, exposure to a drug seems to initiate the disease. A range of severity is seen, with milder forms designated as *erythema multiforme minor*, when only the skin or oral mucosa is involved; more severe cases are termed *erythema multiforme major*, when the skin is involved in addition to at least two mucosal sites.

The onset of this condition is usually relatively rapid, with lesions developing within a day or two. The cutaneous lesions are red, palpable, and usually round, initially developing on the extremities. Variation in the appearance of the lesions may be seen (thus the term "multiforme" = "many forms"), with some being macular and some slightly elevated. The target or bull's-eye lesion is considered a classic sign of erythema multiforme, appearing as concentric red circles, reminiscent of a target. The oral lesions usually present as large, shallow ulcers with irregular margins and an erythematous periphery. These affect the nonkeratinized mucosa primarily, with only rare examples described as involving the attached gingivae or hard palate. Patients are quite uncomfortable and have trouble eating and drinking, so dehydration may develop.

The diagnosis is based on the clinical features, especially if target lesions are present. Although the rapid onset is less characteristic of other immunobullous and erosive conditions, biopsy is often done to rule out these conditions. The microscopic features of erythema multiforme are suggestive but not pathognomonic and require clinical correlation to arrive at the diagnosis.

This condition is typically self-limiting, and usually the lesions resolve over a period of several weeks. Chronic erythema multiforme has been described, and this may respond to antiviral medication, presumably because the triggering herpesvirus is suppressed. A short course of systemic corticosteroids at a moderate dose may hasten healing for some individuals. Recurrences happen occasionally, and for unknown reasons, these tend to develop in the spring and autumn.

Stevens-Johnson syndrome and **toxic epidermal necrolysis** (TEN) were once thought of as representing severe forms of erythema multiforme, but current opinion places these two conditions in a separate category. The triggering agent for these disorders is usually a drug, rather than infection. These conditions may be preceded by fever or flulike illness, followed by development of nonpalpable erythematous lesions that initially develop on the trunk. Oral ulcers are common, appearing similar to those of erythema multiforme. TEN is characterized by large cutaneous bullae that slough rapidly, resulting in significant areas of denuded skin. Patients are susceptible to infection and electrolyte imbalance and typically are managed in the burn unit of a tertiary care center. The mortality rate of TEN often approaches 30% despite such care.

■ **Figure 16.39**
Erythema Multiforme
Characteristic hemorrhagic crusting of the lips.

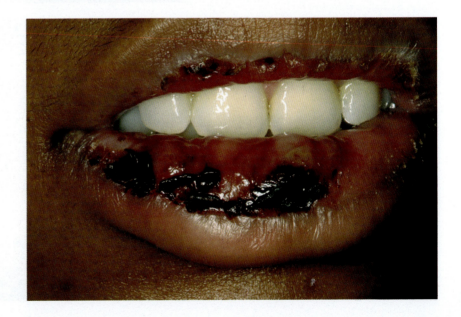

■ Figure **16.40**
Erythema Multiforme
Erythematous round macular lesions of the palmar skin.

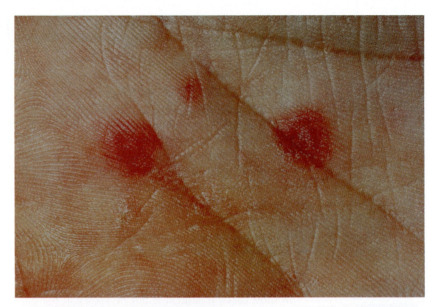

■ Figure **16.41**
Erythema Multiforme
Shallow ulcers with ragged borders, primarily affecting nonkeratinized mucosa. This patient had a history of sulfa drug exposure 1 week earlier.

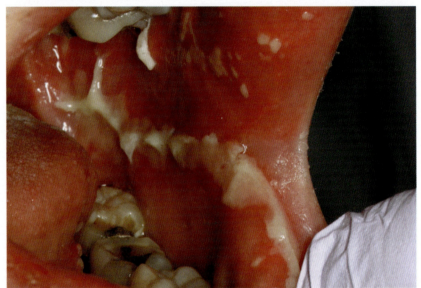

■ Figure **16.42**
Erythema Multiforme
Same patient as Fig. 16.41 after 1 week of treatment with prednisolone syrup.

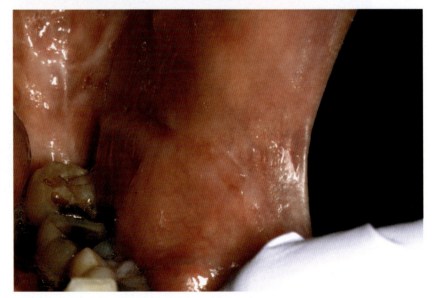

Figs. **16.43–16.46**

Erythema migrans (benign migratory glossitis; geographic tongue) is a common inflammatory condition of unknown etiology. The lesions microscopically resemble those of cutaneous psoriasis, and some studies suggest that patients with psoriasis may have an increased prevalence of oral erythema migrans.

The diagnosis of erythema migrans usually does not require biopsy because of its very characteristic clinical features. The lesions appear as sharply demarcated erythematous patches of atrophy of the filiform papillae of the dorsal tongue, with a tendency to involve the lateral aspects of the dorsum. Each patch usually has a linear yellow-white border by which it is either partially or completely encompassed. The lesional areas persist for a variable period, then the inflammation subsides and the papillae regenerate. Other sites of the dorsal tongue then may develop lesions. Although the dorsal tongue is the most common site of involvement, the lateral and ventral tongue mucosa also are affected rather frequently. Very uncommonly, the soft palate, buccal mucosa, or labial mucosa may develop these lesions, which are characterized by demarcated red patches that are partially or completely surrounded by linear yellow-white borders. In most instances, the lesions are asymptomatic, but some individuals may complain of a mild burning sensation with hot, spicy, or acidic foods when the lesions are active.

In most cases, treatment is not necessary. If the burning sensation is severe enough, application of a thin film of one of the stronger topical corticosteroid gel preparations may provide some relief.

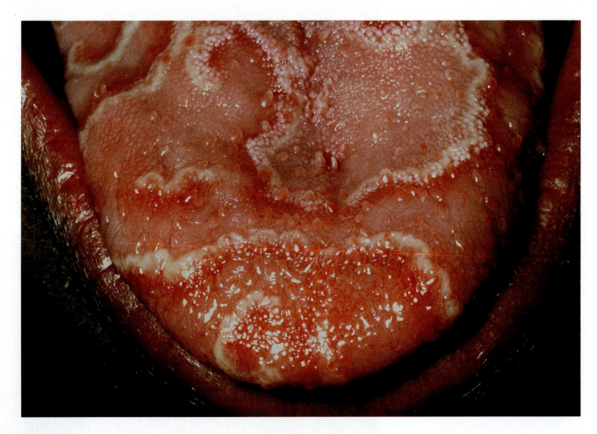

■ Figure **16.43**
Erythema Migrans
Erythematous atrophic patches surrounded by yellow-white linear borders.

■ Figure 16.44
Erythema Migrans
Ovoid erythematous lesions with slightly raised yellow-white borders on the ventral tongue and floor of the mouth.

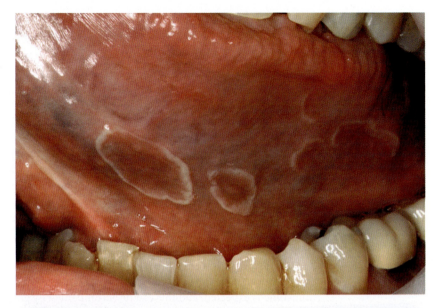

■ Figure 16.45
Erythema Migrans
Involvement of the mandibular labial mucosa.

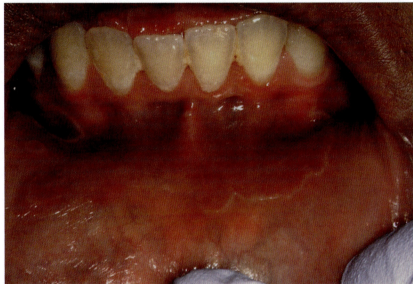

■ Figure 16.46
Erythema Migrans
Semicircular and ringlike lesion of the soft palate mucosa. (Courtesy Dr. Walter Colon.)

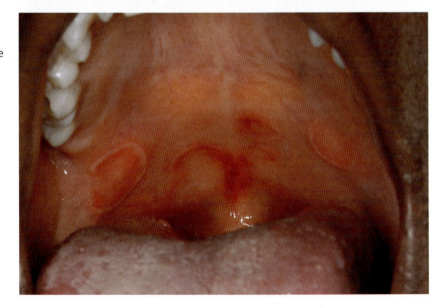

Lichen planus is an immune-mediated disease that was originally described as a skin condition in 1869. The cause is essentially unknown, although there has been much research performed with respect to the pathogenesis of the disorder. The cutaneous lesions appear as purple, polygonal, pruritic papules that affect the skin of the ankles, base of the spine, and wrists most frequently.

Oral involvement can essentially be categorized as reticular and erosive lesions, which probably reflect the intensity of the immunologic reaction. Reticular lichen planus is characterized by the symmetric distribution of interlacing white lines, sometimes with small white papule or plaques, on the posterior buccal mucosa. In addition to these sites, the gingivae and dorsal or lateral tongue are common areas of involvement. Less frequently, the vermilion zone of the lips, the labial mucosa, floor of the mouth, and the palatal mucosa may be affected, but the characteristic bilateral buccal mucosal lesions also should be evident. If they are not evident, then other "lichenoid" conditions (things that clinically mimic oral lichen planus) should be considered.

Oral lichen planus in the erosive phase is seen as shallow ulcers that can vary in size, surrounded by a zone of erythema with fine radiating white striae at the periphery. Symmetric distribution on the buccal mucosae is expected, and this can be accompanied by gingival involvement (a clinical pattern of so-called desquamative gingivitis) or tongue involvement. As with most immune-mediated disorders, the condition may wax and wane in severity without treatment, and it is not unusual for patients to have reticular lichen planus at one appointment and erosive lichen planus at the next one a few weeks later.

Biopsy is often performed to rule out other immune-mediated disorders and potentially cancerous conditions. Although the microscopic features of oral lichen planus are characteristic, they are not pathognomonic, and a variety of other diseases may resemble the pattern of hyperkeratosis, irregular thickness of the spinous layer, pointed rete ridges, disruption of the basal cell layer, and intense subepithelial chronic inflammatory infiltrate. Clinical correlation is often required to rule out conditions such as lichenoid amalgam reaction, lichenoid foreign body gingivitis, lichenoid drug reaction, contact stomatitis, graft-versus-host disease, lupus erythematosus, or an early, lichenoid presentation of proliferative verrucous leukoplakia. Direct immunofluorescence studies would be necessary to rule out chronic ulcerative stomatitis as well.

Whether treatment of lichen planus is necessary depends on the patient's symptoms. Most cases of reticular lichen planus are asymptomatic and require no treatment. Approximately 25% of oral lichen planus cases will have superimposed candidiasis, and this may cause a burning sensation, as well as blurring of the reticular striae. Treatment with a course of clotrimazole oral troches should relieve symptoms within 1 to 2 days after initiating a 10-day course of medication, and often no further treatment is needed. Many patients with erosive lichen planus are symptomatic due to their ulcerations, and they typically complain of pain associated with salty, acidic, or alcoholic foods and drinks. Treatment with one of the stronger topical corticosteroid gel preparations, applied as a thin film only to the areas that are sore, 4 times daily (after meals and at bedtime) usually results in resolution of the ulcers. However, periodic re-treatment of lesions usually is necessary because of the recurrent nature of the disease.

■ Figure **16.47**
Lichen Planus
Close-up image of a lesion of cutaneous lichen planus. Note the white lines (Wickham striae) on the surface of the erythematous plaque.

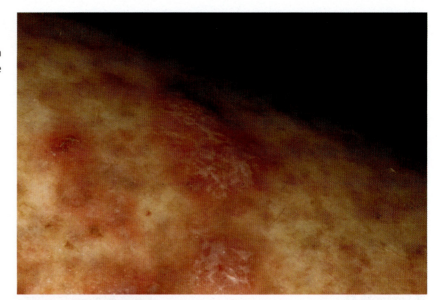

■ Figure **16.48**
Lichen Planus
Classic example of oral lichen planus in a reticular phase. Bilateral involvement would be expected.

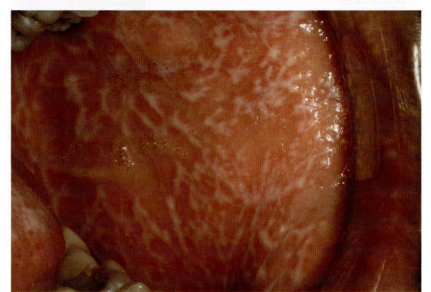

■ Figure **16.49**
Lichen Planus
Interlacing white linear lesions (reticular phase) that tend to have a fine radiating pattern peripherally in some areas. This process affected the buccal mucosa of a person of color, and benign reactive melanosis is noted.

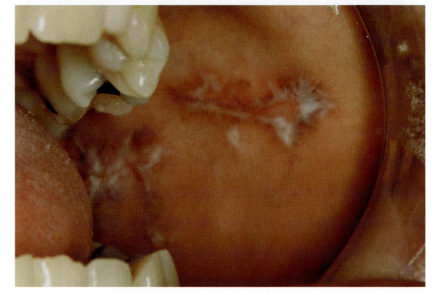

■ Figure **16.50**
Lichen Planus
Dorsal tongue involvement, characterized by flat white plaques and peripheral striae.

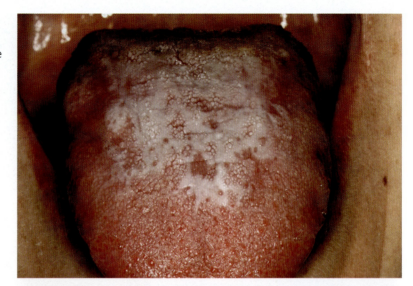

■ Figure **16.51**
Lichen Planus
Reticular white striae involving the vermilion zone of the lower lip.

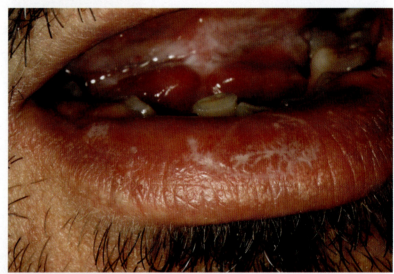

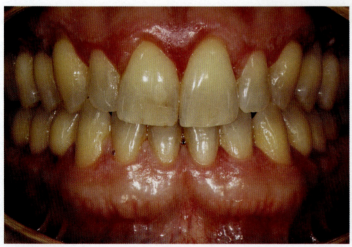
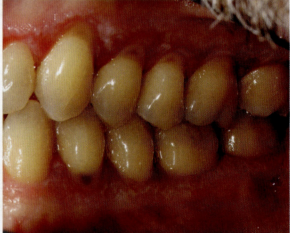

■ Figure **16.52**
Lichen Planus
Gingival lesions showing erythematous zones with peripheral radiating striae. Buccal mucosal involvement also would be expected. If not, then conditions such as lichenoid foreign body gingivitis or contact stomatitis may have to be considered in the differential diagnosis.

■ Figure **16.53**
Lichen Planus

White striations with central erosions on the right buccal mucosa.

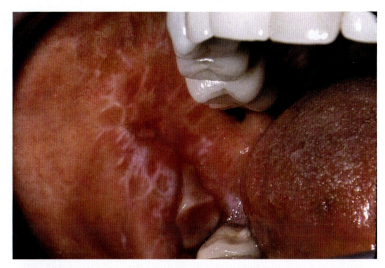

■ Figure **16.54**
Lichen Planus

Same patient as Fig. 16.53 showing similar lesions on the left buccal mucosa.

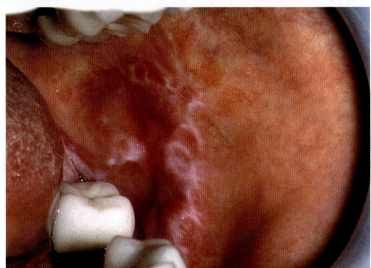

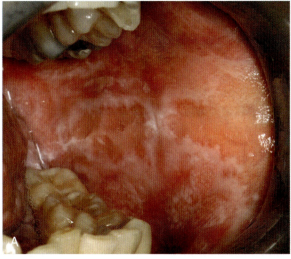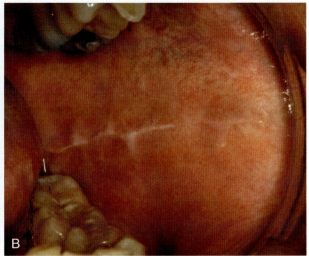

■ Figure **16.55**
Lichen Planus

(A) Relatively severe reticular and erosive lichen planus involving the buccal mucosa. (B) Same patient 1 month after applying a superpotent topical corticosteroid gel preparation to the lesions four times daily for several weeks. A linea alba is present, but the lichen planus has resolved.

Fig. **16.56**

Chronic ulcerative stomatitis, first described in 1989, is a relatively rare, immune-mediated lichenoid process that primarily affects oral mucosa, although skin involvement also has been described. The condition is often confused clinically and histopathologically with erosive lichen planus or other lichenoid conditions, and direct immunofluorescence studies are necessary to make the diagnosis.

This disorder has an adult female predilection and typically involves the tongue, buccal mucosa, and/ or the gingivae. A pattern of desquamative gingivitis is not uncommon, but any intraoral site may be affected. Atrophic, eroded, and ulcerated areas with fine peripheral white striae are seen, although usually the striae are not as crisply defined as in lichen planus. These lesions wax and wane in severity, and tend to heal without scarring in one area, only to develop in another area. Often the symmetric pattern of distribution seen with oral lichen planus is not present.

The diagnostic work-up for this condition often is initiated when a patient presents with oral lesions that seem resistant to topical corticosteroid therapy. Histopathologic findings have been reported to be inadequate to distinguish between oral lichen planus and chronic ulcerative stomatitis. When biopsy for direct immunofluorescence is performed, there is positive immunoreactivity of the stratified squamous epithelial cell nuclei in the basal and parabasal regions. Indirect immunofluorescence studies, using guinea pig or monkey esophagus as a substrate, can provide additional support for the diagnosis.

Although some patients may respond sufficiently to topical application of one of the stronger corticosteroid gel preparations, this is not always the case. In such situations, consideration should be given to treatment with hydroxychloroquine, an antimalarial drug that is often used for management of other immune-mediated conditions. Periodic ophthalmologic examination and hematologic studies are necessary if this medication is used, due to its potential side effects.

Figs. **16.57 and 16.58**

Graft-versus-host disease (GVHD) is a condition that is seen in a significant number of patients who have undergone an allogenic bone marrow or stem cell transplant, usually as part of therapy for leukemia or other life-threatening disorders. Cytotoxic drugs and radiation are typically used to destroy the malignant cells, but in the process, the patient's own hematopoietic cells are wiped out. To restore the patient's hematopoietic cells, bone marrow or stem cells from an human leukocyte antigen (HLA)-matched donor are obtained and infused into the patient (host). Unfortunately, such matches are often not perfect. The engrafted immune cells can then detect surface antigens of the cells of the host, recognizing them as being "foreign" and subsequently mounting an attack on the host cells. Thus, the term "graft-versus-host disease" was applied to the disorder that resulted from this attack.

Although any tissues of the host patient may be affected, the skin and oral mucosa are commonly involved, producing a pattern that may mimic lichen planus or systemic sclerosis. At times, the oral lesions may be the only manifestation of this disease, presenting in several patterns, including fine white striae or pinpoint white dots that typically affect the labial mucosa, tongue, or buccal mucosa. Erosions and ulcerations also may develop within the areas of white striae, similar to erosive lichen planus; however, various infections, including herpesvirus and deep fungal organisms, may need to be ruled out because of the patient's immune suppression. Ulceration and crusting of the lips may develop, especially in acute GVHD. In addition, these patients will have an increased risk of developing oral squamous cell carcinoma, so biopsy may be necessary to rule out that process. Patients may complain of a dry mouth, typically as a result of the attack of salivary gland tissue by the engrafted immune cells.

The diagnosis of oral GVHD is based on the clinical history in conjunction with the histopathologic findings of lichenoid mucositis, although the intensity of the inflammatory infiltrate is not as great in GVHD as it is in oral lichen planus. Salivary gland involvement may also be seen, causing destruction of the acinar structures, followed by fibrosis.

Prevention of GVHD is perhaps the best treatment, and closely matching the HLA types of the donor and recipient will decrease the severity of the condition. Patients who develop GVHD are treated with systemic corticosteroids and various steroid-sparing agents, as well as with immune-modulating drugs such as mycophenolate mofetil and cyclosporine. Oral lesions of GVHD are usually treated with one of the stronger topical corticosteroids, and if ulcers are present, then topical anesthetics may be used to allay pain until healing ensues. With significant involvement of the salivary apparatus, over-the-counter oral lubricants may bring some relief. Salivary stimulants may be useful if enough intact salivary tissue remains. Topical 1% neutral sodium fluoride solution should be applied daily to inhibit cervical dental caries.

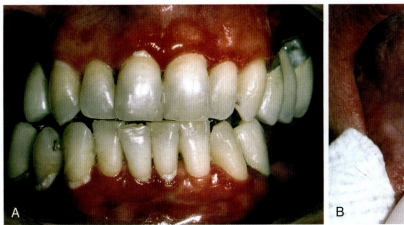
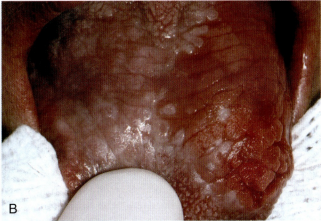

■ Figure **16.56**
Chronic Ulcerative Stomatitis
(A) The erythematous gingival mucosa could suggest pemphigoid or lichen planus, although direct immunofluorescence studies confirmed the diagnosis of chronic ulcerative stomatitis. (B) Atrophic and keratotic changes of the dorsal tongue are also somewhat lichenoid, requiring direct immunofluorescence studies to make the diagnosis.

■ Figure **16.57**
Graft-Versus-Host Disease
Lichenoid changes are present on the buccal mucosa and tongue.

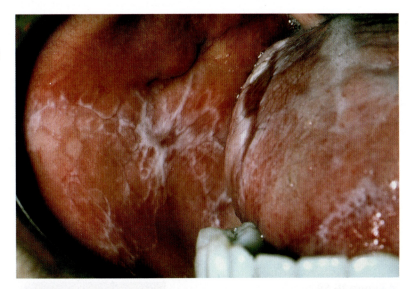

■ Figure **16.58**
Graft-Versus-Host Disease
Diffuse ulcerations of the hard palate.

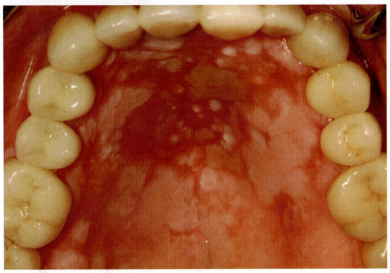

Figs. **16.59–16.62**

Lupus erythematosus is an immune-mediated disorder that may present as a relatively mild skin disease (**chronic cutaneous lupus erythematosus [CCLE]**), a serious systemic disease (**systemic lupus erythematosus [SLE]**), or an intermediate disease (**subacute cutaneous lupus erythematosus [SCLE]**). SLE is characterized by dysregulation of both the T- and B-cell limbs of the immune system, resulting in significant damage to a wide range of organ systems, including the skin, kidneys, heart, blood vessels, and joints. CCLE primarily attacks the skin, producing red, scaly patches that may heal with scarring. The features of SCLE lie somewhere between the other two forms.

SLE tends to affect young women predominantly, and signs and symptoms can be relatively nonspecific in the initial stages of the disease. Fever, malaise, arthritis, weight loss, and fatigue are often noted, as well as a characteristic erythematous patch that involves the malar skin and bridge of the nose, termed a "butterfly rash." Kidney involvement develops in 30% to 40% of these patients and may lead to kidney failure. Pericarditis and vegetative endocarditis affect the heart in approximately 50% of SLE patients. The scaly, erythematous patches of CCLE often appear on the facial skin and frequently worsen with sun exposure. The oral lesions of SLE and CCLE can appear very similar to erosive lichen planus, although in SLE, the lesions may have a nonspecific, or even granulomatous, character. Such lesions occur in a significant percentage of SLE patients, affecting the lips, tongue, buccal mucosa, and hard palate primarily.

The diagnosis of SLE can be challenging in its initial phases, and the American Rheumatism Association has developed a list of laboratory and clinical findings that, in the appropriate context, could indicate a diagnosis of SLE. The characteristic but not pathognomonic histopathologic features typically show a lichenoid mucositis with perivascular inflammation. Serologic studies frequently identify elevated levels of autoantibodies, some of which are nonspecific; however, if autoantibodies directed against double-stranded DNA or Sm protein are identified, this is rather specific for a diagnosis of SLE. These serologic findings are usually not present in CCLE or SCLE.

Patients with any form of lupus erythematosus should avoid sun exposure if possible. Mild cases of SLE may be managed with nonsteroidal antiinflammatory agents in conjunction with hydroxychloroquine, an antimalarial drug that seems to modulate the inflammatory response. More severe cases of SLE may require treatment with more potent immune-modulating and immunosuppressive medications. Most cases of CCLE and SCLE can be managed with topical corticosteroids.

The prognosis of SLE can vary considerably from person to person, although 95% of these patients are alive 5 years after their diagnosis. However, by 20 years, the survival rate drops to 75%. The prognosis of CCLE and SCLE is much better, and some of these cases may resolve completely after several years.

■ Figure **16.59**
Lupus Erythematosus
Red, scaly plaques with areas of regression and postinflammatory melanosis involving sun-exposed skin.

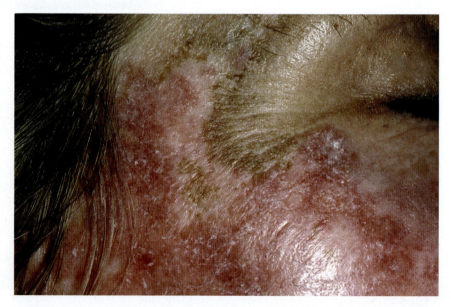

■ Figure **16.60**
Lupus Erythematosus

Scaly, erythematous round ("discoid") plaques of chronic cutaneous lupus erythematosus.

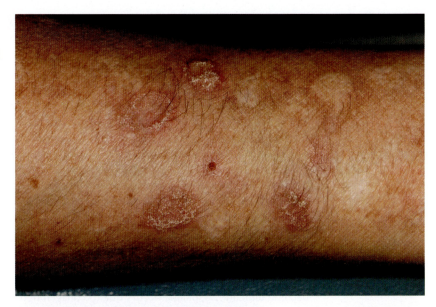

■ Figure **16.61**
Lupus Erythematosus

Oral mucosal lesions often appear similar to those of lichen planus, showing areas of erythema in conjunction with white plaques and striae affecting the buccal mucosa.

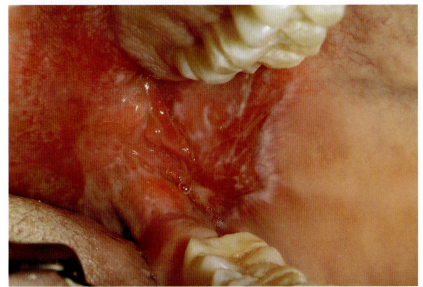

■ Figure **16.62**
Lupus Erythematosus

Characteristic lesion showing a mixed red and white plaque involving the mid-posterior hard palate.

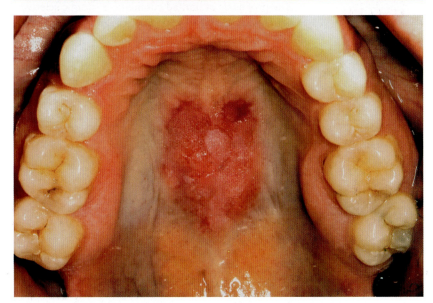

Figs. 16.63–16.66

Systemic sclerosis is an uncommon immune-mediated disorder that is characterized by the abnormal deposition of collagen in a variety of anatomic regions of the body. The precise pathogenesis of systemic sclerosis is unknown. Sometimes the condition seems to remain limited to the skin of the face and extremities and is designated as *limited cutaneous systemic sclerosis*. In other cases the collagen deposition begins in the skin but becomes more widespread, and this is termed *diffuse cutaneous systemic sclerosis*.

Systemic sclerosis commonly affects middle-aged or older women and often is first detected due to cutaneous changes that are characterized by very firm, inelastic skin. If the hands are affected, the fingers become fixed in a claw-shaped deformity known as sclerodactyly (literally, "hard fingers"). Raynaud phenomenon often develops in these patients. Renal failure with attendant hypertension is seen with kidney involvement. Collagen deposition in the lungs results in loss of pulmonary elasticity, causing pulmonary hypertension and subsequent cardiac failure.

When the facial skin is involved, the face has a smooth appearance with atrophy of the nasal alae and development of microstomia. The skin around the mouth may develop a drawn "purse-string" pattern of radiating furrows. Patients may have trouble inserting dental appliances, and oral hygiene procedures become difficult. Dysphagia occurs due to collagen deposition in the wall of the esophagus, and the rest of the gastrointestinal tract also may be involved.

Radiographs typically show generalized widening of the periodontal ligament space. Occasionally resorption of the chin, condyle, coronoid process, or posterior ramus of the mandible is identified.

The diagnosis of systemic sclerosis is based on the clinical features, including skin changes and presence of Raynaud phenomenon, combined with the histopathologic and serologic findings. Biopsy of involved skin or mucosa identifies extensive deposition of dense collagen in the superficial connective tissue. Serologic studies may show anticentromere antibodies, consistent with limited cutaneous systemic sclerosis (as well as CREST syndrome), whereas antitopoisomerase antibodies are seen more often in diffuse cutaneous systemic sclerosis.

Treatment of this condition can be challenging, and currently there are no medications that will reverse the disease. The complications are generally addressed as they develop. For example, dysphagia is treated with periodic esophageal dilation; Raynaud phenomenon is treated with vasodilators, such as calcium channel blocking drugs, or by discontinuing habits such as cigarette smoking. Antihypertensive medications that are directed at inhibiting angiotensin can be used for treating high blood pressure caused by renal impairment.

Oral hygiene procedures can be difficult due to immobility of the fingers and microstomia, so use of an electric toothbrush is recommended. Occasionally specialized dental prosthetic devices are fabricated with features such as hinges to ease their insertion and removal.

The prognosis of limited cutaneous systemic sclerosis is better than the diffuse form, with 75% to 80% of patients surviving 10 years after diagnosis, on average. Approximately 55% to 60% of patients with the diffuse form can expect to survive 10 years. Mortality is typically related to pulmonary or cardiac complications of the disease.

■ Figure **16.63**
Systemic Sclerosis
Masklike facies, atrophy of the nasal alae, and the "purse-string" perioral wrinkling that typify changes in the facial skin. (Courtesy Dr. Malcolm Miracle.)

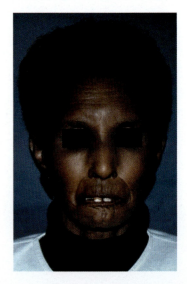

■ Figure **16.64**
Systemic Sclerosis
Sclerodactyly and the claw-like deformity of the fingers. (Courtesy Dr. Malcolm Miracle.)

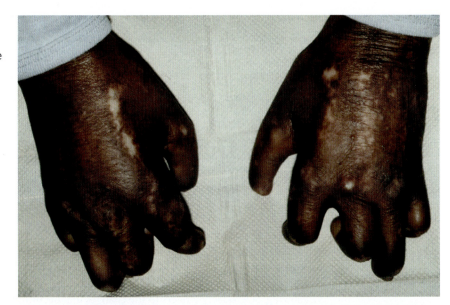

■ Figure **16.65**
Systemic Sclerosis
Generalized widening of the periodontal ligament space. (Courtesy Dr. Michele Ravenel.)

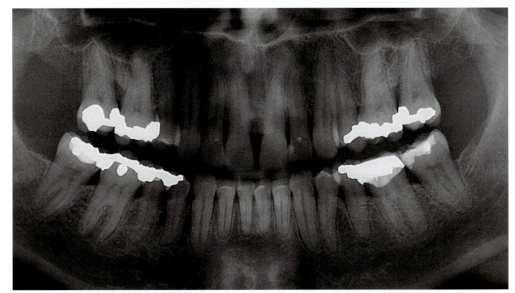

■ Figure **16.66**
Systemic Sclerosis
Marked resorption of the mandibular ramus and coronoid process bilaterally, in addition to generalized widening of the periodontal ligament spaces.

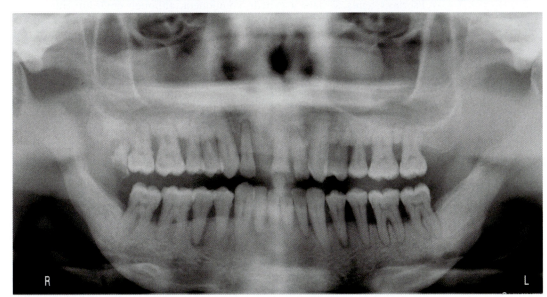

Figs. **16.67 and 16.68**

CREST syndrome is an uncommon condition that is related to systemic sclerosis, and some investigators feel that this is a form of limited cutaneous systemic sclerosis. The acronym stands for **C**alcinosis cutis, **R**aynaud phenomenon, **E**sophageal dysfunction, **S**clerodactyly, and **T**elangiectasias, which are the hallmark features of the disorder. Calcinosis cutis refers to nontender collections of dystrophic calcifications in the superficial dermis. On palpation, these lesions are movable and resemble pebbles, ranging from 0.5 to 2.0 cm, underneath the skin. Raynaud phenomenon is a condition that can occur as an isolated problem but is seen with increased frequency in several immune-mediated disorders. Upon exposure to cold temperatures, vasoconstriction occurs in the arteries that supply the hands, cutting off the blood flow almost completely and causing the fingers to lose their color and turn a pale white. After a few minutes, the arterial walls relax, and blood rushes into the fingers, causing congestion that clinically appears bluish. After several more minutes of warming, the blood vessels have increased blood flow, resulting in a dusky red color. Varying degrees of pain may accompany the process. Esophageal dysfunction is caused by deposition of collagen in the wall of the esophagus, thereby disrupting normal swallowing. Early stages can be identified with a barium swallow study, and in more advanced cases, the patient has difficulty swallowing. Sclerodactyly refers to the changes that occur in the fingers of these patients. The skin becomes tight and shiny, and the fingers curl into a fixed claw-like deformity. The telangiectasias that develop in this condition appear similar to those seen in hereditary hemorrhagic telangiectasia, presenting as flat or slightly red lesions that are usually only 2 to 3 mm in diameter. These are often distributed on the lips and facial skin but also can involve the skin of the fingers.

The diagnosis is usually based on the clinical features, although this can be supported by serologic studies that identify characteristic anticentromere antibodies associated with this condition.

Management of CREST syndrome is similar to that of localized cutaneous systemic sclerosis. Sometimes the lesions of calcinosis cutis become symptomatic and require excision. Monitoring for pulmonary hypertension and primary biliary cirrhosis is prudent, although these occur less frequently and later in the course of disease, compared with systemic sclerosis.

Psoriasis

Fig. **16.69**

Psoriasis is one of the most common conditions seen in dermatologic practice, affecting approximately 2% of the US population. This disease can range in severity, with the cutaneous lesions sometimes being quite problematic. The cause is unknown, but according to current concepts, both autoimmune and autoinflammatory factors play a role in its pathogenesis, resulting in increased turnover of the epidermis. Psoriasis tends to have a genetic component, although environmental factors also play a role in its pathogenesis.

Clinically, the principal lesion of psoriasis consists of an erythematous plaque with a silvery keratotic scale on its surface. The elbows, knees, and scalp are frequently affected, although in some patients the lesions may be more extensive. Pruritus may be a prominent symptom for some patients. In addition, as many as 30% of affected patients will develop psoriatic arthritis, typically approximately one decade after the skin lesions appear. Oral lesions are quite uncommon and generally asymptomatic. Often they wax and wane in conjunction with the skin lesions.

In most cases, the diagnosis of psoriasis is made clinically, based on the characteristic cutaneous findings. If the diagnosis is in question, then biopsy shows a characteristic pattern. Intraorally, the lesions may microscopically resemble psoriasis of the skin, but other lesions, such as erythema migrans and cinnamon reaction, also can display a psoriasiform mucositis. For this reason, clinical correlation is necessary, showing the expected waxing and waning that mirrors the activity of the skin lesions.

A variety of treatments are available for psoriasis, depending on the severity of involvement. Exposure to sunlight (ultraviolet; UV) may help milder cases, but topical corticosteroids and vitamin D_3 analogues are the mainstay of treatment. Systemic therapy may be required for moderate to severe psoriasis, including retinoids, cyclosporine, psoralen and ultraviolet A (PUVA) therapy, or methotrexate. Several new biologic agents (e.g., etanercept, adalimumab, infliximab, ixekizumab) have been developed to block different inflammatory pathways. Oral lesions of psoriasis usually require no treatment, but therapy for the cutaneous lesions has been reported to improve the oral lesions as well.

■ Figure **16.67**
CREST Syndrome

Pale appearance of the distal phalanges, characteristic of Raynaud phenomenon. (Courtesy Dr. Brent Martin.)

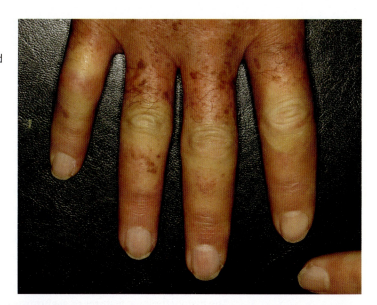

■ Figure **16.68**
CREST Syndrome

Multiple erythematous macules, representing mat-like telangiectasias that have developed on the vermilion zone of the lips.

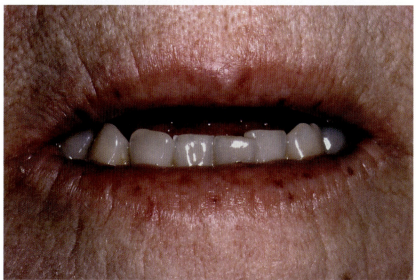

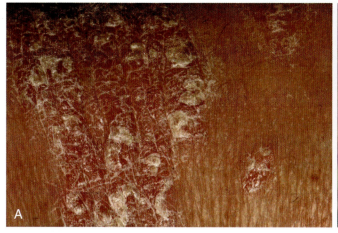

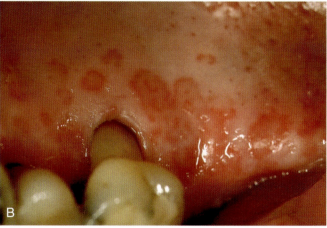

■ Figure **16.69**
Psoriasis

(A) Cutaneous lesions characterized by erythematous plaques surmounted by silvery keratotic scale. (B) Oral lesions characterized by round to serpiginous, faintly erythematous macules with more strikingly red borders involving the keratinized mucosa. (Courtesy Dr. Robert T. Jensen.)

Acanthosis nigricans is a cutaneous process that occurs in both benign and malignant forms. Benign acanthosis nigricans is seen commonly in patients who are obese or diabetic, typically affecting the intertriginous areas of the body. Oral lesions are not found in this form of the condition. Malignant acanthosis nigricans also involves the skin but develops in association with internal malignancy, usually a gastrointestinal adenocarcinoma. Malignant acanthosis nigricans occurs much less commonly than the benign form of the condition. Unlike benign acanthosis nigricans, oral lesions have been described in 40% to 50% of the reported cases of malignant acanthosis nigricans.

The cutaneous lesions of acanthosis nigricans typically present as velvety areas with a tan, brown, or black color. In the setting of diabetes or obesity, they usually develop in the body folds (intertriginous areas), such as the axillae or groin. Malignant acanthosis nigricans appears identical to benign acanthosis nigricans but can be more widespread. Oral lesions appear as finely papillary areas of the labial and buccal mucosa that show minimal or no pigmentation compared with their cutaneous counterpart. Occasionally the patient is unaware that they have cancer, and for this reason, acanthosis nigricans has been said to represent a cutaneous marker of internal malignancy.

The histopathologic features of acanthosis nigricans consist of a papillary pattern of hyperkeratosis and acanthosis, perhaps accompanied by variable degrees of melanin pigmentation. These findings should be correlated with the clinical setting of the skin and oral lesions to arrive at the correct diagnosis.

Although the process may appear innocuous, it must be determined whether it represents the more common form of acanthosis nigricans that is associated with diabetes mellitus and obesity or if it is an example of malignant acanthosis nigricans. Treatment of the underlying cause (diabetes or obesity) may result in resolution of benign acanthosis nigricans. If malignant acanthosis nigricans is suspected, evaluation to find a malignancy is appropriate. Some resolution of malignant acanthosis nigricans may be seen after the malignancy is treated. Often the responsible tumor is relatively advanced, so the prognosis for these individuals unfortunately is poor.

■ Figure 16.70
Acanthosis Nigricans

Velvety brown cutaneous alteration of the posterior neck in a woman with malignant acanthosis nigricans. (Courtesy Dr. Robert Roddy.)

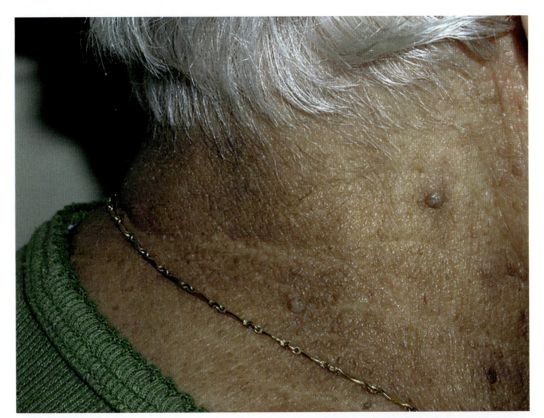

■ Figure 16.71
Acanthosis Nigricans

Same patient as Fig. 16.70 with a diffuse, finely papillary alteration of the buccal mucosa. Subsequent to the recognition of her oral lesions, the patient was diagnosed with endometrial adenocarcinoma, which was treated with surgical excision and chemotherapy. However, the tumor quickly recurred and the patient died 11 months later. (Courtesy Dr. Robert Roddy.)

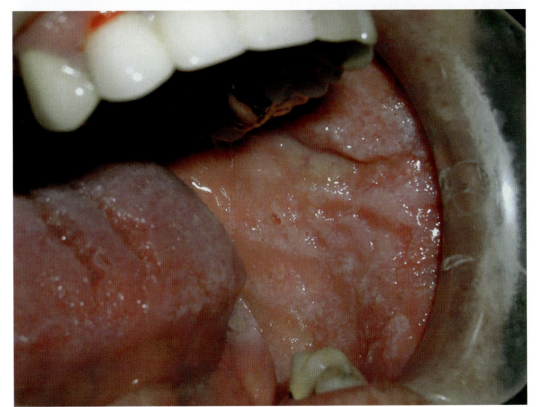

Bibliography

Ectodermal Dysplasia

Bergendal B. Orodental manifestations in ectodermal dysplasia – a review. *Am J Med Genet Part A*. 2014;164A:2465–2471.

Itin PH. Etiology and pathogenesis of ectodermal dysplasias. *Am J Med Genet Part A*. 2014;164A:2472–2477.

Koyuncuoglu CZ, Metin S, Saylan I, et al. Full-mouth rehabilitation of a patient with ectodermal dysplasia with dental implants. *J Oral Implantol*. 2014;40:715–721.

Pagnan NAB, Visinoni ÁF. Update on ectodermal dysplasias clinical classification. *Am J Med Genet Part A*. 2014;164A:2415–2423.

Trzeciak WH, Koczorowski R. Molecular basis of hypohidrotic ectodermal dysplasia: an update. *J Appl Genetics*. 2016;57:51–61.

Visinoni ÁF, Lisboa-Costa T, Pagnan NAB, et al. Ectodermal dysplasias: clinical and molecular review. *Am J Med Genet Part A*. 2009;149A:1980–2002.

Wu Y, Zhang C, Squarize CH, et al. Oral rehabilitation of adult edentulous siblings severely lacking alveolar bone due to ectodermal dysplasia: a report of 2 clinical cases and a literature review. *J Oral Maxillofac Surg*. 2015;73:1733.e1–1733.e12.

White Sponge Nevus

Cai W, Chen Z, Jiang B, et al. Keratin 13 mutations associated with oral white sponge nevus in two Chinese families. *Meta Gene*. 2014;2: 374–383.

Kimura M, Nagao T, Machida J, et al. Mutation of keratin 4 gene causing white sponge nevus in a Japanese family. *Int J Oral Maxillofac Surg*. 2013;42:615–618.

Martelli H, Mourão-Pereira S, Martins-Rocha T, et al. White sponge nevus: report of a three-generation family. *Oral Surg Oral Med Oral Pathol Oral Radiol Endod*. 2007;103:43–47.

Hereditary Benign Intraepithelial Dyskeratosis

Bui T, Young JW, Frausto RF, et al. Hereditary benign intraepithelial dyskeratosis: report of a case and reexamination of the evidence for locus heterogeneity. *Ophthalmic Genet*. 2016;37:76–80.

Cummings TJ, Dodd LG, Eedes CR, et al. Hereditary benign intraepithelial dyskeratosis. An evaluation of diagnostic cytology. *Arch Pathol Lab Med*. 2008;132:1325–1328.

Haisley-Royster CA, Allingham RR, Klintworth GK, et al. Hereditary benign intraepithelial dyskeratosis: report of two cases with prominent oral lesions. *J Am Acad Dermatol*. 2001;45:634–636.

Pachyonychia Congenita

Forrest CE, Casey G, Mordaunt DA, et al. Pachyonychia congenita: a spectrum of KRT6a mutations in Australian patients. *Pediatric Dermatol*. 2016;33:337–342.

Gönül M, Gül Ü, Arzu Kılıç A, et al. A case of pachyonychia congenita with unusual manifestations: an unusual type or a new syndrome? *Int J Dermatol*. 2015;54:334–337.

Jiráková A, Rajská L, Rob F, et al. First case of pachyonychia congenital in the Czech Republic. *Dermatol Ther*. 2015;28:10–12.

Wilson NJ, O'Toole EA, Milstone LM, et al. The molecular genetic analysis of the expanding pachyonychia congenita case collection. *Br J Dermatol*. 2014;171:343–355.

Dyskeratosis Congenita

Alter BP, Giri N, Savage SA, et al. Squamous cell carcinomas in patients with Fanconi anemia and dyskeratosis congenita: a search for human papillomavirus. *Int J Cancer*. 2013;133:1513–1515.

Barbaro PM, Ziegler DS, Reddel RR. The wide-ranging clinical implications of the short telomere syndromes. *Intern Med J*. 2016;46:393–403.

Gramatges MM, Bertuch AA. Short telomeres: from dyskeratosis congenita to sporadic aplastic anemia and malignancy. *Transl Res*. 2013;162: doi:10.1016/j.trsl.2013.05.003.

Xeroderma Pigmentosum

Black JO. Xeroderma pigmentosum. *Head Neck Pathol*. 2016;10:139–144.

Bodner L, Manor E, Friger MD, et al. Oral squamous cell carcinoma in patients twenty years of age or younger – review and analysis of 186 reported cases. *Oral Oncol*. 2014;50:84–89.

Dupuya A, Sarasina A. DNA damage and gene therapy of xeroderma pigmentosum, a human DNA repair-deficient disease. *Mutat Res*. 2015;776:2–8.

Karass M, Naguib MM, Elawabdeh N, et al. Xeroderma pigmentosa: three new cases with an in depth review of the genetic and clinical characteristics of the disease. *Fetal Pediatr Pathol*. 2015;34:120–127.

Mareddy S, Reddy J, Babu S, et al. Xeroderma pigmentosum: man deprived of his right to light. *Sci World J*. 2013;2013:8. Article ID 534752.

Hereditary Mucoepithelial Dysplasia

Boralevi F, Haftek M, Vabres P, et al. Hereditary mucoepithelial dysplasia: clinical, ultrastructural and genetic study of eight patients and literature review. *Br J Dermatol*. 2005;153:310–318.

Halawa M, Abu-Hasan MN, ElMallah MK. Hereditary mucoepithelial dysplasia and severe respiratory distress. *Respiratory Medicine Case Reports*. 2015;15:27–29.

Hernández-Martin A, Colmenero I, Torrelo A. Hereditary mucoepithelial dysplasia: report of two sporadic cases. *Pediatr Dermatol*. 2012;29: 311–315.

Darier Disease

Anuset D, Goutorbe C, Bernard P, et al. Efficacy of oral alitretinoin for the treatment of Darier disease: a case report. *J Am Acad Dermatol*. 2014;71:e46–e48.

Takagi A, Kamijo M, Ikeda S. Darier disease. *J Dermatol*. 2016;43:275–279.

Vender R, Vender R. Acral hemorrhagic Darier's disease: a case report. *J Cutan Med Surg*. 2016;20:478–480.

Warty Dyskeratoma

Allon I, Buchner A. Warty dyskeratoma/focal acantholytic dyskeratosis – an update on a rare oral lesion. *J Oral Pathol Med*. 2012;41:261–267.

Peters SM, Roll KS, Philipone EM, et al. Oral warty dyskeratoma of the retromolar trigone: an unusual presentation of a rare lesion. *JAAD Case Reports*. 2017;3:336–338.

Peutz-Jeghers Syndrome

Chan TC, Sirlin C. Abdominal pain in a young man with oral pigmentations. *J Emergency Med*. 2016;50:335–336.

Duan S-X, Wang G-H, Zhong J, et al. Peutz-Jeghers syndrome with intermittent upper intestinal obstruction: a case report and review of the literature. *Medicine (Baltimore)*. 2017;96:17.

Meserve EEK, Nucci MR. Peutz-Jeghers syndrome pathobiology, pathologic manifestations, and suggestions for recommending genetic testing in pathology reports. *Surg Pathol*. 2016;9:243–268.

Ponti G, Tomasi A, Manfredini M, et al. Oral mucosal stigmata in hereditary-cancer syndromes: from germline mutations to distinctive clinical phenotypes and tailored therapies. *Gene*. 2016;582:23–32.

Shaco-Levy R, Jasperson KW, Martin K, et al. Morphologic characterization of hamartomatous gastrointestinal polyps in Cowden syndrome, Peutz-Jeghers syndrome, and juvenile polyposis syndrome. *Human Pathol*. 2016;49:39–48.

Hereditary Hemorrhagic Telangiectasia

Albiñana V, Zafra MP, Colau J, et al. Mutation affecting the proximal promoter of *Endoglin* as the origin of hereditary hemorrhagic telangiectasia type 1. *BMC Med Genet*. 2017;18:20.

Chin CJ, Rotenberg BW, Witterick IJ. Epistaxis in hereditary hemorrhagic telangiectasia: an evidence based review of surgical management. *J Otolaryngol Head Neck Surg*. 2016;45:3.

Geisthoff UW, Nguyen H-L, Röth A, et al. How to manage patients with hereditary haemorrhagic telangiectasia. *Br J Haematol*. 2015;171: 443–452.

Hopp RN, Cardoso de Siqueira D, Sena-Filho M, et al. Oral vascular malformation in a patient with hereditary hemorrhagic telangiectasia: a case report. *Spec Care Dentist*. 2013;33:150–153.

Parambil JG. Hereditary hemorrhagic telangiectasia. *Clin Chest Med*. 2016;37:513–521.

Sautter NB, Smith TL. Treatment of hereditary hemorrhagic telangiectasia–related epistaxis. *Otolaryngol Clin N Am*. 2016;49:639–654.

Tuberous Sclerosis

Araújo Lde J, Muniz GB, Santos E, et al. Tuberous sclerosis complex diagnosed from oral lesions. *Sao Paulo Med J*. 2013;131:351–355.

Chernoff KA, Schaffer JV. Cutaneous and ocular manifestations of neurocutaneous syndromes. *Clin Dermatol*. 2016;34:183–204.

DiMario FJ Jr, Sahin M, Ebrahimi-Fakhari D. Tuberous sclerosis complex. *Pediatr Clin N Am*. 2015;62:633–648.

Ebrahimi-Fakhari D, Meyer S, Vogt T, et al. Dermatological manifestations of tuberous sclerosis complex (TSC). *J Dtsch Dermatol Ges*. 2017;15(7):695–700.

Islam MP, Roach ES. Tuberous sclerosis complex. In: *Handbook of Clinical Neurology*. Vol. 132. 3rd series. 2015:98–109, [Chapter 6].

Magliocca KR, Bhattacharyya I, Wolfrom RB, et al. Multiple impacted teeth and associated pericoronal tissue abnormality in tuberous sclerosis complex. *J Oral Maxillofac Surg*. 2012;70:2581–2584.

Multiple Hamartoma Syndrome

Gosein MA, Narinesingh D, Nixon CA, et al. Multi-organ benign and malignant tumors: recognizing Cowden syndrome: a case report and review of the literature. *BMC Res Notes*. 2016;9:388.

Luana Flores I, Aranda Romo S, Tejeda Nava FJ, et al. Oral presentation of 10 patients with Cowden syndrome. *Oral Surg Oral Med Oral Pathol Oral Radiol*. 2014;117:e301–e310.

Mukamal LV, Ferreira AF, Jacques Cde, et al. Cowden syndrome: review and report of a case of late diagnosis. *Int J Dermatol*. 2012;51:1494–1499.

Ponti G, Tomasi A, Manfredini M, et al. Oral mucosal stigmata in hereditary-cancer syndromes: from germline mutations to distinctive clinical phenotypes and tailored therapies. *Gene*. 2016;582:23–32.

Epidermolysis Bullosa

Fine J-D, Bruckner-Tuderman L, Eady RAJ, et al. Inherited epidermolysis bullosa: updated recommendations on diagnosis and classification. *J Am Acad Dermatol*. 2014;70:1103–1126.

Gonzalez ME. Evaluation and treatment of the newborn with epidermolysis bullosa. *Sem Perinatol*. 2013;37:32–39.

Kummer TR, Müller Nagano HC, Schaefer Tavares S, et al. Oral manifestations and challenges in dental treatment of epidermolysis bullosa dystrophica. *J Dent Child*. 2013;80:97–100.

Laimer M, Prodinger C, Bauer JW. Hereditary epidermolysis bullosa. *J Dtsch Dermatol Ges*. 2015;13(11):1125–1133.

McPhie A, Merkel K, Lossius M, et al. Newborn infant with epidermolysis bullosa and ankyloglossia. *J Pediatr Health Care*. 2016;30:390–395.

Pemphigus

Cholera M, Chainani-Wu N. Management of pemphigus vulgaris. *Adv Ther*. 2016;33:910–958.

Magliocca KR, Fitzpatrick SG. Autoimmune disease manifestations in the oral cavity. *Surg Pathol*. 2017;10:57–88.

McMillan R, Taylor J, Shephard M, et al. World Workshop on Oral Medicine VI: a systematic review of the treatment of mucocutaneous pemphigus vulgaris. *Oral Surg Oral Med Oral Pathol Oral Radiol*. 2015;120:132–142.

Santoro FA, Stoopler ET, Werth VP. Pemphigus. *Dent Clin North Am*. 2013;57:597–610.

Svecova D. Pemphigus vulgaris: a clinical study of 44 cases over a 20-year period. *Int J Dermatol*. 2015;54:1138–1144.

Paraneoplastic Pemphigus

Al Zamel G, Micheletti RG, Nasta SD, et al. The importance of multidisciplinary healthcare for paraneoplastic pemphigus. *Spec Care Dentist*. 2015;35:143–147.

Broussard KC, Leung TG, Moradi A, et al. Autoimmune bullous diseases with skin and eye involvement: cicatricial pemphigoid, pemphigus vulgaris, and pemphigus paraneoplastica. *Clin Dermatol*. 2016;34:205–213.

Ghandi N, Ghanadan A, Azizian M-R, et al. Paraneoplastic pemphigus associated with inflammatory myofibroblastic tumour of the mediastinum: a favourable response to treatment and review of the literature. *Australas J Dermatol*. 2015;56:120–123.

Healy WJ, Peters S, Nana-Sinkam SP. A middle-aged man presenting with unexplained mucosal erosions and progressive dyspnea. *BMJ Case Rep*. 2015;doi:10.1136/bcr-2014-208677.

Ohzono A, Sogame R, Li X, et al. Clinical and immunological findings in 104 cases of paraneoplastic pemphigus. *Br J Dermatol*. 2015;173:1447–1452.

Su Z, Liu G, Liu J, et al. Paraneoplastic pemphigus associated with follicular dendritic cell sarcoma: report of a case and review of literature. *Int J Clin Exp Pathol*. 2015;8:11983–11994.

Wieczorek M, Czernik A. Paraneoplastic pemphigus: a short review. *Clin Cosmet Investig Dermatol*. 2016;9:291–295. eCollection 2016.

Yong AA, Tey HL. Paraneoplastic pemphigus. *Australasian J Dermatol*. 2013;54:241–250.

Mucous Membrane Pemphigoid

Broussard KC, Leung TG, Moradi A, et al. Autoimmune bullous diseases with skin and eye involvement: cicatricial pemphigoid, pemphigus vulgaris, and pemphigus paraneoplastica. *Clin Dermatol*. 2016;34:205–213.

Di Zenzo G, Carrozzo M, Chan LS. Urban legend series: mucous membrane pemphigoid. *Oral Dis*. 2014;20:35–54.

Maley A, Warren M, Haberman I, et al. Rituximab combined with conventional therapy versus conventional therapy alone for the treatment of mucous membrane pemphigoid (MMP). *J Am Acad Dermatol*. 2016;74:835–840.

Queisi MM, Zein M, Lamba N, et al. Update on ocular cicatricial pemphigoid and emerging treatments. *Survey Ophthalmol*. 2016;61:e314–e317.

Taylor J, McMillan R, Shephard M, et al. World Workshop on Oral Medicine VI: a systematic review of the treatment of mucous membrane pemphigoid. *Oral Surg Oral Med Oral Pathol Oral Radiol*. 2015;120:161–171.

Xu HH, Werth VP, Parisi E, et al. Mucous membrane pemphigoid. *Dent Clin North Am*. 2013;57:611–630.

Yasukochi A, Teye K, Ishii N, et al. Clinical and immunological studies of 332 Japanese patients tentatively diagnosed as anti-BP180-type mucous membrane pemphigoid: a novel BP180 C-terminal domain enzyme-linked immunosorbent assay. *Acta Derm Venereol*. 2016;96:762–767.

Erythema Multiforme

Brown RS. Oral erythema multiforme: trends and clinical findings of a large retrospective: European case series. *Oral Surg Oral Med Oral Pathol Oral Radiol*. 2016;121:681.

Celentano A, Tovaru S, Yap T, et al. Oral erythema multiforme: trends and clinical findings of a large retrospective European case series. *Oral Surg Oral Med Oral Pathol Oral Radiol*. 2015;120:707–716.

Farquharson AA, Stoopler ET, Houston AM, et al. Erythema multiforme major secondary to a cosmetic facial cream: first case report. *Oral Surg Oral Med Oral Pathol Oral Radiol*. 2016;121:e10–e15.

Hsu DY, Brieva J, Silverberg NB, et al. Morbidity and mortality of Stevens-Johnson syndrome and toxic epidermal necrolysis in United States adults. *J Invest Dermatol*. 2016;136:e1387–e1397.

Kohanim S, Palioura S, Saeed HN, et al. Stevens-Johnson syndrome/toxic epidermal necrolysis - a comprehensive review and guide to therapy. I. Systemic disease. *Ocul Surf*. 2016;14:2–19.

Langley A, Anooshiravani N, Kwan S, et al. Erythema multiforme in children and *Mycoplasma pneumoniae* aetiology. *J Cutan Med Surg*. 2016;20:453–457.

Samim F, Auluck A, Zed C, et al. Erythema multiforme: a review of epidemiology, pathogenesis, clinical features, and treatment. *Dent Clin N Am*. 2013;57:583–596.

Sawada T, Suehiro M. Erythema multiforme associated with *Chlamydophila pneumoniae* infection: a report of two cases and a mini-literature review. *J Dermatol*. 2015;42:336–337.

Spencer S, Buhary T, Coulson I, et al. Mucosal erosions as the presenting symptom in erythema multiforme: a case report. *Br J Gen Pract*. 2016;doi:10.3399/bjgp16X684205.

Yamane Y, Matsukura S, Watanabe Y, et al. Retrospective analysis of Stevens-Johnson syndrome and toxic epidermal necrolysis in 87 Japanese patients - Treatment and outcome. *Allergol Int*. 2016;65:e74e81.

Erythema Migrans

Alikhani M, Khalighinejad N, Ghalaiani P, et al. Immunologic and psychologic parameters associated with geographic tongue. *Oral Surg Oral Med Oral Pathol Oral Radiol.* 2014;118:68–71.

Cigic L, Galic T, Kero D, et al. The prevalence of celiac disease in patients with geographic tongue. *J Oral Pathol Med.* 2016;45:791–796.

Mangold AR, Torgerson RR, Rogers RS. Diseases of the tongue. *Clin Dermatol.* 2016;34:458–469.

Picciani BL, Domingos TA, Teixeira-Souza T. Geographic tongue and psoriasis: clinical, histopathological, immunohistochemical and genetic correlation - a literature review. *An Bras Dermatol.* 2016;91:410–421.

Picciani BLS, Souza TT, de Carla B, et al. Geographic tongue and fissured tongue in 348 patients with psoriasis: correlation with disease severity. *Sci World J.* 2015;2015:7. http://dx.doi.org/10.1155/2015/564326. Article ID 564326.

Rezaei F, Safarzadeh M, Mozafari H, et al. Prevalence of geographic tongue and related predisposing factors in 7-18 year-old students in Kermanshah, Iran 2014. *Glob J Health Sci.* 2015;7(5):ISSN 1916-9736 E-ISSN 1916-9744.

Scariot R, Dias Batistab TB, Olandoskic M, et al. Host and clinical aspects in patients with benign migratory glossitis. *Arch Oral Biol.* 2017;73:259–268.

Zadik Y, Drucker S, Pallmon S. Migratory stomatitis (ectopic geographic tongue) on the floor of the mouth. *J Am Acad Dermatol.* 2011;65:459–460.

Lichen Planus

Aghbari SMH, Abushouk AI, Attia A, et al. Malignant transformation of oral lichen planus and oral lichenoid lesions: a meta-analysis of 20095 patient data. *Oral Oncol.* 2017;68:92–102.

Alrashdan MS, Cirillo N, McCullough M. Oral lichen planus: a literature review and update. *Arch Dermatol Res.* 2016;308:539–551.

Cheng Y-SL, Gould A, Kurago Z, et al. Diagnosis of oral lichen planus: a position paper of the American Academy of Oral and Maxillofacial Pathology. *Oral Surg Oral Med Oral Pathol Oral Radiol.* 2016;122:332–354.

De Rossi SS, Ciarrocca K. Oral lichen planus and lichenoid mucositis. *Dent Clin N Am.* 2014;58:299–313.

Fitzpatrick SG, Hirsch SA, Gordon SC. The malignant transformation of oral lichen planus and oral lichenoid lesions. A systematic review. *JADA.* 2014;145:45–56.

Kurago ZB. Etiology and pathogenesis of oral lichen planus: an overview. *Oral Surg Oral Med Oral Pathol Oral Radiol.* 2016;122:72–80.

Mravak-Stipetić M, Lončar-Brzak B, Bakale-Hodak I, et al. Clinicopathologic correlation of oral lichen planus and oral lichenoid lesions: a preliminary study. *Sci World J.* 2014;2014:6. http://dx.doi.org/10.1155/2014/746874. Article ID 746874.

Olson MA, Rogers III RS, Bruce AJ. Oral lichen planus. *Clin Dermatol.* 2016;34:495–504.

Chronic Ulcerative Stomatitis

Qari H, Villasante C, Richert J, et al. The diagnostic challenges of separating chronic ulcerative stomatitis from oral lichen planus. *Oral Surg Oral Med Oral Pathol Oral Radiol.* 2015;120:622–627.

Solomon LW, Aguirre A, Neiders M, et al. Chronic ulcerative stomatitis: clinical, histopathologic, and immunopathologic findings. *Oral Surg Oral Med Oral Pathol Oral Radiol Endod.* 2003;96:718–726.

Graft-Versus-Host Disease

Chaudhry HM, Bruce AJ, Wolf RC, et al. The incidence and severity of oral mucositis among allogeneic hematopoietic stem cell transplantation patients: a systematic review. *Biol Blood Marrow Transplant.* 2016;22:e605–e616.

Ion D, Stevenson K, Woo S-B, et al. Characterization of oral involvement in acute graft-versus-host disease. *Biol Blood Marrow Transplant.* 2014;20:e1717–e1721.

Jamil MO, Mineishi S. State-of-the-art acute and chronic GVHD treatment. *Int J Hematol.* 2015;101:452–466.

Kuten-Shorrer M, Woo S-B, Treister NS. Oral graft-versus-host disease. *Dent Clin N Am.* 2014;58:351–368.

Weng X, Xing Y, Cheng B. Multiple and recurrent squamous cell carcinoma of the oral cavity after graft-versus-host disease. *J Oral Maxillofac Surg.* 2017;75:1899–1905.

Yuan A, Chai X, Martins F, et al. Oral chronic GVHD outcomes and resource utilization: a subanalysis from the chronic GVHD consortium. *Oral Dis.* 2016;22:235–240.

Psoriasis

Brooks JK, Kleinman JW, Modly CE, et al. Resolution of psoriatic lesions on the gingiva and hard palate following administration of adalimumab for cutaneous psoriasis. *Cutis.* 2017;99:139–142.

Kim WB, Jerome D, Yeung J. Diagnosis and management of psoriasis. *Can Fam Physician.* 2017;63:278–285.

Liang Y, Sarkar MK, Tsoi LC, et al. Psoriasis: a mixed autoimmune and autoinflammatory disease. *Curr Opin Immunol.* 2017;49:1–8.

Mattsson U, Warfvinge G, Jontell M. Oral psoriasis - a diagnostic dilemma: a report of two cases and a review of the literature. *Oral Surg Oral Med Oral Pathol Oral Radiol.* 2015;120:e183–e189.

Picciani BL, Domingos TA, Teixeira-Souza T. Geographic tongue and psoriasis: clinical, histopathological, immunohistochemical and genetic correlation - a literature review. *An Bras Dermatol.* 2016;91:410–421.

Picciani BLS, Souza TT, de Carla B, et al. Geographic tongue and fissured tongue in 348 patients with psoriasis: correlation with disease severity. *Sci World J.* 2015;2015:7. http://dx.doi.org/10.1155/2015/564326. Article ID 564326.

Lupus Erythematosus

Chowdhary VR. Broad concepts in management of systemic lupus erythematosus. *Mayo Clin Proc.* 2017;92:744–761.

Khatibi M, Shakoorpour AH, Jahromi ZM, et al. The prevalence of oral mucosal lesions and related factors in 188 patients with systemic lupus erythematosus. *Lupus.* 2012;21:1312–1315.

Nico MMS, Bologna SB, Lourenço SV. The lip in lupus erythematosus. *Clin Exp Dermatol.* 2014;39:563–569.

Simões DM, Fava M, Figueiredo MA, et al. Oral manifestations of lupus erythematosus – report of two cases. *Gerodontology.* 2013;30:303–308.

Thong B, Olsen NJ. Systemic lupus erythematosus diagnosis and management. *Rheumatol.* 2017;56:i3–i13.

Systemic Sclerosis

Baron M, Hudson M, Dagenais M, et al. Relationship between disease characteristics and oral radiologic findings in systemic sclerosis: results from a Canadian oral health study. *Arthritis Care Res.* 2016;68:673–680.

Baron M, Hudson M, Tatibouet S, et al. Relationship between disease characteristics and orofacial manifestations in systemic sclerosis: Canadian systemic sclerosis oral health study III. *Arthritis Care Res (Hoboken).* 2015;67:681–690.

Gyger G, Baron M. Systemic sclerosis. Gastrointestinal disease and its management. *Rheum Dis Clin N Am.* 2015;41:459–473.

Pope JE, Johnson SR. New classification criteria for systemic sclerosis (scleroderma). *Rheum Dis Clin N Am.* 2015;41:383–398.

Simeón-Aznar CP, Fonollosa-Plá V, Tolosa-Vilella C, et al. Registry of the Spanish Network for Systemic Sclerosis: survival, prognostic factors, and causes of death. *Medicine (Baltimore).* 2015;94:1–9.

Stern EP, Denton CP. The pathogenesis of systemic sclerosis. *Rheum Dis Clin N Am.* 2015;41:367–382.

Volkmann ER, Furst DE. Management of systemic sclerosis-related skin disease. A review of existing and experimental therapeutic approaches. *Rheum Dis Clin N Am.* 2015;41:399–417.

CREST Syndrome

Bonnecaze AK. Raynaud's phenomenon in limited cutaneous systemic sclerosis. *BMJ Case Rep.* 2015;doi:10.1136/bcr-2015-212911.

Chamberlain AJ, Walker NPJ. Successful palliation and significant remission of cutaneous calcinosis in CREST syndrome with carbon dioxide laser. *Dermatol Surg.* 2003;968–970.

Daoussis D, Antonopoulos I, Liossis S-NC, et al. Treatment of systemic sclerosis-associated calcinosis: a case report of rituximab-induced regression of CREST-related calcinosis and review of the literature. *Semin Arthritis Rheum.* 2012;41:822–829.

Acanthosis Nigricans

Bustan RS, Wasim D, Yderstræde KB, et al. Specific skin signs as a cutaneous marker of diabetes mellitus and the prediabetic state - a systematic review. *Dan Med J*. 2017;64:A5316.

Chu H-W, Li J-M, Chen G-F, et al. Oral malignant acanthosis nigricans associated with endometrial adenocarcinoma. *Int J Oral Science*. 2014;6:247–249.

Kutlubay Z, Engin B, Bairamov O, et al. Acanthosis nigricans: a fold (intertriginous) dermatosis. *Clin Dermatol*. 2015;33:466–470.

Ramirez-Amador V, Esquivel-Pedraza L, Caballero-Mendoza E, et al. Oral manifestations as a hallmark of malignant acanthosis nigricans. *J Oral Pathol Med*. 1999;28:278–281.

Zhang N, Qian Y, Feng AP. Acanthosis nigricans, tripe palms, and sign of Leser-Trélat in a patient with gastric adenocarcinoma: case report and literature review in China. *Int J Dermatol*. 2015;54:338–342.

17

Oral Manifestations of Systemic Disease

Fig. 17.1

Jaundice is the term used to describe increased bilirubin (>3 mg/dL) in the circulation, with higher levels producing a yellowish cast to the skin and oral mucosa. Bilirubin is the normal breakdown product of hemoglobin, which is released from degenerating erythrocytes at the end of their 120-day life span. Hemoglobin is taken up by macrophages, converting it to biliverdin. Biliverdin is then converted to unconjugated bilirubin, which is lipid soluble and easily absorbed by the cell membranes of hepatocytes. Hepatocytes convert unconjugated bilirubin to conjugated bilirubin, which is water soluble, and this is collected in the gallbladder as a component of bile. Bile is then released into the small intestine during digestion and eventually is excreted in stool.

If the levels of bilirubin in the serum are increased sufficiently, this compound is deposited in various tissues, including the skin and sclera. This results in a yellowish color, also known as *icterus*. This should not be confused with *hypercarotenemia*, an increase in levels of carotene, a dietary pigment found in yellow or orange fruits and vegetables. This may result in a yellow skin color, but it spares the sclera.

Although in some cases elevated bilirubin levels may be normal for a particular individual, the presence of jaundice should be of some concern, and evaluation to identify the cause should be undertaken. A variety of hematologic studies should be performed, including determining levels of unconjugated and conjugated bilirubin. If elevated unconjugated bilirubin levels are found, then conditions that cause premature destruction of erythrocytes may be responsible, including various hemolytic anemias (autoimmune diseases, thalassemia, sickle cell anemia) and other erythrocyte abnormalities. If increased levels of conjugated bilirubin are identified, then conditions that are associated with damage to the liver itself should be considered as potential causes. Various forms of hepatitis (e.g., viral, alcohol related, other toxins) and cirrhosis, as well as other problems that may cause biliary obstruction, such as malignancy in this anatomic site, would result in elevated levels of conjugated bilirubin in the circulation.

Therefore, treatment of jaundice is directed at correcting the underlying cause of the elevated bilirubin levels in the bloodstream.

Lipoid Proteinosis

Figs. 17.2 and 17.3

Lipoid proteinosis, also known as *hyalinosis cutis et mucosae*, is a rare autosomal recessive disorder that is caused by mutation of the *ECM1* gene, which encodes for extracellular matrix protein 1, a glycoprotein. Deposition of an acellular, hyalinized material in the vocal cords during infancy causes the baby's cries to be hoarse and may lead to initial discovery of the disorder. Later in life, the affected individual will develop acneiform facial lesions, as well as very small papules along the margins of the eyelids. Eventually the oral mucosa and skin may develop yellowish, waxy papular and nodular changes. Intraorally, the tongue is often affected, in addition to the lips, buccal mucosa, and tonsillar pillars. In some patients, intracranial calcifications may form in the temporal lobes of the brain, and these calcifications may be responsible for seizure disorders that are occasionally experienced. The precise nature of the hyalinized material is unknown, but it seems to be composed of basement-related compounds, including laminin and types IV and V collagen.

Genetic counseling is appropriate for parents of persons with this disorder. Treatment is limited to surgical reduction of those lesions that cause significant functional problems, such as vocal cord enlargement that impairs the airway. Surgical recontouring for aesthetic purposes can sometimes be performed, usually on a limited basis. The life span of these patients is typically not reduced significantly.

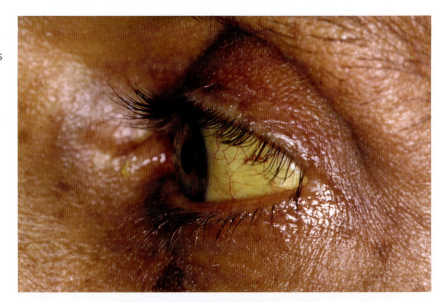

■ Figure **17.1**
Jaundice
Yellow sclera of a patient with sclerosing cholangitis of the liver.

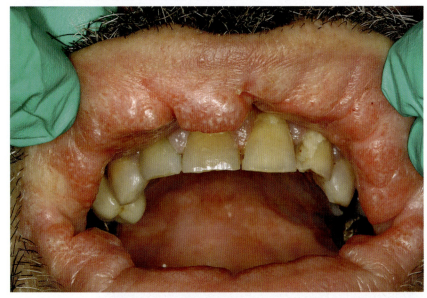

■ Figure **17.2**
Lipoid Proteinosis
Submucosal nodules of the labial mucosa.

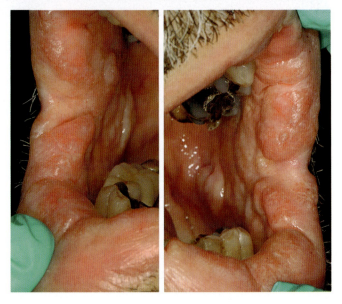

■ Figure **17.3**
Lipoid Proteinosis
Bilateral submucosal nodules of the buccal mucosa.

Amyloidosis

Fig. **17.4**

Amyloidosis is a group of conditions that are characterized by the deposition of an insoluble fibrillary protein, primarily in the soft tissues of the body. Approximately 30 different proteins have been associated with this process, and each type of amyloidosis is associated with a specific protein. Some forms of amyloidosis are inherited, whereas others are acquired. In all cases the deposits of the protein have a molecular structure that has been described as a beta pleated sheet arrangement. Because of this stereochemical structure, Congo red dye preferentially binds to the amyloid material and uniquely will exhibit a glowing apple-green birefringence when viewed with polarized light, confirming the diagnosis of amyloidosis.

The type of amyloidosis that is most frequently seen intraorally is caused by deposition of monoclonal light chain components of the immunoglobulin molecule, which are usually produced by abnormal plasma cells. This presentation is known as AL amyloidosis, and it is often associated with multiple myeloma. Diffuse deposition within the tongue, producing macroglossia, is the most common oral feature of AL amyloidosis, but the labial and buccal mucosa also may be involved. In addition, biopsy of labial salivary glands will often demonstrate amyloid deposition in cases of systemic amyloidosis.

After amyloid is confirmed microscopically, further analysis is required to determine the precise molecular diagnosis because the various types of amyloidosis have predilections for deposition at different sites and have different treatments and prognoses. Patients affected by systemic amyloidosis typically have a poor prognosis because amyloid accumulates in the heart and kidneys, disrupting the function of these vital organs and resulting in death.

Xanthelasma

Fig. **17.5**

The cutaneous xanthomata comprise a variety of yellowish skin lesions that are characterized by accumulations of lipid-laden macrophages in the superficial dermis. The most common of these conditions is known as **xanthelasma**. Xanthelasma develops on the periorbital skin of adults, and the lesions typically present as bilateral, coalescing, soft papules and plaques. The upper eyelid is involved more often than the lower. Periorbital amyloid deposits may mimic xanthelasma clinically, but those lesions are firm and are not yellow.

Treatment usually is initiated for cosmetic reasons. Surgical excision or laser ablation may be performed, although recurrence of the lesions is rather common.

Some studies have found that affected patients may have hyperlipidemia more frequently than a control-matched population. Therefore, referral of the patient for medical evaluation may be appropriate.

Scurvy

Fig. **17.6**

Scurvy is a condition that results from prolonged dietary deficiency of vitamin C (ascorbic acid). Vitamin C is necessary for normal synthesis and maintenance of collagen, a significant constituent of most connective tissues. Although scurvy is relatively uncommon today, certain populations are at risk, including autistic children, alcoholics, psychiatric patients, and the elderly, all of whom may have a limited dietary repertoire. Patients with graft-versus-host disease may develop scurvy because acidic foods irritate their oral mucosa. Furthermore, patients with conditions that are associated with iron overload, such as sickle cell anemia and thalassemia, may acquire this condition because excess iron in the tissues increases the degradation of vitamin C.

The initial symptoms of scurvy can be nonspecific, including irritability, fatigue, and malaise. With persistent deficiency, perifollicular keratosis, petechial hemorrhages, and joint pain develop. Diffuse gingival hyperplasia with gingival hemorrhage and ulceration is also among the earlier signs of scurvy. Periodontal bone loss and exfoliation of teeth eventually occur. Subperiosteal hematomas, delayed wound healing, and ecchymoses caused by minor trauma represent clinical findings later in the course of disease.

A careful dietary history that demonstrates a significant lack of vitamin C–rich foods often will be highly suggestive of this disease in the appropriate clinical setting. If the diagnosis is in doubt, serum ascorbic acid levels can be ordered. With vitamin C supplementation, dramatic improvement typically is seen within a few weeks.

■ Figure **17.4**
Amyloidosis
Firm diffuse swelling of the tongue, resulting in a scalloped appearance of the lateral borders. (Courtesy Dr. Gregory Erena.)

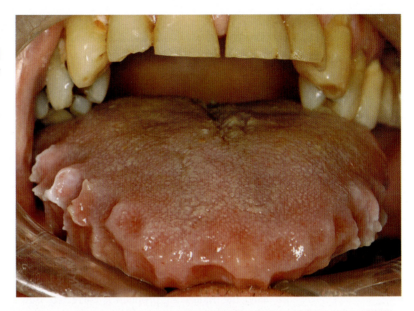

■ Figure **17.5**
Xanthelasma
Soft yellow plaques affecting the periorbital skin.

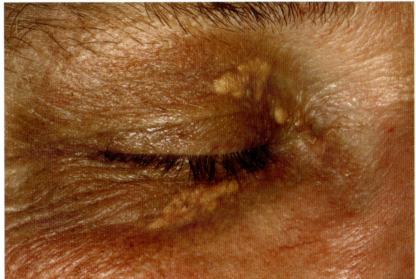

■ Figure **17.6**
Scurvy
Spontaneous gingival hemorrhage with oral mucosal ecchymoses and hematoma formation. (Courtesy Dr. James Hargan.)

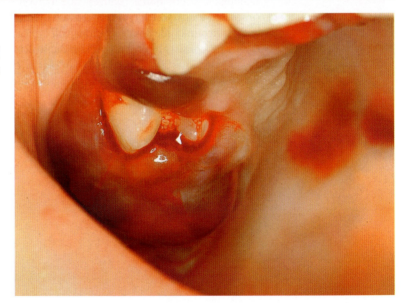

Iron Deficiency Anemia

Figs. **17.7 and 17.8**

Iron deficiency anemia is the most common form of anemia, and in the United States, it is estimated that 1% to 2% of adult men and 10% of adult women may be affected. Iron is a necessary component of oxygen-carrying hemoglobin, and the deficiency may result from reduced absorption of iron or increased demand for iron related to destruction of erythrocytes.

As with any anemia, the signs and symptoms reflect the reduced oxygen-carrying capability of the blood, resulting in fatigue, pallor of the mucous membranes, and shortness of breath. Oral signs and symptoms include angular cheilitis, atrophy of the dorsal tongue papillae, and burning sensation of the tongue.

The diagnosis of iron deficiency anemia is based on hematologic studies, including complete blood count with erythrocyte parameters, hemoglobin, hematocrit, serum ferritin levels, and iron-binding capacity. Once the diagnosis is established, the cause should be investigated to determine whether the deficiency is related to dietary factors, iron absorption problems, or increased erythrocyte turnover. Increased erythrocyte turnover increases demand for iron when erythrocytes are lost through hemorrhage (e.g., gastric ulcer, ulcerated colon carcinoma, menorrhagia) and have to be replaced. Only after the specific cause is identified can appropriate therapy be instituted.

After the underlying problem is corrected, iron stores typically have to be restored by administering supplemental iron, either orally or intravenously.

Pellagra

Fig. **17.9**

A deficiency of niacin (vitamin B_3; nicotinic acid) results in the condition known as **pellagra**. Niacin is an essential component of nicotinamide adenine dinucleotide (NAD^+) and nicotinamide adenine dinucleotide phosphate ($NADP^+$), which are critical enzymes for a variety of vital oxidation-reduction reactions. This vitamin is found in beans, eggs, milk, and vitamin-enriched flour, and small amounts are stored in the liver, although the body can synthesize niacin from dietary tryptophan. Therefore, a diet that is deficient in this vitamin will result in pellagra in a relatively short time. The most important features of pellagra are designated by "the 4 Ds": diarrhea, dermatitis, dementia, and death. Dementia often encompasses irritability, depression, and delusions. The dermatitis that develops is usually more severe in sun-exposed areas.

Stomatitis and glossitis can be noted intraorally, with the tongue appearing erythematous and raw or smooth.

Although this condition is relatively rare in developed countries, individuals whose diets consist primarily of corn-based foods, which typically contain minimal niacin and tryptophan, can develop pellagra. Urinary N-methyl-nicotinamide concentrations will typically be reduced significantly, confirming the diagnosis.

Treatment consists of oral nicotinamide, which is an amide of niacin that, when taken orally, usually has fewer gastrointestinal side effects than niacin itself. The pellagra-related dermatitis will typically begin resolving within a few days after beginning this therapy.

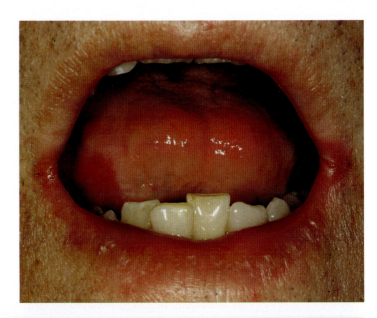

■ Figure **17.7**
Iron Deficiency Anemia
Bilateral angular cheilitis.

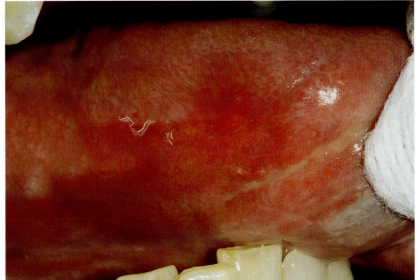

■ Figure **17.8**
Iron Deficiency Anemia
Erythematous patches with blending margins, affecting the lateral and ventral tongue mucosa.

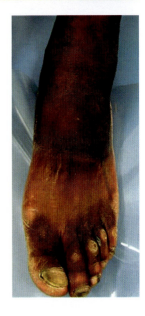

■ Figure **17.9**
Pellagra
Roughened, scaly skin with hyperpigmentation of sun-exposed areas. The pale band across the dorsum of the foot was covered by a sandal strap. (Courtesy Dr. Sylvie Brener.)

Figs. **17.10–17.12**

Pernicious anemia is an immune-mediated condition that is characterized by low levels of cobalamin (vitamin B_{12}), which is necessary for nucleic acid synthesis and, therefore, normal cell division. Thus, deficiency of this vitamin results in impaired hematopoiesis, as well as impacting any tissue that normally has a rapid turnover, such as the gastrointestinal lining cells. Cobalamin (or *extrinsic factor*) is found in foods derived from animals, and it is necessary for normal cell division to take place. Extrinsic factor binds to *intrinsic factor*, which is produced by the *parietal cells* of the stomach lining, and the cobalamin-intrinsic factor complex is preferentially absorbed by the lining cells of the small intestine, after which it is disseminated throughout the body by the bloodstream. Autoantibodies directed against the parietal cells and intrinsic factor result in inhibition of cobalamin absorption, and with reduced levels of this critical molecule, there is impaired mitotic activity of the hematopoietic cells. The hematopoietic cells that are produced appear abnormal and include hypersegmented neutrophils and enlarged erythrocytes. The term *megaloblastic anemia* is applied to this condition because of these large erythrocytes (which are also seen in folate deficiency).

The initial symptoms of pernicious anemia usually include fatigue, weakness, and shortness of breath, but eventually neurologic symptoms, such as symmetric paresthesias and numbness, develop. Central nervous system involvement may also eventuate in difficulty walking and dementia.

Oral signs and symptoms may include neurologic components, such as oral mucosal pain or a burning sensation. This may be accompanied by red macular patches and atrophic glossitis.

Evaluation of a patient suspected of having pernicious anemia includes a complete blood count with erythrocyte parameters. If a megaloblastic anemia is identified, then serum cobalamin and folate levels can be ordered. If serum cobalamin levels are low, then anti-parietal cell and anti-intrinsic factor antibody assays should be obtained. Although anti-parietal cell antibodies may be found in as high as 90% of patients with pernicious anemia, they are not specific, because they can be found in a number of other autoimmune diseases as well. Anti-intrinsic factor antibodies are found in approximately 70% of affected patients, and they are quite specific for pernicious anemia.

Treatment generally consists of intramuscular injections of cobalamin at regular intervals because the presence of intrinsic factor antibodies in the gastrointestinal tract could inhibit absorption. Some studies have found that large doses of cobalamin given orally can overcome the lack of intrinsic factor because of the overwhelming concentration of the vitamin. It is important to distinguish pernicious anemia from folate deficiency because folate supplementation will improve the hematologic status but the neurologic issues associated with pernicious anemia will worsen. Monitoring these patients for gastric carcinoma is prudent because some studies have suggested that the incidence of this malignancy is increased in the areas of atrophic gastritis that develop in pernicious anemia.

■ Figure **17.10**
Pernicious Anemia
Erythematous patches with ill-defined borders affecting the right lateral tongue.

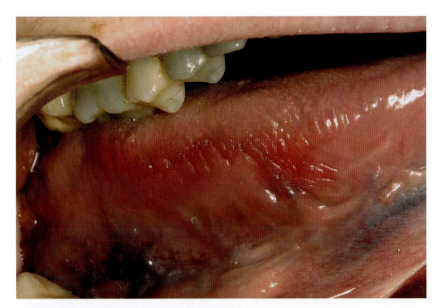

■ Figure **17.11**
Pernicious Anemia
Same patient as Fig. 17.10, showing a similar erythematous patch affecting the left lateral tongue. Such lesions are often multiple and can affect any oral mucosal site.

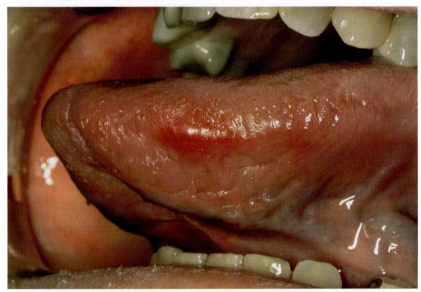

■ Figure **17.12**
Pernicious Anemia
Erythematous patch involving the maxillary labial mucosa.

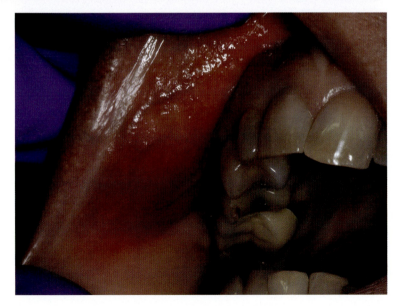

Figs. **17.13–17.15**

Inadequate vitamin D levels during the early years of development lead to the condition known as **rickets**. The manifestations of this disorder initially may be noted by age 2 or 3 years, when affected children develop widened, enlarged epiphyseal plates throughout the skeleton because the trabeculae of osteoid that are forming in these areas lacks calcium for appropriate mineralization. Because vitamin D is necessary for absorption of calcium from the gut, inadequate vitamin D results in reduced calcium in the bloodstream, which impacts the developing calcified structures of the body, including the teeth. Calcium metabolism and the role that vitamin D plays in maintaining appropriate calcium levels in the body represent a complex array of checks and balances. Most investigators classify vitamin D as a hormone rather than a true vitamin. In most instances, vitamin D deficiency is not related to diet, because the precursor is produced in the skin by the action of ultraviolet light on 7-dehydrocholesterol. This results in formation of previtamin D_3, which is then converted to vitamin D_3 (cholecalciferol). In the liver, vitamin D_3 is transformed to 25-hydroxy-vitamin D_3 (25-OH-vitamin D_3), which is then altered in the cells of the kidney to its final active form, $1\alpha,25$-dihydroxy-vitamin D_3. Active vitamin D_3 is necessary for absorption of calcium from the gut and interacts with parathyroid hormone to ensure that proper levels of calcium are present in the bloodstream.

In most cases of rickets, lack of adequate sun exposure leads to reduced levels of vitamin D. Factors such as dark skin (melanin absorbs ultraviolet [UV] light), illness that requires confinement indoors, higher latitudes geographically, and garments that cover most of the skin contribute to vitamin D deficiency. In most developed countries, milk and cereal are fortified with vitamin D, although rickets may develop in children who are exclusively breast-fed for an extended period of time and do not receive adequate sunlight exposure.

Reduced calcium absorption results in poorly calcified osteoid in developing bone, and the resulting bone is quite weak. When the child begins to walk, either bowing or "knock-kneed" distortion of the legs develops. Hypotonia and muscle weakness, both of which are related to decreased serum calcium, also signal vitamin D deficiency. Active growth centers of the skeleton are enlarged, resulting in prominent swellings of the costochondral junctions (so-called rachitic rosary, because it resembles a string of beads draped on the chest). The anterior fontanelle of the skull often remains open in infants with rickets. Vitamin D deficiency during early childhood, when the teeth are developing, causes significant hypocalcified defects in the teeth.

Treatment consists of daily oral supplementation with cholecalciferol. If calcium deficiency appears to be contributing to the patient's rickets, calcium supplements should also be administered.

■ Figure **17.13**
Rickets

Enamel hypoplasia in a patient affected by rickets. In this case the child had been exclusively breast-fed and had little exposure to sunlight. (Courtesy Dr. Pamela McDonald.)

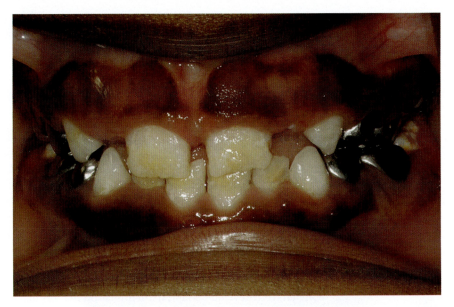

■ Figure **17.14**
Rickets

Radiograph of the same patient in Fig. 17.13 identifying enamel hypoplasia of the central incisors. The enamel of these teeth is formed early in childhood and therefore was most affected by the dietary vitamin D deficiency. (Courtesy Dr. Pamela McDonald.)

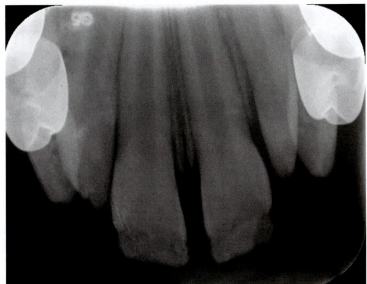

■ Figure **17.15**
Rickets

Radiograph of the same patient in Fig. 17.13 showing enamel hypoplasia and hypocalcification of the crown of the mandibular permanent first molar. (Courtesy Dr. Pamela McDonald.)

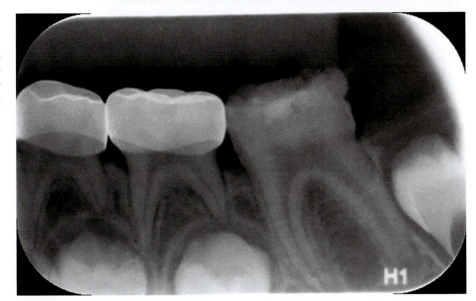

Figs. **17.16 and 17.17**

Vitamin D–resistant rickets (VDRR), also known as *familial hypophosphatemic rickets*, represents a group of heritable conditions that are characterized by loss of phosphate in the urine (leading to reduced serum phosphate levels), low to normal vitamin D levels, and elevated levels of FGF23 (fibroblast growth factor 23). Patients develop many of the signs of rickets, including bowing of the lower limbs in childhood, reduced height, and bone pain. Most cases of VDRR are inherited as an X-linked dominant trait, caused by mutation of the *PHEX (phosphate-regulating gene with endopeptidase activity on the X chromosome)* gene. When *PHEX* is mutated, levels of FGF23 are increased, and this increases the loss of phosphate by the kidney. X-linked dominant VDRR occurs with a frequency of 1 in 20,000, but less common autosomal dominant and recessive forms are also described and involve mutations of different genes.

The oral findings are significant because the dentition exhibits a variety of abnormalities, including thin enamel and defects in the dentin that may extend to the dentinoenamel junction. An ill-defined lamina dura is often seen radiographically, as well as abbreviated roots. The teeth have enlarged pulp chambers, and the lengthened pulp horns reach into the cusps of the teeth. This results in susceptibility of the teeth to pulpal exposure and necrosis, either spontaneous or caused by attrition and abrasion. The nonvital teeth develop periapical inflammation that results in abscess formation and multiple sinus tracts. This can be puzzling for the clinician because the teeth are not carious. Some investigators also have suggested that periodontitis is more prevalent and severe in patients affected by VDRR.

Treatment of the skeletal manifestations of VDRR includes administration of oral phosphate supplements in conjunction with calcitriol, the active form of vitamin D. This therapy improves some of the serologic parameters, but modest impact on growth and development is usually seen, and some patients may not respond at all.

Management of the dental problems includes careful periodic clinical and radiographic examination, and dental sealants have been recommended by some investigators to prevent pulpal exposure. Endodontic treatment of teeth showing signs of pulpal necrosis or periapical inflammatory disease also is recommended. Full crown restorations may be challenging because of the reduced amount of dentin that comprises the crowns of the teeth. With respect to periodontitis, studies have found that adult VDRR patients who have taken phosphate and active vitamin D supplements from the time of childhood seem to have less periodontal destruction.

Fig. **17.18**

Hypophosphatasia represents a group of heritable disorders that are characterized by a decrease in tissue nonspecific alkaline phosphatase. Both autosomal dominant and autosomal recessive inheritance patterns have been described, and because of the variety of mutations responsible for this condition, the spectrum of clinical features and severity of involvement is wide ranging. Detailed discussion of each of these varieties—odontohypophosphatasia, adult, childhood, infantile, perinatal, pseudohypophosphatasia, and benign prenatal hypophosphatasia—is beyond the scope of this text.

Odontohypophosphatasia is probably the most common variant and has the least impact on the overall health of the patient. Affected individuals experience premature loss of the deciduous dentition, typically the incisor teeth. No other significant problems arise, and a normal life span is expected. Perinatal and infantile hypophosphatasia are serious conditions that appear early in life. Perinatal hypophosphatasia is evident at birth, and severe hypomineralization of the skeleton is present. These patients typically die soon after birth. Infantile hypophosphastasia can be identified by 6 months of age and is characterized by skeletal deformities related to hypomineralization of bone. Approximately 50% mortality can be expected. The childhood form of hypophosphatasia is typically identified after 6 months of age and can show a range of expression from mild to severe. In the severe form, there is premature loss of all of the deciduous dentition, whereas with mild cases only a few teeth are lost prematurely. Many of the skeletal features seen in rickets may be evident in severe examples.

Diagnosis of hypophosphatasia depends on identifying decreased serum alkaline phosphatase in the appropriate clinical setting (medical history, physical examination, routine laboratory findings, radiographic features). Because alkaline phosphatase levels vary during life, age- and sex-adjusted reference ranges should be used. Blood and urine samples can be tested for increased phosphoethanolamine, which is another feature of hypophosphatasia. Deciduous teeth that are shed prematurely can be examined histo-pathologically for evidence of reduced or absent cementum.

■ Figure **17.16**
Vitamin D–Resistant Rickets
Widened, elongated pulp chambers characteristic of vitamin D–resistant rickets. Note the teeth that have become nonvital due to this condition, necessitating endodontic therapy. (Courtesy Dr. Pamela McDonald.)

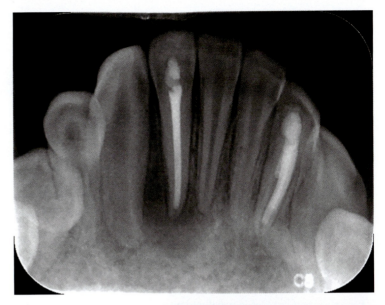

■ Figure **17.17**
Vitamin D–Resistant Rickets
The widened, elongated pulp chambers often extend far into the coronal portion of the dentin, increasing the risk of pulpal exposure related to minor trauma. (Courtesy Dr. Pamela McDonald.)

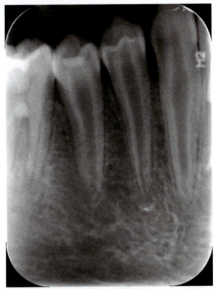

■ Figure **17.18**
Hypophosphatasia
Premature loss of the mandibular anterior dentition.

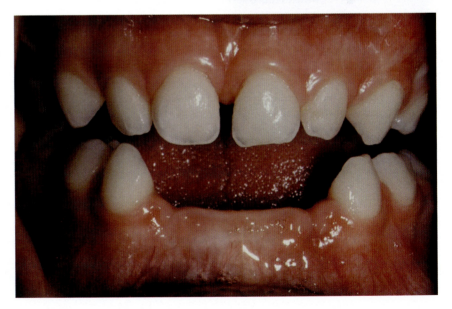

Management consists of genetic counseling for the parents and patient. Treatment is essentially focused on symptomatic care, such as orthopedic surgery to help correct skeletal deformities and fractures. Prosthetic replacement of lost dentition is also appropriate.

Hyperparathyroidism

Figs. **17.19–17.22**

Excess parathyroid hormone production, whether autonomous or physiologic, is termed **hyperparathyroidism** (HPT). *Primary HPT* represents autonomous production of parathyroid hormone, usually by a parathyroid adenoma (80% to 85% of cases), although parathyroid hyperplasia (10% to 15%) or parathyroid carcinoma (1%) may be responsible. A physiologic reason for HPT is seen in patients with end-stage renal disease because they typically have low serum calcium levels. The low calcium levels are related to loss of calcium by the kidney and lack of absorption of calcium from the gut, the latter caused by lack of production of active vitamin D by damaged kidneys. This parathyroid hormone production that is stimulated by low calcium levels is termed *secondary HPT*. Parathyroid hormone interacts with osteoblasts to stimulate the differentiation of osteoclasts. The osteoclasts then resorb bone, releasing calcium into the bloodstream. Under such continuous stimulation, the parathyroid glands usually become hyperplastic, and occasionally they can develop into autonomously functioning adenomas. This condition is termed *tertiary HPT*, and it is usually identified after the patient is treated by kidney transplantation and the calcium levels do not return to normal.

Most cases of HPT are asymptomatic and are identified by routine laboratory studies that are ordered during annual physical examinations, usually in patients older than 60 years. There are signs and symptoms of this condition that are considered characteristic, including the findings of "stones, bones, and abdominal groans," referring to increased prevalence of renal calculi (kidney stones); a variety of osseous alterations, such as brown tumors of bone; and duodenal ulcers.

Radiographic changes seen in the jaws include generalized loss of the lamina dura, which represents one of the first skeletal changes seen with imaging studies. The terminal phalanges are also affected early in this process. The trabecular pattern of the bone often takes on a fine opaque appearance that has been described as a "ground-glass" pattern. Brown tumors tend to occur later in the course of this disorder and can cause a radiolucent defect in any bone, including the jaws. These lesions represent a reactive process composed of vascular granulation-type tissue, osteoclast-type giant cells, and abundant hemorrhage with hemosiderin. The formalin-fixed erythrocytes and hemosiderin have a brown color, thus the term "brown tumor."

Treatment of primary or tertiary HPT consists of surgical removal of the offending lesional parathyroid tissue, which is identified by means of a nuclear medicine imaging study termed a *sestamibi scan*. Secondary HPT is treated with calcium supplements, active vitamin D analogues, and non–calcium phosphate binders, which reduce serum phosphate levels. At times, surgical excision of hyperplastic parathyroid glands also is necessary in this situation.

■ Figure **17.19**
Hyperparathyroidism
Initial presentation of a patient with a parathyroid adenoma that was producing parathyroid hormone. The left facial swelling is caused by an intraoral mass, representing a brown tumor of hyperparathyroidism.

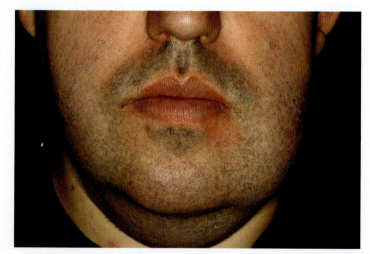

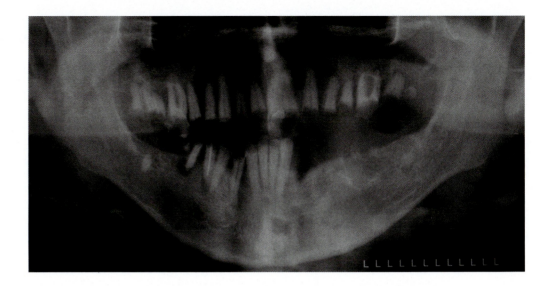

■ Figure **17.20**
Hyperparathyroidism

A panoramic radiograph of the same patient seen in Fig. 17.19 demonstrating an ill-defined radiolucency of the left body of the mandible. Biopsy showed a giant cell lesion, and serologic studies identified increased levels of parathyroid hormone produced by a parathyroid adenoma.

■ Figure **17.21**
Hyperparathyroidism

Same patient as in Fig. 17.20 showing an ulcerated mass that represents a parathyroid adenoma-related brown tumor of hyperparathyroidism that has broken out of bone.

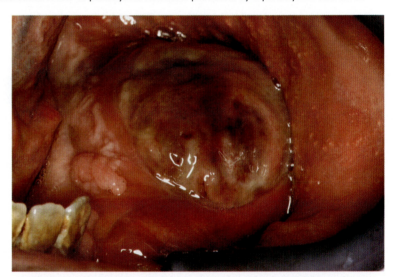

■ Figure **17.22**
Hyperparathyroidism

Same patient as in Fig. 17.20 several weeks after removal of the parathyroid adenoma, showing intact oral mucosa and reduction in the size of the lesion.

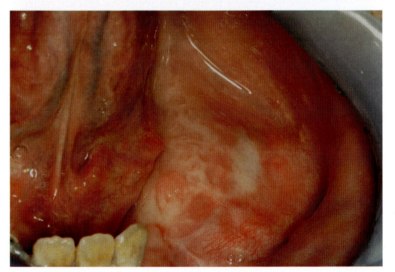

Renal Osteodystrophy

Renal osteodystrophy (ROD) is a significant and common complication of chronic kidney disease (CKD), and just one component of CKD mineral bone disorder (MBD). The pathogenesis of ROD is complex, involving abnormal interactions and imbalances among parathyroid hormone, vitamin D metabolites, serum calcium and phosphate levels, the kidneys, and fibroblast growth factor 23, resulting in the disruption of normal bone physiology. Affected children will show stunted growth and distortion of the long bones, and adults will have an increased incidence of fractures, in addition to expansion of affected bones.

Involvement of the facial bones by ROD is frequently observed, but the extent can vary considerably. These lesions usually have a high rate of turnover of the osseous tissue. In early cases, a "salt and pepper" radiographic pattern may develop due to scattered foci of osteoclastic activity and osteoblastic activity. This pattern is particularly evident in skull films. The marrow spaces are usually replaced by fibrous connective tissue, and the term *osteitis fibrosa cystica* has been applied to the radiographic changes, although the "cystica" portion of the name refers only to the areas of bone resorption and not true cyst formation. Other patients may develop a diffuse, ground-glass appearance of the bone, including resorption of the lamina dura, as described with hyperparathyroidism. A smaller percentage of patients, most of whom have had poorly controlled CKD, will develop osseous expansion, characterized by diffuse enlargement of the jaws. Although historically this has been termed *leontiasis ossea* (literally "lion bones"), some investigators have suggested that a more appropriate term would be *expansive renal osteitis fibrosa*.

Renal transplant is the ideal treatment for this condition, but a lack of matched donors and previous failed transplants are significant barriers. Patients are usually managed by administering a reduced-phosphate diet, calcium-free phosphate binders, and active vitamin D supplementation in an attempt to correct the serologic balance between calcium and phosphate ions.

Addison Disease

Fig. **17.25**

Addison disease, also known as *hypoadrenocortism* or *primary adrenal insufficiency*, is a condition that is characterized by destruction of the adrenal cortex, with subsequent reduction in the production of steroid hormones. Prior to the synthesis of cortisone by biochemists in 1949, this disease was uniformly fatal. In industrialized countries, 80% to 90% of cases are caused by autoimmune attack of the glandular tissue, but in less developed parts of the world, tuberculosis is the principal cause. Although heritable conditions can result in adrenal hypofunction, these are rare; nevertheless, if Addison disease occurs in a child, genetic causes should be considered.

The initial manifestations of Addison disease can be quite nonspecific, and delayed diagnosis of this condition is common. The reduced production of glucocorticoid and mineralocorticoid hormones results initially in signs and symptoms that are rather nonspecific, including fatigue, vomiting, loss of appetite, weight loss, and abdominal pain. If salt craving or increased skin pigmentation ("bronzing" of the skin) are among the early symptoms, these may suggest the diagnosis. Pigmentation occurs because circulating steroid levels are reduced, and the anterior pituitary is stimulated to produce adrenocorticotropic hormone (ACTH). ACTH also reacts with a receptor on melanocytes to stimulate melanin production. Oral pigmentation also may develop, primarily affecting the lips, buccal mucosa, and gingiva. The diagnosis is confirmed by the standard-dose corticotropin test, by which synthetic ACTH is injected and the cortisol level is measured. If no significant rise in cortisol production is seen, the diagnosis of primary Addison disease is confirmed.

If the condition is not diagnosed, the patient may experience acute adrenal insufficiency, also known as an *addisonian crisis*, which is a life-threatening event. This may develop while the patient is under treatment as well, and typically is identified when the patient experiences symptoms of vomiting, abdominal pain, severe hypotension, and shock. This represents a medical emergency and should be managed in the hospital.

Treatment consists of lifelong hormone replacement therapy, including a glucocorticoid, such as hydrocortisone, potentially combined with a mineralocorticoid, such as fludrocortisone. Because the adrenal cortex normally is responsible for all of the androgenic hormone production in women, those women who have reduced libido or symptoms of depression may benefit from treatment with an androgen, such as dehydroepiandrosterone (DHEA). Careful monitoring of the hormone levels and routine blood parameters is necessary, and hydrocortisone should be increased during periods of stress, such as during significant illness or major surgery.

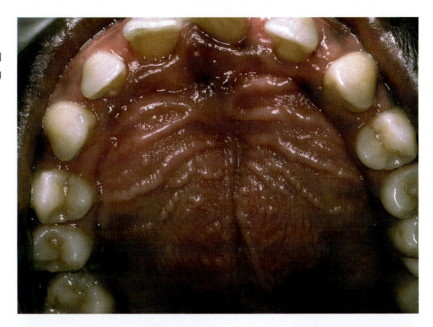

■ Figure **17.23**
Renal Osteodystrophy
Expansion of the maxilla in a patient with renal osteodystrophy, resulting in a bony hard, bulging palatal mass.

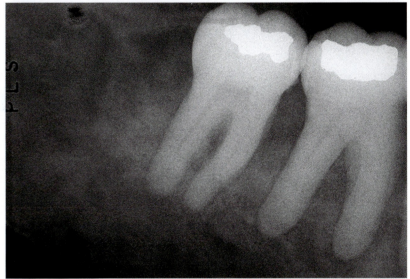

■ Figure **17.24**
Renal Osteodystrophy
Radiograph demonstrating the fine, ground-glass pattern associated with renal osteodystrophy. Note the loss of lamina dura around the teeth.

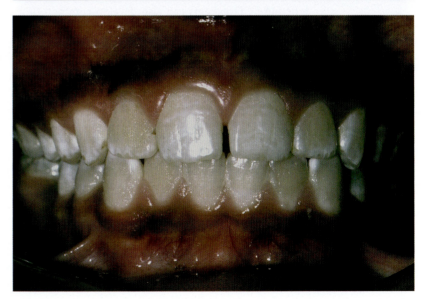

■ Figure **17.25**
Addison Disease
Diffuse brown pigmentation of the attached gingiva in a white patient with Addison disease.

Fig. **17.26**

Diabetes mellitus (DM) is considered to be a group of disorders that are caused by altered carbohydrate metabolism, resulting in chronically elevated levels of blood glucose (hyperglycemia). Most cases of DM are related to either a decrease in insulin production (type 1 DM, representing 5% to 10% of all diabetics) or a reduced impact of insulin on the target tissues, known as insulin resistance (type 2 DM). Type 1 DM is often caused by immunologic attack of the insulin-producing beta cells of the pancreatic islets, whereas type 2 DM is usually associated with obesity. An in-depth discussion of DM is beyond the scope of this text. However, the impact of this common systemic disease is tremendous, as reflected in the fact that its complications are the leading cause of end-stage kidney disease, adult blindness, and lower limb amputations that are not related to trauma. Significant acceleration of peripheral vascular disease and coronary artery disease is associated with this condition, as well as susceptibility to infection. The diagnosis is based on fasting blood glucose levels, glucose tolerance testing, and levels of hemoglobin A1c (glycated hemoglobin).

Although no oral lesions that are specific for DM are currently recognized, many authors have identified oral mucosal and periodontal alterations that seem to be more prevalent and more severe in patients with DM. Periodontitis is seen more frequently in DM, and the severity is usually worse than in a non-DM control population. Gingival inflammation also appears to be more pronounced in diabetic patients, compared with nondiabetic patients with similar plaque control. Modest improvements in the hemoglobin A1c levels of diabetic patients have been shown when their periodontitis is treated and gingival health is maintained.

Crohn Disease

Figs. **17.27 and 17.28**

Crohn disease (CD), also known as *regional ileitis*, is an inflammatory bowel disease of uncertain etiology. The condition is seen primarily in industrialized countries and can present at any age, although two peaks in frequency—the second to third decade and the sixth decade—are identified in most large series. Although the most common site of involvement with CD is the terminal segment of the ileum, any portion of the gastrointestinal tract, from the mouth to the anus, can be affected.

Patients may have nonspecific signs and symptoms, including abdominal cramping, diarrhea, nausea, weight loss, vomiting, and fever. Persistence of these problems will usually trigger investigation to rule out CD.

Oral lesions are found in some patients with CD, although the precise frequency is difficult to assess because CD patients can also develop common oral lesions that may not be related to their systemic disease. In addition, the oral lesions may develop prior to the diagnosis of CD. A variety of oral mucosal alterations have been described, including ulcers, a "cobble-stone" appearance of the mucosa, swelling of the lips, mucosal tags, and erythematous enlargement of the gingivae. Some investigators have described the oral ulcers as resembling aphthous ulcerations. In many cases the ulcers have a linear, fissured configuration, lying at the depth of the buccal vestibule, and these seem to be more suggestive of CD. Parallel hyperplastic folds of tissue that resemble epulis fissuratum have also been described in the buccal vestibules of these patients. In addition, pyostomatitis vegetans (see next topic) may develop in CD, but this uncommon condition is more frequently associated with ulcerative colitis.

Histopathologic findings are characteristic but not pathognomonic. Nonnecrotizing granulomatous inflammation may be found, although this is not identified in every gastrointestinal biopsy sample. Often the granulomatous inflammation will be seen in biopsies of the oral lesions. The diagnosis of CD is based primarily on the clinical presentation, combined with endoscopic, histopathologic, and radiologic findings. Serologic studies are often helpful in ruling out other conditions, but no specific tests are diagnostic for CD.

Medical treatment is generally used initially, with systemic corticosteroids being given to suppress the abnormal inflammatory process, followed by a variety of different classes of medication designed to maintain remission. Most patients with CD will eventually require surgery for resection of an involved bowel segment that has developed a stricture or for correction of a cutaneous or vaginal fistula.

Figure **17.26**
Diabetes Mellitus

Bright red, hyperplastic gingival lesions, characteristic of poorly controlled diabetes mellitus.

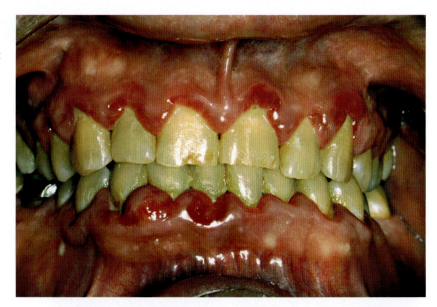

Figure **17.27**
Crohn Disease

Bilateral corrugated, cobblestone changes of the buccal mucosa in a patient with Crohn disease. (Courtesy Dr. John Lovas.)

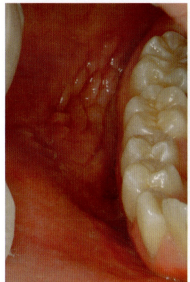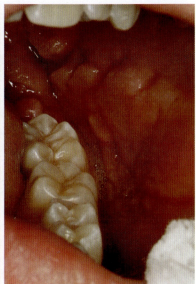

Figure **17.28**
Crohn Disease

Erythematous gingival enlargement with aphthous-like ulceration involving the mandibular anterior labial vestibule in a 20-year-old female. Multiple biopsies of her gastrointestinal tract identified nonnecrotizing granulomatous inflammation in two sites only: the gingivae and the terminal ileum.

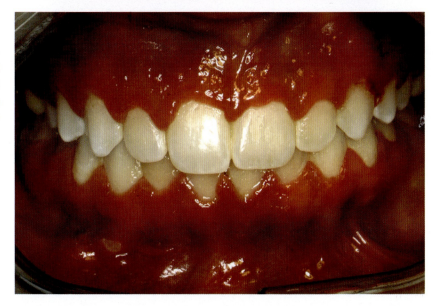

Figs. **17.29 and 17.30**

Pyostomatitis vegetans is an uncommon manifestation of inflammatory bowel disease, with most cases being associated with ulcerative colitis. Some patients with Crohn disease may also present with pyostomatitis vegetans. A similar skin condition, known as *pyodermatitis vegetans*, may develop simultaneously in some instances.

Pyostomatitis vegetans appears as yellow-white, slightly elevated, circinate mucosal lesions that can affect most oral mucosal sites, although the buccal mucosa, labial mucosa, gingivae, and palate seem to be favored. The lesions are often described as having a "snail-track" appearance clinically. For some patients the lesions are relatively asymptomatic, but others may complain of pain or tenderness.

The diagnosis is sometimes made on the basis of the characteristic clinical appearance of the lesions. Biopsy will show a unique pattern of microabscesses that are primarily composed of eosinophils in the spinous layer of the surface epithelium. Varying degrees of intraepithelial edema may be present, simulating an intraepithelial cleft.

Usually pyostomatitis vegetans will resolve when the inflammatory bowel disease is treated. Occasionally this process may develop prior to diagnosis of inflammatory bowel disease, in which case the lesions will respond to application of one of the stronger topical corticosteroid gel preparations.

Uremic Stomatitis

Fig. **17.31**

Uremic stomatitis is a rare condition that develops in patients with end-stage renal disease. Patients who are not receiving adequate hemodialysis will typically have markedly elevated levels of urea in their blood. This is thought to be secreted in the saliva of affected patients. The lesions are thought to be caused by the action of urease, produced by some of the oral microflora, on the urea in the saliva, liberating ammonia and causing chemical injury to the oral mucosa.

Patients with uremic stomatitis complain of diffuse oral mucosal pain and loss of taste or development of dysgeusia. Loosely adherent white plaques are found primarily on the tongue and buccal mucosa. Microscopic descriptions of this process are uncommon, but most describe a peculiar hyperparakeratosis with acanthosis and minimal inflammation.

Treatment consists of renal dialysis, which corrects the blood urea levels and eliminates the urea substrate from the saliva. The oral lesions typically resolve in a few days.

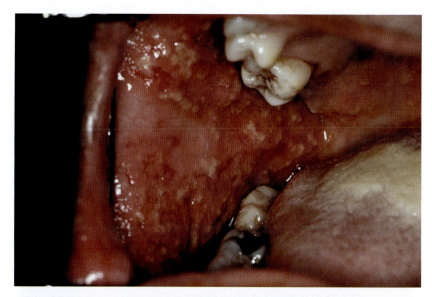

■ Figure **17.29**
Pyostomatitis Vegetans
Superficial pustules, some of which suggest a "snail-track" pattern.

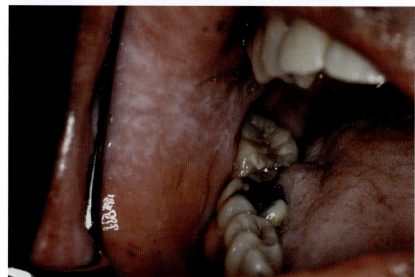

■ Figure **17.30**
Pyostomatitis Vegetans
Same patient as in Fig. 17.29 5 days after systemic corticosteroid therapy.

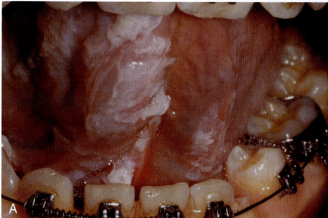
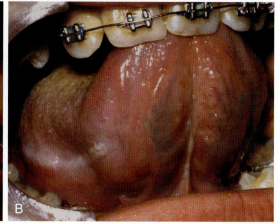

■ Figure **17.31**
Uremic Stomatitis
(A) White plaques of the ventral tongue in a patient suffering from chronic renal failure. (B) Same patient, showing resolution of the white plaques following renal dialysis. (Courtesy Dr. William Ross.)

Bibliography

Jaundice

Carroll WJ, Peck T, Jenkins TL. Periocular, periorbital, and orbital pathology in liver disease. *Surv Ophthalmol.* 2017;62:e134–e149.

Fargo MV, Grogan SP, Saguil A. Evaluation of jaundice in adults. *Am Fam Physician.* 2017;95:164–168.

Pratt DS, Kaplan MM. Jaundice. In: Longo DL, Fauci AS, Kasper DL, et al, eds. *Harrison's Principles of Internal Medicine.* 18th ed. New York: McGraw-Hill; 2012:324–329.

Winger J, Michelfelder A. Diagnostic approach to the patient with jaundice. *Prim Care.* 2011;38:469–482.

Lipoid Proteinosis

Callizo M, Ibáñez-Flores N, Laue J, et al. Eyelid lesions in lipoid proteinosis or Urbach-Wiethe disease: case report and review of the literature. *Orbit.* 2011;30:242–244.

Kartal D, Çınar SL, Kartal L, et al. Lipoid proteinosis. *Acta Dermatovenerol APA.* 2016;25:19–21.

Molina-Ruiz AM, Cerroni L, Kutzner H, et al. Cutaneous deposits. *Am J Dermatopathol.* 2014;36:1–48.

Ranjan R, Goel K, Sarkar R, et al. Lipoid proteinosis: a case report in two siblings. *Dermatol Online J.* 2015;21:20.

Amyloidosis

Ankarcrona M, Winblad B, Monteiro C, et al. Current and future treatment of amyloid diseases. *J Intern Med.* 2016;280:177–202.

Gertz M. CME information: immunoglobulin light chain amyloidosis: 2016 update on diagnosis, prognosis, and treatment. *Am J Hematol.* 2016;91:947–956.

Mangold AR, Torgerson RR, Rogers III RS. Diseases of the tongue. *Clin Dermatol.* 2016;34:458–469.

Pau M, Reinbacher KE, Feichtinger M, et al. Surgical treatment of macroglossia caused by systemic primary amyloidosis. *Int J Oral Maxillofac Surg.* 2013;42:294–297.

Suzuki T, Kusumoto S, Yamashita T, et al. Labial salivary gland biopsy for diagnosing immunoglobulin light chain amyloidosis: a retrospective analysis. *Ann Hematol.* 2016;95:279–285.

Wechalekar AD, Gillmore JD, Hawkins PN. Systemic amyloidosis. *Lancet.* 2016;387:2641–2654.

Xanthelasma

Dey A, Aggarwal R, Dwivedi S, et al. Cardiovascular profile of xanthelasma palpebrarum. *Biomed Res Int.* 2013;3. Article ID 932863.

Frew JW, Murrell DF, Haber RM. Fifty shades of yellow: a review of the xanthodermatoses. *Int J Dermatol.* 2015;54:1109–1123.

Heng JK, Chua SH, Goh CL, et al. Treatment of xanthelasma palpebrarum with a 1064-nm, Q-switched Nd:YAG laser. *J Am Acad Dermatol.* 2017;77:728–734.

Kavoussi H, Ebrahimi A, Rezaei M, et al. Serum lipid profile and clinical characteristics of patients with xanthelasma palpebrarum. *An Bras Dermatol.* 2016;91:468–471.

Sayin I, Ayli M, Oğuz AK, et al. Xanthelasma palpebrarum: a new side effect of nilotinib. *BMJ Case Rep.* 2016;doi:10.1136/bcr-2015-213511.

Scurvy

Golriz F, Donnelly LF, Devaraj S, et al. Modern American scurvy—experience with vitamin C deficiency at a large children's hospital. *Pediatr Radiol.* 2017;47:214–220.

Hafez D, Saint S, Griauzde J, et al. A deficient diagnosis. *N Engl J Med.* 2016;374:1369–1374.

Harrison LB, Nash MJ, Fitzmaurice D, et al. Investigating easy bruising in an adult. *BMJ.* 2017;356:j251. doi:10.1136/bmj.j251. Published 9 February 2017.

Kletzel M, Powers K, Hayes M. Scurvy: a new problem for patients with chronic GVHD involving mucous membranes; an easy problem to resolve. *Pediatr Transplant.* 2014;18:524–526.

Ma NS, Thompson C, Weston S. Brief report: scurvy as a manifestation of food selectivity in children with autism. *J Autism Dev Disord.* 2016;46:1464–1470.

Singh S, Richards SJ, Lykins M, et al. An underdiagnosed ailment: scurvy in a tertiary care academic center. *Am J Med Sci.* 2015;349:372–373.

Iron-Deficiency Anemia

Betesh AL, Santa Ana CA, Cole JA, et al. Is achlorhydria a cause of iron deficiency anemia? *Am J Clin Nutr.* 2015;102:9–19.

Cascio MJ, DeLoughery TG. Anemia: evaluation and diagnostic tests. *Med Clin N Am.* 2017;101:263–284.

DeLoughery TG. Iron deficiency anemia. *Med Clin N Am.* 2017;101:319–332.

Lu S-Y. Perception of iron deficiency from oral mucosa alterations that show a high prevalence of *Candida* infection. *J Formosan Med Assoc.* 2016;115:e619–e627.

Powell DJ, Achebe MO. Anemia for the primary care physician. *Prim Care Clin Office Pract.* 2016;43:527–542.

Wu Y-C, Wang Y-P, Chang JY-F, et al. Oral manifestations and blood profile in patients with iron deficiency anemia. *J Formosan Med Assoc.* 2014;113:e83–e87.

Pellagra

Crook MA. The importance of recognizing pellagra (niacin deficiency) as it still occurs. *Nutrition.* 2014;30:729–730.

Gupta Y, Shah I. Ethionamide-induced pellagra. *J Tropical Pediatr.* 2015;61:301–303.

Kitamura S, Hata H, Shimizu H. Dark-violaceous lesions on the dorsa of both hands. *Clin Exp Dermatol.* 2015;40:941–942.

Mooney SJ, Knox J, Morabia A. The Thompson-McFadden Commission and Joseph Goldberger: contrasting 2 historical investigations of pellagra in cotton mill villages in South Carolina. *Am J Epidemiol.* 2014; 180:235–244.

Terada N, Kinoshita K, Taguchi S, et al. Wernicke encephalopathy and pellagra in an alcoholic and malnourished patient. *BMJ Case Rep.* 2015;doi:10.1136/bcr-2015-209412.

Pernicious Anemia

Bizzaro N, Antico A. Diagnosis and classification of pernicious anemia. *Autoimmun Rev.* 2014;13:565–568.

Couderc A-L, Camalet J, Schneider S, et al. Cobalamin deficiency in the elderly: aetiology and management: a study of 125 patients in a geriatric hospital. *J Nutr Health Aging.* 2015;19:234–239.

Green R. Vitamin B12 deficiency from the perspective of a practicing hematologist. *Blood.* 2017;129:2603–2611.

Green R, Mitra AD. Megaloblastic anemias: nutritional and other causes. *Med Clin N Am.* 2017;101:297–317.

Powell DJ, Achebe MO. Anemia for the primary care physician. *Prim Care Clin Office Pract.* 2016;43:527–542.

Shipton MJ, Thachil J. Vitamin B12 deficiency – a 21st century perspective. *Clin Med.* 2015;15:145–150.

Rickets

DeLuca HF. Vitamin D: historical overview. *Vitamins Hormones.* 2016;100.

Gittoes NJL. Vitamin D – what is normal according to latest research and how should we deal with it? *Clin Med.* 2016;16:171–174.

Kalra S. Vitamin D deficiency: pragmatic suggestions for prevention and treatment. *J Pak Med Assoc.* 2017;67:1116–1118.

Prentice A. Nutritional rickets around the world. *J Steroid Biochem Mol Biol.* 2013;136:201–206.

Reid IR. What diseases are causally linked to vitamin D deficiency? *Arch Dis Child.* 2016;101:185–189.

Vitamin D-Resistant Rickets

Biosse-Duplan M, Coyac BR, Bardet C, et al. Phosphate and vitamin D prevent periodontitis in X-Linked hypophosphatemia. *J Dent Res.* 2017;96:388–395.

Capelli S, Donghi V, Maruca K, et al. Clinical and molecular heterogeneity in a large series of patients with hypophosphatemic rickets. *Bone.* 2015;79:143–149.

Che H, Roux C, Etcheto A, et al. Impaired quality of life in adults with X-linked hypophosphatemia and skeletal symptoms. *Eur J Endocrinol*. 2016;174:325–333.

Li S-S, Gu J-M, Yu W-J, et al. Seven novel and six *de novo PHEX* gene mutations in patients with hypophosphatemic rickets. *Int J Mol Med*. 2016;38:1703–1714.

Sabandal MMI, Robotta P, Bürklein S, et al. Review of the dental implications of X-linked hypophosphataemic rickets (XLHR). *Clin Oral Invest*. 2015;19:759–768.

Souza AP, Kobayashi TY, Lourenço-Neto N, et al. Dental manifestation of patient with vitamin D-resistant rickets. *J Appl Oral Sci*. 2013;21:601–606.

Hypophosphatasia

Foster BL, Ramnitz MS, Gafni RI, et al. Rare bone diseases and their dental, oral, and craniofacial manifestations. *Crit Rev Oral Biol Med*. 2014;93:7S–19S.

Hollis A, Arundel P, High A, et al. Current concepts in hypophosphatasia: case report and literature review. *Int J Paediatr Dent*. 2013;23:153–159.

Whyte MP. Hypophosphatasia: enzyme replacement therapy brings new opportunities and new challenges. *J Bone Mineral Res*. 2017;32:667–675.

Whyte MP. Hypophosphatasia: an overview for 2017. *Bone*. 2017;102:15–25.

Hyperparathyroidism

Duan K, Gomez-Hernandez K, Mete O. Clinicopathological correlates of hyperparathyroidism. *J Clin Pathol*. 2015;68:771–787.

Dulfer RR, Franssen GJH, Hesselink DA, et al. Systematic review of surgical and medical treatment for tertiary hyperparathyroidism. *Br J Surg*. 2017;104:804–813.

Guarnieri V, Seaberg RM, Kelly C, et al. Large intragenic deletion of CDC73 (exons 4-10) in a three-generation hyperparathyroidism-jaw tumor (HPT-JT) syndrome family. *BMC Med Genet*. 2017;18:83.

Mathews JW, Winchester R, Alsaygh N, et al. Hyperparathyroidism-jaw tumor syndrome: an overlooked cause of severe hypercalcemia. *Am J Med Sci*. 2016;352:302–305.

Rodríguez-Portillo M, Rodríguez-Ortiz ME. Secondary hyperparathyroidism: pathogenesis, diagnosis, preventive and therapeutic strategies. *Rev Endocr Metab Disord*. 2017;18:79–95.

Salam SN, Khwaja A, Wilkie ME. Pharmacological management of secondary hyperparathyroidism in patients with chronic kidney disease. *Drugs*. 2016;76:841–852.

Stephen AE, Mannstadt M, Hodin RA. Indications for surgical management of Hyperparathyroidism. A review. *JAMA Surg*. 2017;152:878–882.

Wilhelm SM, Wang TS, Ruan DT, et al. The American Association of Endocrine Surgeons guidelines for definitive management of primary hyperparathyroidism. *JAMA Surg*. 2016;151:959–968.

Yang Q, Sun P, Li J, et al. Skeletal lesions in primary hyperparathyroidism. *Am J Med Sci*. 2015;349:321–327.

Yuen NK, Ananthakrishnan S, Campbell MJ. Hyperparathyroidism of renal disease. *Perm J*. 2016;20:79–83.

Renal Osteodystrophy

Baracaldo RM, Bao D, Iampornpipopchai P, et al. Facial disfigurement due to osteitis fibrosa cystica or brown tumor from secondary hyperparathyroidism in patients on dialysis: a systematic review and an illustrative case report. *Hemodialysis Int*. 2015;19:583–592.

Guimarães-Henriques JC, de Melo Castilho JC, Jacobs R, et al. Severe secondary hyperparathyroidism and panoramic radiography parameters. *Clin Oral Invest*. 2014;18:941–948.

Kemper MJ, van Husen M. Renal osteodystrophy in children: pathogenesis, diagnosis and treatment. *Pediatrics*. 2014;26:180–186.

Lundquist AL, Nigwekar SU. Optimal management of bone mineral disorders in chronic kidney disease and ESRD. *Curr Opin Nephrol Hypertens*. 2016;25:120–126.

Raubenheimer EJ, Noffke CE, Hendrik HD. Recent developments in metabolic bone diseases: a gnathic perspective. *Head Neck Pathol*. 2014;8:475–481.

Raubenheimer EJ, Noffke CE, Mohamed A. Expansive jaw lesions in chronic kidney disease: review of the literature and a report of two cases. *Oral Surg Oral Med Oral Pathol Oral Radiol*. 2015;119:340–345.

Rodríguez-Portillo M, Rodríguez-Ortiz ME. Secondary hyperparathyroidism: pathogenesis, diagnosis, preventive and therapeutic strategies. *Rev Endocr Metab Disord*. 2017;18:79–95.

Addison Disease

Bain A, Stewart M, Mwamure P, et al. Addison's disease in a patient with hypothyroidism: autoimmune polyglandular syndrome type 2, Bain A, et al. *BMJ Case Rep*. 2015;doi:10.1136/bcr-2015-210506.

Bensing S, Hulting A-L, Husebye ES, et al. Epidemiology, quality of life and complications of primary adrenal insufficiency: a review. *Eur J Endocrinol*. 2016;175:R107–R116.

Burton C, Cottrell E, Edwards J. Addison's disease: identification and management in primary care. *Br J Gen Practice*. 2015;65:488–490.

Charmandari E, Nicolaides NC, Chrousos GP. Adrenal insufficiency. *Lancet*. 2014;383:2152–2167.

Gondak R-O, da Silva-Jorge R, Jorge J, et al. Oral pigmented lesions: clinicopathologic features and review of the literature. *Med Oral Patol Oral Cir Bucal*. 2012;17:e919–e924.

Michels A, Michels N. Addison disease: early detection and treatment principles. *Am Fam Physician*. 2014;89:563–568.

Diabetes Mellitus

Fierabracci A. Type 1 Diabetes in autoimmune polyendocrinopathy-candidiasis-ectodermal dystrophy syndrome (APECED): a "rare" manifestation in a "rare" disease. *Int J Mol Sci*. 2016;17:1106.

Gilbert MP. Screening and treatment by the primary care provider of common diabetes complications. *Med Clin N Am*. 2015;99:201–219.

González-Serrano J, Serrano J, López-Pintor RM, et al. Prevalence of oral mucosal disorders in diabetes mellitus patients compared with a control group. *J Diabetes Res*. 2016;2016:11. Article ID 5048967.

López-Pintor RM, Casañas E, González-Serrano J, et al. Xerostomia, hyposalivation, and salivary flow in diabetes patients. *J Diabetes Res*. 2016;2016:15. Article ID 4372852.

Meah F, Juneja R. Insulin tactics in type 2 diabetes. *Med Clin N Am*. 2015;99:157–186.

Preshaw PM, Bissett SM. Periodontitis oral complication of diabetes. *Endocrinol Metab Clin N Am*. 2013;42:849–867.

Stephens E. Insulin therapy in type 1 diabetes. *Med Clin N Am*. 2015;99:145–156.

Thomas CC, Philipson LH. Update on diabetes classification. *Med Clin N Am*. 2015;99:1–16.

Crohn Disease

Alawi F. An update on granulomatous diseases of the oral tissues. *Dent Clin North Am*. 2013;57:657–671.

Feuerstein JD, Cheifetz AS. Crohn disease: epidemiology, diagnosis, and management. *Mayo Clin Proc*. 2017;92:1088–1103.

Laass MW, Roggenbuck D, Conrad K. Diagnosis and classification of Crohn's disease. *Autoimmun Rev*. 2014;13:467–471.

Laranjeira N, Fonseca J, Meira T, et al. Oral mucosa lesions and oral symptoms in inflammatory bowel disease patients. *Arq Gastroenterol*. 2015;52:105–110.

Muhvić-Urek M, Tomac-Stojmenović M. Mijandrušić-Sinčić B: Oral pathology in inflammatory bowel disease. *World J Gastroenterol*. 2016;22:5655–5667.

Pereira MS, Munerato MC. Oral manifestations of inflammatory bowel diseases: two case reports. *Clin Med Res*. 2016;14:46–52.

Pyostomatitis Vegetans

Clark LG, Tolkachjov SN, Bridges AG, et al. Pyostomatitis vegetans (PSV)-pyodermatitis vegetans (PDV): a clinicopathologic study of 7 cases at a tertiary referral center. *J Am Acad Dermatol*. 2016;75:578–584.

Magliocca KR, Fitzpatrick SG. Autoimmune disease manifestations in the oral cavity. *Surg Pathol*. 2017;10:57–88.

Thrash B, Patel M, Shah KR, et al. Cutaneous manifestations of gastrointestinal disease - part II. *J Am Acad Dermatol.* 2013;68: 211.e1–211.e33.

Wu YH, Chang JYF, Chen H-M, et al. Pyostomatitis vegetans: an oral manifestation of inflammatory bowel disease. *J Formosan Med Assoc.* 2015;114:672–e673.

Uremic Stomatitis

Leão JC, Gueiros LAM, Segundo AVL, et al. Uremic stomatitis in chronic renal failure. *Clinics.* 2005;60:259–262.

Liao C-Y. Uremic stomatitis. *Quarterly J Med.* 2017;110:247–248.

Proctor R, Kumar N, Stein A, et al. Oral and dental aspects of chronic renal failure. *J Dent Res.* 2005;84:199–208.

Index

Page numbers followed by "*f*" indicate figures.